SOCIOECONOMIC STATUS AND HEALTH IN INDUSTRIAL NATIONS

SOCIAL, PSYCHOLOGICAL, AND BIOLOGICAL PATHWAYS

ANNALS OF THE NEW YORK ACADEMY OF SCIENCES
Volume 896

SOCIOECONOMIC STATUS AND HEALTH IN INDUSTRIAL NATIONS

SOCIAL, PSYCHOLOGICAL, AND BIOLOGICAL PATHWAYS

Edited by Nancy E. Adler, Michael Marmot,
Bruce S. McEwen, and Judith Stewart

The New York Academy of Sciences
New York, New York
1999

Library of Congress Cataloging-in-Publication Data

Socioeconomic status and health in industrial nations : social, psychological, and
biological pathways / edited by Nancy E. Adler ... [et al.].
    p. cm. — (Annals of the New York Academy of Sciences, ISSN 0077-8923 ;
    v. 896)   Includes bibliographical references and index.
  ISBN 1-57331-211-8 (cloth : alk. paper). — ISBN 1-57331-212-6 (paper : alk. paper)
    1. Social medicine—Congresses. 2. Public health—Economic aspects—Congresses.
    3. Social status—Health aspects—Congresses. 4. Economic status x Health aspects
    — Congresses. 5. Diseases—Causes and theories of causation—Congresses.
    I. Adler, Nancy E. II. Series.
    Q11 .N5   vol. 886
    [RA418]
    500 s—dc21
    [362.1]

    99-052320
    CIP

K-M Research/PCP
Printed in the United States of America
ISBN 1-57331-211-8 (cloth)
ISBN 1-57331-212-6 (paper)
ISSN 0077-8923

ANNALS OF THE NEW YORK ACADEMY OF SCIENCES

Volume 896

SOCIOECONOMIC STATUS AND HEALTH IN INDUSTRIAL NATIONS

SOCIAL, PSYCHOLOGICAL, AND BIOLOGICAL PATHWAYS[a]

Editors and Conference Organizers
NANCY E. ADLER, MICHAEL MARMOT,
BRUCE S. MCEWEN, AND JUDITH STEWART

CONTENTS

[a]This volume is the result of a conference entitled **Socioeconomic Status and Health in Industrial Nations: Social, Psychological, and Biological Pathways**, which was sponsored by the John D. and Catherine T. MacArthur Foundation Research Network on Socioeconomic Status and Health and the New York Academy of Sciences and held on May 10–12, 1999 in Bethesda, Maryland.

Part III. Effects of the Social Environment

Part IV. Psychobiological and Psychosocial Pathways and Mechanisms to Disease

Part V. Aspects of Policy Implications for Health and Research

Part VI. Poster Papers

Financial assistance was received from:

- THE JOHN D. AND CATHERINE T. MACARTHUR FOUNDATION RESEARCH NETWORK ON SOCIOECONOMIC STATUS AND HEALTH
- THE ROBERT WOOD JOHNSON FOUNDATION
- OFFICE OF BEHAVIORAL AND SOCIAL SCIENCES RESEARCH, OFFICE OF THE DIRECTOR, NATIONAL INSTITUTES OF HEALTH
- NATIONAL INSTITUTE OF ENVIRONMENTAL HEALTH SCIENCES, NIH

Preface

NANCY E. ADLER[a,b] AND JUDITH STEWART[a]

[a]MacArthur Network for Socioeconomic Health, 3333 California Street,
Suite 465, Box 0848, San Francisco, California 94143-0848, USA

[b]Department of Psychiatry, University of California, San Francisco,
San Francisco, California 94143, USA

Understanding the association of socioeconomic status (SES) and health is of scientific, applied, and political interest. As a scientific question, it challenges researchers to understand how a socially defined variable such as SES gets into the body in ways that can profoundly affect mental and physical health, functioning, and longevity. It is clearly a question that cannot be answered without a fundamental understanding not only of the mind–body relationship, but also of how this relationship is molded by social context. As an applied question, it challenges the health care system to reduce the additional burden of disease that is associated with lower socioeconomic status. SES is one of the strongest and most consistent predictors of health, and it will not be possible to achieve the goal of maximizing health without addressing the increased risk of disease, disability, and premature death imposed by lower socioeconomic status. Identifying the mechanisms by which SES influences health can provide additional targets of intervention to buffer the effects of existing socioeconomic differences as well as addressing more macro determinants. Finally, the relationship between SES and health is also a political issue. Just as political and economic policies in recent years have led to greater disparities in income and health, new policies could work to reduce such disparities. Whether one is primarily interested in scientific, applied, or political issues, good empirical data are central to achieving the relevant goals.

The New York Academy of Sciences and the John D. and Catherine T. MacArthur Foundation Research Network on Socioeconomic Status and Health jointly sponsored a meeting at the National Institutes of Health in Bethesda on May 11–12, 1999 to provide a forum for the review of empirical findings related to the SES–health association. The meeting was also supported by the Robert Wood Johnson Foundation, and the Office of Behavioral and Social Sciences Research and the National Institute of Environmental Health Sciences, both of the National Institutes of Health. The breadth and depth of the papers that resulted from the conference, Socioeconomic Status and Health in Industrial Nations: Social, Psychological, and Biological Pathways, and appear in this volume attest to the wide interest in understanding the SES–health relationship. The researchers who participated came from a wide range of disciplines and backgrounds as reflects the diversity of interest noted above. Some have been drawn to the study of socioeconomic factors because of their interest in a specific disease and their realization that understanding how SES influences etiology or progression is necessary to reduce its incidence or impact. Others have been drawn to the area because of their interest in a given mechanism, seeing that the associations with SES and with health provide a new window on how the mechanism may function. Still others have a commitment to reducing the social inequalities in health represented by the SES–health gradient and are particularly troubled by ethnic differences in health, which are entwined with socioeconomic factors.

The papers contained in this volume, along with the many posters, provide impressive documentation about the pervasiveness of the SES–health gradient across diseases and populations. They provide important lessons drawn from both animal research and human populations. One lesson is the importance of early environments; both animal research presented by Michael Meaney and longitudinal research (see chapters by Hertzman and by Singer and Ryff) demonstrate that experiences early in life, in human experiences that are associated with the socioeconomic position of one's family, can set trajectories in later life. Among the things shaped by childhood experiences may be health behaviors and psychological responses, which later can play a role in health (see chapters by Winkleby *et al.*, Taylor and Seeman, and Gallo and Matthews). At the same time, contemporaneous experiences in adult life are strongly linked to health. There is compelling evidence of the impact on health of conditions in work environments associated with the occupational component of SES. These involve physical exposures to toxins and to risk of injury, as well as conditions in the social environment at work, particularly low levels of control (see chapters by Lundberg and Marmot).

A second lesson is that individuals' experiences are embedded in a social context. A key context for ethnic minorities is a culture of racism. As Williams discusses in his paper, it is not simply that people of color are overrepresented at lower socioeconomic levels but that institutional barriers and discrimination create added burdens that impair health. These effects are important not only for those who experience discrimination, but also for the whole society. As Kawachi discusses in his chapter, communities (be they states or countries) that have greater income disparities also have less social capital, which in turn influences the health and well-being of the entire community. Wilkinson provides a broad-ranging review of related factors, such as respect in the social context that are associated with health outcomes.

A third lesson relates to a theme that arises across multiple chapters, that differential exposure to stress plays an important role in health outcomes. McEwen and Seeman present animal and human data showing how the adaptive responses of the body to short-term acute stressors can become problematic when the organism is exposed to long-term chronic stressors, and they review a model that captures this interaction. The lower individuals are on the SES hierarchy, the more likely they are to be exposed to chronic stressors (see chapter by Baum) and the fewer resources they may have to address these threats (see chapter by Taylor and Seeman). Low social status itself may be a stressor for both human and nonhuman primates as shown by the work reported by Kaplan and Manuck and by Cohen. Proximal pathways that have been suggested as possible avenues for SES-related stress to affect the body, such as deficits in sleep and post-work relaxation related to shift work and nonrestful home environments, were described by Van Cauter and Spiegel, Pickering, and Lundberg. Policies to reduce social inequalities and to improve health need to be informed by our understanding of the various pathways by which socioeconomic factors act to influence health. Tarlov and Lee point to strategies for developing policies for reducing these social inequalities in health; and Anderson, in his contribution to the volume, lays out a framework for developing interdisciplinary, multilevel research.

The conference illustrated that SES-related health disparities exist and that we know a significant amount about possible mechanisms and pathways whereby SES affects the body. It is now time for us to begin to weave the different levels together. The need for interdisciplinary, multilevel research was the overall message of this conference. We need continued research on specific pathways and mechanisms. But this research needs to take account of wide individual variation and of the role of social contexts in developing, fostering, and sustaining individual variation. A complete understanding of the association between social status and health is not likely to emerge from an additive model, but rather a complex multiplicative model, involving interactions among social, psychological, and biological mechanisms. At this conference the majority of the presentations were focused on specific levels and mechanisms. On the basis of this good foundation, we hope that the next such conference will be able to present research showing how these levels act together to influence health.

The scheduling of the conference was timely. There has been a marked increase in scientific interest in SES and health in the past two decades (see Adler and Ostrove). Many of the NIH institutes are developing research agendas to address social disparities in health, particularly those associated with SES and ethnicity. Within NIH, NIEHS has taken an active role in examining community influences in health disparities, and as noted above, the OBSSR under the leadership of Norman Anderson is underscoring the need for research programs that are multilevel and interdisciplinary. Data that was released shortly after the conference was held and that received wide coverage in the popular press showed that income disparity in the United States is increasing, a state of affairs that is likely to exacerbate health disparities. As policies are developed at the local, state, and federal levels, we hope that the research presented at this conference and further research that may be stimulated by this volume will be useful as applied and policy-based attempts to reduce social disparities in health are crafted.

This is an exciting body of work focused on pathways and mechanisms that are implicated in the production of health disparities. Together these papers set the stage for the multilevel, interdisciplinary work that is the next step in unraveling and hopefully diminishing the social gradient.

Part I Summary: Overview

MICHAEL MARMOT

International Centre for Health and Society, University College London,
1-19 Torrington Place, London WC1E 6BT, United Kingdom

The fact that people of lower socioeconomic status have worse health than people of higher status was for a long time not an object of legitimate study. It seemed somehow to be taken for granted that people in poverty had worse health without particularly questioning why. It was only necessary to control for the effects of socioeconomic status in an analysis, in order to rule out confounding. When it came to "important" diseases such as coronary heart disease, these were known as the diseases of affluence.

The papers in this section document a complete shift in view. It is now abundantly clear that, in affluent countries, the so-called diseases of affluence are in general more common among those in lower socioeconomic groups. This represents a new challenge for understanding. It is not difficult to list reasons why people suffering from absolute deprivation should have greater likelihood of succumbing to diseases associated with unsanitary conditions, crowding or inadequate housing, malnutrition, and lack of access to medical care. It is less obvious why people in deprivation should have higher rates of coronary heart disease and stroke, of many cancers, of gastrointestinal disease and renal disease, of accidents and violence.

The widespread finding, crossing cultures, of different rates of disease in different socioeconomic groups is an important part of the search for causes. It might be thought, for example, that the long documented social inequalities in health in Britain are the product of the class system or that socioeconomic differences in health, now well documented in the United States, are the result of inequalities in access to high-quality medical care. The finding of similar inequalities in health in countries with historically different approaches to social class and those with and without a National Health Service cast doubt on too simple explanations. These papers begin the task of setting out a framework for understanding how these patterns come about.

There is a second challenge documented in these papers: that of the social gradient. The Whitehall and other studies make plain that the problem is not a dichotomous one: worse health in the deprived, better health for everyone else. There is a social gradient in health and that gradient applies to people who are not poor. It is unlikely that the type of explanation applied to the health disadvantage of those in absolute deprivation will apply to people in the middle of the socioeconomic range who have worse health than those at the top. These papers pick up and develop the hypothesis that psychosocial factors, "stress," may be important links between position in the hierarchy and ill health. In each of the papers, aspects of this are developed.

The strands of investigation cover different levels: social, individual behavior and psychological function, biological. All are necessary to understand how social inequalities relate to health inequalities. Wilkinson argues that societies characterized by high status differentials are likely to be societies with low levels of social cohesion that induce social anxiety in its members lower in the hierarchy. This social anxiety in turn may relate to the type of pathway that McEwen and Seeman discuss in their exposition of allostatic load. Whether social anxiety is *the* unifying pathway or some of the other psychosocial factors such as low control (as I suggest in my chapter) remains to be worked out by further research. This uncertainty does not, by itself, detract from the overall thesis that psychosocial factors may be important links in the chain from social position to ill health. This is a fertile area for investigation, and we can expect much in the next few years. If the initial support for this hypothesis is maintained, a crucial question will then be how it feeds into the policy process.

Socioeconomic Status and Health: What We Know and What We Don't

NANCY E. ADLER[a,b] AND JOAN M. OSTROVE[c]

[b]Health Psychology Program, Center for Health and Community,
University of California, SF, San Francisco, California 94143-0844, USA

[c]Department of Psychology, Macalester College, St. Paul, Minnesota 55105, USA

ABSTRACT: In the past 15 years, we have seen a marked increase in research on socioeconomic status (SES) and health. Research in the first part of this era examined the nature of the relationship of SES and health, revealing a graded association; SES is important to health not only for those in poverty, but at all levels of SES. On average, the more advantaged individuals are, the better their health. In this paper we examine the data regarding the SES–health gradient, addressing causal direction, generalizability across populations and diseases, and associations with health for different indicators of SES. In the most recent era, researchers are increasingly exploring the mechanisms by which SES exerts an influence on health. There are multiple pathways by which SES determines health; a comprehensive analysis must include macroeconomic contexts and social factors as well as more immediate social environments, individual psychological and behavioral factors, and biological predispositions and processes.

Our perceptions of the world are biased, and one source of bias is selective attention. Selective attention leads us to pay greater attention to certain aspects of our environment and, as a result, to overestimate the prevalence or importance of these aspects. Soon after buying a given model of a car, for example, we are attuned to how many such models are on the road, giving us the impression that almost everyone seems to have made the same choice we have. Our perception that there has been an explosion of interest in the association of socioeconomic status (SES) and health could be the result of biased perception. Having begun our work in this field in the mid-1990s, it could be that our perception of growing interest simply reflects this egocentric bias. However, a review of MEDLINE citations of studies suggests that this is not the case, or at least is not wholly the case. FIGURE 1 presents the number of articles published annually on SES and health. As the figure shows there has, indeed, been a substantial increase in the number of articles appearing on socioeconomic status and health in recent years. The increase has been especially marked in the last few years. In this paper we will examine the three "eras" of research represented in FIGURE 1.

[a]Address for correspondence: Nancy E. Adler, Health Psychology Program, Center for Health and Community, University of California San Francisco, 3333 California Street, Suite 465, California 94143-0844, USA. 415-476-7759 (voice); 415-476-7744 (fax).
e-mail: nadler@itsa.ucsf.edu

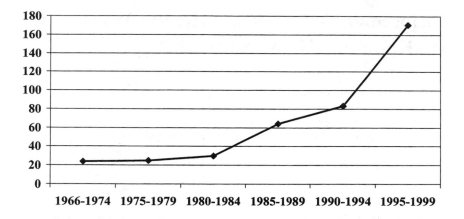

FIGURE 1. Trends in articles on "SES and health" in MEDLINE.

PRE-1985: THE POVERTY ERA

Before the mid-1980s, SES was notable largely in terms of its absence in research on health except as a control variable. Researchers were aware of the power of SES to swamp the effects of the variables in which they were interested. As a result, researchers either used subjects who were homogeneous in terms of SES, or they statistically controlled for SES before entering their variable of interest.

The most frequent measure of SES used in research was poverty status. Individuals were characterized in terms of being either above or below the poverty line. The underlying assumption appeared to be a threshold model (see FIGURE 2). Such a model assumes that increasing levels of income below the poverty line would contribute to improved health. Above the poverty line, however, increasing income would not to be expected to make a significant contribution to improved health status.

During this time there was a good deal of research on the health effects of poverty, which has continued. FIGURE 3 adds to our initial figure of publications on SES, the number of publications in MEDLINE on poverty and health for the same years. As the figure illustrates, there has been substantially more interest in poverty and health than in SES and health, both before and since 1985. Since 1985, as with SES and health, there has also been a marked increase in articles on poverty and health in the medical literature.

1985–1995: DECADE OF THE GRADIENT

A key event in the mid-1980s was a conference organized by Dr. Alvin Tarlov at the Kaiser Family Foundation, resulting in the publication of the volume, *Pathways to Health*.[5] That volume brought together papers from a number of researchers who were suggesting that the impact of socioeconomic factors on health was broader and

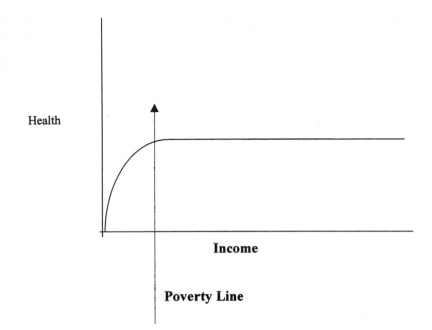

FIGURE 2. Threshold model of poverty.

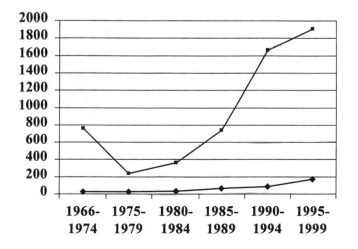

FIGURE 3. Trends in articles on "SES and health" and "Poverty and health" in MED-LINE. ◆, SES and health; ■, poverty and health.

more pervasive than the poverty threshold model represented. Their research was showing that the health effects of SES were not only due to the adversities of extreme poverty, but continued at higher levels of SES as well.

The threshold model was challenged most forcefully by the Whitehall study.[28] This research (which is described in more detail by Michael Marmot in this volume) looked at morbidity and 10-year mortality among British civil servants at each of the occupational grades within the civil service. The research revealed a gradient pattern—health improved and mortality decreased at each higher step of occupational grade. Not only did those at the bottom of the occupational grades have worse health and greater mortality than those above, but there was improvement in health status at each successive step of occupational grade up to the very top. This finding contradicted a threshold model. Not only were all the subjects employed, but also they all had access to health care. Moreover, those in the middle and higher ranks were clearly above the poverty line, yet higher occupational grade, even at this segment of the SES hierarchy, was associated with better health.

One might try to explain away the findings of the Whitehall study by arguing that the British (and especially British civil servants) are so attuned to social class differences in occupational grade or other SES indicators that they would be more profoundly affected by these differences than would individuals in the United States. The Whitehall study challenged us to see whether we could find data to test the gradient in the U.S. Such data were not easy to find, because obtaining them required

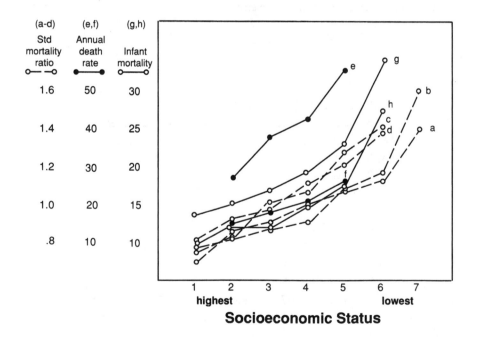

FIGURE 4. Mortality rate by socioeconomic status level. (Taken from the *American Psychologist,* January, 1994, **49**(1): 15–24; used with permission.)

reporting health outcomes at several levels of SES, not simply at the poverty level. Fortunately, several such studies existed. The data, summarized in Adler *et al.*,[1] showed a gradient effect for both mortality and morbidity. FIGURE 4 presents findings from four studies of mortality at different levels of SES. Each study used a different indicator of mortality and different SES measures. As a result, the specific numbers on the *x*-axis do not have real meaning, and their absolute value may be different across studies. Nevertheless the figure clearly shows a gradient relationship between different levels of SES and mortality. The gradient is not perfectly linear, particularly for infant mortality; there is a sharper drop in infant mortality with increases in SES at the lower end of the hierarchy than at the upper end. However, it is clear that even infant mortality continues to drop as one goes up the SES ladder to the highest levels.

The relationship between prevalence of chronic diseases and SES shows an even clearer linear gradient. FIGURE 5 shows data from four studies on prevalence of various chronic diseases by SES level. At each higher level of SES, prevalence of chronic disease decreases. As SES increases, there are drops in the prevalence of osteoarthritis, hypertension, cervical cancer, and having any chronic disease. In addition to morbidity and mortality, risk factors for disease also show a gradient with SES. Rates of smoking, cholesterol levels, and prevalence of sedentary lifestyle are lower the higher one goes on the SES hierarchy, and these occur in a gradient relationship[39] (see also Winkleby[40]).

Research in this decade addressed several questions about the nature of the relationship between SES and health. One question had to do with causal direction—

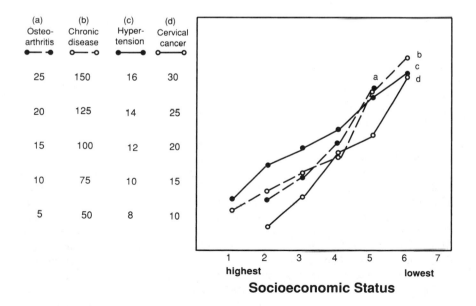

FIGURE 5. Prevalence of chronic diseases by socioeconomic status level. (Taken from the *American Psychologist,* January, 1994, **49**(1): 15–24; used with permission.)

whether SES influences health or vice versa. Other questions had to do with the generalizability of the gradient: Does it occur for all diseases? Does it occur for all populations? Does it occur for all indicators of SES? Each of these questions is discussed briefly below.

Causal Direction

There are two alternative explanations for the association of SES and health. One is that SES influences health status (social causation). The other is that health status contributes to socioeconomic status (social drift or selection). Social drift is more likely for diseases with early onset that have more profound effects on life trajectories (e.g., schizophrenia). Although there is some reciprocal influence of SES and health,[36] the data are more compelling for social causation than for social drift[13,15] For example, we find effects of education acquired through young adulthood on health problems that emerge many years later, suggesting that educational attainment is determining later health. We also find effects of childhood SES on adult health, apart from adult socioeconomic level.[41] Although some childhood diseases are sufficiently debilitating that childhood health may determine educational attainment and later socioeconomic status, these are sufficiently rare that they are unlikely to account for the substantial SES association later in life in general populations. One aspect of the research agenda on SES and health should be to understand how SES plays a role in health across the life cycle and how the cumulative effect of socioeconomic disadvantage operates to influence health.

Diseases

The answer to the question of whether one finds an SES gradient for all diseases is "no." It does not occur for all diseases, but does occur across a wide range of diseases and for many diseases that carry a heavy burden of morbidity and premature mortality. In terms of specific diseases and syndromes, there is a strong and consistent SES gradient for cardiovascular disease, diabetes, metabolic syndrome, arthritis, tuberculosis chronic respiratory disease, gastrointestinal disease, and adverse birth outcomes as well as for accidental and violent deaths.[6,8,18,29,32,35]

There are complicated relationships between SES and cancer. The direction and strength of the association depends on the type of cancer and whether one is looking at incidence or survival. Two diseases for which the gradient in incidence is in the opposite direction (i.e., rates are higher among higher SES individuals) are breast cancer and malignant melanoma. In both cases, behaviors that differ by SES play a role in the reversal of the gradient: delayed childbearing in relation to breast cancer and recreational tanning in relation to malignant melanoma.[10,16] For breast cancer, the familiar SES gradient reappears in looking at survival; once diagnosed, higher SES women show better survival. Longer survival is only partly a function of early diagnosis; the survival advantage for higher SES women remains even when controlling for histology and stage of disease.[7,9]

Lung cancer associations with SES differ by age and gender, reflecting the changing patterns of smoking. Smoking used to be more common among higher SES individuals. As the health effects of smoking became known, particularly through publication of the Surgeon General's report, smoking rates dropped. The decline was greatest among higher SES men so that there are now higher rates of smoking among lower SES individuals, particularly among men.[35] Lung cancer mortality is now greater among lower SES men than higher SES men, and the association is stronger for those under age 65. The gradient of lung cancer by SES is weaker for women; among women over age 65 there is actually higher mortality among higher SES women.[35]

Looking at the difference in associations of SES with incidence versus survival, there are some suggestions that SES plays a different role in survival for those cancers for which health care makes more of a difference. Research in Canada reveals that the association of SES with survival is strongest for cancers of the head and neck region, uterus and cervix, and bladder. These are cancers in which local symptoms often antedate development of metastatic disease and allow early treatment. In contrast, SES is less strongly related to survival for cancer of the lung and pancreas where diagnosis often comes with systemic symptoms, at which time the disease may be incurable.[27] Kogevinas and Porta[22] reviewed over 40 studies of cancer survival, finding both consistent SES differences in survival and greater differences for cancers in which prognosis is more favorable (e.g., breast, bladder and colon cancer, and cancer of the corpus uteri).

Total mortality from any given disease will reflect both incidence and survival. Analyses of which diseases show the SES gradient in mortality and the extent to which this reflects SES differences in incidence and/or in survival may help identify the more specific pathways by which SES increases premature mortality. Differences in incidence are unlikely to be related to differences in medical care. Currently, most medical care systems allocate relatively few resources to prevention and so access to care in these systems will do little to prevent onset of disease. To the extent that prevention becomes a greater focus of medical care and such care is more available to higher SES individuals, differential access will contribute more to SES gradients in incidence of disease. SES differences in survival may be more closely linked to health care disparities. Even here, health care may play only a partial role. Our research agenda needs to include both studies of the pathways by which SES influences etiology of diseases and their incidence, as well as studies of differential recovery and survival that may involve other pathways and mechanisms.

Populations

The second issue of generalizability has to do with the populations in which the SES gradient has been found: Is it the same in all populations? A gradient between SES and health has been found in almost every industrialized nation in which it has been studied. However, the strength of the association is not uniform. The gradient has been shallower in more egalitarian countries such as the Scandinavian countries,[12] although recent data presented by Mackenbach, Kunst, Cavelaars et al.[26] show more complicated patterns of differences across countries in Western Europe. In addition, the familiar gradient may not be found in nonindustrialized countries, at least in terms of cardiovascular disease.[30] For example, research on Nigerian civil servants parallel to the Whitehall studies of British civil servants found a reversal of the gradient. Among the Nigerian civil servants, it was those at higher rank who had a greater incidence of risk factors for cardiovascular disease such as obesity, high-fat diet, and high blood pressure.[4]

Even within the United States, there may be differences in the strength and shape of the gradient in different populations, particularly by race/ethnicity and gender. There is a large literature on racial and ethnic differences in health and within that literature there has been increasing attention to SES.[20,37] Reflecting the history of discrimination in this country, African-Americans and other people of color are more heavily concentrated at lower socioeconomic levels. Some studies have examined and discussed racial differences in health without considering the extent to which these might reflect socioeconomic differences. This attribution to race rather than to socioeconomic differences has been fostered by the nature of available data, particularly in the area of mortality. It is only in recent years that information on education was collected on death certificates in addition to information on race; some states still do not collect data on education. Analyses based on earlier death certificates and those from states that do not collect information on education can therefore only address racial differences. Attributions of differences to race may ignore the contribution of socioeconomic status to differences in health of various racial/ethnic groups.

Not all differences in health among racial/ethnic groups are necessarily due to socioeconomic differences. Members of minority groups face substantial discrimination (see Williams[43]). Personal experiences of discrimination have been found to be associated with greater prevalence of hypertension.[23] In addition, economic and social discrimination may change the association of traditional socioeconomic indicators with health. Additional years of education, particularly at the upper level, appear to "buy" more improvement in health for white men than for white women or for African-American men or women.[3]

We still have very little understanding of how SES is both affected by race/ethnicity and gender or how aspects of SES may operate in conjunction with race/ethnicity and gender to influence health. Thus, another part of the research agenda for the future is developing a greater understanding of the joint and separate functioning of SES, gender, and race/ethnicity in influencing health.

SES Indicators

A final issue of generalizability of the SES–health gradient has to do with the components of SES. SES reflects different aspects of social stratification, and the traditional indicators at the individual level have been income, education, and occupation. These are often used interchangeably even though they are only moderately correlated with one another.[33,39] In some studies in which more than one SES indicator is used, health outcomes may be more highly correlated with one indicator than another. Such studies are useful in identifying specific resources associated with education, income, or occupation that have implications for health. At the same time, similar associations with health have been found no matter which SES indicator is used. Together with the animal literature on the effects of dominant versus subordinate status (see Kaplan and Manuck[43]), this suggests that there may be some common element of social ordering that may be operating to influence health.

One common element among the SES indicators is social status, and a direct measure of subjective social standing may capture this. We have been testing a new measure of subjective social standing and are finding that it has very strong associations with health outcomes, even stronger than the associations of health with objective indicators of SES.[2,4,34]

The measures described above are all individual indicators, but SES also operates at the social level. The interesting work on income inequality has shown that the distribution of income within areas, be they countries, states, or cities, is associated with mortality.[19,21,38] Populations living in areas with greater income inequality have shorter life expectancies, independent of median levels of income. Other studies have shown that the socioeconomic characteristics of neighborhoods in which individuals are living (e.g., the average income of residents, percent unemployed, and residence in a poverty area) predicts morbidity and mortality above and beyond individual SES characteristics.[11,14] Another part of the research agenda is understanding how these multiple levels of influence work together and separately to influence health. These are not alternative explanations but, rather, begin to fill in the complex puzzle of how health is affected by both individual characteristics and the environments in which individuals are living.

1995 AND BEYOND: DECADE OF MECHANISMS

Finally, we come to the most recent era, where there has been another inflection point in publications (see FIG. 1). This might be termed the beginning of the decade of mechanisms. The more recent studies have been addressing the pathways by which SES influences health, examining social, psychological, behavioral, and biological mechanisms. One example of a conceptual model setting out possible pathways was developed by the MacArthur Network on SES and Health. This was done to guide our research on the mechanisms by which SES can get "under the skin" to influence health (see FIG. 6).

The figure indicates that one pathway from SES to health is through exposure to different environments and adaptations to these environments. One aspect of environments with health consequences is differential exposure to pathogens and carcinogens. Equally important are the social and interpersonal aspects of environments, particularly differential exposure to threat and stress in both the work and the home environment. Environments associated with different SES levels may vary in how much control is afforded to individuals, the degree of emotional and instrumental support provided, and exposure to conflict and threat.

Environmental demands and supports can shape psychological responses that, in turn, become more frequent modes of responding. For example, individuals in social environments that are consistently threatening are more likely to develop a sense of distrust and fear of others. Over time this may develop into a more chronic sense of hostility that can place the individual at increased risk for cardiovascular disease (see, e.g., Helmers, Posluszny, and Krantz[17] for evidence on the association of hostility and cardiovascular disease).

The environment also shapes health behaviors. For example, low income neighborhoods have more liquor stores and afford fewer opportunities for exercise and less access to nutritious foods.[25] The combination of individual characteristics and the environmental demands and constraints will affect the likelihood of enacting health-related behaviors such as tobacco use, alcohol use, exercise, and dietary practice.

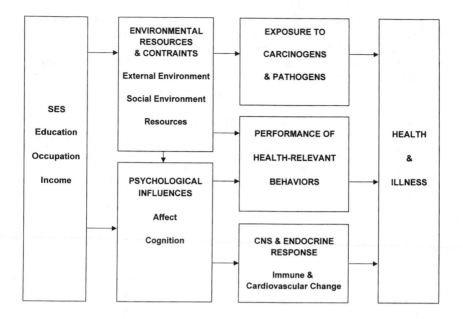

FIGURE 6. Model of the pathways by which SES influences health.

The combination of environmental and individual factors will determine the extent to which the individual experiences repeated stress responses. The CNS and endocrine responses associated with repeated exposures to stress may have long-term effects on the immune and cardiovascular systems, leading to an increased risk of disease onset or more rapid progression of diseases once established. These processes are described in McEwen's chapter in this volume, which examines the development of allostatic load.[44]

The impact of environmental threats and individual responses may be modified by the same health behaviors that are also shaped by socioeconomic forces. For example, exercise may reduce some of the adverse biological effects of stress exposure.[31] At lower positions on the SES hierarchy, one may not only be more subject to chronic stressors that can lead to allostatic load, but also may have fewer opportunities to engage in exercise that could help to buffer the adverse effects of stress responses. Thus, enhanced risk of disease at lower levels of SES is due both to greater exposure to stress and reduced resources for buffering its impact.

This model is oversimplified. The arrows have been drawn in one direction to suggest the pathways by which socioeconomic factors can play out in various ways to influence onset and progression of disease. In fact, there are likely to be feedback loops and interaction effects (e.g., interaction of exercise, stress exposure, and hostility). As research accumulates in this field, we will be better able to establish the pathways and refine our models.

Research on the gradient in the second half of the decade will add to our knowledge of the mechanisms by which SES influences health. Research establishing the pathways from SES to health will be important for developing policies and interventions at the federal, state, or local level to reduce SES disparities in health; some potential approaches are addressed in the final section of this volume (see chapters by Anderson,[45] Lee,[46] and Tarlov[47]). Mechanisms that emerge out of the social environment and broader economic context (e.g., income distribution) may be most effectively addressed by legislation. Other mechanisms may emerge out of more immediate social environments and require more direct action (e.g., building social institutions, empowering communities, modifying working conditions). Still other mechanisms may be at the individual level, so interventions aimed at individual-level change (e.g., health behavior change, parenting support) could help ameliorate some of the adverse effects of SES differentials. Ideally, change can be undertaken at all of these levels to reduce the disparities in health associated with the various determinants. Such change will benefit from a strong science base, and it is our hope that this volume will help to build that foundation.

REFERENCES

1. ADLER, N.E., T. BOYCE, M.A. CHESNEY, S. COHEN, S. FOLKMAN, R.L. KAHN & S.L. SYME. 1993. Socioeconomic status and health: the challenge of the gradient. Am. Psychol. **49:** 15–24.

2. ADLER, N.E. & E. EPEL. 1999. Relationship of subjective and objective social status with psychological and physical health in healthy white women. Under review.

3. ADLER, N.E. B. SINGER & M. CORIELL. 1999. SES and health: for who the gradient holds. In preparation.

4. BUNKER, C.H., F.A.M. UKOLI, M.U. NWANKWO et al. 1992. Factors associated with hypertension in Nigerian civil servants. Prevent. Med. **21:** 710–722.

5. BUNKER, J.P., D.S. GOMBY & B.H. KEHRER, Eds. 1989. Pathways to health: the role of social factors. The Henry J. Kaiser Family Foundation, Menlo Park, CA.

6. CANTWELL, M.F., M.T. McKENNA, E. McCRAY & I.M. ONORATO. 1998. Tuburculosis and race/ethnicity in the United States: impact of socioeconomic status. Am. J. Respir. Crit. Care Med. **157:** 1016–1020.

7. CARNON, A.G. et al. 1994. Relation between socioeconomic deprivation and pathological prognostic factors in women with breast cancer. Br. Med. J. **309:** 1054–1057.

8. CUNNINGHAM, L.S. & J.L. KELSEY. 1984. Epidemiology of musculoskeletal impairments and associated disability. J. Pub. Health **74:** 574–579.

9. DAYAL, H.H., R.N. POWER & C. CHIU. 1982. Race and socio-economic status in survival from breast cancer. J. Chronic Dis. **35:** 675–683.

10. DEVESSA, S.S. & E.L. DIAMOND. 1980. Association of breast cancer and cervical cancer incidences with income and education among whites and blacks. J. Nat. Cancer Inst. **65**(3): 515–528.

11. DIEZ-ROUX, A.V. et al. 1997. Neighborhood environments and coronary heart disease: a multilevel analysis. Am. J. Epidemiol. **146:** 48–63.

12. FEINSTEIN, J.S. 1993. The relationship between socioeconomic status and health: a review of the literature. Milbank Q. **71:** 279–322.

13. FOX, A.J., P.O. GOLDBLATT & D.R. JONES. 1985. Social class mortality differentials: artefact, selection, or life circumstance. J. Epidemiol. Commun. Health **39:** 1–8.

14. HAAN, M., G.A. KAPLAN & T. CAMACHO. 1987. Poverty and health: prospective evidence from the Alameda County Study. Am. J. Epidemiol. **125:** 989–998.

15. HAAN, M.N., G.A. KAPLAN & S.L. SYME. 1989. Socioeconomic status and health: old observations and new thoughts. *In* Pathways to Health: The Role of Social Factors. J.P. Bunker, D.S. Gomby & B.H. Kehrer, Eds.: 76–117. The Henry J. Kaiser Family Foundation, Menlo Park.

16. HAKAMA, M., T. HAKULINEN, E. PUKKALA, E. SAXEN & L. TEPPO. 1982. Risk indicators of breast cancer and cervical cancer on ecologic and individual levels. Am. J. Epidemiol. **116**(6): 990–1000.

17. HELMERS, K., D. POSLUSZNY & D.S. KRANTZ. 1994. Associations of hostility and cor-onary artery disease: a review of studies. *In* Anger, Hostility, and the Heart. A. Siegman & T. Smith, Eds. Erlbaum, Hillsdale.

18. KAPLAN, G.A. & J.E. KEIL. 1993. Socioeconomic factors and cardiovascular disease: a review of the literature. Circulation **88**: 1973–1998.

19. KAPLAN, G.A., E.R. PAMUK, J.W. LYNCH, R.D. COHEN & J.L. BALFOUR. 1996. Inequality in income and mortality in the United States: analysis of mortality and potential pathways. Br. Med. J. **312**: 999–1003.

20. KAUFMAN, J.S., R.S. COOPER & D.L. MCGEE. 1997. Socioeconomic status and health in blacks and whites: the problem of residual confounding and the resiliency of race. Epidemiology **8**: 621–628.

21. KENNEDY, B.P., I. KAWACHI & D. PROTHROW-STITH. 1996. Income distribution and mortality: cross-sectional ecological study of the Robin Hood index in the United States. Br. Med. J. **312**: 1004–1007.

22. KOGEVINAS, M. & M. PORTA. 1997. Socioeconomic differences in cancer survival: a review of the evidence. IARC Sci. Pub. **138**: 177–206.

23. KRIEGER, N. & S. SIDNEY. 1996. Racial discrimination and blood pressure: the CARDIA Study of young black and white adults. Am. J. Pub. Health **86**: 1370–1378.

24. KUNST, A.E., C.W.N. LOOMAN & J.P. MACKENBACH. 1990. Socioeconomic mortality differences in the Netherlands in 1950-1984: A regional study of cause specific mortality. Soc. Sci. Med., **31**: 141–152.

25. MACINTYRE, S., S. MACIVER & A. SOOMAN. 1993. Area, class and health: should we be focusing on places or people? J. Soc. Pol. **22**: 213–234.

26. MACKENBACH, J.P., A.E. KUNST, A.E. CAVELAARS, F. GROENHOF, J.J. GEURTS & EU WORKING GROUP ON SOCIOECONOMIC INEQUALITIES IN HEALTH. 1997. Socioeconomic inequalities in morbidity and mortality in Western Europe. Lancet **349**: 1655–1659.

27. MACKILLOP, W.J., J. ZHANG-SALOMONS, P.A. GROOME, L. PASZAT & E. HOLOWATY. 1997. Socioeconomic status and cancer survival in Ontario. J. Clin. Oncol. **15**: 1680–1689.

28. MARMOT, M.G., M.J. SHIPLEY & G. ROSE. 1984. Inequalities in death: specific explanations of a general pattern? Lancet **1**: 1003–1006.

29. MATTHEWS, K.A., S.F. KELSEY, E.N. MEILAHN, L.H. KULLER & R.R. WING. 1989. Educational attainment and behavioral and biologic risk factors for coronary heart disease in middle-aged women. Am. J. Epidemiol. **129**: 1132–1144.

30. MARMOT, M. 1992. Coronary heart disease: rise and fall of a modern epidemic. *In* Coronary Heart Disease Epidemiology. M. Marmot & P. Elliott, Eds.: 3–19. Oxford University Press, New York.

31. MCEWEN, B.S. 1998. Protective and damaging effects of stress mediators. N. Engl. J. Med. **338**: 171–179.

32. O'CAMPO, P., X. XUE, M.C. WANG & M. CAUGHY. 1997. Neighborhood risk factors for low birthweight in Baltimore: a multilevel analysis. Am. J. Pub. Health **87**: 1113–1118.

33. OSTROVE, J.M. & N.E. ADLER. 1998. The relationship of socioeconomic status, labor force participation, and health among men and women. J. Health Psychol. **3**: 451–463.

34. OSTROVE, J.M., N.E. ADLER, M. KUPPERMANN & A.E. WASHINGTON. Resources and rankings: alternative assessments of socioeconomic status and their relationship to health in an ethnically diverse sample of women. Under review.

35. PAMUK, E., D. MAKUC, K. HECK, C. REUBEN & K. LOCHNER. 1998. Socioeconomic Status and Health Chartbook. Health, United States, 1998. National Center for Health Statistics, Hyattsville, MD.
36. WADSWORTH, M.E.J. 1986. Serious illness in childhood and its association with later-life achievement. *In* Class and Health. Research and Longitudinal Data. R.G. Wilkinson, Ed.: 50–74. Tavistock Publications, New York.
37. WILLIAMS, D.R. & C. COLLINS. 1995. U.S. socioeconomic and racial differentials in health: patterns and explanations. Annu. Rev. Sociol. **21:** 349–386.
38. WILKINSON, R.G. 1992. Income distribution and life expectancy. Br. Med. J. **304:** 165–168.
39. WINKLEBY, M.A., D.E. JATULIS, E. FRANK & S.P. FORTMANN. 1992. Socioeconomic status and health: how education, income, and occupation contribute to risk factors for cardiovascular disease. Am. J. Pub. Health **82:** 816–820.
40. WINKLEBY, M.A., C. CUBBIN, D.K. AHN & H.C. KRAEMER. 1999. Pathways by which SES and ethnicity influence cardiovascular disease risk factors. Ann. N.Y. Acad. Sci. **896:** this volume.
41. HERTZMAN, C. 1999. The biological embedding of early experience and its effects on health in adulthood. Ann. N.Y. Acad Sci. **896:** this volume.
42. WILLIAMS, D.R. 1999. Race, socioeconomic status, and health: the added effects of racism and discrimination. Ann. N.Y. Acad. Sci. **896:** this volume.
43. KAPLAN, J.R. & S.B. MANUCK. 1999. Status, stress, and atherosclerosis: the role of environment and individual behavior. Ann. N.Y. Acad. Sci. **896:** this volume.
44. McEWEN, B.S. & T. SEEMAN. 1999. Protective and damaging effects of mediators of stress: elaborating and testing the concepts of allostasis and allostatic load. Ann. N.Y. Acad. Sci. **896:** this volume.
45. ANDERSON, N.B. 1999. Solving the puzzle of SES and health: the need for interdisciplinary, multilevel research. Ann. N.Y. Acad. Sci. **896:** this volume.
46. LEE, P.R. 1999. Socioeconomic status and health: policy implications in research, public health, and medical care. Ann. N.Y. Acad. Sci. **896:** this volume.
47. TARLOV, A.R. 1999. Public policy frameworks for improving population health. Ann. N.Y. Acad. Sci. **896:** this volume.
48. COHEN, S. 1999. Social status and susceptibility to respiratory infections. Ann. N.Y. Acad. Sci. **896:** this volume.

Epidemiology of Socioeconomic Status and Health: Are Determinants Within Countries the Same as Between Countries?

MICHAEL MARMOT[a,b]

Department of Epidemiology and Public Health, University College London, 1-19 Torrington Place, London WC1E 6BT, United Kingdom

ABSTRACT: Within societies, health and ill-health follow a social gradient: lower socioeconomic position, worse health. The slope of the gradient has varied over time. It is likely that social and economic circumstances play a role in this changing slope. Within Europe, differences in health between East and West have also varied in magnitude. The advantage in the West increased through the 1970s and 1980s. Although similar in their health trends up to 1989, the countries of central and eastern Europe have diverged quite sharply subsequently. It is again likely that changing social and economic fortunes account for these trends. There is evidence to support the role of psychosocial factors in relating to socioeconomic differences within and between countries.

INTRODUCTION

Researchers interested in inequalities in health are wont to quote data from the Titanic disaster. The fatality rates from drowning were comparatively low among first class passengers, were higher among second class passengers, and higher still among passengers in the third class.[1] Perhaps it is not too fanciful to use these data on inequalities in rates of drowning to illustrate different approaches to dealing with the problem of inequalities in health. A typical medical response might be better treatment for hypothermia and more rapid response units. The holistic primary care response might be to deal with the feelings of unhappiness induced by the experience. An orientation that emphasizes the individualistic approach to prevention, namely that individuals have it within their own power to choose healthy ways of living, might focus on swimming lessons. An approach that emphasized the environmental causes of illness might focus on safe navigation. In this instance, whatever power individuals may have had over their own ability to survive the catastrophe, had the catastrophe not occurred no-one would have drowned. This would have been of great advantage, but it is a reasonable prediction that there still would have

[a]Address for correspondence: 44-171-391-1680 (voice); 44-171-813-0242 (fax).
e-mail: m.marmot@public-health.ucl.ac.uk

[b]This article, with some modifications, was first presented at the Kansas Conference on Health and it Determinants, in Wichita, Kansas, USA, April 20–21, 1998 and published as a chapter in The Society and Population Health Reader, Alvin R. Tarlov and Robert F. St. Peter, Eds. The New Press, New York, late 1999. It is published here with permission of the editors and the publishers of the New Press volume.

been inequalities in health. The third class passengers would have died at a younger age than the first class passengers, but of other causes.

This is the theme of my contribution. There is a gradient in health outcome running from the most to the least advantaged members of society; these health outcomes are not specific to any particular cause; a medical response will not solve the problem; nor will a response that emphasizes individual choices over lifestyle. Inequalities in health are a manifestation of the social determinants of health. While it does not follow automatically that if the causes are social in origin, the solutions need necessarily to be social—aspirin can relieve headache, even if the cause is poverty—it is likely that an understanding of causes of inequality has the possibility to lead to policies that can make a fundamental contribution to improving health in society.

THE PROBLEM OF INEQUALITIES IN HEALTH

Social Inequalities Within Countries

My approach to this problem starts with the Whitehall study.[2-4] FIGURE 1, from the 25-year follow-up of British civil servants in the original Whitehall study, shows the social gradient in all-cause mortality. These men were all in stable employment, and none was in poverty in any absolute sense of that word, yet there is a gradient in mortality. Each grade in the civil service has higher mortality rates than the grade above it in the hierarchy. This figure shows the data for all-cause mortality, but there are similar gradients for all the major causes of death.

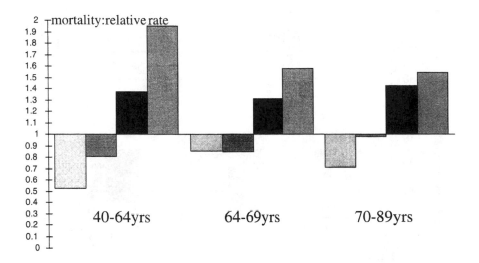

FIGURE 1. All-cause mortality by grade of employment. Whitehall men 25-year follow-up. ▢, administrative; ▪, professional/executive; ▪, clerical; ▨, other.

The gradient is relevant to the later policy discussion. Poverty is a major public health problem, and policies to reduce poverty are likely to have an impact on the health consequences of poverty. These data illustrate a different problem: that of inequality. Inequality is likely to relate to relative, rather than absolute deprivation. This is likely to require a different policy response.

The magnitude of the social gradient in mortality is not constant but has been changing over time. FIGURE 2 shows national data for England and Wales over the

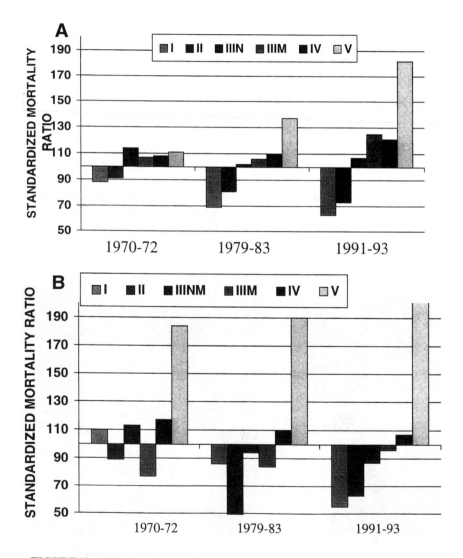

FIGURE 2. (A) Ischemic heart disease and (B) suicide, by social class in England and Wales. Males, 1970–1993. (For B 1970–1972 does not include undetermined.) (Data from Drever et al.[5])

time period 1970 to 1993. Both for ischemic heart disease and suicide the social gradient became considerably steeper over the last 20 years.[5]

These social gradients are not confined to the UK. The Panel Study of Income Dynamics in the USA showed a similar gradient in mortality with respondents classified according to household income.[6] This study, too, illustrates that inequalities in health run across the whole of society. People in the lowest income category, less than $15,000 average household income in 1993, had 3.9 times the risk of dying of people in the highest income category (greater than $70,000). But, only about 7% of the population fell into this poverty category. Nearly 25% of the population were in the second highest income bracket, and they had 34% higher mortality than the top group. Nearly 30% fell into the third income bracket and they had 59% higher mortality. The implication is clear: poverty is potentially fatal for the worst off members of society, but inequality has a major impact on mortality even among those who are relatively well off but still not among the most fortunate.

Inequalities Between Countries

We have been concerned with East–West differences in mortality in Europe,[7] as FIGURE 3 illustrates. It shows life expectancy at age 15, thereby removing the effect of infant and child mortality. In 1970 the differences in life expectancy between the Nordic and European Union countries on the one hand and the communist countries of Central and Eastern Europe on the other, was relatively small. The Soviet Union lagged behind the other countries, and the difference in life expectancy for men at age 15 was 4 years compared with the European Union. Over the next 25 years life expectancy improved steadily in the Nordic and European Union countries and stag-

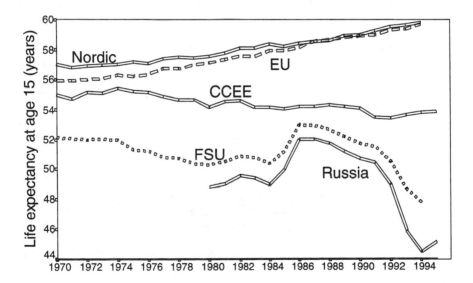

FIGURE 3. Life expectancy at age 15 in Europe, men. Abbreviations: EU, European Union; CCEE, countries of Central and Eastern Europe; FSU, former Soviet Union.

TABLE 1. Structure of mortality in middle income countries

	Infant Mortality per 1,000	Prob. (%) of Death 15–60 males	IHD	Life expectancy at birth, males
South Africa	53	30.8	Low	60
Hungary	15	27.7	High	65
Costa Rica	14	14.5	Low	74

nated or declined in the countries of Central and Eastern Europe. By 1994 the gap in life expectancy at age 15 between Russia and the European Union was about 10 years—a dramatic widening of inequalities across Europe in a relatively short time. The causes of death that contribute most to the East–West difference in mortality are cardiovascular disease and external causes of death.[8] Interestingly, these particular causes make a major contribution to inequalities in mortality within the UK and the USA. This has led us to speculate that the causes of inequalities in health within countries may be similar to the causes of international differences.[7] This is similar to the implication of Wilkinson's work summarized in another chapter in this volume.[9]

The worsening mortality pattern has not affected all groups equally within Central and Eastern European countries. In general, there has been a widening social gradient within those countries.[10]

The fact that, in addition to poverty, other more general social factors may also be operating is illustrated by the comparison of three countries that all had an equivalent gross national product in the early 1990s of around $2000 (TABLE 1). The high infant mortality in South Africa is related to poverty as is the high probability of death between the ages of 15 and 60, given that ischemic heart disease mortality is low. The relatively favorable infant mortality in Hungary and Costa Rica is, in a sense, better than one would have predicted from their GNP. The difference between these two countries is in the mortality among middle-aged men, high in Hungary, largely due to ischemic heart disease, which results in a dramatic difference in life expectancy. There is something about society in Hungary, which cannot be summed up under the rubric "poverty," that relates to the high mortality among middle-aged men. If the above speculation is correct, an understanding of what this factor(s) might be could help us understand the causes of inequalities in health within our own societies.

EXPLANATIONS FOR INEQUALITIES IN HEALTH

Social Causes of Disease Rates in Society

In paying a tribute to the work of Geoffrey Rose,[11] I illustrated his insight, along with Durkheim, that the causes of disease rates of a population may be different from the causes of individual differences in disease occurrence.[12] (TABLE 2 illustrates.) We tend to think of accidental deaths as accidents, but the relative constancy of their rate of occurrence suggests that each population has a characteristic accident rate.

TABLE 2. "Accidental" deaths in Engand and Wales[a]

	Male		Female	
	1993	1994	1993	1994
Motor vehicle traffic accidents	2,395	2,287	1,039	998
Accidental falls	1,517	1,481	2,400	2,189
Suicide and self-inflicted injury	2,875	2,838	866	803

[a]Mortality statistics, ONS 1996.

The figures on suicide are quite remarkable. The number of suicide deaths appears to be relatively constant year on year. There are, of course, long-term secular trends, but not wide fluctuations from one year to the next. This suggests, following Durkheim and Rose, that populations have a characteristic rate of occurrence of causes of death. As the characteristics of populations change, so the death rates may change. We will not, however, necessarily discover the causes of the population rate of occurrence by studying the differences among individuals within a population.

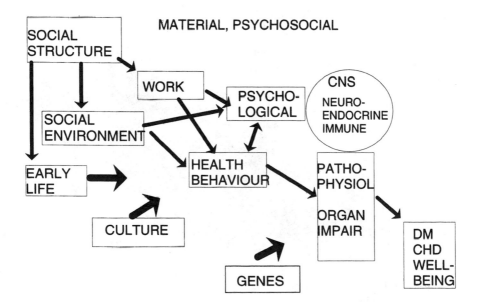

FIGURE 4. Simplified causal model of inequalities in health. Abbreviations: CNS, central nervous system; DM, diabetes mellitus; CHD, coronary heart disease.

A Causal Model

We have been working with a simplified causal model of inequalities in health (FIG. 4). At the right-hand end of this figure, it shows the health outcomes that have been the focus of much of our research: diabetes mellitus (DM), coronary heart disease, and measures of well-being; and at the upper left, aspects of the social structure that manifest themselves as social inequalities. The boxes in between are an oversimplified way of representing the causal pathways. This could be made impossibly complex, but in this simple version, it allows us to study how, for example, individual risk factors might relate to circumstances from early life or the conditions in adulthood in which people live and work, and hence the potential role of these individual factors in mediating the relation between social factors and disease outcome.

FIGURE 5 illustrates that individual risk factors do not help greatly in understanding the Whitehall gradient in mortality. It shows that within each employment grade plasma total cholesterol is a predictor of CHD mortality. Within each quintile of cholesterol level the social gradient in mortality is evident. Plasma cholesterol is a predictor of coronary heart disease mortality, but it does not account for the social gradient. Smoking shows a clear social gradient, but the social gradient in CHD mortality was similar in nonsmokers to that in smokers.[3]

However much of the social gradient is explained by risk factors, we must bear in mind that individual behaviors are affected by the environment. In the case of alcohol, for example, the evidence shows that the higher the mean consumption of a population, the greater the prevalence of heavy drinkers.[12,13] The clear implication is that a societal intervention might be more effective in reducing the harm associated with alcohol, than a program targeting individual heavy drinkers.

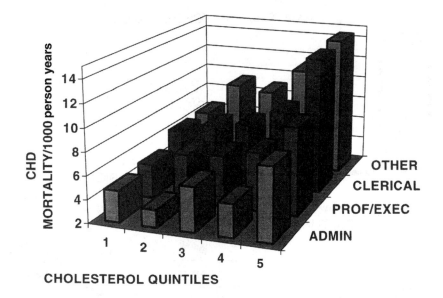

FIGURE 5. Twenty-five-year coronary heart disease mortality by employment grade, Whitehall men.

Psychosocial or Material Causes of Inequalities

In Britain, there has been lively debate about what proportion of the causes of inequalities in health are material or psychosocial. There is a good case to be made that material deprivation in one way or another accounts for the link between poverty and ill health. Even here, material deprivation may have an important psychosocial component. The ways of doing without in Britain, at least, have changed (Alan Marsh, personal communication). Whereas in the past, material deprivation meant inadequate housing, under-nutrition, inadequate clothing, and risky work places, now the definition of what it means to be on the "bread line" has broadened. It also means inability to entertain children's friends, buy children new clothes, go on holiday, and pursue a hobby or leisure activity. In other words, material deprivation in a modern context may mean inability to participate fully in society and to control one's life.

Thus, there is a link with the concept of relative deprivation that may underlie the social gradient. The mechanisms linking social position to health, across the whole social gradient, are likely to involve psychosocial factors. Among the psychosocial factors with the strongest evidence to support their role in generating inequalities in health are: social supports/social integration, the psychosocial work environment, control/mastery, hostility, and parenting.

Social Supports/Integration

Lisa Berkman has reviewed the evidence for the strong and consistent protective effect of participation in social networks and of social supports.[14] Evidence from the Whitehall II study shows that the lower the position on the hierarchy, the less participation in social networks outside the family, and the more negative the degree of social support.[15]

Data from Central and Eastern European countries show that the adverse trend in mortality has particularly affected men who were single, widowed, or divorced.[16,17] The adverse effect was not seen in women. One possible explanation for this is that marriage provided the main source of support for men in societies where other forms of social participation were weak.[18] Women, on the other hand, were more likely to participate in informal social networks, at least in part, because barter and other forms of informal exchange were mechanisms that allowed families to function.

There is a clear potential link between social ties and social capital as reviewed in this volume by Kawachi.[19]

Psychosocial Work Environment

The two dominant models in the field of the psychosocial work environment are the demand/control model[20] and that of effort reward imbalance.[21]

In the Whitehall II study, along with a number of other studies[22] the demand dimension did not predict coronary heart disease. Low control in the workplace was an important predictor of CHD incidence rates.[23] FIGURE 6, from the Whitehall II study, shows the social gradient in the occurrence of incident CHD events[24] and the contribution of three sets of factors, taken one at a time, to explaining this social gradient. Short height, as a measure of early life effects, is a predictor of coronary heart disease incidence and makes a small contribution to explaining the social gradient. As in Whitehall I, the standard coronary risk factors, serum cholesterol, blood pres-

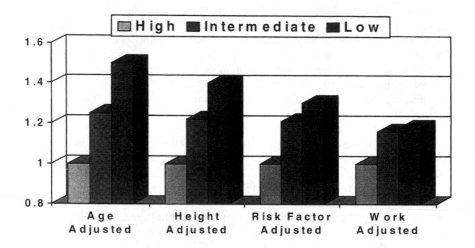

FIGURE 6. Odds ratio for new CHD in Whitehall II by employment grade, men.[24]

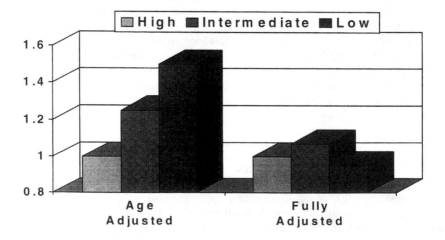

FIGURE 7. Odds ratio for new CHD in Whitehall II by employment grade, men.[24] (Fully adjusted for height, risk factors, and low control.)

sure, smoking, body mass index, and physical activity accounted for between a quarter and a third of the social gradient. More than half the gradient appeared to be accounted for by low control in the workplace. FIGURE 7 shows that, in multivariate analysis, the combination of height, coronary risk factors, and low control in the workplace appear to provide a complete explanation for the social gradient in occurrence of CHD.

Using the same methods but in a very different population in the Czech Republic, we had remarkably similar findings. A combination of coronary risk factors and low control in the workplace provided an explanation for the association between low education and risk of myocardial infarction.[25]

In discussing these findings we noted that there are, of course, social gradients in the occurrence of coronary heart disease among people who are not working. However, if low control is important, it does not derive only from the workplace. It may be a feature of the social conditions under which people live, as well as work.

Control/Mastery

There is a large literature on this subject.[26] It tends to view low control as a characteristic of individuals. Indeed, our work from Central and Eastern Europe would confirm that individuals who report low control have worse health.[27] It may be possible to characterize whole societies on degree of control. FIGURE 8 plots mean control for population subgroups against coronary heart disease rates for whole populations in an "ecological" analysis. It shows the higher the mean level of control of a society the lower the coronary heart disease rates.

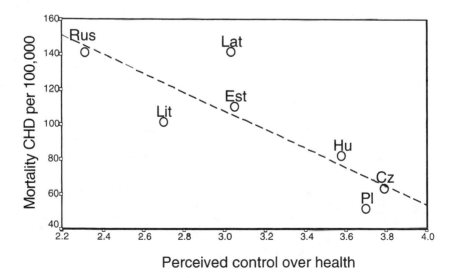

FIGURE 8. Standardized mortality from coronary heart disease, 0–64 years. Abbreviations: Rus, Russia; Lat, Latvia; Lit, Lithuania; Est, Estonia; Hu, Hungary; Cz, Czech Republic; Pl, Poland.

Hostility

Redford Williams has produced similar findings for hostility.[28] He and others have shown that hostile persons have higher risk of coronary heart disease than those who are not hostile. If hostility is viewed as a stable trait of individuals, there is no particular reason why it should be related to the environment. Williams did a Gallup survey of 10 American cities and showed that they differed in mean hostility levels. He showed further that there was a direct correlation between mean hostility of a city and that city's mortality from coronary heart disease (FIG. 9).

Parenting

Barker's group in the UK have provided strong evidence for the programming hypothesis.[29] The *in-utero* environment programs organ systems of the developing fetus that change the individual's likelihood of developing chronic disease later in life. The British Birth Cohorts confirm that there are substantial effects of early life that continue to influence disease risk later in life.[30–32] Working with data from the 1958 Birth Cohort, Power shows that it is accumulation of advantage and disadvantage throughout the lifecourse that accounts for inequalities in health in adulthood.[33]

Nevertheless, what happens in early life is likely to be crucial. A review by Fonagy[34] shows the substantial effect that quality of parenting and relationships within families has on the health and well-being of children. Put this together with the reviews by Hertzman[35] and Mustard[36] of what happens to children from disordered families when they enter the school system and evidence from the longitudinal studies, and one can build a case for the impact of parenting on the health of adults.

Biological Pathways

It could be argued that we did not need to know what the biological effects were of smoking to reach conclusions about its health effects. However, the criteria for as-

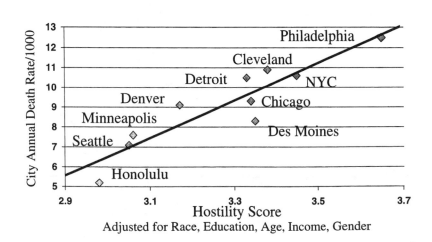

FIGURE 9. Hostility and coronary heart disease mortality by city.[40]

sessing causation developed by Bradford-Hill and the U.S. Surgeon General had much to do with the controversy around smoking and health. One of these criteria is biological plausibility. The argument was that, without a biologically plausible mechanism, the causal nature of epidemiological association remains suspect.

When we reported our findings suggesting that low control in the workplace was an important contributor to the social gradient in coronary heart disease, we asked ourselves why pick on low control in the workplace?[24] After all, a number of factors showed a social gradient, why incriminate this particular feature of the workplace? Part of our answer was that low control was related to levels of plasma fibrinogen[3] and that plasma fibrinogen in turn is a predictor of coronary heart disease. We do not think that plasma fibrinogen is necessarily "the answer" to the question of biological mechanisms. Plasma fibrinogen is an acute-phase protein and is correlated with the metabolic syndrome of insulin resistance.[38] This is an active area of research, and it is important for those of us concerned with social and psychological causes of illness not to be ignorant of modern biology.

Insights about biological pathways linking social status to cardiovascular risk come from the animal work. Shively recently reviewed the work on nonhuman primates showing the importance of the hypothalamic pituitary and sympatho-adrenal medullary axis.[39]

IMPLICATIONS FOR POLICY

The view exists that observational evidence is an inadequate basis for formulation of health policies. The only reliable guide, in this view, is the evidence that an intervention works. The best evidence for this is likely to come from a randomized controlled trial. For years, critics of the dietary fat/plasma cholesterol theory of the etiology of coronary heart disease claimed that (a) there was no evidence that lowering plasma cholesterol would produce benefit, and (b) there was concern that it might produce harm. This was in the face of a wealth of evidence from observational studies that argued for the safety and efficacy of lowering plasma cholesterol. With the advent of the 4S and WOSCOPS studies showing that lowering plasma cholesterol by treatment with statins produced a predictable reduction in primary and secondary occurrence of CHD, most critics of cholesterol converted. In passing, it might be noted that much of this conversion was not to a public health approach to reducing coronary heart disease but to a medical approach that relied on choosing which individuals should receive prescriptions for cholesterol-lowering drugs.

The randomized, controlled trial is the best tool we have for evaluating medical interventions on individual patients. The further upstream we go in our search for causes (see FIG. 4), the less applicable is the randomized, controlled trial. A randomized, controlled trial to improve social capital and evaluate its effect on mortality is difficult to conceive of, and perhaps impossible to execute.

We must therefore rely on observational evidence and judgment in formulating policies to reduce inequalities in health. In this process, the best should not be the enemy of the good. Although we should not formulate policies in the absence of evidence to support them, we must not be paralyzed into inaction while we wait for the evidence to be absolutely unimpeachable. The evidence in this volume provides ample basis for formulating policies to address the social determinants of health.

ACKNOWLEDGMENTS

MM is supported by an MRC Research Professorship and by the John D. and Catherine T. MacArthur Foundation Research Networks on Socioeconomic Status and Health and Successful Midlife Development.

REFERENCES

1. BROOM, L. & P. SELZNICK. 1968. Sociology. Harper International Edition. Harper & Row and John Weatherhill, Tokyo. 562pp.
2. MARMOT, M.G., G. ROSE, M. SHIPLEY & P.J.S. HAMILTON. 1978. Employment grade and coronary heart disease in British civil servants. J. Epidemiol. Community Health 32: 244–249.
3. MARMOT, M.G., M.J. SHIPLEY & G. ROSE. 1984. Inequalities in death—specific explanations of a general pattern. Lancet i: 1003–1006.
4. MARMOT, M.G. & M.J. SHIPLEY. 1996. Do socioeconomic differences in mortality persist after retirement? 25 year follow up of civil servants from the first Whitehall study. Br. Med. J. 313: 1177–1180.
5. DREVER, F., M. WHITEHEAD & M. RODEN. 1996. Current patterns and trends in male mortality by social class (based on occupation). Population Trends 86: 15–20.
6. MCDONOUGH, P., G.J. DUNCAN, D. WILLIAMS & J.S. HOUSE. 1997. Income dynamics and adult mortality in the United States, 1972 through 1989. Am. J. Public Health 87: 1476–1483.
7. BOBAK, M. & M.G. MARMOT. 1996. East–West mortality divide and its potential explanations: proposed research agenda. Br. Med. J. 312: 421–425.
8. BOBAK, M. & M. MARMOT. 1996. East–West health divide and potential explanations. In East–West Life Expectancy Gap in Europe. Environmental and Non-environmental Determinants. C. Hertzman, S. Kelly & M. Bobak, Eds.: 17–44. Kluwer Academic Publishers, Dordrecht.
9. WILKINSON, R.G. 1999. Health, hierarchy, and social anxiety. Ann. N.Y. Acad. Sci. 896: this volume.
10. MARMOT, M. & M. BOBAK. 1997. Psychosocial and biological mechanisms behind the recent mortality crisis in central and eastern Europe. In The Mortality Crisis in Transitional Economies. A.G. Cornia & R. Panicci, Eds. Oxford University Press, Oxford.
11. ROSE, G. 1992. The Strategy of Preventive Medicine. Oxford University Press, Oxford.
12. MARMOT, M.G. 1998. Improvement of social environment to improve health. Lancet 351: 57–60.
13. COLHOUN, H., Y. BEN-SHLOMO, W. DONG, L. BOST & M. MARMOT. 1997. Ecological analysis of collectivity of alcohol consumption in England: importance of average drinker. Br. Med. J. 314: 1164–1168.
14. BERKMAN, L. 1999. In The Society and Population Health Reader. Alvin R. Tarlov & Robert F. St. Peter, Eds. The New Press, New York.
15. STANSFELD, S.A. & M.G. MARMOT. 1992. Deriving a survey measure of social support: the reliability and validity of the Close Persons Questionnaire. Soc. Sci. Med. 35: 1027–1035.
16. HAJDU, P., M. MCKEE & F. BOJAN. 1995. Changes in premature mortality differentials by marital status in Hungary and in England and Wales. Eur. J. Pub. Health 5: 259–264.

17. WATSON, P. 1995. Explaining rising mortality among men in Eastern Europe. Soc. Sci. Med. **41:** 923–934.
18. ROSE, R. 1995. Russia as an hour-glass society: a constitution without citizens. East Eur. Constit. Rev. **4:** 34–42.
19. KAWACHI, I. 1999. Social capital and community effects on population and individual health. Ann. N.Y. Acad. Sci. **896:** this volume.
20. KARASEK, R. & T. THEORELL. 1990. Healthy Work: Stress, Productivity, and the Reconstruction of Working Life. Basic Books, New York.
21. SIEGRIST, J. 1996. Adverse health effects of high-effort/low-reward conditions. J. Occupat. Health Psychol. **1:** 27–41.
22. HEMINGWAY, H. & M. MARMOT. 1999. Evidence based cardiology: psychosocial factors in the aetiology and prognosis of coronary heart disease. Systematic review of prospective cohort studies. Br. Med. J. **38:** 1460–1467.
23. BOSMA, H., M.G. MARMOT, H. HEMINGWAY, A. NICHOLSON, E.J. BRUNNER & S. STANSFELD. 1997. Low job control and risk of coronary heart disease in the Whitehall II (prospective cohort) study. Br. Med. J. **314:** 558–565.
24. MARMOT, M., H. BOSMA, H. HEMINGWAY, E.J. BRUNNER & S.A. STANSFELD. 1997. Contribution of job control and other risk factors to social variations in coronary heart disease incidence. Lancet **350:** 235–239.
25. BOBAK, M., C. HERTZMAN, Z. SKODOVA & M. MARMOT. 1998. Association between psychosocial factors at work and non-fatal myocardial infarction in a population based case-control study in Czech men. Epidemiology **9:** 43–47.
26. SKINNER, E.A. 1996. A guide to constructs of control. J. Pers. Soc. Psychol. **71:** 549–570.
27. BOBAK, M., H. PIKHART, C. HERTZMAN, R. ROSE & M. MARMOT. 1998. Socioeconomic factors, perceived control and self-reported health in Russia. A cross-sectional survey. Soc. Sci. Med. **47**(2): 269–279.
28. WILLIAMS, R., T. HANEY, K. LEE, Y. KONG, J. BLUMENTHAL & R. WHALEN. 1980. Type A behavior, hostility and coronary heart disease. Psychosom. Med. **42:** 539–549.
29. BARKER, D.J. 1990. The fetal and infant origins of adult disease. Br. Med. J. **301:** 1111.
30. WADSWORTH, M.E.J. 1991. The Imprint of Time: Childhood, History and Adult Life. Clarendon Press, Oxford.
31. WADSWORTH, M.E.J. 1997. Changing social factors and their long term implications for health. Br. Med. Bull. **53:** 170–184.
32. POWER, C., O. MANOR & J. FOX. 1991. Health and Class: The Early Years. Chapman & Hall, London.
33. POWER, C., S. MATTHEWS & O. MANOR. 1998. Inequalities in self-rated health: explanations from different stages of life. Lancet **351:** 1009–1014.
34. FONAGY, P. 1999. In The Society and Population Health Reader. Alvin R. Tarlov & Robert F. St. Peter, Eds. The New Press, New York.
35. HERTZMAN, C. 1999. In The Society and Population Health Reader. Alvin R. Tarlov & Robert F. St. Peter, Eds. The New Press, New York.
36. MUSTARD, F. 1999. In The Society and Population Health Reader. Alvin R. Tarlov & Robert F. St. Peter, Eds. The New Press, New York.
37. BRUNNER, E., G. DAVEY SMITH, M. MARMOT, R. CANNER, M. BEKSINSKA & J. O'BRIEN. 1996. Childhood social circumstances and psychosocial and behavioural factors as determinants of plasma fibrinogen. Lancet **34:** 1008–1013.
38. BRUNNER, E.J., M.G. MARMOT, K. NANCHAHAL, et al. 1997. Social inequality in coronary risk: central obesity and the metabolic syndrome. Evidence from the Whitehall II study. Diabetologia **40:** 1341–1349.
39. SHIVELEY, C.A. In The Society and Population Health Reader. Alvin R. Tarlov & Robert F. St. Peter, Eds. The New Press, New York.
40. WILLIAMS, R.B., et al. 1995. Psychosom. Med. **57:** 57–96.

Protective and Damaging Effects of Mediators of Stress

Elaborating and Testing the Concepts of Allostasis and Allostatic Load

BRUCE S. McEWEN[a,b] AND TERESA SEEMAN[c]

[b]*Laboratory of Neuroendocrinology, The Rockefeller University, 1230 York Avenue, Box 165, New York, New York 10021, USA*

[c]*Division of Geriatrics, Department of Medicine, UCLA School of Medicine, Los Angeles, California, USA*

ABSTRACT: Stress is a condition of human existence and a factor in the expression of disease. A broader view of stress is that it is not just the dramatic stressful events that exact their toll but rather the many events of daily life that elevate activities of physiological systems to cause some measure of wear and tear. We call this wear and tear "allostatic load," and it reflects not only the impact of life experiences but also of genetic load; individual habits reflecting items such as diet, exercise, and substance abuse; and developmental experiences that set life-long patterns of behavior and physiological reactivity (see McEwen[1]). Hormones associated with stress and allostatic load protect the body in the short run and promote adaptation, but in the long run allostatic load causes changes in the body that lead to disease. This will be illustrated for the immune system and brain. Among the most potent of stressors are those arising from competitive interactions between animals of the same species, leading to the formation of dominance hierarchies. Psychosocial stress of this type not only impairs cognitive function of lower ranking animals, but it can also promote disease (e.g. atherosclerosis) among those vying for the dominant position. Social ordering in human society is also associated with gradients of disease, with an increasing frequency of mortality and morbidity as one descends the scale of socioeconomic status that reflects both income and education. Although the causes of these gradients of health are very complex, they are likely to reflect, with increasing frequency at the lower end of the scale, the cumulative burden of coping with limited resources and negative life events and the allostatic load that this burden places on the physiological systems involved in coping and adaptation.

INTRODUCTION

There are gradients of health, when groups of people are classified according to their socioeconomic status, that reflect both income and level of education. The poor suffer earlier mortality and worse health, on the average, than the middle class, which, in turn, is not as healthy as those who are wealthier and/or better educated.

[a]Address for correspondence: 212-327-8624 (voice); 212-327-8634 (fax).
e-mail: mcewen@rockvax.rockefeller.edu

Attempts to explain these gradients on the basis of access to health care or such behaviors as smoking have failed to explain the gradient.[2,3] Instead there is a need to understand more comprehensively how various aspects of life impact collectively on health, involving such factors as living environment, work, relationships, community, and knowledge and practice of health-promoting or health-damaging behaviors including diet and exercise. In order to do this, we must move from groups to individuals and understand how behavior and biology interact.

Often, we use the word "stress" to refer to these biological factors, but this is an oversimplification because they are more than "stress" and include many aspects of lifestyle and daily experience and behavior, including the adjustments to the circadian light–dark cycle. Moreover, the widespread use of the term "stress" in popular culture has made this word an ambiguous term to describe the ways in which the body copes with psychosocial, environmental, and physical challenges. Thus we have been in search of a more comprehensive term for the role of biological mediators in adaptation and maladaptation of the individual to the circumstances of life.

WHERE STRESS FITS IN

The body responds to the external and internal environment by producing hormonal and neurotransmitter mediators that set in motion physiological responses of cells and tissues throughout the body, leading to a coordination of physiological responses to the current circumstances. The measurement of the physiological responses of the body to environmental challenges constitutes the primary means of connecting experience with resilience or the risk for disease. Because the subjective experience of stress does not always correlate with the output of physiological mediators of stress,[4] the measurement of the physiological responses of the body to environmental challenges constitutes the primary means of connecting experience with resilience or the risk for disease. The so-called "stress mediators," hormones such as cortisol and catecholamines, also vary in their basal secretion according to a diurnal rhythm that is coordinated by the light–dark cycle and sleep–waking patterns, a fact that reinforces the inadequacy of the popular use of the term "stress" as a useful descriptor of the source of all biological dysregulations. For example, the internal biological clock of the hypothalamic suprachiasmatic nucleus regulates cyclicity of sleep and waking and the production of adrenocortical hormones that are entrained by the light–dark cycle; shifting the light–dark cycle, as by trans-Atlantic jet airplane travel, results in disregulation of adrenocortical hormone and contributes to disruption of sleep, activity, appetite, and cognitive function.

With regard to stress, the sudden occurrence of danger, as for a gazelle being chased by a lion or a person confronted by a threat to physical safety, calls forth release of both adrenalin and adrenocortical hormones ("fight or flight" response) that help the body survive the immediate crisis. Indeed, new research has reinforced the fact that the so-called "stress mediators" have protective and adaptive as well as damaging effects, and the search for biological mechanisms that determine protective versus damaging effects of these mediators is a theme in biobehavioral research.[1] This search has also led to a new formulation of the relationship between environmental challenge and biological responses.

ALLOSTASIS AND ALLOSTATIC LOAD

Rather than referring to everything dealing with responses to environmental and psychosocial situations as "stress," we have provided a new formulation using two new terms, "allostasis" and "allostatic load." Allostasis, meaning literally "maintaining stability (or homeostasis) through change" was introduced by Sterling and Eyer[5] to describe how the cardiovascular system adjusts to resting and active states of the body. This notion can be applied to other physiological mediators, such as the secretion of cortisol as well as catecholamines, and the concept of "allostatic load" was proposed to refer to the wear and tear that the body experiences due to repeated cycles of allostasis as well as the inefficient turning-on or shutting-off of these responses.[1,6] As an example of allostatic load, the persistent activation of blood pressure in dominant male cynomologus monkeys vying for position in an unstable dominance hierarchy is reported to accelerate atherosclerotic plaque formation.[7] Blood pressure surges accompany the social confrontations, and catecholamines are elevated during those surges. Together, the blood pressure and catecholamine elevations accelerate atherosclerosis, as shown by the fact that the acceleration of atherosclerosis in dominant monkeys was prevented by beta-adrenergic blocking, drugs.[8]

The concept of allostasis and allostatic load envisions a cascade of cause and effect that begins with primary stress mediators, such as catecholamines and cortisol, and leading to primary effects and then to secondary and tertiary outcomes, as will be described below. In order to begin to understand this formulation, FIGURE 1 summarizes four key features of the model. First, the brain is the integrative center for coordinating the behavioral and neuroendocrine responses (hormonal, autonomic) to challenges, some of which qualify as "stressful" but others of which are related to the diurnal rhythm and its ability to coordinate waking and sleeping functions with

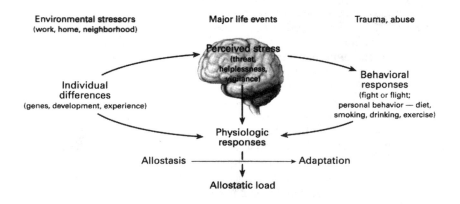

FIGURE 1. The stress response and development of allostatic load. Perception of stress is influenced by one's experiences, genetics, and behavior. When the brain perceives an experience as stressful, physiologic and behavioral responses are initiated leading to allostasis and adaptation. Over time, allostatic load can accumulate, and the overexposure to neural, endocrine, and immune stress mediators can have adverse effects on various organ systems, leading to disease. (Reprinted from McEwen[1] by permission from the *New England Journal of Medicine.*)

the environment. Second, there are considerable individual differences in coping with challenges, based on interacting genetic, developmental, and experiential factors. There is a cascading effect of genetic predisposition and early developmental events, such as abuse and neglect or other forms of early life stress, to predispose the organism to overreact physiologically and behaviorally to events throughout life. Third, inherent within the neuroendocrine and behavioral responses to challenge is the capacity to adapt (allostasis, meaning to achieve stability, or homeostasis, through change); and, indeed, the neuroendocrine responses are set up to be protective in the short run. For the neuroendocrine system, turning on and turning off responses efficiently is vital (see FIG. 2); inefficiency in allostasis leads to cumulative effects over long time intervals, as will be described below.

Fourth, allostasis has a price (allostatic load, referring, to cumulative negative effects, or the price the body pays for being forced to adapt to various psychosocial

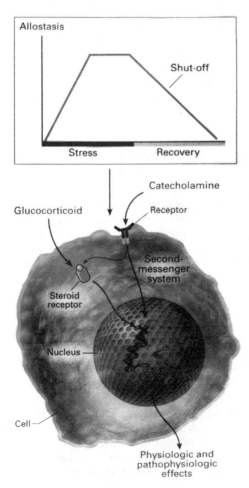

FIGURE 2. Allostasis in the autonomic nervous system and the hypothalamic–pituitary–adrenal axis.
Allostatic systems respond to stress (*upper panel*) by initiating the adaptive response, sustaining it until the stress ceases, and then shutting it off (recovery). Allostatic responses are initiated (*lower panel*) by an increase in circulating catecholamines from the autonomic nervous system and glucocorticoids from the adrenal cortex. This sets into motion adaptive processes that alter the structure and function of a variety of cells and tissues. These processes are initiated via intracellular receptors for steroid hormones, plasma membrane receptors, and second messenger systems for catecholamines. Cross-talk between catecholamines and glucocorticoid receptor signaling systems can occur (see text). (Reprinted from McEwen[1] by permission from the *New England Journal of Medicine*.)

challenges and adverse environments) that is related to how inefficient the response is, or how many challenges an individual experiences (i.e., a lot of stressful events). Thus allostatic load is more than "chronic stress" and encompasses many aspects of an individual's life that affect the regulation and level of the mediators of allostasis. Among the many factors that contribute to allostatic load are genes and early development, as well as learned behaviors reflecting life style choices of diet, exercise, smoking, and drinking. All of these factors influence the reactivity of the systems that produce the physiological stress mediators. Thus allostatic load reflects, in part, genetically or developmentally programmed inefficiency in handling, the normal challenges of daily life related to the sleep–wake cycle and other daily experiences, as well as the adverse physiological consequences of a fat-rich diet, drinking, or smoking.

Many of the same considerations apply to behavioral, as opposed to physiological, responses to challenge, and there are also protective and damaging aspects to one's behavior. Individuals can act to increase or decrease further risk for harm or disease—for example, antisocial responses such as hostility and aggression versus cooperation and conciliation; risk-taking behaviors such as smoking, drinking, and physical risk-taking versus self-protection; poor diet and health practices versus good diet, exercise, etc. The linkage of "allostasis" and "allostatic load" probably applies to behavioral responses as well to physiological responses to challenge insofar as the behavioral response, such as smoking or alcohol consumption, may have at least perceived adaptive benefits in the short run but produce damaging effects in the long run.

ALLOSTATIC LOAD REQUIRES UNDERSTANDING OF PHYSIOLOGICAL MECHANISMS

Although allostasis and allostatic load are general concepts to be applied across physiological and behavioral responses, they require in each case an understanding of underlying mechanisms in each system of the body. This understanding begins with the mediators that produce organ- and tissue-specific effects by acting via receptors that are common throughout the body (see FIG. 2). The mediators of allostasis include adrenal steroids and catecholamines, primarily, but also other hormones like DHEA, prolactin, growth hormones, and the cytokines related to the immune system, as well as local tissue mediators like the excitatory amino acids. In FIGURE 2, the actions of two mediators, the glucocorticoids and the catecholamines, are shown, acting via receptors that trigger changes throughout the target cell in processes, including both rapid effects and changes in gene expression that have long-lasting consequences for cell function. Thus, whenever a hormone is secreted, both the short-term and long-term consequences of hormone action on cell function are to be considered.

For each system of the body, there are both short-term adaptive actions (allostasis) that are protective and long-term effects that can be damaging (allostatic load). For the *cardiovascular system*, a prominent example of *allostasis* is the role of catecholamines in promoting adaptation by adjusting heart rate and blood pressure to sleeping, waking, and physical exertion.[5] Yet, repeated surges of blood pressure in

the face of job stress or the failure to shut off blood pressure surges efficiently accel-
erates atherosclerosis and synergizes with metabolic hormones to produce Type II
diabetes, and this constitutes a type of *allostatic load* (see McEwen[1]). Closely related to this is the role of adrenal steroids in *metabolism.* Whereas adrenal steroids promote allostasis by enhancing food intake and facilitating the replenishment of energy
reserves, the overactivity of this system involving repeated HPA activity in stress or
elevated evening, cortisol leads to allostatic load in terms of insulin resistance, accelerating progression towards Type II diabetes, including abdominal obesity, atherosclerosis, and hypertension.[9,10]

In the *brain,* actions of adrenal steroids and catecholamines that are related to allostasis include promoting retention of memories of emotionally charged events,
both positive and negative. Yet, overactivity of the HPA axis together with overactivity of the excitatory amino acid neurotransmitters promotes a form of allostatic load,
consisting of cognitive dysfunction by a variety of mechanisms that involve reduced
neuronal excitability, neuronal atrophy, and, in extreme cases, death of brain cells,
particularly in the hippocampus.[11,12]

For the *immune system,* adrenal steroids promote allostasis together with catecholamines by promoting "trafficking" (i.e., movement) of immune cells to organs
and tissues where they are needed to fight an infection or other challenge, and they
also modulate the expression of the hormones of the immune systems, the cytokines
and chemokines.[13] With chronic overactivity of these same mediators, allostatic load
results, consisting of immunosuppressive effects when these mediators are secreted
chronically or not shut off properly.[13] Yet, some optimal levels of these mediators is
required to maintain a functional balance within the competing forces of the immune
system, and the absence of sufficient levels of glucocorticoids and catecholamines
allows other immune mediators to overreact and increases the risk of autoimmune
and inflammatory disorders.[14] Therefore, an inadequate response of the HPA axis
and autonomic nervous system is another type of allostatic load, in which the disregulation of other mediators, normally contained by cortisol and catecholamines, is a
primary factor in a disorder.

Thus, allostatic load may be subdivided into at least four subtypes, as summarized in FIGURE 3. The first type is simply too much "stress" in the form of repeated,
novel events that cause repeated elevations of stress mediators over long, periods of
time. For example, the amount and frequency of economic hardship predicts decline
of physical and mental functioning as well as increased mortality.[15] Yet not all types
of allostatic load deal with chronic stress. A second type of allostatic load depicted
in FIGURE 3 involves a failure to habituate or adapt to the same stressor. This leads
to the overexposure to stress mediators because of the failure of the body to dampen
or eliminate the hormonal stress response to a repeated event. An example of this is
the finding that repeated public speaking, challenges, in which most individuals ha-
bituated their cortisol response, led a significant minority of individuals to fail to habituate and continue to show cortisol response.[16]

A third and related type of allostatic load, also depicted in FIGURE 3, involves the
failure to shut off either the hormonal stress response or to display the normal trough
of the diurnal cortisol pattern. One example of this is blood pressure elevations in
work-related stress which turn off slowly in some individuals with a family history
of hypertension.[17] Another example of perturbing the normal diurnal rhythm is that

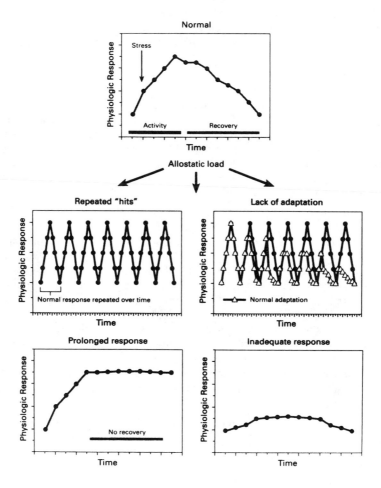

FIGURE 3. Four types of allostatic load. The *top panel* illustrates the normal allostatic response, in which a response is initiated by a stressor, sustained for an appropriate interval, and then turned off. The remaining panels illustrate four conditions that lead to allostatic load: (1) repeated "hits" from multiple novel stressors, (2) lack of adaptation, (3) prolonged response due to delayed shut down, and (4) inadequate response leading to compensatory hyperactivity of other mediators (e.g., inadequate secretion of glucocorticoid, resulting in increased levels of cytokines that are normally counterregulated by glucocorticoids). Figure drawn by Dr. Firdaus Dhabhar, The Rockefeller University, New York. (Reprinted from McEwen[1] by permission from the *New England Journal of Medicine.*)

of sleep deprivation leading to elevated evening cortisol and hyperglycemia within five days[18] and depressive illness leading to chronically elevated cortisol and loss of bone mineral mass.[19]

The fourth type of allostatic load depicted in FIGURE 3 involves an inadequate hormonal stress response that allows other systems, such as the inflammatory cytokines, to become overactive. The Lewis rat is an example of an animal strain in which increased susceptibility to inflammatory and autoimmune disturbances is related to inadequate levels of cortisol.[14,20]

VALIDATION OF ALLOSTATIC LOAD

Assessment of allostatic load would optimally incorporate information on "resting" or "usual" levels of allostatic mediators for each individual, as well as assessments of system dynamics (i.e., alterations in the "operating range" of the system parameters in response to stimulation, so as to tap into the four types of allostatic load depicted in FIG. 3); and it would include information for parameters of all major physiological regulatory systems. Such a goal is rather ambitious, but a first step was made in that direction using available data from the MacArthur Successful Aging Study. Using this data, we previously reported on an initial operational measure of allostatic load that reflects information on levels of physiologic activity across a range of important regulatory systems, including the hypothalamic–pituitary–adrenal and sympathetic nervous systems as well as the cardiovascular system and metabolic processes.[21] Our measure of allostatic load reflects only one of the two aspects of physiologic activity postulated to contribute to allostatic load, namely, higher, chronic, steady-state levels of activity related to the diurnal variation as well as any residual activity reflecting chronic stress or failure to shut off responses to acute stressors. Specifically, available data on physiologic activity represent single measures of activity levels rather than assessments of the dynamics of these systems in response to challenge.

Available data from the MacArthur Study provided information on the following parameters[21]:

- Systolic and diastolic blood pressure, indices of cardiovascular activity.

- Waist–hip ratio, an index of more chronic levels of metabolism and adipose tissue deposition, thought to be influenced by increased glucocorticoid activity.

- Serum HDL and total cholesterol, related to the development of atherosclerosis—increased risks being seen with higher levels in the case of total cholesterol and lower levels in the case of HDL.

- Blood plasma levels of glycosylated hemoglobin, an integrated measure of glucose metabolism over several days' time.

- Serum dihydroepiandrosterone sulfate (DHEA-S), a functional HPA axis antagonist.

- Overnight urinary cortisol excretion, an integrated measure of 12-hour HPA axis activity.

- Overnight urinary norepinephrine and epinephrine excretion levels, integrated indices of 12-hour SNS activity.

Our initial measure of allostatic load was created by summing across indices of subjects' status with respect to these 10 components of allostatic load. For each of the 10 indicators, subjects were classified into quartiles based on the distribution of scores in the high function cohort (see Seeman et al.[21]). The decision to use distributions in the high-function cohort was based on the fact that analyses of relationships between allostatic load and health outcomes were based on longitudinal data for this latter group. Allostatic load was measured by summing the number of parameters for which the subject fell into the "highest" risk quartile (i.e., top quartile for all parameters except HDL cholesterol and DHEA-S for which membership in the lowest quartile corresponds to highest risk).

Several alternative criteria for calculating allostatic load were also examined. One such alternative using a stricter criterion was based on a sum of the number of parameters for which the subject fell into the top (or bottom) 10% of the distribution (i.e., the group at highest "risk"). Another measure of allostatic load was based on averaging z-scores for each of the parameters. In each case, analyses yielded essentially the same results as the measure based on the quartile criteria, though the latter showed the strongest effects. These concurrent results suggest to us that the disease risks associated with allostatic load derive (as the original conceptualization would argue) from being, relatively higher on various measures of physiologic regulation rather than only at the most extreme levels. At the same time, simply averaging levels of activity across systems may tend to obscure the impact of elevations in a subset of systems that contribute to higher allostatic load. Thus, we selected an algorithm for allostatic load that avoids the problem of averaging, using instead a count of the number of parameters for which subjects exhibited relatively elevated levels. The 10 components were equally weighted because, based on factor analysis, indicators from physiologic systems defined different factors, and the component loadings on the relevant factors were virtually the same. This measure of allostatic load was then examined for its ability to predict health outcomes over a 2.5-year follow-up. Higher baseline allostatic load scores were found to predict significantly increased risks for incident cardiovascular disease as well as increased risks for decline in physical and cognitive functioning and for mortality.[21]

FURTHER REFINEMENT OF ALLOSTATIC LOAD

One of the problems with the original conceptualization of allostatic load and its measurement is that the components were not organized and categorized with regard to what each measure represents in the cascade of events that lead from allostasis to allostatic load. Nor was there any suggested organization in choosing, those original measures that would facilitate systematically relating measures to specific disease outcomes or systematically adding, new measures. Allostasis and allostatic load are concepts that are mechanistically based and only as good as the information about mechanisms that lead to disease. A new way of classifying the measures must provide a handle for relating what is measured to a pathophysiological process and allow for the incorporation of new measures as more is known about underlying mechanisms leading to disease. Below, we summarize a new formulation, based on the notion of *primary mediators* leading to *primary effects* and then to *secondary outcomes,* which lead, finally, to *tertiary outcomes* that represent actual diseases.

Primary Mediators: Chemical Messengers That Are Released as Part of Allostasis

At present, we have four such mediators (cortisol, noradrenalin, epinephrine, and DHEA). In general, the primary mediators have widespread influences throughout the body and are very useful, when measured correctly, in predicting, a variety of secondary and tertiary outcomes. Cortisol is a glucocorticoid with wide-ranging effects throughout the body. Glucocorticoid receptors are present in virtually every tissue and organ in the body and mediate effects ranging from induction of liver enzymes involved in energy metabolism to regulating the trafficking of immune cells and cytokine production to facilitating formation of fear-related memories.[22,23] DHEA is a functional antagonist of cortisol[24,25] that may also have effects via other signalling pathways[26]; generally, low DHEA is considered deleterious, as is chronically high cortisol.[27] As already noted, it is important to emphasize that the acute effects of stress mediators are generally adaptive (allostasis) and it is the chronic elevation or disregulation of these mediators over long times that causes problems, that is, allostatic load.

Catecholamines (adrenalin, noradrenalin) are released by the adrenal medulla and sympathetic nervous system, respectively, and they produce widespread effects throughout the body, ranging from vasoconstriction and acceleration of heart rate to trafficking of immune cells to targets, as well as enhancement of fear-related memory formation.[28] Adrenergic receptors are widespread throughout the body, in blood vessels and target organs such as the liver, pancreas, and the brain, which is not accessible to circulating catecholamines. However, catecholamines signal the brain through the sensory vagus and the nucleus of the solitary tract, as in learned fear.[28]

Primary Effects: Cellular Events, Like Enzymes, Receptors, Ion Channels, or Structural Proteins Induced Genomically or Phosphorylated via Second-Messenger Systems, That Are Regulated as Part of Allostasis by the Primary Mediators

We do not presently measure primary effects, and it may be desirable to study primary effects as the basis for the secondary and tertiary outcomes—this, in fact, is the mechanistic research that is supported by the NIH! Glucocorticoids regulate gene expression via several pathways, involving interactions with DNA via the glucocorticoid response elements (GREs) and also via protein–protein interactions with other transcriptional regulators.[29] As noted above, DHEA antagonizes glucocorticoid actions in a number of systems. Catecholamines act via alpha and beta adrenergic receptors, and beta receptors stimulate the formation of the intracellular second messenger, cyclic AMP (cAMP), which, in turn, regulates intracellular events via phosphorylation, including, transcription regulators via the CREB family of proteins.[30]

In some cases, the glucocorticoid and cAMP pathways converge at the level of gene expression (e.g, see Yamada[31]). Therefore it is not surprising that secondary outcomes (see below) are the result of more than one primary mediator. Primary effects are organ- and tissue-specific in many cases. Hence, at this level, and even more for the secondary and tertiary outcomes, we *must* become more organ and disease specific!

Secondary Outcomes: Integrated Processes That Reflect the Cumulative Outcome of the Primary Effects in a Tissue/Organ-Specific Manner in Response to the Primary Mediators, Often Reflecting the Actions of More Than One Primary Mediator, Including the Ones Described above as Well as Others Not Yet Measured

As already noted above, we measured the following secondary outcomes, which are all related to abnormal metabolism and risk for cardiovascular disease: WHRI blood pressure, glycosylated hemoglobin, cholesterol/HDL ratio, HDL cholesterol. As noted above, WHR and glycosylated hemoglobin both reflect the effects of sustained elevations in glucose and the insulin resistance that develops as a result of elevated cortisol and elevated sympathetic nervous system activity. Blood pressure elevation is part of the pathophysiological pathway of the metabolic syndrome, but is also a more primary indication of the allostatic load that can lead to accelerated atherosclerosis as well as insulin resistance. Cholesterol and HDL cholesterol are measures of metabolic imbalance in relation to obesity and atherosclerosis and also reflect the operation of the same primary mediators as well as other metabolic hormones.

In general, in the future, we feel that we need to expand the secondary outcomes in two directions. First, there is need for more specific outcomes related to the damage pathway in cardiovascular disease and risk for myocardial infarction (e.g., nitric oxide, fibrinogen). Fibrinogen has already been used as an allostatic load measure in relation to job stress and socioeconomic status.[32] Second, we need outcomes related to other systems such as the brain and the immune system. For the brain, assessments of declarative and spatial memory have been employed to see individual differences in brain aging, reflecting atrophy of the hippocampus and progressive elevation of cortisol.[33] For the immune system, integrated measures of the immune response such as delayed-type hypersensitivity[34,35] and immunization challenge[36] should reveal the impact of allostatic load on cellular and humoral immune function and help distinguish between the immunoenhancing effects of acute stress and immunosuppressive effects of chronic stress. Moreover, assessment of the frequency and severity of the common cold[37,38] is another indirect way of assessing immune function, and this might be considered a secondary outcome.

Tertiary Outcomes: Actual Diseases or Disorders That Are the Result of the Allostatic Load That Is Predicted from the Extreme Values of the Secondary Outcomes and of the Primary Mediators

Thus far, we have used cardiovascular disease, decreased physical capacity, and severe cognitive decline as outcomes in the successful aging studies,[21,39] but some redefinition of outcomes is needed. That is, a stricter criterion based on the new definitions of primary, secondary, and tertiary outcomes would assign cognitive decline as a secondary outcome, although Alzheimer's disease or vascular dementia would be tertiary outcomes when there is clearly a serious and permanent disease. By the same token, cancer would be a tertiary outcome, whereas the common cold would be a secondary outcome and an indirect measure, in part, of immune system efficacy, as discussed above.

This new classification of the existing measures of allostatic load should permit the following next steps:

1. relating progression of pathophysiology from primary mediators to secondary outcomes and then to tertiary, that is, disease outcomes;

2. identifying clusters of secondary outcomes that are relevant to particular diseases; and

3. moving to earlier ages in measuring allostatic load by relying more on secondary outcomes that are known to be risk factors for later disease; tertiary outcomes generally appear later in life, at least for dementia and cardiovascular disease, and an important question for future studies is whether secondary outcomes in younger subjects can be used as a surrogate for tertiary outcomes.

EARLY LIFE INFLUENCES ON LIFE-LONG PATTERNS OF BEHAVIOR AND HEALTH

One of the very most important factors affecting life-long health is the stability of a child's early life, and cold or unstable parent–child relationships and outright abuse in childhood lead to behavioral and physical problems in childhood that continue throughout adult life. Increased mortality and morbidity from a wide variety of common diseases are reported in individuals who were abused as children.[40] Other, less extreme characteristics of the family environment have also been shown to result in increased physical and mental health risks for children. As outlined in a recent review,[41] families characterized by a lack of warmth and support, or by parental overregulation or underregulation of children's behavior, are also associated with increased physical and mental health risks for children. In addition to the immediate health risks associated with such family environments, the physiological effects of such environments may have long-term effects on adult health and well-being.

As shown in several nonhuman primate and rodent models, early environmental exposures can alter physiological regulator systems in permanent ways. Early life experiences play a powerful role in determining allostatic load over a lifetime in experimental animals, and these animal models provide an attractive model for understanding some environmental and developmental influences on individual differences in human stress reactivity. Neonatal "handling" of newborn rats produces animals that have lower HPA reactivity and slower rates of brain aging measured in terms of loss of cognitive function, whereas prenatal or postnatal stress is suspected of causing increased HPA reactivity over a lifetime and leading to increased rates of brain aging (see Refs. 42–44). There are individual differences in human brain aging related to elevated cortisol levels (see Refs. 33, 39, and 44), although their connection to early life events is unknown.

Nevertheless, phenomena such as low birthweight and various types of early life trauma may influence stress hormone responsiveness over a lifetime. Evidence that low birth weight, which may be caused by stress to the mother, is a risk factor for Type II diabetes is one indication of a life-long influence of early life events (see

Refs. 42–48). Moreover, experiences in childhood have other, deleterious consequences: for example, a history of sexual and physical abuse in childhood is a risk factor not only for posttraumatic stress disorder but also for hippocampal atrophy and cognitive impairment in adulthood (see Bremner[48]). As noted above, in clinical studies, new evidence for the consequences of child abuse and dysfunction of the family in early life points to substantial increases in substance abuse, depression, and suicide, as well as sexual promiscuity and in increased incidence of heart disease, cancer, chronic lung disease, extreme obesity, skeletal fractures, and liver disease.[40] Abuse and neglect during early childhood also links to the neurochemical imbalances that are associated with low serotonin and risk for hostility, aggression, substance abuse, and suicide, as discussed earlier in this section. Studies in infrahuman primates have shown that early maternal deprivation reduces brain serotonin levels and increases alcohol preference and aggressive behavior and decreases affiliative behaviors, thus increasing the risk for elevated allostatic load[50] (for discussion see Higley et al.[51]).

Evidence from human studies indicates similar patterns of altered physiological regulation in children exposed to "risky families" (i.e., families characterized by aggression, lack of warmth, or over/under-regulation). In these latter studies, children from such families exhibit dysregulated HPA axis activity, characterized primarily by higher levels of activity (see Repetti et al.[41]). There is also evidence suggesting dysregulation of serotonergic function, especially among children exposed to abuse[52] and to deficient nurturing.[53] To the extent that such dysregulations are experienced chronically by these children, they would be hypothesized to contribute to more rapid cumulation of allostatic load and its resulting health risks.

In general, the health effects of trauma and other childhood adversities are very broad and do not appear to be specific for any one type of psychiatric or other disorder[40,54]; the breadth and strength of the effects of such trauma is reminiscent of the broad systemic effects of alterations of the responsiveness of physiological mediators that is embodied in the concept of allostatic load.

APPLICATION TO SOCIOECONOMIC STATUS GRADIENTS

The concepts of allostasis and allostatic load and their measurement by the collection of physiological measures constitutes a means to assess the collective impact of the many environmental and behavioral factors that constitute differences in "socioeconomic status" or SES. What we have emphasized thus far is what happens to the individual and how the individual's behavioral and neuroendocrine responses and risk for disease are determined by aenetic, developmental, and experiential factors. However, all of this occurs within the broader social and economic context of the individual's socioeconomic status, and this broader context has significant impacts on the biobehavioral consequences of the individual's interaction with his or her environment.

Thus we move from individuals back to populations and consider the average properties of groups of individuals classified according to measures of income and education. SES appears to be an important factor in disease, and new evidence points to gradients of health across SES in the British Civil Service as well as in other

Western countries. (See Refs. 2, 3, and 55; also chapters by Marmot, Adler, and others in this volume.) It should be emphasized that these are true gradients, operating over the full range of SES and not just a phenomenon of the poorest or lowest end of the scale. Indeed, the measurement of allostatic load, involving secondary outcome measures such as waist–hip ratio[55] and fibrinogen[32] has revealed gradients that parallel the gradients for cardiovascular disease and mortality, indicating that the further application of these measures to different populations should enrich our knowledge of the underlying biological risk factors. Analysis of data from a longitudinal cohort study in Finland has also shown that biological risk factors account for at least part of the association between lower SES and mortality risk, since previously significant SES differences in risks are reduced to nonsignificance with controls for a range of biological parameters including fibrinogen, lipids, blood pressure, glucose, and BMI.[57]

Although it is important to measure allostatic load as a function of SES in different populations, we continue to look for social and cultural factors that have an impact on individual health and provide insights into the driving forces behind allostatic load and poorer health. For example, economic hardship, defined in purely economic terms, has been shown independently of SES gradients to compromise health, including cognitive and physical function and mental health (see Lynch et al.[15]), although there has been little attention to possible physiological mediators of these relationships. And social upheaval in a society is also associated with poorer health. The collapse of communism resulted in worse health in Eastern Europe, and particularly in Russia, between 1989 and 1993; and behavioral problems—alcoholism, suicide, homicide, and cardiovascular disease—accounted for much of the increased mortality (see Refs. 58–60).

CONCLUSIONS

Allostatic load appears to be a useful construct for conceptualizing how "wear and tear" and increased morbidity and mortality are caused over long, time intervals, not only by the more dramatic stressful life events but also by the many events of daily life that elevate activities of physiological systems. Allostatic load reflects the impact not only of life experiences but also of genetic load; individual habits reflecting items such as diet, exercise, and substance abuse; and developmental experiences that set life-long patterns of behavior and physiological reactivity. All of these factors influence the temporal patterning and efficiency of turning on and turning off the hormonal mediators of stress, primarily the catecholamines and glucocorticoids. These hormones protect the body in the short run and promote adaptation, but in the long run allostatic load causes changes in the body that lead to disease. Factors in early life that increase allostatic load include childhood abuse and neglect.

Throughout life, the most potent influences arise from competitive interactions between animals of the same species, leading to the formation of dominance hierarchies. Psychosocial stress of this type not only impairs cognitive function of lower ranking animals, but it can also promote disease (e.g., atherosclerosis) among those vying for the dominant position. Social ordering in human society is also associated with gradients of disease, with an increasing frequency of mortality and morbidity as one descends the scale of socioeconomic status that reflects both income and education. Social ordering in humans may also be associated with gradients of such factors as early life abuse and neglect, as well as prenatal influences that increase the risk for low birthweight, which is itself a risk factor for obesity and cardiovascular disease. Although the causes of these gradients of health are very complex, they are likely to reflect, with increasing frequency at the lower end of the scale, the cumulative burden of coping with limited resources and negative life events and the allostatic load that this burden places on the physiological systems involved in coping and adaptation.

REFERENCES

1. McEwen, B.S. 1998. Protective and damaging effects of stress mediators. N. Engl. J. Med. **338:** 171–179.
2. Adler, N., W.T. Boyce, M. Chesney, S. Folkman & L. Syme. 1993. Socioeconomic inequalities in health: no easy solution. J. Am. Med. Assoc. **269:** 3140–3145.
3. Adler, N.E., T. Boyce, M.A. Chesney, S. Cohen, S. Folkman, R.L. Kahn & L.S. Syme. 1994. Socioeconomic status and health: the challenge of the gradient. Am. Psychol. **49:** 15–24.
4. Kirschbaum, C., B.M. Kudielka, J. Gaab, N.C. Schommer & D.H. Hellhammer. 1999. Impact of gender, menstrual cycle phase and oral contraceptive use on the activity of the hypothalamo–pituitary–adrenal axis. Psychosom. Med. **61:** 154–162.
5. Sterling, P. & J. Eyer. 1988. Allostasis: a new paradigm to explain arousal pathology. In Handbook of Life Stress, Cognition and Health. S. Fisher & J. Reason, Eds.: 629–649. John Wiley & Sons, New York.
6. McEwen, B.S. & E. Stellar. 1993. Stress and the individual: mechanisms leading to disease. Arch. Int. Med. **153:** 2093–2101.
7. Manuck, S.B., J.R. Kaplan, M.R. Adams & T.B. Clarkson. 1995. Studies of psychosocial influences on coronary artery atherosclerosis in cynomolgus monkeys. Health Psychol. **7:** 113–124.
8. Manuck, S.B., J.R. Kaplan, M.F. Muldoon, M.R. Adams & T.B. Clarkson. 1991. The behavioral exacerbation of atherosclerosis and its inhibition by propranolol. In Stress, Coping and Disease. P.M. McCabe, N. Schneiderman, T.M. Field & J.S. Skyler, Eds.: 51–72. Lawrence Erlbaum Associates, Hove and London.
9. Brindley, D.N. & Y. Rolland. 1989. Possible connections between stress, diabetes, obesity, hypertension and altered lipoprotein metabolism that may result in atherosclerosis. Clin. Sci. **77:** 453–461.
10. Bjorntorp, P. 1990. Editorial: "Portal" adipose tissue as a generator of risk factors for cardiovascular disease and diabetes. Atherosclerosis **10:** 493–496.
11. McEwen, B.S. 1997. Possible mechanisms for atrophy of the human hippocampus. Mol. Psychiatry **2:** 255–262.
12. McEwen, B.S. 1999. Stress and hippocampal plasticity. Annu. Rev. Neurosci. **22:** 105–122.
13. McEwen, B.S., C.A. Biron, K.W. Brunson, K. Bulloch, W.H. Chambers, F.S. Dhabhar, R.H. Goldfarb, R.P. Kitson, A.H. Miller, R.L. Spencer & J.M. Weiss. 1997. Neural–endocrine–immune interactions: the role of adrenocorticoids as modulators of immune function in health and disease. Brain Res. Rev. **23:** 79–133.
14. Sternberg, E.M. 1997. Neural-immune interactions in health and disease. J. Clin. Invest. **100:** 2641–2647.
15. Lynch, J.W., G.A. Kaplan & S.J. Shema. 1997. Cumulative impact of sustained economic hardship on physical, cognitive, psychological, and social functioning. N. Engl. J. Med. **337:** 1889–1895.

16. KIRSCHBAUM, C., J.C. PRUSSNER, A.A. STONE, 1. FEDERENKO, J. GAAB, D. LINTZ, N. SCHOMMER & D.H. HELLHAMMER. 1995. Persistent high cortisol responses to repeated psychological stress in a subpopulation of healthy men. Psychosom. Med. **57:** 468–474.

17. GERIN, W. & T.G. PICKERING. 1995. Association between delayed recovery of blood pressure after acute mental stress and parental history of hypertension. J. Hypertension **13:** 603–610.

18. VAN CAUTER, E., K.S. POLONSKY & A.J. SCHEEN. 1997. Roles of circadian rhythmicity and sleep in human glucose regulation. Endocrinol. Rev. **18:** 716–738.

19. MICHELSON, D., C. STRATAKIS, L. HILL, J. REYNOLDS, E. GALLIVEN, G. CHROUSOS & P. GOLD. 1996. Bone mineral density in women with depression. N. Engl. J. Med. **335:** 1176–1181.

20. STERNBERG, E.M., J.M. HILL & G.P. CHROUSOS. 1996. Inflammatory mediator-induced hypothalamic–pituitary–adrenal axis activation is defective in streptococcal cell wall arthritis susceptible Lewis rats. Proc. Natl. Acad. Sci. **86:** 2374–2378.

21. SEEMAN, T.E., B.H. SINGER, J.W. ROWE, R.I. HORWITZ & B.S. MCEWEN. 1997. Price of adaptation—allostatic load and its health consequences: MacArthur studies of successful aging. Arch. Intern. Med. **157:** 2259–2268.

22. MCEWEN, B.S., R.R. SAKAI & R.L. SPENCER. 1993. Adrenal steroid effects on the brain: versatile hormones with good and bad effects. *In* Hormonally-Induced Changes in Mind and Brain. J. Schulkin, Ed.: 157–189. Academic Press, San Diego.

23. QUIRARTE, G.L., B. ROOZENDAAL & J.L. MCGAUGH. 1997. Glucocorticoid, enhancement of memory storage involves noradrenergic activation in the basolateral amygdala. Proc. Natl. Acad. Sci. USA **94:** 14048–14053.

24. MAY, M., E. HOLMES, W. ROGERS & M. POTH. 1990. Protection from glucocorticoid induced thymic involution by dehydroepiandrosterone. Life Sci. **46:** 1627–1631.

25. WRIGHT, B.E., J.R. PORTER, E. BROWNE & F. SVEC. 1992. Antiglucocorticoid action of dehydroepiandrosterone in young obese Zucker rats. Int. J. Obesity **16:** 579–593.

26. ARANEO, B. & R. DAYNES. 1995. Dehydroepiandrosterone functions as more than an antiglucocorticoid in preserving immunocompetence after thermal injury. Endocrinology **136:** 393–401.

27. MORALES, A.J., J.J. NOLAN, J.C. NELSON & S.S.C. YEN. 1994. Effects of replacement dose of dehydroepiandrosterone in men and women of advancing age. J. Clin. Endocrinol. Metab. **78:** 1360–1367.

28. CAHILL, L., B. PRINS, M. WEBER & J.L. MCGAUGH. 1994. Beta-adrenergic activation and memory for emotional events. Nature **371:** 702–704.

29. MINER, J.N., M.I. DIAMOND & K.R. YAMAMOTO. 1991. Joints in the regulatory lattice: composite regulation by steroid receptor–AP I complexes. Cell Growth Differ. **2:** 525–530.

30. SIEGEL, G.J., B.W. AGRANOFF, R.W. ALBERS, S.K. FISHER & M.D. UHLER. 1999. Basic Neurochemistry. Sixth edit. Lippincott-Raven, New York.

31. YAMADA, K., D.T. DUONG, D.K. SCOTT, J.-C. WANG & D.K. GRANNER. 1999. CCAAT/Enhancer-binding protein is an accessory factor for the glucocorticoid response from the cAMP response element in the rat phosphoenolpyruvate carboxykinase gene promoter. J. Biol. Chem. **274:** 5880–5887.

32. MARKOWE, H.L.J., M.G. MARMOT, M.J. SHIPLEY, C.J. BULPITT, T.W. MEADE, Y. STIRLING, M.V. VICKERS & A. SERNMENCE. 1985. Fibrinogen: a possible link between social class and coronary heart disease. Br. Med. J. **291:** 1312–1314.

33. LUPIEN, S.J., M.J. DELEON, S. DE SANTI, A. CONVIT, C. TARSHISH, N.P.V. NAIR, M. THAKUR, B.S. MCEWEN, R.L. HAUGER & M.J. MEANEY. 1998. Cortisol levels during human aging predict hippocampal atrophy and memory deficits. Nature Neurosci. **1:** 69–73.

34. DHABHAR, F.S. & B.S. MCEWEN. 1996. Moderate stress enhances, and chronic stress suppresses, cell-mediated immunity in vivo. Soc. Neurosci. **22:** 536.3–p1350. (Abstr.).

35. DHABHAR, F. & B. MCEWEN. 1999. Enhancing versus suppressive effects of stress hormones on skin immune function. Proc. Natl. Acad. Sci. USA **96:** 1059–1064.

36. KIECOLT-GLASER, J.K., R. GLASER, S. GRAVENSTEIN, W.B. MALARKEY & J. SHERIDAN. 1996. Chronic stress alters the immune response to influenza virus vaccine in older adults. Proc. Natl. Acad. Sci. USA **93:** 3043–3047.
37. COHEN, S., S. LINE, S.B. MANUCK, B.S. RABIN, E.R. HEISE & J.R. KAPLAN. 1997. Chronic social stress, social status, and susceptibility to upper respiratory infections in nonhuman primates. Psychosomat. Med. **59:** 213–221.
38. COHEN, S., D.A.J. TYRRELL & A.P. SMITH. 1991. Psychological stress and susceptibility to the common cold. N. Engl. J. Med. **325:** 606–612.
39. SEEMAN, T.E., B.S. McEWEN, B.H. SINGER, M.S. ALBERT & J.W. ROWE. 1997. Increase in urinary cortisol excretion and memory declines: MacArthur studies of successful aging. J. Clin. Endocrinol. Metab. **82:** 2458–2465.
40. FELITTI, V.J., R.F. ANDA, D. NORDENBERG, D.F. WILLIAMSON, A.M. SPITZ, V. EDWARDS, M.P. KOSS & J.S. MARKS. 1998. Relationship of childhood abuse and household dysfunction to many of the leading causes of death in adults. The adverse childhood experiences (ACE) study. Am. J. Prev. Med. **14:** 245–258.
41. REPETTI, R.L., S. TAYLOR & T SEEMAN. 1999. Risky families: family social environments and the mental and physical health of offspring. Submitted.
42. MEANEY, M., D. AITKEN, H. BERKEL, S. BHATNAGER & R. SAPOLSKY. 1988. Effect of neonatal handling of age-related impairments associated with the hippocampus. Science **239:** 766–768.
43. DELLU, F., W. MAYO, M. VALLEE, M. LEMOAL & H. SIMON. 1994. Reactivity to novelty during youth as a predictive factor of cognitive impairment in the elderly: a longitudinal study in rats. Brain Res. **653:** 51–56.
44. LIU, D., J. DIORIO, B. TANNENBAUM, C. CALDJI, D. FRANCIS, A. FREEDMAN, S. SHARMA, D. PEARSON, P.M. PLOTSKY & M.J. MEANEY. 1997. Maternal care, hippocampal glucocorticoid receptors, and hypothalamic–pituitary–adrenal responses to stress. Science **277:** 1659–1662.
45. LUPIEN, S., A.R. LECOURS, 1. LUSSIER, G. SCHWARTZ, N.P.V. NAIR & M.J. MEANEY. 1994. Basal cortisol levels and cognitive deficits in human aging. J. Neurosci. **14:** 2893–2903.
46. WADHWA, P.D., C.A. SANDMAN, M. PORTO, C. DUNKEL-SCHETTER & T.J. GARITE. 1993. The association between prenatal stress and infant birth weight and gestational age at birth: a prospective investigation. Am. J. Ob. Gyn. **169:** 858–865.
47. BARKER, D.J.P. 1997. The fetal origins of coronary heart disease. Acta. Paediatr. Suppl. **422:** 78–82.
48. WADHWA, P.D., C.A. SANDMAN, A. CHICZ-DEMET & M. PORTO. 1997. Placental CRH modulates maternal pituitary–adrenal function in human pregnancy. Neuropeptides Dev. Aging **814:** 276–281.
49. BREMNER, J.D., P. RANDALL, E. VERMETTEN, L. STAIB, R.A. BRONEN, C. MAZURE, S. CAPELLI, G. McCARTHY, R.B. INNIS & D.S. CHARNEY. 1997. Magnetic resonance imaging-based measurement of hippocampal volume in posttraumatic stress disorder related to childhood physical and sexual abuse—a preliminary report. Biol. Psychiatry **41:** 23–32.
50. HIGLEY, J.D., M.F. HASERT, S.J. SUOMI & M. LINNOILA. 1991. Nonhuman primate model of alcohol abuse: effects of early experience, personality, and stress on alcohol consumption. Proc. Natl. Acad. Sci. USA **88:** 7261–7265.
51. HIGLEY, J.D., W.W. THOMPSON, M. CHAMPOUX, D. GOLDMAN, M.F. HASERT, G.W. KRAEMER, J.M. SCANLAN, S.J. SUOMI & M. LINNOILA. 1993. Paternal and maternal genetic and environmental contributions to cerebrospinal fluid monoamine metabolites in Rhesus monkeys (*Macaca mulatta*). Arch. Gen. Psychiatry **50:** 615–623.
52. KAUFMAN, J., B. BIRMAHER, J. PEREL, R.E. DAHL, S. STULL, D. BRENT, L. TRUBNICK, M. AL-SHABBOUT & N.D. RYAN. 1998. Serotonergic functioning in depressed abused children: clinical and familial correlates. Biol. Psychiatry **44:** 973–981.
53. PINE, D.S., J.D. COPLAN, G.A. WASSERMAN, L.S. MILLER, J.E. FRIED, M. DAVIES, T.B. COOPER, L. GREENHILL, D. SHAFFER & B. PARSONS. 1998. Neuroendocrine response to D,1-fenfluramine challenge in boys. Associations with aggressive behavior and adverse rearing. Arch. Gen. Psychiatry **54:** 785–789.

54. KESSLER, R.C., C.G. DAVIS & K.S. KENDLER. 1997. Childhood adversity and adult psychiatric disorder in the US National Comorbidity Survey. Psychol. Med. **27:** 1101–1119.
55. MARMOT, M.G., G. DAVEY SMITH, S. STANSFELD, C. PATEL, F. NORTH, J. HEAD, I. WHITE, E. BRUNNER & A. FEENEY. 1991. Health inequalities among British civil servants: the Whitehall 11 study. Lancet **337:** 1387–1393.
56. BRUNNER, E.J., M. MARMOT, K. NANCHAHAL, M.J. SHIPLEY, S.A. STANSFELD, M. JUNEJA & K.G.M.M. ALBERTI. 1997. Social inequality in coronary risk: central obesity and the metabolic syndrome. Evidence from the Whitehall 11 study. Diabetologia **40:** 1341–1349.
57. LYNCH, J.W., G.A. KAPLAN, R.D. COHEN, J. TUOMILEHTO & J.T. SALONEN. 1996. Do cardiovascular risk factors explain the relation between socioeconomic status, risk of all-cause mortality, cardiovascular mortality, and acute myocardial infarction? Am. J. Epidemiol. **144:** 934–942.
58. BOBAK, M. & M. MARMOT. 1996. East–West mortality divide and its potential explanations: proposed research agenda. Br. Med. J. **312:** 421–425.
59. NOTZON, F.C., Y.M. KOMAROV, S.P. ERMAKOV, C.T. SEMPOS, J.S. MARKS & E.V. SEMPOS. 1998. Causes of declining life expectancy in Russia. JAMA **279:** 793–800.
60. BOBAK, M., H. PIKHART, C. HERTZMAN, R. ROSE & M. MARMOT. 1998. Socioeconomic factors, perceived control and self-reported health in Russia. A cross-sectional survey. Soc. Sci. Med. **47:** 269–279.

Health, Hierarchy, and Social Anxiety

RICHARD G. WILKINSON[a]

*Trafford Centre for Medical Research, University of Sussex,
Brighton BN1 9RY, United Kingdom*

ABSTRACT: This paper suggests that the main reasons why populations with narrower income differences tend to have lower mortality rates are to be found in the psychosocial impact of low social status. There is now substantial evidence showing that where income differences are greater, violence tends to be more common, people are less likely to trust each other, and social relations are less cohesive. The growing impression that social cohesion is beneficial to health may be less a reflection of its direct effects than of its role as a marker for the underlying psychological pain of low social status. Low social status affects patterns of violence, disrespect, shame, poor social relations, and depression. In its implications for feelings of inferiority and insecurity, it interacts with other powerful health variables such as poor emotional attachment in early childhood and patterns of friendship and social support. Causal pathways are likely to center on the influence that the quality of social relations has on neuroendocrine pathways.

INTRODUCTION:
FROM MATERIAL TO PSYCHOSOCIAL PATHWAYS

Our understanding of the determinants of population health has undergone a profound change over the last couple of decades. In the judgement of most people working in this field, the accumulated research evidence at the end of the 1980s seemed to show: (1) that medical services were not a major determinant of population health—and certainly not of the substantial social gradient in health found even in countries providing universal access to medical care; (2) that the well-known behavioral risk factors left most of the social gradient in health unexplained; and (3) that social selection—or reverse causality—made only a minor contribution to health inequalities. On that basis most people in the research community, myself included, assumed the task before us was to identify which aspects of people's material circumstances were responsible for the social gradient in health. Was it the occupational hazards to which people were exposed, the differences in diets, in housing, air pollution, or what? Growing interest in the problem reflected not only a concern for social justice but also the hope that health inequalities were an epidemiological clue: that the factors causing them would emerge as more general determinants of population health.

The biggest change in understanding since then has been our growing knowledge of the power of psychosocial influences on health. Few of us had imagined that the most important etiological factors could be anything but the direct effects of expo-

[a]Address for correspondence: 44-1273-877231 (voice); 44-1273-623714 (fax).
e-mail: R.G.Wilkinson@Sussex.ac.uk

sure to different material circumstances and standards. Of course early studies such as those on the effects of bereavement on risk of death among surviving spouses or relatives had provided evidence that psychosocial factors could, at least in these special situations, be important influence on health.[1] But it took factory closure studies to show us that psychosocial factors might be important contributors to the social gradient in health. These studies showed that health deteriorated not only when people actually became unemployed, but often from much earlier—when jobs first became insecure and people knew that there were going to be redundancies.[2–4]

At the same time there was growing evidence that "life events," social support, and sense of control were also closely associated with health. And just as epidemiologists began to wonder how we might identify the particular ideational states that were damaging to health, the picture emerging from biological research seemed to suggest that anything contributing to chronic anxiety was likely to affect health.[5,6]

It was easy to see how life events and job insecurity might increase anxiety, while a sense of control and social support would decrease it. Although these all seemed to be powerful influences on health, with so many exposed that population-attributable risk might be very high indeed, it was not until the arrival of two further pieces of evidence that it seemed possible that psychosocial pathways may make the largest single contribution to the socioeconomic gradient in health. One of these concerned the income–health relation. Because income was related to health within developed countries (or U.S. states) but not between them, it seemed likely that the relationship was not so much a relationship between health and absolute living standards or material circumstances—regardless of the rest of society, so much as a relationship with relative standards or with relative income serving as a marker for social status.[7]

Apparently providing independent confirmation of this view was the evidence that, although mortality rates in developed countries were not closely related to average income, they were related to income distribution. Measures of income inequality can plausibly be interpreted as measures of the burden of relative deprivation on health in each society. Associations between income inequality and population health have now been reported on numerous different bases: across developed and developing countries, in Eastern and Western Europe, cross-sectionally as well as when looking at changes over time, and also within large areas within countries.[8]

The possibility that we were dealing with the effects of social status itself also received powerful support from studies of the biological effects of social status among nonhuman primates. Sapolsky's studies of wild baboons and Shively's of maquaques in captivity showed that a number of physiological risk factors had similar associations with social status among animals as among humans. Sapolsky was able to rule out reverse causality as an explanation by examining the effects of changing social circumstances. Shively was able to do so by manipulating social status experimentally, by transferring animals between cages to form new social groups. Because Shively was able to control diet and the environment while manipulating social status, there was little else but the changes in social status themselves with which to explain the changes in risk factors she has reported.

These animal studies would be less compelling for those of us interested in human health if the physiological risk factors associated with social status among animals and people were quite different. However, worse HDL:LDL ratios, central obesity, glucose intolerance, increased atherosclerosis, raised basal cortisol levels, and attenuated cortisol responses to experimental stressors have all been reported to be associated with social status among people and among animals.[6,5,9,10]

Similar effects are likely to have similar causes. The animal studies describe the causal processes unambiguously in terms of the psychosocial anxiety of animals in low social status positions. The suggested mechanisms center on sustained activation of the hypothalamus–pituitary–adrenal axis and the sympathetic nervous system.

INEQUALITY AND THE SOCIAL ENVIRONMENT

But before we get further into the links between social status and health, let us return to the relationship between income distribution and health mentioned earlier. It provides a useful perspective on some of the same issues because income distribution captures the extent of social status differences in a society. The most plausible attempts to explain why more egalitarian societies tend to be healthier have focused on the way the social environment is affected by inequality. Examples of a number of unusually healthy and egalitarian societies had provided circumstantial evidence that more egalitarian countries were more socially cohesive than less egalitarian ones.[11] Since then, data from several sources has strongly confirmed this pattern. Kawachi and Kennedy[12] found that people were much more likely to feel trustful towards others in those U.S. states in which income differences were smaller ($r = 0.73$). Similarly, the hostility scores for 10 U.S. cities that Williams *et al.*[13] found were related to city mortality rates ($r = 0.9$) have also been found to be related to the extent of income inequality in those cities (Wilkinson, unpublished). In addition, in his study of the functioning of regional governments in Italy, Putnam[14] notes that his index of "civic community" (a measure of the strength of people's involvement in community life) was closely correlated with the extent of income inequality ($r = -0.81$). Speaking of social attitudes, Putnam says, "Citizens in the more civic regions, like their leaders, have a pervasive distaste for hierarchical authority patterns" (p. 104). "Political leaders in the civic regions are more enthusiastic supporters of political equality than their counterparts in less civic regions" (p. 102). Indeed, he goes as far as to say that "Equality is an essential feature of the civic community" (p. 105). Lastly, there is evidence from a large number of studies that homicide and violent crime are substantially more common in less egalitarian countries.[15]

This evidence strongly suggests that as social status differences in a society increase, the quality of social relations deteriorates. This appears to be a very general human phenomenon. Rather than being confined to one country, the evidence cited above comes from the United States, Britain, Italy, Japan, and Eastern Europe. On top of that, the meta-analysis of Hsieh and Pugh's[15] showing that violent crime and homicide rates are related to income inequality covers some 34 studies including some that use international data from both developed and developing countries.

The combination of increasing social status differentials and deteriorating social relations could hardly be a more potent mix for population health. Social status and social support or social affiliation are—at least in the developed world—perhaps the two most important risk factors for population health. Both have been associated with two, three, or even fourfold mortality differences. While there are other factors that carry a larger relative risk, there must be few with such a high-population attributable risk.

But what is it about social status and social integration that makes them so important to health? Interestingly, Putnam refers to them as vertical and horizontal relations: he contrasts the more egalitarian horizontal relations of the regions where the "civic community" is stronger with the vertical "patron–client" relations of the less civic regions. In an important sense perhaps social hierarchy and social affiliation are not two quite separate variables. Instead they are linked as two sides of the same coin, as the two alternative forms of social interaction and forms of social organization. Social hierarchy is the human equivalent of pecking order or dominance hierarchy. Though institutionalized to minimize open conflict, it is nevertheless a ranking based on power, coercion, and access to resources regardless of other's needs. Friendship, on the other hand, is marked by reciprocity, mutuality, and a recognition of the needs of others. The alternative to hierarchical power relations is some form of egalitarian cooperation. Among human and nonhuman primates, these contrasting bases of social organization have been referred to as "agonic" (those social systems based on power and dominance hierarchies) and "hedonic" (those based on more egalitarian cooperation).[16]

Although we are familiar with the agonic forms of social organization that have been predominant since class societies began, we are less familiar with the hedonic. It is therefore worth noting that egalitarian forms of social organization were dominant during most of human hunting and gathering prehistory. In a recent review of over 100 anthropological accounts covering some 24 recent hunter and gatherer societies spread over four continents, Erdal and Whiten[17] conclude that these societies were characterized by "egalitarianism, cooperation and sharing on a scale unprecedented in primate evolution" (p. 140). "They share food, not simply with kin or even just with those who reciprocate, but according to need even when food is scarce" (p. 142). "There is no dominance hierarchy among hunter-gatherers. No individual has priority of access to food which...is shared. In spite of the marginal female preference for the more successful hunters as lovers, access to sexual partners is not a right which correlates with rank. In fact rank is simply not discernible among hunter-gatherers. This is a cross cultural universal, which rings out unmistakably from the ethnographic literature, sometimes in the strongest terms" (p. 144).

In an important sense, friendship is naturally egalitarian. It was Plato[18] who said "How correct the old saying is, that 'equality leads to friendship'! It's right enough and it rings true..." (p. 229). This is so taken for granted that in the Cambridge Scale, which is used to classify occupations into a social hierarchy, friendship patterns serve as a measure of equality or social distance.[19] People interviewed in a sample survey are asked to name their own occupation and the occupation of six friends. Occupations linked by many friendships are regarded as being of similar social status, while occupations linked by few are regarded as being socially distant from each other.

From the discussion above, it looks as if health and the quality of social relations in a society vary inversely with how hierarchical the social hierarchy is. We can see that the link between health and both social capital and egalitarianism is underpinned by the epidemiological findings testifying to the importance of social status and social relations. As a result there is now a growing literature suggesting that social cohesion is beneficial to health. But despite having helped draw attention to the tendency for more egalitarian societies to be more cohesive and have higher standards of health, I suspect that—at least in terms of the causation of health and illness—social capital may be largely an epiphenomenon and that we still have to identify the causal factors underlying it.

THE EXPLANATORY PROBLEM

No one has yet provided a plausible explanation of why either social cohesion/capital or friendship and the quality of social relations are important to health. Good social relations of all kinds—from close "confiding" relationships, to having more friends, to involvement in community associations—all seem to be beneficial to health. Although it seems plausible that having a close confidant with whom to discuss problems may make some difference to health, it is harder to believe that going to a weekly or monthly meeting of a local club, or greeting neighbors when passing on the street, could make much difference. This is, however, the rather weak stuff of which social cohesion seems to be made.

In an attempt to give the benefits of friendship a material rather than a psychosocial interpretation, it is sometimes suggested that friendship may benefit health because of the material support friends provide for each other. But when you actually think what friends give or share with each other, it is not a healthy list. Friends buy each other drinks, they offer each other cigarettes, and—at least in England—the material resource that neighbors proverbially borrow from each other is "a cup of sugar". And now, increasingly, friends give each other AIDS. This is hardly the mixture to explain two- to fourfold decreases in morbidity and mortality rates among people who have more friends compared to those who have few. We need to think through psychosocial explanations of the health benefits of friendship.

Rather the same difficulties arise when we start to ask about the direct effects of social status among humans. The fact that a number of the same physiological risk factors are associated with low social status among humans as have been reported among monkeys means that they are unlikely to be explained by smoking, unemployment, bad housing, and the like. Among monkeys the physiological risk factors associated with low social status can be confidently attributed to the chronic anxiety that comes from the constant threat of being attacked and bitten by superiors. But the sources of the chronic anxiety inherent in low social status among people are rather different and usually more subtle.

Thus we have a fundamental area of doubt at the center of what appear to be some of the most important determinants of population health. We do not really know why social affiliation matters to health; we do not know why social cohesion is associated with better health; and we have not yet identified what is inherently stressful about low social status. I want to use the remainder of this paper to suggest how we might fill these gaps in our understanding.

Although not the subject of this paper, nevertheless we can be confident that once we have identified the main sources of chronic anxiety, there are a variety of plausible biological pathways from there to physiological illness and death. When a state of physiological arousal—the so called "fight or flight" response—is activated for brief emergencies, little or no harm is done. But when the anxiety and worry lasts for months and years, and the body is frequently in a high state of arousal, there are likely to be a variety of health costs. Sapolsky describes how, when the body is mobilizing resources for muscular activity, other system-maintenance and repair processes not relevant to our response to the short-term emergency (such as growth, tissue repair and maintenance, immunity, digestion, reproductive functions) "are put on hold."[6] In addition, as well as increasing the risks of blood clots and so of heart attacks, if the energy resources that are mobilized are not used, they increase the accumulation of cholesterol in blood vessels.[5] The variety of physiological processes affected by chronic anxiety mean that its health effects are in many respects analogous to more rapid aging. Our aim then is to understand the central sources of chronic anxiety related to the main risk factors for population health in the developed world.

VIOLENCE

A useful starting point is the association between income inequality and homicide. The association between income inequality and homicide is not only robust (as described above[15]) but among the 50 states of the U.S.A. it seems to account for half of the very large variations in homicide rates between states. Income inequality is related to homicide in much the same way as it is related to death rates from all other causes. Indeed the relationship between income inequality and all other causes of death disappears when it is controlled either by the distribution of homicide or by other measures of the social environment such as social trust.[12,20] This, and the close association between the distribution of homicide and death rates from all other causes, suggests that if we knew the social milieu that produced high homicide rates we would also know the social milieu which raised death rates from other causes. In a recent paper in which we explored these issues and reviewed some of the literature on the causes of violence, we concluded that the central issue was respect.[20] There is a remarkable degree of agreement among violent men and those who have worked with them that violence is very frequently a response to people feeling they are being disrespected. Gilligan,[21] who was a prison psychiatrist for 25 years before becoming director of the Center for the Study of Violence at the Harvard School of Public Health, said "I have yet to see a serious act of violence that was not provoked by the experience of feeling shamed and humiliated, disrespected and ridiculed, and that did not represent the attempt to prevent or undo this 'loss of face'—no matter how severe the punishment" (p.110). The same emphasis also comes from people who have been imprisoned for violence. The central importance of respect is confirmed by people with records for violence. In his autobiography, McCall[22] writes "...the underlying issue was always respect. You could ask a guy, 'Damn, man, why did you bust that dude in the head with a pipe?' And he might say, 'The mothafucka disrespected me!' That was explanation enough. It wasn't even necessary to explain how the guy had disrespected him. It was universally understood that if a dude got disrespected, he had to do what he had to do" (p.52). (A fuller discussion of these connections can be found in Wilkinson et al.[20])

It may seem surprising that the higher levels of violence in societies where in-come differences are greater is not (short of revolutionary uprisings) violence be-tween rich and poor. Instead, the violence associated with greater inequality occurs largely among the most deprived. The role of respect not only explains why this is so, but it also explains the statistical relationship between violence and inequality. It is understandable, where income inequalities are greater and more people are denied access to the conventional sources of respect and status in terms of jobs and money, that people become increasingly vulnerable to signs of disrespect, that they are being treated or regarded as inferior, insignificant, and worthless.

SOCIAL STATUS

What is important about this picture of violence in the present context is perhaps that it suggests how much social status matters to people. The resort to violence to defend one's dignity and honor, to gain respect, to avoid loss of face, and the con-nection between violence and greater inequality, shows how low social status gets to people so intensely. Perhaps what hurts most about relative poverty is not so much the lack of material possessions itself, but the affront to one's dignity that it repre-sents. Living standards are, after all, frequently talked about in terms of maintaining respectability, and low standards as an affront to people's dignity and sense of de-cency.

This begins to illustrate how low social status may be a direct source of anxiety. Another element in the picture comes from the growing health interest in emotional development in early life. Poor attachment and emotional trauma in early childhood cast a long shadow forward affecting health in later life.[23–27] Why early emotional development should affect health is again not clear. But just as the associations be-tween health and both friendship and low social status may reflect some similar underlying sources of anxiety, perhaps the importance of poor early emotional de-velopment may tell us more about the same underlying picture. We do, after all, use terms like insecurity, lack of confidence, fear of personal inadequacy, to talk both about the effects of the personal insecurities that can come from early life and about the effects of low social status and status insecurities in society at large. What is more, friends—or lack of friends—can have similar effects. Having friends gives a sense of confidence, of reassurance and self-confirmation, whereas being rejected or not having friends fills one with self-doubt and causes confidence to evaporate. As every worried parent of a child going to a new school knows only too well, the big question affecting happiness is always: Will he or she make friends?

All too easily the social hierarchy presents itself to us as if it were a hierarchy from the most capable, intelligent, and successful people at the top to the most inca-pable and inadequate at the bottom. Indeed, there is a substantial literature in soci-ology and social psychology that suggests that we infer ability partly from institutional position.[28,29] As creatures whose behavior is very largely determined by learning rather than instinct, we are obliged constantly to monitor our behavior. We learn primarily through processes of social comparison: by comparing our behavior with that of others, by monitoring how others perceive us and making corrections where necessary. No doubt closely related to this is one of the most powerfully social features of our brains: that as well as our direct knowledge of ourselves, we are also reflexive beings who know and experience ourselves partly through the eyes of others. We fear rejection and negative evaluations from others. Monitoring our behavior and how we appear to others can be a considerable source of social anxiety. Indeed, if we are looking for a source of chronic anxiety acting on health in a way that would giving rise to the observed associations (i) between health and social status, (ii) between health and friendship, and (iii) between health and early emotional development, these sources of social anxiety must be prime candidates.

Some of our sensitivity to these sources of anxiety may reflect evolved human sensitivities to particular features of our social environment. We have to ask why it is so difficult just to shrug off being treated as inferior or not having friends. Why are we so sensitive—it often appears irrationally sensitive—to some features of our social environment?

Too often we picture human characteristics as having evolved simply in relation to the natural environment. But, as Alexander[30] argued, the "primary hostile force of nature" which, as human beings, we have always faced, was other human beings. Other human beings have the potential to compete with us for everything: food, clothes, sexual partners, housing, jobs, etc. But as well as being our most feared competitor, other people are also the greatest source of comfort, love, help, friendship, assistance, and learning. Getting relationships with other people right has always been absolutely crucial to human welfare—even to our basic material welfare. This is so much the case that some of the leading theories of the growth of the human brain suggest that the crucial selective environmental stimulus to its rapid growth may have been the demands of having to deal with the complexity of social life.[31] Intriguing aspects of this approach include not only evidence that among primates the size of the neocortex relative to the rest of the brain is related to the size of the social group, but also suggestions that the capacity for language developed primarily for its social functions[32] rather than for practical tasks such as coordinating hunting (which, after all, lions manage to do with great sophistication without language). In order to understand the psychological importance of social status and friendship, perhaps we need to think of the brain as a much more social organ than we usually do.

There are a good many indications that we are more sensitive and attentive to issues to do with social status than is often recognized. The literature on "white coat hypertension" (the tendency for blood pressure to be higher when measured by a doctor) developed initially simply as a result of the desire to get more accurate clinical measures of blood pressure. But it is paralleled by work from social psychologists who have shown that blood pressure tends to rise when people are interviewed by a higher rather than an equal or lower status interviewer.[33,34] There is little doubt that they are both a reflection of the response of the sympathetic nervous system to the social anxiety induced by interacting with someone who is of higher social status.

The salience of social status is shown in many different ways. Adam Smith[35] believed it was one of the main driving forces behind economic activity. In his *Theory of the Moral Sentiments,* he asks: "What is the end of avarice and ambition, of the pursuit of wealth, of power and pre-eminence? Is it to supply the necessities of nature? The wages of the meanest labourer can supply them…. What are the advantages which we would propose to gain by that great purpose of human life which we call bettering our condition? To be observed, to be attended to, to be taken notice of with sympathy, complacency, and approbation, are all the advantages which we can propose to derive from it" (p. 50).

Several modern economists have developed this theme, suggesting that an important part of people's desire for higher incomes and consumption is a concern to maintain or improve their social status, that it is ultimately a form of social competition and that in the end people are (often without recognizing it) effectively concerned with relative income and relative standards.[36–38] As Schor said, "We live with high levels of psychological denial about the connection between our buying habits and the social statements they make."

Bourdieu's[39] empirical research has also shown how we use aesthetic taste and an important area of cultural life to maintain and express social distinctions, and, despite changes in the way it is expressed, there can be little doubt of the importance of snobbishness in everyday life.

Our sensitivity and attentiveness to social status is likely to be an evolved human characteristic. Position in the dominance hierarchy was important in determining access to resources and reproductive success both before and after our existence in egalitarian hunting and gathering societies. We should note in passing that Erdal and Whiten[17] do not suggest that our early egalitarianism was based on any sudden change to selflessness in our genetic makeup. Instead, they say that sharing was "vigilant" sharing with people watching to make sure they got a fair deal, and that equality is likely to have been based on what they call a generalized "counter dominance strategy" derived from the ways in which nonhuman primates use alliances to oust— or defend themselves from—dominant animals. Indeed, rather than implying that people are unconcerned with social status, the maintenance of equality in prehistoric societies should probably be seen as an indication of the importance of avoiding the social costs of inequality.

It might be useful in passing to point out that suggesting some characteristics are genetic does not reduce the scope for environmental influence on behavior. Rather than reducing our interaction with the environment, it tells us more about the elements we might bring to our interaction with particular features of the environment. Just as we may be genetically sensitive to a particular infectious disease to which various other animals may be insensitive, how much we get that disease will still be affected by exposure to the infective agent and a range of other factors affecting our resistance. Take an example like TB, for which there were known to be important genetic differences in people's susceptibility. It was nevertheless environmental change that led first to its rapid decline in developed countries and then to its subsequent re-emergence as poverty increased. So hypotheses about our genetic characteristics are not about whether the environment is important, but about how we interact with our environment. Perhaps, if we knew more about our genetic characteristics, we would know more about the importance of the environment. Indeed, one of the conclusions of this area of work on the socioeconomic determinants of health is likely to be that our sensitivity to social hierarchy means that the costs of socioeconomic inequality are higher than we may have realized.

SOCIAL ANXIETY

Scheff *et al.*[40] and others have suggested that shame is the social emotion. He says "there has been a continuing suggestion in the literature that shame is *the* primary social emotion, generated by the virtually constant monitoring of the self in relation to others" (p.79).[41] Among the literature he cites are both Goffman,[42] who said that embarrassment plays a prominent role in every social encounter, and Darwin,[43] who, in his chapter on blushing, argues that shame "depends in all cases on...a sensitive regard for the opinion, more particularly the depreciation of others."

However, Scheff uses shame to cover a wide range of social anxieties, suggesting that when we talk about "having low self-esteem, feeling foolish, stupid, ridiculous, inadequate, defective, incompetent, awkward, exposed, vulnerable, insecure, helpless," we are usually talking about experiences of shame (p.181).[40] Its intimate relation with social status is clear. Scheff[44] regards it as part of what he calls the "deference–emotion system," and Gilbert and McGuire[45] say, "Shame is nearly always associated with depictions of loss of status...of being devalued, disgraced, demoted, and dishonoured" (p.111). Elsewhere, Gilbert[46] emphasizes how feelings of shame are related to ways of "processing socially threatening information— particularly in the domains of social rank/status and social exclusions/rejection" (p.17).

Illustrating its importance in social life, Scheff[40] cites its role both in social conformity and in obedience to authority. He discusses Asch's[47] experiments in which fear of looking stupid, or others thinking you can't see straight, made people reluctant even to say which of two lines was the same length as another if their judgment stood out from the group. On voluntary obedience to authority, Scheff discusses Milgram's[48] experiments in which people voluntarily administered what they were led to believe were very painful and life-threatening electric shocks to students in what they took to be a learning experiment, simply because they were instructed to do so by a supervisor.

Thinking about this literature from the point of view of health and the need to identify the most powerful sources of chronic anxiety related to low social status, lack of friends, to lack of secure early attachment and to violence, the literature on shame should probably not be treated as distinct from much work on social anxiety, most of which centers on what could be called "evaluation anxiety." The "social anxiety" literature embraces work on the links between shyness and fear of social evaluation, on embarrassment, "fear of negative evaluation," "social-evaluative disorder," "behavioral inhibition," "fear of failure," "approval motivation," "self-conscious affect," "interpersonal competence," "self-presentational predicament," "sense of inferiority," and "inferiority complex"—to name but a few.

Schore[49] argues that the shame response develops, simultaneously with the growth of the prefrontal cortex of the brain, towards the end of the first year of life in the interaction between parent and child following attachment. Soon after the infant has become used to the pleasurable attention and eye contact during the first year, parents start shaping the child's behavior through expressions of disapproval. The pleasurable face-to-face interactions of attachment are frequently replaced by the caregivers expressions of disgust. Hence Lewis[50] called shame the "attachment emotion."

There is widespread agreement that the capacity for shame is innate, and Gilbert and McGuire[45] have argued that it plays a central role in dominance hierarchies. As they point out, if conflict is to be avoided, dominance hierarchies require that dominance is matched by submissiveness. In their words: "Shame signals (e.g., head down, gaze avoidance, and hiding) are generally regarded as submissive and appeasement displays, designed to de-escalate and/or escape from conflict. Thus insofar as shame is related to submissiveness and appeasement behavior, then it is a damage limitation strategy, adopted when continuing in a shameless, nonsubmissive way might provoke very serious attacks or rejections from others" (p. 102).

Leary and Kowalski[51] write, "we favor the idea that social anxiety evolved as a mechanism for fostering social inclusion and minimizing the possibility of rejection or exclusion…. The most parsimonious evolutionary explanation of social anxiety is that it evolved as a mechanism for fostering and maintaining one's membership in supportive (i.e., mutually interdependent) groups and relationships" (p. 27).

Central to these social anxieties are processes of social comparison and fears of inferiority and inadequacy in relation to others. Trower et al.[16] said: "socially anxious people…perceive themselves as subordinates in hostile hierarchies and utilize submissiveness and other 'reverted escape' behaviors to minimize loss of status and rejection" (p. 39). What Leary and Kowalski[51] describe as the "sociometer theory of self-esteem" links self-esteem, social anxiety, and rejection. They argue (in rather mechanistic terms) that "the self-esteem system functions as a 'sociometer' that monitors the individual's behavior and the social environment (particularly other's reactions) for indications that the person may experience social disapproval or rejection. When cues connoting rejection are detected, the system alerts the individual via negative affect and motivates behavior to restore one's standing with other people. The self-esteem system may have evolved as a mechanism for minimizing the likelihood of social exclusion" (p. 113).

The link between social anxiety and violence is enshrined in the common origin of the words anguish, anxiety, and anger. The connection with social anxiety and shame explains why violence is related to inequality in much the same way as is mortality from other causes. As Gilbert[46] says, "anger and…aggression can substitute for shame" (p 23). He writes that "covering shame with anger is often referred to as a 'face saving' strategy, known to be a typical source of male violence" (p. 8). Similarly Scheff et al.[40] point to the affinity between shame and anger: "…hostility can be viewed as an attempt to ward off feelings of humiliation (shame) generated by inept, ineffectual moves, a sense of incompetence, insults, and a lack of power to defend against insults" (p. 188). Indeed, central to his view of the "deference emotion system" is the "shame-rage spiral" (p. 183).[44] "As humiliation increases, rage and hostility increases proportionally to defend against loss of self-esteem….In our theory, rage is used as a defence against a threat to self, that is, feeling shame, a feeling of vulnerability of the whole self. Anger can be a protective measure to guard against shame, which is experienced as an attack on self. As humiliation increases, rage and hostility increases proportionally to defend against loss of self-esteem" (p. 188). On the relationship between violence, disrespect, and social status that we discussed earlier, Scheff et al.[40] write "…pride and shame states almost always depend on the levels of deference accorded a person: pride arises from deferential treatment by others ('respect'), and shame from lack of deference ('disrespect')" (p. 184).

As well as explaining the relationships between violence, inequality, and health, these social anxieties also contribute to the relationship between friendship and health. In a brief review of numerous studies of social anxiety and social affiliation, Leary and Kowalski[51] write, "People who feel socially anxious tend to disaffiliate" (p.157). The empirical research shows that socially anxious people report less contact with friends, have fewer casual conversations, and are less likely to initiate conversations. "Socially anxious people who hold negative expectancies regarding the outcomes of interactions have shorter conversations, speak more quietly, and engage in less eye contact with other interactants" (p.158). Leary and Kowalski point out that this less sociable behavior is a form of avoidance linked specifically to social anxiety. In contrast, when facing some nonsocial source of anxiety, people prefer to have friends with them. They also emphasize that it is not a matter of a lower desire for social contact: socially anxious people wish they could participate more fully in social encounters.

Lastly, social anxiety is also linked to depression. According to Leary and Kowalski[51]: "The most common emotional concomitant of social anxiety is depression" (p.137). Gilbert[52] argues persuasively that depression is derived from psychological processes that have evolved from responses related to defeat and submission—again having to do with self-evaluation. The point of mentioning the possible evolutionary link in the present context is that it shows its relationship both to social evaluation anxieties and to dominance and subordination. That we should be so prone to such an incapacitating condition as serious depression inevitably poses an evolutionary puzzle: is it just a biological mistake or does it have some value? Dominance behavior would, as we said earlier, lead to continuous conflict were it not matched by a capacity to accept subordinate status and submission. It is then plausible that a mindset consisting of a low self-evaluation, which leads the depressed person to present themselves as downcast, unchallenging, and unthreatening, would have survival value if it served to extricate someone from conflicts that seemed unwinnable.

Gilbert[53] lists the various kinds of situations known to cause depression in which people feel defeated, devalued, or suffer setbacks and loss of control. He, of course, also emphasizes that among humans the sense of being defeated, of a failed struggle, does not usually come from involvement with direct social conflict, but may involve a wide range of evaluative domains—from insoluble family problems to failure to get promotion—in which the depressed person makes "unfavorable judgements about their relative rank, in terms of their attractiveness, talents, competencies, desirability to others or 'power.'" As Gilbert[53] says, low self-confidence is affected by unfavorable social comparisons and "can be seen as 'involuntary subordinate self perception.'"

CONCLUSION

We can now see how social anxiety, shame, depression, and violence may all involve evaluative social comparisons and represent various accommodations to, or protests against, perceptions of inferiority, unattractiveness, failure, or rejection. Sometimes the salient social comparisons are in relation to the society at large, and sometimes in relation to a more immediate social circle. Not only are these very common and intense sources of chronic anxiety of a kind that we might expect to make a difference to health, but they explain why health is so closely related to lack of friends, low social status, violence, and poor early emotional attachment.

Evidence that comes tantalizingly close to clinching the argument are the findings that not only low social status, but also lack of friends and poor early attachment are all associated with similar patterns of raised basal cortisol levels and attenuated responses to experimental stressors.[25,54–56] Both in terms of its likely intensity and the large proportion of the population exposed to it, social anxiety is a very plausible central source of the chronic anxiety that depresses health standards and feeds into the socioeconomic gradient in health.

There is a danger that some readers will take the levels of social anxiety experienced by individuals as fixed and relatively unaffected by environmental factors. Although I have discussed the possibility of an evolved genetic human potential for these kinds of anxiety, when that potential is brought into play, when we actually feel shame, social inferiority, insecurity, lack of control, depression, rejection, or anger is clearly highly responsive to environmental circumstances. I have been concerned to suggest why, as human beings, we may be sensitive to particular features of our social environment so that we can understand the remarkable salience of social comparisons, social evaluations, status, inferiority, etc. As Gilbert[46] writes "There is now increasing evidence that social intelligence is not simply general intelligence directed to social problems. Rather there are probably specific information processing routines for dealing with social information" (p.17). While it is true that some of the psychological research on social anxiety is concerned with individual differences, there is a growing body of research looking at the effects of environmental factors that can be experimentally controlled, and there is little doubt that differences in the social environment are absolutely crucial to how much social anxiety people experience. Having friends or being rejected by people is something to which we are all highly sensitive, and the same is true of having a job or not having one, being appreciated at work or being ignored, of having high or low social status, and so on.

If the social insecurities we have described are an important part of the link between socioeconomic circumstances and health, then the fact that health is responsive to changes in circumstances, that it varies with income distribution, that it is damaged by job loss and responds to friendship, is all evidence that levels of social anxiety are also responsive to environmental factors.

One of the associations that I set out to explain at the beginning of this paper was the association between health and social cohesion. The most intuitively plausible explanation of this relationship came from evidence suggesting that improved social networks are beneficial to health. Indeed, because narrower income differences appear to be closely associated with social cohesion, it looked as if better social networks explained why more egalitarian societies were healthier. However, we might now move to a more complicated model. The hypothesis is that the most important psychosocial determinant of population health are the levels of the various forms of social anxiety in the population, and these in turn are determined by income distribution, early childhood, and social networks. Where levels of social anxiety are low, the quality of social interaction (and measures of social cohesion) improve, and a better, more supportive social environment then feeds back to produce a more widespread lowering of levels of social anxiety in a population. In this context, social cohesion is partly an epiphenomenon: it is related to health partly because it is a reflection of an underlying pathway between health and a more egalitarian, less socially anxious, and more socially confident population, which is therefore also less violent and more socially affiliative.

Social anxiety has been discussed here as a suggested explanation for the links between health and friendship, health and early emotional development, health and the direct psychosocial effects of low social status, the patterning of violence and health in relation to inequality, and of the association between health and social cohesion. Psychologists have long recognized the central importance of insecurity, poor early attachment, lack of confidence, and so forth to mental and emotional welfare throughout life. However, the links between them and social hierarchy have received insufficient attention: as a result their political implications have gone unrecognized. The links with health will serve to draw attention to them. The emphasis given here to the evolutionary sources of social anxieties is intended to show both why we are so highly sensitive to particular aspects of the social environment and to which aspects we are highly sensitive.

Despite the attention we have given to social anxieties in understanding population health, it is not intended to exclude an important role for a wide range of other risk factors, both material and psychosocial. Indeed, rather than discounting the health effects of unemployment, loss of income, or debt, the issues we have discussed may throw additional light on why these things can be so traumatic: they do, after all, carry a burden of stigma and threaten loss of status and respect.

REFERENCES

1. REES, W.D. & S.G. LUTKINS. 1967. Mortality of bereavement. Br. Med. J. **4:** 13–16.
2. COBB, S. & S.C. KASL. 1977. Termination: the consequences of job loss. Department of Health, Education and Welfare. Publication no. 77-224. US National Institutes for Occupational Safety and Health. Cincinnati, OH.
3. IVERSEN, L. & H. KLAUSEN. 1981. The closure of the Nordhavn shipyard. Institute of Social Medicine. Kobenhavns Universitet Publikation 13 FADL. Copenhagen.
4. BEALE, N. & S. NETHERCOTT. 1985. Job-loss and family morbidity: a study of factory closure. J. R. Coll. Gen. Pract. **35:** 510–514.
5. BRUNNER, E. & M. MARMOT. 1999. Social organization, stress, and health. *In* The Social Determinants of Health. M.G. Marmot & R.G. Wilkinson, Eds. Oxford University Press, Oxford.
6. SAPOLSKY, R.M. 1998. Why Zebras Don't Get Ulcers. A Guide to Stress, Stress-Related Disease and Coping. 2nd edit. W.H. Freeman, New York.
7. WILKINSON, R.G. 1997. Health inequalities: relative or absolute material standards? Br. Med. J. **314:** 591–595.
8. KAWACHI, I., B. KENNEDY & R.G. WILKINSON, Eds. 1999. Income Inequality and Health. Vol. 1, The Society and Population Health Reader. New Press, New York.
9. BRUNNER, E. 1997. Stress and the biology of inequality. Br. Med. J. **314:** 1472–1476.
10. KRISTENSON, M. *et al.* 1998. Attenuated cortisol response to a standardised stress test in Lithuanian versus Swedish men: the LiVicordia Study. Int. J. Behav. Med. **5**(1): 17–30.
11. WILKINSON, R.G. 1996. Unhealthy Societies: The Afflictions of Inequality. Routledge, London.
12. KAWACHI, I., B.P. KENNEDY, K. LOCHNER & D. PROTHEROW-STITH. 1997. Social capital, income inequality and mortality. Am. J. Pub. Health **87:** 1491–1498.

13. WILLIAMS, R.B., J. FEAGANES & J.C. BAREFOOT. 1995. Hostility and death rates in 10 US cities. Psychosom. Med. **57**(1): 94.
14. PUTNAM, R.D., R. LEONARDI & R.Y. NANETTI. 1993. Making Democracy Work: Civic Traditions in Modern Italy. Princeton University Press, Princeton.
15. HSIEH, C.C. & M.D. PUGH. 1993. Poverty, income inequality, and violent crime: a meta-analysis of recent aggregate data studies. Criminal Justice Rev. **18**: 182–202.
16. TROWER, P., P. GILBERT & G. SHERLING. 1990. Social anxiety, evolution and self-presentation. *In* Handbook of Social and Evaluation Anxiety. H. Leitenberg, Ed.: 11–45. Plenum Press, New York.
17. ERDAL, D. & A. WHITEN. 1996. Egalitarianism and Machiavellian intelligence in human evolution *In* Modelling the Early Human Mind. P. Mellars & K. Gibson, Eds.: 139–160. McDonald Institute Monographs. Cambridge, England.
18. PLATO (trans. T.J. SAUNDERS). 1970. The Laws. Penguin.Harmondsworth, England.
19. PRANDY, K. 1990. The revised Cambridge scale of occupations. Sociology **24**(4): 629–655.
20. WILKINSON, R.G., I. KAWACHI & B. KENNEDY. 1998. Mortality, the social environment, crime and violence. Sociol. Health Illness **20**(5): 578–597.
21. GILLIGAN, J. 1996. Violence: Our Deadly Epidemic and its Causes. G.P. Putnam, New York.
22. MCCALL, N. 1994. Makes Me Wanna Holler. A Young Black Man in America. Random House, New York.
23. LUNDBERG, O. 1993. The impact of childhood living conditions on illness and mortality in adulthood. Soc. Sci. Med. **36**: 1047–1052.
24. POWER, C. & C. HERTZMAN. 1977. Social and biological pathways linking early life and adult disease. Br. Med. Bull. **53**(1): 210–221.
25. FONAGY, P. 1999. Early influences on development and social inequalities: an attachment theory perspective. *In* The Society and Population Health Reader. Vol. II: A State Perspective. A.R. Tarlov, Ed.: New Press, St. Peter RF.
26. MONTGOMERY, S.M., M.J. BARTLEY & R.G. WILKINSON. 1997. Family conflict and slow growth. Arch. Dis. Child. **77**: 326–330.
27. WADSWORTH, M.E.J. 1984. Early stress and associations with adult health, behaviour and parenting. *In* Stress and Disability in Childhood. N.R. Butler & B.D. Corner, Eds. Wright, Bristol.
28. SENNETT, R. & J. COBB. 1973. The Hidden Injuries of Class. Knopf, New York.
29. ROSS, L. 1978. The intuitive psychologist and his shortcomings: distortions in the attribution process. *In* Cognitive Theories in Social Psychology. L. Berkowitz, Ed. Academic Press, New York.
30. ALEXANDER, R.D. 1987. The biology of moral systems. Aldine de Gruyter, New York.
31. WHITEN, A. & R. BYRNE, Eds. 1997. Machiavellian Intelligence II. Extensions and Evaluations. Cambridge University Press, Cambridge.
32. DUNBAR, R. 1996. Grooming, Gossip and the Evolution of Language. Faber and Faber, London.
33. LONG, J.M., J.J. LYNCH, N.M. MACHIRAN, S.A. THOMAS & K. MALINOW. 1982. The effect of status on blood pressure during verbal communication. J. Behav. Med. **5**: 165–172.
34. KLEINKE, C.I. & G. WILLIAMS. 1994. Effects of interviewer status, touch, and gender on cardiovascular reactivity. J. Soc. Psychol. **134**(2): 247–249.
35. SMITH, A. 1982. The Theory of the Moral Sentiments. Liberty Classics, Indianapolis.
36. FRANK, R. 1999. Luxury Fever. Free Press, New York.
37. SCHOR, J. 1998. The Overspent American: When Buying Becomes You. Basic Books, New York.
38. FRANK, R.H. 1985. Choosing the Right Pond: Human Behaviour and the Quest for Status. Oxford University Press, Oxford.
39. BOURDIEU, P. 1984. Distinction: A Social Critique of the Judgement of Taste. Routledge, London.
40. SCHEFF, T.J., S.M. RETZINGER & M.T. RYAN. 1989. Crime, violence, and self-esteem: review and proposals. *In* The Social Importance of Self-Esteem. A.M. Mecca, N.J. Smelser & J. Vasconcellos, Eds. University of California Press, Berkeley.

41. SCHEFF, T.J. 1990. Microsociology: Discourse, Emotion and Social Structure. University of Chicago Press, Chicago.
42. GOFFMAN, E. 1967. Interaction Ritual. Anchor Doubleday, Garden City.
43. DARWIN, C. 1872. The Expression of Emotion in Men and Animals. John Murray, London.
44. SCHEFF, T.J. 1988. Shame and conformity: the deference–emotion system. Am. Sociol. Rev. **53:** 395–406.
45. GILBERT, P & M.T. MCGUIRE. 1998. Shame, status, and social roles: psychobiology and evolution. *In* Shame: Interpersonal Behavior, Psychopathology, and Culture. P. Gilbert & B. Andrews, Eds. Oxford University Press, New York.
46. GILBERT, P. 1998. What is shame? Some core issues and controversies. *In* Shame: Interpersonal Behaviour, Psychopathology and Culture. P. Gilbert & B. Andrews, Eds. Oxford University Press, New York.
47. ASCH, S.E. 1952. Social Psychology. Prentice-Hall, New York.
48. MILGRAM, S. 1969. Obedience to Authority. Harper, New York.
49. SCHORE, A.N. 1998. Early shame experiences and infant brain development. *In* Shame: Interpersonal Behavior, Psychopathology and Culture. P. Gilbert & B. Andrews, Eds. Oxford University Press, New York.
50. LEWIS, H.B. 1980. "Narcissistic personality" or "shame-prone superego mode." Comp. Psychother. **1:** 59–80.
51. LEARY, M.R. & R.M. KOWALSKI. 1995. Social Anxiety. Guilford Press, New York.
52. GILBERT, P. 1992. Depression: The Evolution of Powerlessness. Lawrence Erlbaum, Hove.
53. GILBERT, P. 1999. Varieties of submissive behavior as forms of social defence: their evolution and role in depression. *In* Subordination: Evolution and Mood Disorders. L. Sloman & P. Gilbert, Eds. Lawrence Erlbaum, Hove. In press.
54. SAPOLSKY, R.M., S.C. ALBERTS & J. ALTMANN. 1997. Hypercortisolism associated with social subordinance or social isolation among wild baboons. Arch. Gen. Psychiatry **54**(12): 1137–1143.
55. LIU, D., J. DIORIO, B. TANNENBAUM, C. CALDJI, D. FRANCIS, A. FREEDMAN, S. SHARMA, D. PEARSON, P.M. PLOTSKY & M.J. MEANEY. 1997. Maternal care, hippocampal glucocorticoid receptors, and hypothalamic–pituitary–adrenal responses to stress. Science **277:** 1659–1662.
56. MEANEY, M.J., D.H. AITKEN, C. VAN BERKEL, S. BHATNAGAR & R.M. SAPOLSKY. 1988. Effect of neonatal handling on age-related impairments associated with the hippocampus. Science **239:** 766–768.
57. SUOMI, S.J. 1991. Early stress and adult emotional reactivity in rhesus monkeys. *In* The Childhood Environment and Adult Disease. Ciba Foundation, Ed.: 171–186. John Wiley & Sons, New York.

Part II Summary: Developmental Influences across the Life Span

TERESA SEEMAN[a]

Division of Geriatrics, Department of Medicine, UCLA School of Medicine, Los Angeles, California 90095, USA

The chapters in this next section discuss early childhood experiences and exposures that may lay the foundations for biological and behavioral patterns that influence health outcomes from childhood through older age. The papers address factors that may be related to socioeconomic status and thus may contribute to observed health disparities across socioeconomic gradients.

As highlighted in a recent paper by Felitti *et al.*,[1] increased mortality and morbidity from a wide variety of common diseases are seen in individuals who report physical and/or psychological abuse as children. Other, less extreme characteristics of children's family environments have also been shown to result in increased physical and mental health risks for children. As outlined in a recent review by Repetti *et al.*,[2] families characterized by a lack of warmth and support, or by parental overregulation or underregulation of children's behavior, are also associated with increased physical and mental health risks for children. In addition to the immediate health risks associated with such family environments, the physiological effects of such environments may have long-term effects on adult health and well-being. As shown in several nonhuman primate and rodent models, early environmental exposures can alter physiological regulatory systems in permanent ways (Suomi[3]; Meany,[4] this volume). Evidence from human studies indicates similar patterns of altered physiological regulation in children exposed to "risk families" (i.e., families characterized by aggression, lack of warmth, or over/underregulation). In these latter studies, children from such families exhibit dysregulated hypothalamic–pituitary–adrenal axis activity, characterized primarily by higher levels of activity (see Repetti *et al.*[2] for review). There is also evidence suggesting dysregulation of serotonergic function, especially among children exposed to abuse (Kaufman *et al.*[5]) and to deficient nurturing (Pine *et al.*[6]). To the extent that such dysregulations are experienced chronically by these children, they would be hypothesized to contribute to more rapid accumulation of allostatic load and its resulting health risks.

The first chapter, by Michael Meany, outlines evidence from animal models where experimental designs permit us to examine the impacts of experimental manipulations of early experiences on subsequent biological mechanisms and behaviors that may be associated with differential health outcomes. The Meany chapter focuses on the impact of different patterns of maternal behavior in terms of the biological and behavioral consequences for the pups. Of considerable interest is the dis-

[a]Address for correspondence: Teresa Seeman, Ph.D., Division of Geriatrics, UCLA School of Medicine, 10945 Le Conte Ave, Suite 2339, Los Angeles, CA 90095-1687, USA. 310-825-8253 (voice); 310-794-2199 (fax).
e-mail: tseeman@medl.medsch.ucla.edu

cussion of the consequences of interactions between these differing maternal "environments" and the pups' genetic inheritance as they impact subsequent biology and behavior.

The second and third chapters in this section examine evidence from human populations for similar impacts of early childhood exposures on subsequent biology, behavior, and health status. The chapter by Clyde Hertzmann discusses several potential models for early childhood influences on subsequent health outcomes over the life course, including latent effects, pathway effects, and cumulative risk models. In the third chapter, Burton Singer uses data from the Wisconsin Longitudinal Study to examine the impact of early childhood SES and subsequent experiences of psychosocial advantage or adversity through adulthood on levels of cumulative biological risk (i.e., allostatic load) measured in late middle age. Specific attention is given to the question of possible modulation of early childhood disadvantage through subsequent experiences of psychosocial advantage in adulthood.

As outlined in these chapters, there is considerable evidence from both animal and human studies that early experiences can have significant and lasting impacts of subsequent health risks. The following sections of this volume examine how these early experiences and exposures may be amplified or modified by subsequent life experiences and exposures.

REFERENCES

1. FELITTI, V.J., R.F. ANDA, D. NORDENBERG, D.F. WILLIAMSON, A.M. SPITZ, V. EDWARDS, M.P. KOSS & J.S. MARKS. 1998. Relationship of childhood abuse and household dysfunction to many of the leading causes of death in adults. The adverse childhood experiences (ACE) study. Am. J. Prev. Med. **14:** 245–259.
2. REPETTI, R., S. TAYLOR & T. SEEMAN. 1999. Risky families: family social environments and the mental and physical health of offspring. Submitted.
3. SUOMI, S.J. 1999. Attachment in rhesus monkeys. *In* Handbook of Attachment: Theory, Research and Clinical Applications. J. Cassidy & P. Shaver, Eds.: 181–197. Guilford Press, New York.
4. MEANY, M.J. 1999. Stress, maternal care, and infant brain development. Ann. N.Y. Acad. Sci. **896:** this volume.
5. KAUFMAN, J., B. BIRMAHER, J. PEREL, R.E. DAHL, S. STULL, D. BRENT, L. TRUBNICK, M. AL-SHABBOUT & N.D. RYAN. 1998. Serotonergic functioning in depressed abused children: clinical and familial correlates. Biol. Psychiatry **44:** 973–981.
6. PINE, D.S., J.D. COPLAN, G.A. WASSERMAN, L.S. MILLER, J.E. FIRED, M. DAVIES, T.B. COOPER, L. GREENHILL, D. SHAFFER & B. PARSONS. 1997 Neuroendocrine response to D,1-fenfluramine challenge in boys: associations with aggressive behavior and adverse rearing. Arch. Gen. Psychiatry **54:** 830–846.

Maternal Care, Gene Expression, and the Development of Individual Differences in Stress Reactivity

DARLENE D. FRANCIS, FRANCES A. CHAMPAGNE, DONG LIU, AND MICHAEL J. MEANEY[a]

Developmental Neuroendocrinology Laboratory, Douglas Hospital Research Center, Departments of Psychiatry and Neurology and Neurosurgery, McGill University, Montréal, Québec, Canada H4H IR3

PARENTAL CARE AND THE HEALTH OF OFFSPRING

The quality of family life influences the development of individual differences in vulnerability to illness throughout later life. As adults, victims of childhood physical or sexual abuse are at considerably greater risk for mental illness, as well as for diabetes and heart disease (e.g., Refs. 1–3). Children need not be beaten to be compromised. Persistent emotional neglect or conditions of harsh, inconsistent discipline serve to increase the risk of depression and anxiety disorders to a level comparable to that observed in cases of abuse.[4] Indeed, for certain outcomes, the consequences of persistent neglect exceed those of abuse.[5,6]

More subtle relationships exist. Low scores on parental bonding scales, reflecting cold, distant parent–child relationships, significantly increase the risk of depression and anxiety in later life (e.g., Refs. 7,8). And the risk is not unique to mental health. Russak and Schwartz[9] found that by midlife those individuals who, as undergraduate students, rated their relationship with parents as cold and detached, had a fourfold greater risk of chronic illness, including depression and alcoholism as well as heart disease and diabetes.

Parental factors also serve to mediate the effects of environmental adversity on development. For example, the effects of poverty on emotional and cognitive development are mediated by parental factors, to the extent that if such factors are controlled, there is no discernible effect of poverty on child development.[10,11] Moreover, treatment outcomes associated with early intervention programs are routinely correlated with changes in parental behavior: In cases where parental behavior proves resistant to change, treatment outcomes are seriously limited. These findings suggest that variations in parental care mediate, in part at least, the effects of environmental adversity on child development. One of the more common findings here is that maternal depression associated with environmental conditions not only compromises parent–child interactions, but also limits the efficacy of early intervention programs.

[a]Address for correspondence: Michael J. Meaney, Douglas Hospital Research Centre, 6875, Boul LaSalle, Montréal, Québec, H4H IR3, Canada.
e-mail: mdmm@ musica.mcgill.ca

The sword cuts both ways. Family life can also serve as a source of resilience in the face of chronic stress.[12] Thus, warm, nurturing families tend to promote resistance to stress and to diminish vulnerability to stress-induced illness.[13]

The critical question concerns the nature of these parental influences on the health of the offspring. What are the factors that mediate such enduring effects? We have argued that the relationship between early life events and health in adulthood is mediated by parental influences on the development of neural systems that underlie the expression of behavioral and endocrine responses to stress (see Ref. 14). There are two critical assumptions here: First, that prolonged activation of neural and hormonal responses to stress can promote illness and second that early environmental events influence the development of these responses. There is strong evidence in favor of both ideas.

RESPONSES TO STRESS

Stress is a risk factor for a variety of illnesses, ranging from autoimmune disorders to mental illness. The pathways by which stressful events can promote the development of such divergent forms of illness involve the same hormones that ensure survival during a period of stress.[15,16] These effects can, in part, be understood in terms of the responses elicited by stressors.[17,18] The increased adrenal release of catecholamines, adrenaline and noradrenaline, as well as the glucocorticoids, orchestrate a move to catabolism, increasing lipolysis and mobilizing glucose reserves and insulin antagonism (see TABLE 1). These actions serve to increase the availability and distribution of energy substrates. At the same time the increase in circulating levels of catecholamines and glucocorticoids is associated with increased cardiovascular tone. Prolonged activation of these pathways provides an obvious risk for decreased sensitivity to insulin and a risk of steroid-induced diabetes, hypertension, hyperlipidemia, hypercholesterolemia, abdominal fat deposition, and arterial

TABLE 1. Summary of major metabolic/cardiovascular effects of stress-induced increases in catecholamines and glucocorticoids[a]

Target	Effect	Function
Liver	Increased gluconeogenesis	Defend blood sugar level
	Decreased HDL synthesis	Increased plasma cholesterol
Selected macromolecular storage sites	Glygogenolysis, lipolysis substrates (glucose, fat metabolites)	Increased available energy
Heart circulatory system	Enhanced AC drive over heart rate, blood pressure	Increased blood flow
GH target tissue	Decreased sensitivity to GH; increase IGF binding protein	Dampened anabolic processes

ABBREVIATIONS: HDL, high density lipoprotein; CA, catecholamine; GH, growth hormone; IGF, insulin-like growth factor.
[a]See references 15–19.

wear and tear (see Ref. 19), all of which are associated with an increased risk for heart disease (see Ref. 20).

There are also cognitive responses to stressors that include systems which mediate attentional processes as well as learning and memory.[21] During stress individuals become hypervigilant; the level of attention directed to the surrounding environment is increased at the expense of our ability to concentrate on a focused set of tasks that are not essential for survival. As a function of these changes in attentional processes, as well as the effects of glucocoticoids on brain structures such as the hippocampus, episodic memory is less functional during periods of stress (see Refs. 22–24). At the same time, glucocorticoids act on areas of the brain such as the amygdala to enhance learning and memory for emotional stimuli (see Refs. 25–27). These changes in psychological arousal are also associated with altered emotional states: Feelings of apprehension and fear predominate during a stressful experience. While these responses are highly adaptive, chronic activation of these systems can promote the emergence of specific forms of congitive impairments, states of anxiety and dysphoria, sleep disorders, and so forth.[28]

Herein lies the dilemma: The same stress hormones that permit survival during stress can ultimately lead to disease. In human and nonhuman populations, individuals that show exaggerated hypothalamic–pituitary–adrenal (HPA) responses to stress are at increased risk for a variety of disorders including heart disease and diabetes, as well as anxiety, depression, and drug addiction.

Corticotropin-Releasing Hormone

In large measure these reactions are governed by central corticotropin-releasing hormone (CRH) systems that coordinate behavioral, emotional, autonomic, and endocrine responses to stressors. There are two major CRH pathways regulating the expression of stress responses. First a CRH pathway from the parvocellular regions of the paraventricular nucleus of the hypothalamus (PVNh) to the hypophysial–portal system of the anterior pituitary, a system that serves as a principal network for the transduction of a neural signal into a pituitary–adrenal response.[29] In responses to stressors, CRH, as well as cosecretagogues such as arginine vasopressin, is released from PVNh neurons into the portal blood supply of the anterior pituitary where it provokes the synthesis and release of adrenocorticotropic hormone (ACTH). Pituitary ACTH, in turn, causes the release of glucocorticoids from the adrenal gland.

CRF neurons in the central nucleus of the amygdala (CnAmy) project to the locus ceruleus (LC) and increase the firing rate of LC neurons, resulting in increased noradrenaline release in the vast terminal fields of this ascending noradrenergic system (see Refs. 30–32). One of the principal noradrenergic targets here is actually the CRF neurons of the PVNh. Noradrenaline is the major known source of driveover CRF release from PVNh neurons during stress.[29,33] The amygdaloid CRF projection to the locus ceruleus[34-36] is also critical for the expression of behavioral responses to stress: Microinjections of the CRF receptor antagonist, α-helical CRF, into the LC attenuate fear-related behaviors.[37-39] Hence, the CRF neurons in the PVNh and the central nucleus of the amygdala serve as important mediators of both behavioral and endocrine responses to stress. Not surprisingly, increased CRF levels have been associated with serious mood disorders.[28]

These findings have provided a basis for understanding how stress can influence health. Yet the influence of stress can only really be fully appreciated when we factor into the equation some appreciation of the individual's response to stress. The hypothesis, which guides a major research effort on the development of psychopathology, focuses on the role of early life events in determining individual differences in vulnerability to stress. This hypothesis rests on the assumption that chronic activation of central and endocrine stress responses can promote illness (see references cited above). Thus, early life events that increase stress reactivity result in a greater vulnerability for stress-induced illness over the lifespan.

Environmental Regulation of HPA and Behavioral Responses to Stress

One of the strongest models for environmental regulation of the development of responses to stress is the postnatal handling research with rodents. Handling involves a brief (i.e., 3–15 min) daily period of separation of the pup from the mother. In the rat and mouse, postnatal handling decreases the magnitude of behavioral and endocrine responses to stress in adulthood.[40–50] In contrast, longer periods (i.e., 3–6 hours) of daily separation from the mother increase behavioral and endocrine responses to stress.[51–53] These effects persist through the life of the animal (e.g., Ref. 54) and are associated with health outcomes.[55,56]

The central CRF systems are critical targets for these effects (see TABLE 2). Predictably, handling decreases and maternal separation increases CRF gene expression in the PVNh and the CnAmy. Moreover, there are also potent effects on systems that

TABLE 2. Summary of the effects of postnatal handling or maternal separation on neural mediators of behavioral and HPA responses to stress in the rat[a]

Target	Postnatal handling	Maternal separation
CRF mRNA (PVNh)	decreased	increased
CRF mRNA (CnAmy)	decreased	increased
CRFir (locus ceruleus)	decreased	increased
CRF rec binding (locus ceruleus, raphé)	decreased	increased
GR mRNA (hippocampus)	increased	decreased
GR mRNA (PVNh)	no effect	decreased
GC feedback inhibition of CRF	increased	decreased
GABAA receptor	increased	decreased
CBZ receptor/g2 mRNA (amygdala, locus ceruleus, nucleus tractus solitarius)	increased	decreased

ABBREVIATIONS: CRF, corticotropin-releasing factor; PVNh, paraventricular nucleus of the hypothalamus; CnAmy, central nucleus of the amygdala; GR, glucocorticoid; CBZ, central benzodiazepine. (The g2 subunit of the GABAA receptor complex is thought to encode for the CBZ receptor site.)
[a]See references 40–55.

are known to regulate CRF gene expression in the PVNh and the CnAmy (see above). These include glucocorticoid receptor systems that serve to inhibit CRF synthesis and release in the PVNh neurons, as well as GABAergic/central benzodiazepine systems that regulate both amygdaloid CRF activity as well as effects at the level of the noradrenergic neurons of the LC and NTS.[57] Predictably, stress-induced activation of ascending noradrenergic systems in adult animals is enhanced by maternal separation and decreased by handling in early life.[53] Thus, environmental manipulations can alter the expression of behavioral and endocrine responses to stress by altering the development of central CRF systems.

In addition, maternal separation in early life alters the development of ascending serotonergic systems in both monkey (see especially the studies of Higley and colleagues[58] and rat.[52] Kraemer *et al.*[59] have shown that repeated periods of maternal separation in early life increase CSF measures of central noradrenaline and serotonin (5-HT) responses to stress in the rhesus monkey. Considering the importance of the ascending NA and 5-HT systems in depression, these findings suggest a mechanism whereby early life events might predispose an individual to depression in later life.

The decreased mother–infant contact resulting from long periods of maternal separation seems likely to be a critical variable in understanding how this procedure increases behavioral and HPA responses to stress. But does this imply that under normal conditions maternal care actively contributes to the development of neural systems that mediate stress responses, or simply that the absence of the mother is so disruptive to pup physiology that it affects the development of these systems? If maternal care is relevant, then what are the relevant features of mother–pup interactions, and how do they influence neural development?

What Are the Critical Features of These Environmental Manipulations?

Handling, although a brief interlude in the routine of mother–pup interactions, does alter the behavior of the mother towards the offspring.[60,61] Overall, mothers of handled (H) pups spend the same amount of time with their litters as mothers of non-handled (NH) pups; however, mothers of H litters spend significantly more time licking/grooming their pups.[61,62] The question, then, is whether this altered pattern of maternal behavior serves as a critical stimulus for the environmental effects on the development of endocrine and behavioral responses to stress.

Interestingly, there are substantial, naturally occurring variations in maternal licking/grooming in rat dams. Maternal licking/grooming of pups occurs most frequently before or during periods in which the mother nurses her young in the arched-back position. As you might imagine, the frequency of the two behaviors are closely correlated ($r = +0.91$[62]) across mothers. Thus, it is feasible to characterize mothers as high or low on licking/grooming and arched-back nursing (LG-ABN). Such naturally occurring variations were first described by Myers and colleagues[63] using behavioral observations of mothers with their pups in the home cages. Moreover, these individual differences are stable across multiple litters.[64]

In one series of studies, mothers were divided into two groups, high or low in licking/grooming and arched-back nursing (LG-ABN), on the basis of behavioral observations performed over the first 10 days of life (6–8 hours of observation per day). It is important to note that there were no differences between these groups in the overall amount of time in contact with pups.[62,64,65] The logic here is simple. If handling-induced differences in licking/grooming or arched-back nursing are relevant for effects on HPA development, then the offspring of high LG-ABN mothers should resemble the H animals. This is exactly what was found.[62] As adults, the offspring of high LG-ABN mothers showed reduced plasma ACTH and corticosterone responses to restraint stress. These animals also showed significantly increased hippocampal GC receptor mRNA expression, enhanced GC negative feedback sensitivity, and decreased hypothalamic CRH mRNA levels. Moreover, the magnitude of the corticosterone response to acute stress was significantly correlated with the frequency of both maternal licking/grooming ($r = 0.61$) and arched-back nursing ($r = -0.64$) during the first 10 days of life, as was the level of hippocampal GC receptor mRNA and hypothalamic CRH mRNA expression (in all cases $r > 0.70$; see Liu *et al.*[62]). In addition, we also found that the adult offspring of low LG-ABN mothers showed significantly increased noradrenergic responses to stress at the level of the PVNh.[66] These studies suggest that the critical feature for the handling effect on HPA development involves an increase in maternal licking/grooming.

The offspring of the high and low LG-ABN mothers also differed in behavioral responses to novelty.[65] As adults, the offspring of the low LG-ABN showed increased startle responses, decreased open-field exploration, and longer latencies to eat food provided in a novel environment. These animals also showed increased CRF receptor levels in the locus ceruleus and decreased CBZ receptor levels in the basolateral and central nucleus of the amygdala, as well as in the locus ceruleus[65] and increased CRF mRNA expression in the CnAmy (D.D. Francis, J. Diorio, and

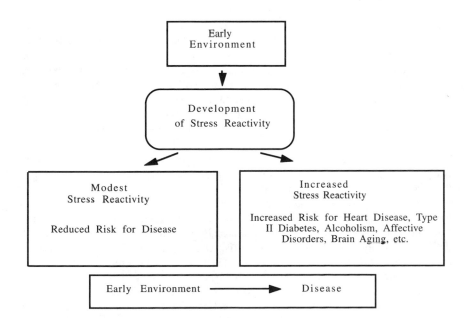

FIGURE 1

Meaney, unpublished). These differences map perfectly onto the differences in H and NH animals and provide support for the idea that the effects of handling are mediated by changes in maternal behavior.

It may surprise the reader that rather subtle variations in maternal behavior have such a profound impact on development. However, for a rat pup, the first weeks of life do not hold a great deal of stimulus diversity. Stability is the theme of the burrow, and the social environment in the first days of life is defined by the mother and littermates. The mother, then, serves as a primary link between the environment and the developing animal. It seems reasonable that variations in mother–pup interaction would serve to carry so much importance for development.

The Transmission of Individual Differences in Maternal Care to the Offspring

Interestingly, individual differences in maternal behavior show intergenerational transmission. The female offspring of high LG-ABN mothers showed significantly more mother licking/grooming and arched-back nursing than did the female offspring of low LG-ABN mothers.[67] The intergenerational transmission of parental behavior has also been reported in primates. In rhesus monkeys there is clear evidence for family lineages expressing child abuse.[68] There is also evidence for transmission of individual differences in parental styles falling within the normal range. Fairbanks[69] found that daughters who were reared by mothers who consistently spent a higher amount of time in physical contact with their offspring became mothers who were similarly more attentive to their offspring. In rhesus monkeys, Berman[70] found that the rate of rejecting the infant by mothers was correlated with the rejection rate of their mothers. In primates, such individual differences in maternal behavior may be revealed in juvenile, nulliparous females. Thus, among juvenile female vervet monkeys, time spent in proximity to nonrelated infants was associated with the maternal behavior of their mothers.[71] In all cases these findings were independent of the social rank of the mother. Equally impressive findings exist in humans, where Miller et al.[72] found that scores on parental bonding measures between a mother and her daughter were highly correlated with the same measures of bonding between the daughter and her child. These findings suggest a perhaps common process of intergenerational transmission of maternal behavior. The critical question here concerns the mechanism underlying this intergenerational transmission of individual differences in behavior.

We[67] have provided evidence for a nongenomic transmission of individual differences in maternal behavior. In one study, we performed reciprocal cross-fostering of the offspring of low and high LG-ABN mothers. The primary concern here was that the wholesale fostering of litters between mothers is known to affect maternal behavior.[73] In order to avert this problem and maintain the original character of the host litter, no more than 2 of 12 pups were fostered into or from any one litter.[74] The critical groups of interest are the biological offspring of low LG-ABN mothers fostered onto high LG-ABN dams, and *vice versa*. The control groups included (1) the offspring of low LG-ABN onto other low LG-ABN mothers as well as offspring of high LG-ABN dams fostered onto other high LG-ABN mothers; (2) sham-adoption animals that were simply removed from the nest and fostered back to their biological mothers; and (3) unmanipulated pups. The limited cross-fostering design did not result in any effect on group differences in maternal behavior. Hence, the frequency of pup licking/grooming and arched-back nursing across all groups of high LG-ABN mothers was significantly higher than that for any of the low LG-ABN dams regardless of litter composition.

The results of the behavioral studies are consistent with the idea that the variations in maternal care are causally related to individual differences in the behavior of the offspring. The biological offspring of low LG-ABN dams reared by high LG-ABN mothers were significantly less fearful under conditions of novelty than were any of the offspring reared by low LG-ABN mothers, including the biological offspring of high LG-ABN mothers. A separate group of female offspring was then mated, allowed to give birth, and observed for differences in maternal behavior. The effect on maternal behavior followed the same pattern as that for differences in fearfulness. As adults, the female offspring of low LG-ABN dams reared by high LG-ABN mothers did not differ from normal, high LG/ABN offspring in the frequency of pup licking/grooming or arched-back nursing. The frequency of licking/grooming and arched-back nursing in animals reared by high LG-ABN mothers was significantly higher than in any of the low LG-ABN groups, and again this included female pups originally born to high LG-ABN mothers but reared by low LG-ABN dams. Individual differences in fearfulness or maternal behavior mapped onto those of the rearing mother, rather than the biological mother.

A second series of studies was designed to examine the intergenerational effects of an "early intervention" program. Handling increases maternal licking/grooming and arched-back nursing. Handling pups, in fact, turns low LG-ABN dams into high LG-ABN mothers.[67] As adults, the handled offspring of such mothers resemble the offspring of high LG-ABN mothers, a finding that is consistent with the nongenomic transmission hypothesis. We then studied the F_3 generation, focusing on the handled and nonhandled offspring of low LG-ABN mothers. These animals were completely unmanipulated. Bear in mind, we refer to these mothers as low LG-ABN because they are derived from low LG-ABN mothers themselves. The low LG-ABN mothers with handled pups behave in a manner that is indistinguishable from high LG-ABN dams. Importantly, their female offspring (F_2 animals) also behave as high LG-ABN.

As shown in TABLE 2, the F_3 offspring of handled/low LG-ABN mothers resemble the offspring of high LG-ABN dams on measures of hypothalamic CRF and hippocampal glucocorticoid receptor mRNA expression, as well as CBZ receptor binding (see also Ref. 67). These findings suggest that individual differences in gene expression in brain regions that result in behavioral and endocrine responses to stress can also be transmitted across generations via a nongenomic mechanism.

These findings are consistent with the results of studies using the cross-fostering technique as a test for maternal-mediation hypotheses. For example, the spontaneously hypertensive rat (SHR) is a strain bred for hypertension, which appears in adolescence. Although the selective breeding suggests a genetic background, the expression of the hypertensive trait is also influenced by epigenetic factors (see Ref. 75). SHR pups reared by wild-type, WKY mothers do exhibit hypertension to the extent of kin reared by SHR dams. When borderline hypertensive rats (BHR), a hybrid formed by SHR-WKY matings, are reared by WKY mothers, they do not express the spontaneous hypertensive phenotype.

The Potential Effects of Maternal Behavior on the Development of Behavior and Endocrine Responses to Stress in BALBc Mice

The BALBc is normally a strain that is very fearful and shows elevated HPA responses to stress. However, BALBc mice cross-fostered to C57 mothers are significantly less fearful, with lower HPA responses to stress.[76] Importantly, C57 mothers normally lick and groom their pups about twice as frequently as BALBc mothers.[77] Comparable findings have emerged with rat strains. Typically, Fisher 344 rats are more responsive to novelty and have increased HPA responses to acute stress in comparison to Long-Evans rats. Moore and Lux[78] reported that Long-Evans darns lick/groom their offspring significantly more often than do Fisher 344 mothers.

Under normal circumstances, of course, BALBc mice are reared by BALBc mothers. The genetic and environmental factors conspire to produce an excessively fearful animal. This is usually the reality of nature and nurture. Genetic and environmental factors work in concert, and are often correlated (see Ref. 79). Because parents provide both genes and environment for their biological offspring, the offspring's environment is therefore, in part, correlated with their genes. The offspring's genes are correlated with those of the parents, and the parents' genes influence the environment they provide for the offspring. The reason why many epidemiological studies based on linear regression models often find that the epigenetic factors, such as parental care, do not add predictive value above that of genetic inheritance is because of this correlation. The environment the parent provides commonly serves to enhance the genetic differences—they are redundant mechanisms. The knowledge of an animal's BALBc pedigree is sufficient to predict a high level of timidity in adulthood. Additional information on maternal care would statistically add little to the predictability—the two factors work in the same direction. But this is clearly different from concluding that the maternal care is not relevant, and the results of the cross-fostering studies attest to the importance of such epigenetic influences.

The value of this process is that it can provide for variation. If the genetically determined trajectory is not adaptive for the animal, then development that can move in the direction of the current environmental signal would be of adaptive value. Hence, environmental events can alter the path of the genetically established trajectory in favor of more adaptive outcomes. This, of course, is the adaptive value of plasticity.

In our minds, these are adaptive processes. Children inherit not only genes from their parents, but also an environment[80]: Englishmen inherit England, as Francis Galton remarked. We believe that the transmission of individual differences in stress reactivity from mother to offspring can provide an adaptive level of "preparedness" for the offspring. Under conditions of increased environmental demand, it is commonly in the animal's interest to enhance behavioral (e.g., vigilance, fearfulness) and endocrine (HPA and metabolic/cardiovascular) responsivity to stress. These responses promote detection of potential threats, avoidance learning, and the mobilization of energy reserves, which are essential under the increased demands of the stressor. Because the offspring usually inhabit a niche that is similar to their parents, the transmission of these traits from parent to offspring could serve to be adaptive. In this context it is understandable that parents inhabiting a very demanding environmental niche might "transmit" a high level of stress reactivity to their offspring.

MATERNAL RESPONSIVITY IN HIGH AND LOW LG-ABN MOTHERS

One question certainly concerns the neural basis for these individual differences in maternal behavior as well as the mechanisms that underlie this apparent transmission of parental behavior from one generation to the next. We believe that these questions can, to some degree, be addressed in nonhuman populations, and the focus of our work lies in the findings of Allison Fleming,[81] showing a direct relationship between fearfulness and maternal behavior.

In the rat, maternal behavior emerges as a resolution of an interesting conflict.[82] Females rats, unless they are in late pregnancy or lactating, exhibit a fearful, neophobic reaction to pups. Habituation through continuous exposure to pups renders females more likely to exhibit maternal behavior. In the classic behavioral test for "maternal responsivity," virgin females are exposed continuously to pups of 3–6 days of age (see Refs. 83, 84). After a number of days most females begin to show active care of the pups, including crouching over the pups in a nursing posture and licking/grooming. Thus, habituation through continuous exposure to pups renders females less neophobic and more likely to exhibit maternal behavior. In general, procedures that reduce fearfulness, including amygdaloid lesions, enhance maternal responsivity, reducing the amount of time for females to exhibit maternal behavior.[85] Such findings may apply to the human condition. Fleming[86] reported that many factors contribute to the quality of the mother's attitude towards her newborn, but none are correlated more highly than the women's level of anxiety. More anxious, depressed mothers are, not surprisingly, less positive towards their babies (also see Ref. 87). Behaviorally, more fearful mothers, such as the low LG-ABN dams, appear to be less maternally responsive towards their offspring.

Considering the differences in fearfulness in the female offspring of high and low LG-ABN, we expected to see differences in the maternal responsivity test in these animals. This was exactly what occurred (Champagne and Meaney, unpublished). The virgin female offspring of high LG-ABN mothers exhibited the full pattern of maternal behavior in about one-half the exposure time of the offspring of low LG-ABN (4.4 vs. 8.9 days exposure). These findings suggest that naturally occurring variations in maternal care are reflected in differences in the maternal responsivity test. Moreover, variations in maternal responsivity in the female offspring of high and low LG-ABN mothers are apparent even in nulipars.

If naturally occurring variations in maternal care are associated with differences in maternal responsivity, then we should be able to screen a population of nulliparous females with the pup sensitization paradigm and use data on individual differences in the latency to express maternal behavior to predict variations in actual maternal care. This admittedly obvious hypothesis has, to the best of our knowledge, never actually been tested. This seems surprising, considering the degree to which our knowledge of the neural basis of maternal behavior rests on the use of the pup-sensitization paradigm. We found that the frequency of licking/grooming over the first 10 days post-partum in primaparous females was highly correlated to the latency in which females exhibited maternal behavior in the maternal responsivity test (Champagne and Meaney, unpublished).

NEURAL BASIS FOR INDIVIDUAL
DIFFERENCES IN MATERNAL BEHAVIOR

The onset of maternal care in the rat is mediated by hormonal events before and during parturition,[82,83] including critical variations in circulating levels of progesterone and estrogen. Estrogen acts at the level of the medial preoptic area (MPOA) to enhance maternal behavior.[82] The MPOA is also a site of action for the effects of placental lactogens, including prolactin, on maternal behavior.[83]

The influence of ovarian hormones on maternal behavior in the rat is mediated, in part, by effects on central oxytocinergic systems (see Ref. 88). Estrogen induces oxytocin receptor gene expression.[89] Administration (i.c.v.) of oxytocin rapidly stimulates maternal behavior in virgin rats.[90,91] The effect of oxytocin is abolished by ovariectomy and reinstated with estrogen treatment. Moreover, treatment with oxytocin antiserum or receptor antagonists blocks the effects of ovarian steroid treatments on maternal behavior.[92,93]

Oxytocin receptor levels are enriched in sites such the MPOA, the ventral tegmental area (VTA) and the CnAmy and increase following parturition in each of these regions.[85,93] Oxytocin infusion into the MPOA or the VTA increases the expression of maternal behavior (e.g., Refs. 88, 90–92). Oxytocinergic neurons that project to the VTA have been located in the ventral bed nucleus of the stria terminalis–lateral preoptic area as well as the PVNh,[88] and lesions of these areas inhibit maternal behavior.[94,95] The VTA is, of course, the source for the mesocorticolimbic dopamine system, and dopamine receptor blockers suppress the expression of pup licking/grooming.[97]

Functionally, the onset of maternal behavior emerges from the decreased fearful response of the female to pups and an increase in the attraction of the mother for her pups (see Refs. 82, 86, and 97 for reviews). The positive cues associated with pups emerge from tactile, gustatory, and auditory stimuli (see Ref. 97). Thus, pup stimuli can either be aversive, eliciting withdrawal, or positive, eliciting approach. The onset of maternal behavior clearly depends on decreasing the negative-withdrawal tendency, and increasing the positive-approach responses.

For virgin females, pups elicit withdrawal and avoidance associated with odor cues transduced via both the vomeronasal and accessory olfactory bulb projections to the MPOA. The vomeronasal projections arise via the amygdala. Thus, anosmic females are more readily maternal,[98] and lesions of the amygdala enhance maternal responsiveness in virgin females[99] (see also Ref. 95). These findings suggest that the cues that elicit withdrawal are transmitted through the amygdala. Morgan et al.[100] found that amygdaloid kindling, which enhances fearfulness in the rat, increases neophobia and decreases approaches to pup-related stimuli in virgin females. Additionally, oxytocin projections to the olfactory bulb may mediate a decrease in odor-induced fear responses to pups (see Ref. 101). Interestingly, Neumann et al.[102] reported that oxytocin infused directly into the CnAmy produced an anxiolytic effect in female rats. These findings suggest that oxytocin might promote the expression of maternal behavior, in part by inhibiting fear-related neural activity.

What is particularly interesting to consider is the possibility that neural systems involved in the expression of fearfulness, notably the CRF systems, can directly influence maternal behavior. Pederson et al.[104] reported that central CRF infusions disrupt maternal behavior in the rat. Such CRF effects could then explain, in part at least, differences in the maternal behavior of high and low LG-ABN mothers. In addition, there may also be effects of maternal care on neural systems mediating attraction to pup-related stimuli. We found significantly reduced oxytocin receptor levels in the CnAmy of low LG-ABN mothers, as well as increased CRF receptors in this same region. Such findings are apparent even in virgin animals and underscore the relationship between neural systems mediating fear and those involved in maternal behavior. In addition to these differences in the amygdala, we also found differences in oxytocin receptors in the MPOA that were evident only during lactation.

Individual differences in maternal care could therefore be derived from early environmental effects on the development of neural systems mediating fearfulness as well as those involved in mediating the attraction of females towards pups. The net effects are differences in maternal responsivity between high and low LG-ABN mothers. These effects, in turn, provide the basis for stable individual differences in stress reactivity and maternal behavior in the offspring. This hypothesis could account, at least in part, for the stable transmission of individual differences in maternal behavior in the rat.

ENVIRONMENTAL REGULATION OF MATERNAL BEHAVIOR

A critical issue here is the relationship between the environment of the mother and the nature of her behavior toward her offspring. We propose that such individual differences are, in turn, functionally related to the level of environmental demand that confronts the animal. Under natural conditions, and the sanctity of the burrow, rat pups have little direct experience with the environment. Instead, conditions such as the scarcity of food, social instability, and low dominance status directly affect the status of the mother and, thus, maternal care. The effects of these environmental challenges on the development of the pups are then mediated by alterations in maternal care, which serve to transduce an environmental signal to the pups (see FIG. 2). The environmentally driven alterations in maternal care then influence the development of neural systems that mediate behavioral and HPA responses to stress. These effects can thus serve to increase or decrease stress reactivity in the offspring. We suggest that more fearful, anxious animals, such as the low LG-ABN mothers, are therefore more neophobic and lower in maternal responsivity to pups than are less fearful animals. Hence, these effects then serve as the basis for comparable patterns of maternal behavior in the offspring and for the transmission of these traits to the subsequent generation (see FIG. 2).

A critical assumption here is that variations in parental behavior are related to the level of environmental demand. Human research suggests that the social, emotional, and socioeconomic context are overriding determinants of the quality of the relationship between parent and child.[80] Human parental care is disturbed under conditions of chronic stress. Conditions that most commonly characterize abusive and neglectful homes involve economic hardship, marital strife, and a lack of social and emotional support (see Ref. 80). Such homes, in turn, breed neglectful parents such that individual differences in parental behavior are reliably transmitted across generations. Although this analysis may seem to be a parental indictment, it is important to note that these same environments are also associated with considerable anxiety and depression. It is important to note that under a high level of environmental demand, increased fearfulness and hypervigilance might well be considered as adaptive. Of course, increased stress reactivity is also associated with enhanced vulnerability to stress-induced illness. Because individual differences in parental care can influence the development of stress reactivity and thus vulnerability for chronic illness in later life, vulnerability for chronic illness is also transmitted across generations. The assumption here is that variations in parental behavior reflect environmental demand.

Perhaps the most compelling evidence for this process emerges from the studies of Rosenblum and colleagues (see Ref. 104 for a review). Bonnet macaque mother–infant dyads were maintained under one of three foraging conditions: low foraging demand (LFD), where food was readily available; high foraging demand (HFD),

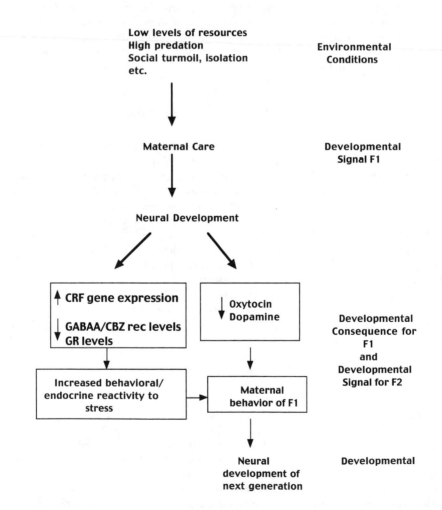

FIGURE 2

where ample food was available but required long periods of searching; and variable foraging demand (VFD), a mixture of the two conditions on a schedule that did not allow for predictability. At the time that these conditions were imposed, there were no differences in the nature of mother–infant interactions. However, after a number of months of these conditions, there were highly significant differences in mother–infant interactions. The VFD condition was clearly the most disruptive. Mother–infant conflict increased in the VFD condition. Infants of mothers housed under these conditions were significantly more timid and fearful. These infants showed signs of depression commonly observed in maternally separated macaque infants—remarkably, even while the infants were in contact with their mothers. As adolescents, the infants reared in the VFD conditions were more fearful and submissive and showed less social play behavior.

More recent studies have demonstrated the effects of these conditions on the development of neurobiological systems that mediate the organisms' behavioral and endocrine/metabolic responses to stress. Coplan *et al.*[105,106] showed that, as adults, monkeys reared under VFD conditions showed increased CSF levels of CRF. Increased central CRF drive would suggest altered noradrenergic and serotonergic responses to stress, and this is exactly what was seen in adolescent VFD-reared animals.[106] Predictably, these animals show increased fearfulness. We would predict that if the environmental conditions remained stable these differences would, in turn, be transmitted to the offspring (see FIG. 2).

These studies underscore two critically important points. First, variations in maternal care falling within the normal range of the species can have a profound influence on development. One does not need to appeal to the more extreme conditions of abuse and neglect to see evidence for the importance of parental care. Second, environmental demands can alter parental care, and thus infant development. Indeed, we hypothesize that environmentally induced alterations in maternal care mediate the effect of variations in the early postnatal environment on the development of specific neural systems that mediate the development of fearfulness. Such individual differences in fearfulness, in turn, influence the parental care of the offspring, providing a neurobiological basis for the intergenerational transmission of specific behavioral traits.

REFERENCES

1. BIFULCO, A., G.W. BROWN & Z. ADLER. 1991. Early sexual abuse and clinical depression in adult life. Br. J. Psychiatry **159:** 115–122.
2. BROWN, G.R. & B. ANDERSON. 1993. Psychiatric morbidity in adult inpatients with childhood histories of sexual and physical abuse. Am. J. Psychiatry **148:** 55–61.
3. FELITTI, V.J., R.F. ANDA, D. NORDENBERG, D.F. WILLIAMSON, A.M. SPITZ, V. EDWARDS, M.P. KOSS & J.S. MARKS. 1998 Relationship of childhood abuse and household dysfunction to many of the leading causes of death in adults. Am. J. Prevent. Med. **14:** 245–258.
4. HOLMES, S.J. & L.N. ROBINS. 1988. The role of parental disciplinary practices in the development of depression and alcoholism. Psychiatry **51:** 24–36.
5. TRICKETT, P.K. & C. MCBRIDE-CHANG. 1995 The developmental impact of different forms of child abuse and neglect. Dev. Rev. **15:** 311–337.
6. AMMERMAN, R.T., J.E. CASSISI, M. HERSEN & V.B. VAN HASSELT. 1986. Consequences of physical abuse and neglect in children. Clin. Psychol. Rev. **6:** 291–310.

7. CANETTI, L., E. BACHAR, E. GALILI-WEISSTUB, A. KAPLAN DE-NOUR & A.Y. SHALEV. 1997. Parental bonding and mental health in adolescence. Adolescence **32:** 381–394.
8. PARKER, G. 1981. Parental representations of patients with anxiety neurosis. Acta Psychiatria Scand. **63:** 33–36.
9. RUSSEK, L.G. & G. SCHWARTZ. 1997. Feelings of parental care predict health status in midlife: a 35 year follow-up of the Harvard mastery of stress study. J. Behav. Med. **20:** 1–11.
10. CONGER, R.D., X. GE, G.H. ELDER, F.O. LORENZ & R.L. SIMONS. 1994. Economic stress, coercive family process, and developmental problems of adolescents. Child Dev. **65:** 541–561.
11. MCLLOYD, V.C. 1998. Socioeconomic disadvantage and child development. Am. Psychol. **53:** 185–204.
12. RUTTER, M. 1979. Protective factors in children's responses to stress and disadvantage. *In* Primary Prevention of Psychopathology, Vol. 3: 49–74. University Press of New England, Hanover, NH.
13. SMITH, J. & M. PRIOR. 1995. Temperament and stress resilience in school-age children: a within-families study. J. Am. Acad. Child Adolesc. Psychiatry **34:** 168–179.
14. FRANCIS, D. & M.J. MEANEY. 1999. Maternal care and the development of stress responses. Curr. Opin. Neurobiol. **9:** 128–134.
15. MCEWEN, B.S. & E. STELLAR. 1993. Stress and the individual: mechanisms leading to disease. Arch. Intern. Med. **153:** 2093–2101.
16. MCEWEN, B.S. 1998. Protective and damaging effects of stress mediators. N. Eng. J. Med. **338:** 171–179.
17. DALLMAN, M.F., S.F. AKANA, K.A. SCRIBNER, M.J. BRADBURY, C.-D. WALKER, A.M. STRACK & C.S. CASCIO. 1993. Stress, feedback and facilitation in the hypothalamo–pituitary–adrenal axis. J. Neuroendocrinol **4:** 517–526.
18. DE KLOET, E.R., E. VREGDENHIL, M.S. OITZL & M. JOELS. 1998. Brain corticosteroid receptor balance in health and disease. Endocrinol. Rev. **19:** 269–301.
19. BRINDLEY, D.N. & Y. ROLLAND. 1989. Possible connections between stress, diabetes, obesity, hypertension and altered lipoprotein metabolism that may result in atherosclerosis. Clin. Sci. **77:** 453–461.
20. SEEMAN, T.E., B.H. SINGER, J.W. ROWE, R.I. HORWITZ & B.S. MCEWEN. 1997. Price of adaptation–allostatic load and its health consequences. Arch. Int. Med. **157:** 2259–2268
21. ARNSTEN, A.F. 1998. The biology of being frazzled. Science **280:** 1711–1712.
22. LUPIEN, S., M. DELEON, S. DESANTI, A. CONVIT, C. TARSHISH, N. NAIR, M. THAKUR, B.S. MCEWEN, R.L. HAUGER & M.J. MEANEY. 1998. Cortisol levels during human aging predict hippocampal atrophy and memory deficits. Nature (Neurosci.) **1:** 69–73.
23. LUPIEN, S.J., N.P.V. NAIR, S. BRIERE, F. MAHEU, M.T. TU, M. LEMAY, B.S. MCEWEN & M.J. MEANEY. 1999. Increased cortisol levels and impaired cognition in human aging: implications for depression and dementia in later life. Rev. Neurosci. **10:** 117–139.
24. NEWCOMER, J.W., G. SELKE, A.K. MELSON, T. HERSHEY, S. CRAFT, K. RICHARDS & A.L. ALDERSON. 1999. Decreased memory performance in healthy humans induced by stress-level cortisol treatment. Arch. Gen. Psychiatry **56:** 527–533.
25. LEDOUX, J.E. 1994. The amygdala: contributions to fear and stress. Sem. Neurosci. **6:** 231–237.
26. DAVIS, M. 1992. The role of the amygdala in fear and anxiety. Ann. Rev. Neurosci. **15:** 353–375.
27. QUIRARTE, G.L., B. ROOZENDAAL & J.L. MCGAUGH. 1997. Glucocorticoid enhancement of memory storage involves noradrenergic activation in the basolateral amygdala. Proc. Natl. Acad. Sci. USA **94:** 14048–14053.
28. ARBORELIUS, L., M.J. OWENS, P.M. PLOTSKY & C.B. NEMEROFF. 1999. The role of corticotropin-releasing factor in depression and anxiety disorders. J. Endocrinol. **160:** 1–12.
29. PLOTSKY, P.M. 1991. Pathways to the secretion of adrenocorticotropin: a view from the portal. J. Neuroendocrinol. **3:** 1–9.

30. GRAY, T.S., M.E. CARNEY & D.J. MAGNUSON. 1989. Direct projections from the central amygdaloid nucleus to the hypothalamic paraventricular nucleus: possible role in stress-induced adrenocorticotropin release. Neuroendocrinology **50:** 433–446.

31. VALENTINO, R.J., A.L. CURTIS, M.E. PAGE, L.A. PAVCOVICH & S.M. FLORIN-LECHNER. 1998. Activation of the locus coeruleus brain noradrenergic system during stress: circuitry, consequences, and regulation. Adv. Pharmacol. **42:** 781–784.

32. LAVICKY, J. & A.J. DUNN. 1993. Corticotropin-releasing factor stimulates catecholamine release in hypothalamus and prefrontal cortex in freely moving rats as assessed by microdialysis. J. Neurochem. **60:** 602–612.

33. PLOTSKY, P.M., E.T. CUNNINGHAM & E.P. WIDMAIER. 1989. Catecholaminergic modulation of corticotropin-releasing factor and adrenocorticotropin secretion. Endo. Rev. **10:** 437–458.

34. MOGA, M.M. & T.S. GRAY. 1989. Evidence for corticotropin-releasing factor, neurotensin, and somatostatin in the neural pathway from the central nucleus of the amygdala to the parabrachial nucleus. J. Comp. Neurol. **241:** 275–284.

35. KOEGLER-MULY, S.M., M.J. OWENS, G.N.E.D. KILTS & C.B. NEMEROFF. 1993. Potential corticotropin-releasing factor pathways in the rat brain as determined by bilateral electrolytic lesions of the central amygdaloid nucleus and the paraventricular nucleus of the hypothalamus. J. Neuroendocrinol. **5:** 95–98.

36. VAN BOCKSTAELE, E., E. COLAGO & R. VALENTINO. 1996. Corticotropin-releasing factor-containing axon terminals synapse onto catecholamine dendrites and may presynaptically modulate other afferents in the rostral pole of the nucleus locus coeruleus in the rat brain. J. Comp. Neurol. **364:** 523–534.

37. BUTLER, P.D., J.M. WEISS, J.C. STOUT & C.B. NEMEROFF. 1990. Corticotropin-releasing factor produces fear-enhancing and behavioural activating effects following infusion into the locus coeruleus. J. Neurosci. **10:** 176–183.

38. SWIERGIEL, A.H., L.K. TAKAHASHI & N.H. KALIN. 1993. Attenuation of stress induced behavior by antagonism of corticotropin-releasing factor receptors in the central amygdala in the rat. Brain Res. **623:** 229–234.

39. ROSEN, J.B. & J. SCHULKIN. 1998 From normal fear to pathological anxiety. Psychol. Rev. **105:** 325–350.

40. LEVINE, S. 1957. Infantile experience and resistance to physiological stress. Science **126:** 405–406.

41. LEVINE, S. 1962. Plasma-free corticosteroid response to electric shock in rats stimulated in infancy. Science **135:** 795–796.

42. MACCARI, S., P.V. PIAZZA, M. KABBAJ, A. BARBAZANGES, H. SIMON & M. LEMOAL. 1995. Adoption reverses the long-term impairment in glucocorticoid feedback induced by prenatal stress. J. Neurosci. **15:** 110–116.

43. LEVINE, S., G.C. HALTMEYER, G. KARAS & V.H. DENENBERG. 1967. Physiological and behavioral effects of infantile stimulation. Physiol. Behav. **2:** 55–63.

44. ADER, R. & L.J. GROTA. 1969. Effects of early experience on adrenocortical reactivity. Physiol. Behav. **4:** 303–305.

45. HESS, J.L., V.H. DENENBERG, M.X. ZARROW & W.D. PFEIFER. 1969. Modification of the corticosterone response curve as a function of handling in infancy. Physiol. Behav. **4:** 109–112.

46. ZARROW, M.X., P.S. CAMPBELL & V.H. DENENBERG. 1972. Handling in infancy: increased levels of the hypothalamic corticotropin releasing factor (CRG) following exposure to a novel situation. Proc. Soc. Exp. Biol. Med. **356:** 141–143.

47. MEANEY, M.J., D.H. AITKEN, S. SHARMA, V. VIAU & A. SARRIEAU. 1989. Postnatal handling increases hippocampal type 11, glucocorticoid receptors and enhances adrenocortical negative-feedback efficacy in the rat. J. Neuroendocrinol. **5:** 597–604.

48. VIAU, V., S. SHARMA, P.M. PLOTSKY & M.J. MEANEY. 1993. The hypothalamic–pituitary-adrenal response to stress in handled and nonhandled rats: differences in stress-induced plasma ACTH secretion are not dependent upon increased corticosterone levels. J. Neurosci. **13:** 1097–1105.

49. BHATNAGAR, S., N. SHANKS & M.J. MEANEY. 1995. Hypothalamic–pituitary–adrenal function in handled and nonhandled rats in response to chronic stress. J. Neuroendocrinol. **7:** 107–119.
50. MEANEY, M., J. DIORIO, J. WIDDOWSON, P. LAPLANTE, C. CALDJI, J.R. SECKL & P.M. PLOTSKY. 1996. Early environmental regulation of forebrain glucocorticoid receptor gene expression: implications for adrenocortical responses to stress. Dev. Neurosci. **18:** 49–72.
51. PLOTSKY, P. & M.J. MEANEY. 1993. Effects of early environment on hypothalamic corticotrophin-releasing factor mRNA, synthesis, and stress-induced release. Mol. Brain Res. **18:** 195–200.
52. LADD, C.O., M.J. OWENS & C.B. NEMEROFF. 1996. Persistent changes in corticotropin-releasing factor neuronal systems induced by maternal deprivation. Endocrinology **137:** 1212–1218.
53. LIU, D., C. CALDJI, S. SHARMA, P.M. PLOTSKY & M.J. MEANEY. 1999. The effects of early life events on in vivo release of norepinepherine in the paraventricular nucleus of the hypothalamus and hypothalamic-pituitary-adrenal responses during stress. J. Neuroendocrinol. In press.
54. MEANEY, M.J., D.H. AITKEN, S. BHATNAGAR, C.V. BERKEL & R.M. SAPOLSKY. 1988. Postnatal handling attenuates neuroendocrine, anatomical, and cognitive impairments related to the aged hippocampus. Science **238:** 766–768.
55. BHATNAGAR, S., N. SHANKS & M.J. MEANEY. 1995. Hypothalamic–pituitary–adrenal function in handled and nonhandled rats in response to chronic stress. J. Neuroendocrinol. **7:** 107–119.
56. LABAN, O., B.M. MARKOVIC, M. DIMITRIJEVIC & B.D. JANKOVIC. 1995. Maternal deprivation and early weaning modulate experimental allergic encephalomyelitis in the rat. Brain Behav. Immun. **9:** 9–19.
57. CALDJI, C., D. FRANCIS, S. SHARMA, P.M. PLOTSKY & M.J. MEANEY. 1999. The effects of early rearing environment on the development of GABA$_A$ and central benzodiazepine receptor levels and novelty-induced fearfulness in the rat. Neuropsychopharmacology, in press.
58. HIGLEY, J.D., M.F. HASER, S.J. SUOMI & M. LINNOILA. 1991 Nonhuman primate model of alcohol abuse: effects of early experience, personality and stress on alcohol consumption. Proc. Natl. Acad. Sci. USA **88:** 7261–7265.
59. KRAEMER, G.W., M.H. EBERT, D.E. SCHMIDT & W.T. MCKINNEY. 1989 A longitudinal study of the effect of different social rearing conditions on cerebrospinal fluinorepinephrine and biogenic amine metabolites in rhesus monkeys. Neuropsychopharmacology **2:** 175–189.
60. BELL, R.W., W. NITSCHKE, T.H. GORRY & T. ZACHMAN. 1971. Infantile stimulation and ultrasonic signaling: a possible mediator of early handling phenomena. Dev. Psychobiol. **4:** 181–191.
61. LEE, M. & D. WILLIAMS. 1974. Changes in licking behaviour of rat mother following handling of young. Anim. Behav. **22:** 679–681.
62. LIU, D., J. DIORIO, B. TANNENBAUM, C. CALDJI, D. FRANCIS, A. FREEMAN, S. SHARMA, D. PEARSON, P.M. PLOTSKY & M.J. MEANEY. 1997. Maternal care, hippocampal glucocorticoid receptors, and hypothalamic–pituitary–adrenal responses to stress. Science **277:** 1659–1662.
63. MEYERS, M., S. BRUNELL, H. SHAIR, J. SQUIRE & M. HOFER. 1989. Relationship between maternal behavior of SHR and WKY dams and adult blood pressures of cross-fostered pups. Dev. Psychobiol. **22:** 55–67.
64. FRANCIS, D.D., A. MAR & M.J. MEANEY. 1999. Naturally-occurring variations in maternal behavior in the rat. Submitted.
65. CALDJI, C., B. TANNENBAUM, S. SHARMA, D. FRANCIS, P.M. PLOTSKY & M.J. MEANEY. 1998. Maternal care during infancy regulates the development of neural systems mediating the expression of behavioral fearfulness in adulthood in the rat. Proc. Natl. Acad. Sci. USA **95:** 5335–5340.
66. CALDJI, C., D. LIU & M.J. MEANEY. 1999. Maternal care alters the development of stress-induced norepinepherine release in the PVNh. Soc. Neurosci. Abstr. In press.

67. FRANCIS, D.D., J. DIORIO, D. LIU & M.J. MEANEY. 1999. Individual differences in responses to stress in the rat are transmitted across generations through variations in maternal care: evidence for a non-genomic mechanism of inheritance. Science, in press.
68. MAESTRIPIERI, D., K. WALLEN & K.A. CARROLL. 1997 Genealogical and demographic influences on infant abuse and neglect in group-lining sooty mangabeys (*Cerocebus atys*). Dev. Psychobiol. **31:** 175–180.
69. FAIRBANKS, L. 1996. Individual differences in maternal style. Adv. Study Behav. **25:** 579–611.
70. BERMAN, C.M. 1990. Intergenerational transmission of maternal rejection rates among free-ranging rhesus monkeys on Cayo Santiago. Anim. Behav. **44:** 247–258.
71. MEANEY, M., J.B. MITCHELL, D.H. AITKEN, S. BHATNAGAR, S. BODNOFF, L.J. INY & A. SARRIEAU. 1991. The effects of neonatal handling on the development of the adrenocortical response to stress: implications for neuropathology and cognitive deficits in later life. Psychoneuroendocrinology **16:** 85–103.
72. MILLER, L., R. KRAMER, V. WARNER, P. WICKRAMARATNE & M. WEISSMAN. 1997. Intergenerational transmission of parental bonding among women. J. Am. Acad. Child Adolesc. Psychiatry. **36:** 1134–1139.
73. MACCARI, S., P.V. PIAZZA, M. KABBAJ, A. BARBAZANGES, H. SIMON & M. LEMOAL. 1995. Adoption reverses the long-term impairment in glucocorticoid feedback induced by prenatal stress. J. Neurosci. **15:** 110–116.
74. MCCARTY, R. & J.H. LEE. 1996. Maternal influences on adult blood pressure of SHRs: a single pup cross-fostering study. Physiol. Behav. **59:** 71–75.
75. MCCARTY, R., M. CIERPIAL, C. MURPHY & J. LEE. 1992. Maternal involvement in the development of cardiovascular phenotype (Review). Experentia **48:** 315–322.
76. ZAHARIA, M.D., N. SHANKS, M.J. MEANEY & H. ANISMAN. 1996. The effects of postnatal handling on Morris water maze acquisition in different strains of mice. Psychopharmacology **128:** 227–239.
77. ANISMAN, H., M.D. ZAHARIA, M.J. MEANEY & Z. MERALIS. 1998. Do early-life events permanently alter behavioral and hormonal responses to stressors? Int. J. Dev. Neurosci. **16:** 149–164.
78. MOORE, C.L. & B.A. LUX. 1998. Effects of lactation on sodium intake in Fischer-344 and Long-Evans Rats. Dev. Psychobiol. **32:** 51–56.
79. SCARR, S. & K. MCCARTNEY. 1983. How people make their on environments. A theory of genotype–environment effects. Child Dev. **54:** 424–435.
80. EISENBERG, L. 1990. The biosocial context of parenting in human families. *In* Mammalian Parenting: Biochemical, Neurobiological, and Behavioral Determinants. N.A. Krasnegor & R.S. Bridges, Eds.: 9–24. Oxford University Press, London.
81. FLEMING, A.S., D.H. O'DAY & G.W. KRAEMER. 1998. Neurobiology of mother–infant interactions: experience and central nervous system plasticity across development and generations. Neurosci. Biobehav. Rev. **16:** 673–685.
82. ROSENBLATT, J. 1994. Psychobiology of maternal behavior: contribution to the clinical understanding of maternal behavior among humans. Acta Paediatr. **397:** 3–8.
83. BRIDGES, R.S. 1994. The role of lactogenic hormones in maternal behavior in female rats. Acta Paediatr. Suppl. **397:** 33–39.
84. STERN, J.M. 1997. Offspring-induced nurtuance: animal–human parallels. Dev. Psychobiol. **31:** 19–37.
85. FLEMING, A.S., U. CHEUNG, M. NATHALIE & K. ZIGGY. 1989. Effects of maternal hormones on "timidity" and attraction to pup-related odors in female rats. Physiol. Behav. **46:** 449–453.
86. FLEMING, A. & C. CORTER. 1988. Factors influencing maternal responsiveness in humans: usefulness of an animal model. Psychoneuroendocrinology **13:** 189–212.
87. FIELD, T. 1998. Maternal depression effects on infants and early interventions. Prev. Med. **27:** 200–203.
88. PEDERSEN, C. 1995. Oxytocin control of maternal behavior. Regulation by sex steroids and offspring stimuli. Ann. N.Y. Acad. Sci. **807:** 126–145.

89. DEKLOET, E.R., T.A.M. VOORHUIS & J. ELANDS. 1986 Estradiol induces oxytocin binding sites in rat hypothalamic ventromedial nucleus. Eur. J. Pharmacol. **118:** 185–186.
90. PEDERSEN, C. & A. PRANGE. 1979. Induction of maternal behavior in virgin rats after intracebroventricular administration of oxytocin. Proc. Natl. Acad. Sci. USA **76:** 6661–6665.
91. FAHRBACH, S.E., J.I. MORRELL & D.W. PFAFF. 1985. Possible role for endogenous oxytocin in estrogen-facilitated maternal behavior in rats. Neuroendocrinology **40:** 526–532.
92. PEDERSEN, C., J. CALDWELL, M. JOHNSON, S. FORT & A. PRANGE. 1985. Oxytocin antiserum delays onset of ovarian steroid-induced maternal behavior. Neuropeptides **6:** 175–182.
93. YOUNG, L.J., S. MUNS, Z. WANG & T.R. INSEL. 1997. Changes in oxytocin receptor mRNA in rat brain during pregnancy and the effects of estrogen and interleukin-6. J. Neuroendocrinol. **9:** 859–865.
94. INSEL, T.R. & C.R. HARBAUGH. 1989. Central administration of corticotropin releasing factor alters rat pup isolation calls. Pharmacol. Biochem. Behav. **32:** 197–201.
95. NUMAN, M. 1994. A neural circuitry analysis of maternal behavior in the rat. Acta Paediatr. Supp. **397:** 19–28.
96. STERN, J.M. & L.A. TAYLOR. 1991. Haloperidol inhibits maternal retrieval and licking, but enhances nursing behavior and litter weight gains in lactating rats. J. Neuroendocrinol. **3:** 591–596.
97. STERN, J.M. 1997. Offspring-induced nurturance: animal–human parallels. Dev. Psychobiol. **31:** 19–37.
98. FLEMING, A.S. 1998. Factors influencing maternal responsiveness in humans: usefulness of an animal model. Psychoneuroendocrinology **13:** 189–212.
99. FLEMING, A., F. VACCARINO & C. LEUBKE. 1980. Amygdaloid inhibition of maternal behavior in the nulliparous female rat. Physiol. Behav. **25:** 731–743.
100. MORGAN, H.D., J.A. WATCHUS & A.S. FLEMING. 1975. The effects of electrical stimulation of the medial preoptic area and the medial amygdala on maternal responsiveness in female rats. Ann. N.Y. Acad. Sci. **807:** 602–605.
101. KENDRICK, K.M. & G. LENG. 1988. Hemorrhage-induced release of noradrenaline, 5-hydroxytryptarnine and uric acid in the supraoptic nucleus of the rat, measured by microdialysis. Brain Res. **440:** 402–411.
102. NEUMANN, I. 1999. Anxiolytic effects of oxytoxin at the level of the amygdala. Paper presented at the Annual Conference of The Maternal Brain, Bristol, United Kingdom.
103. PEDERSEN, C.A., J.D. CALDWELL, M. MCGUIRE & D.L. EVANS. 1991. Corticotropin releasing hormone inhibits maternal behavior and induces pup-killing. Life Sci. **48:** 1537–1546.
104. ROSENBLUM, L., J. COPLAN, S. FREIDMAN, T. BASSOFF, J. GORMAN & M. ANDREWS. 1999. Adverse early experiences affect noradrenergic and serotonergic functioning in adult primates. Biol. Psychol. In press.
105. COPLAN, J.D., M.W. ANDREWS, L.A. ROSENBLUM, M.J. OWENS, S. FRIEDMAN, J.M. GORMAN & C.B. NEMEROFF. 1996. Persistent elevations of cerebrospinal fluid concentrations of corticotropin-releasing factor in adult non-human primates exposed to early-life stressors: implications for psychopathology of mood and anxiety disorders. Proc. Natl. Acad. Sci. USA **93:** 1619–1623.
106. J. COPLAN, R. TROST, M. OWENS, T. COOPER, J. GORMAN, C. NEMEROFF & L. ROSENBLUM. 1998. Cerobrospinal fluid concentrations of somatostatin and biogenic amines in grown primates reared by mothers exposed to manipulated foraging conditions. Arch. Gen. Psychiatry **55:** 473–477.

The Biological Embedding of Early Experience and Its Effects on Health in Adulthood

CLYDE HERTZMAN[a]

Department of Health Care and Epidemiology, University of British Columbia, 5804 Fairview Avenue, Vancouver, British Columbia, Canada, V6T 1Z3

ABSTRACT: Explanations of the socioeconomic gradient in health status must account for the observations that the gradient cuts across a wide range of disease processes and is capable of replicating itself on new disease processes as they emerge in society. Understanding this pattern requires an understanding of how human organisms can become generally vulnerable or resilient to disease over time: a huge collation task across different disciplines. The hypothesis that best fits current evidence is that the gradient is an "emergent property" of the interaction between the developmental status of people and the material and psychosocial conditions they encounter over their life course. Within this broad formulation, special attention is given to child development, and the prospect that socioeconomic differences in the quality of early life experiences contribute to subsequent gradients in health status through socioeconomic differences in brain sculpting and the conditioning of host defense systems that depend on communication with the developing brain. The contribution to the gradient in health is theorized to occur through a combination of latent effects, pathway effects, and cumulative disadvantage.

INTRODUCTION

Can the ubiquitous socioeconomic gradient in health status be explained primarily by differences in life circumstances in adulthood? There are reasons to think that it can. The diseases that contribute to socioeconomic differentials in morbidity and mortality have their onset in adulthood. Societies do tend to create "niches" for adults that, like the "ecological niches" in nature, are more or less hostile to human well-being. Dramatic declines in adult health status in the short term were shown to occur in Central and Eastern Europe in response to disruptions in the socioeconomic environment.[1]

In the West, higher income, better education, and jobs with more status, prestige, and decision latitude provide the most hospitable ecological niches for adult life. If what is true for plants and animals in the wild is also true for humans in society, a socioeconomic gradient in health status would be a natural consequence. Those whose circumstances most closely approximate the hospitable niche would enjoy the longest, healthiest lives and those whose lives diverge the most from it would live lives that were increasingly unhealthy and short. Yet, this view downplays the con-

[a]Address for correspondence: 604-822-3002 (voice); 604-822-4994 (fax).
e-mail: hertzman@unixg.ubc.ca

tribution of life course influences and the special role of child development, in producing socioeconomic gradients in adult health.

A LIFE COURSE PERSPECTIVE

To date, it has not been resolved how the life course perspective fits with explanations of the gradient that focus exclusively on contemporary adult circumstances. There are three reasons to believe that this is a shortcoming that should be corrected. First, the gradient is found, to a greater or lesser degree, for most major causes of morbidity and mortality. It has shown the potential to replicate itself on new conditions, such as heart disease (during the mid-century) and HIV (at the end of the century) soon after they become endemic in society. Thus, explaining the gradient requires recognizing a general resilience and vulnerability, *in addition to* factors that exclusively affect specific diseases. It is exceedingly difficult to conceive of pan-pathological vulnerability or resilience without focusing on the developmental biology of host resistance, which, in turn, requires a focus on life course development.

Second, the socioeconomic gradient in health status found in adult life is paralleled by socioeconomic gradients in cognitive and behavioral development in early life. In Canada and the United States, these gradients are consistent by kindergarten age and are related to differential access, by socioeconomic status, to "developmental priming mechanisms" for healthy child development: encouragement of exploration; mentoring in basic skills; celebration of developmental advances; guided rehearsal and extension of new skills; protection from inappropriate disapproval, teasing, or punishment; and a rich and responsive language environment.[2]

Finally, evidence from longitudinal studies shows that early child development and the socioeconomic and psychosocial environment of childhood are empirically linked to adult health status.

Recently, attention has been paid to the ways in which this last link occurs. Investigators have postulated three different processes: first, latent effects by which the early life environment affects adult health independent of intervening experience; second, pathway effects, through which the early life environment sets individuals onto life trajectories that in turn affect health status over time; and, third, cumulative effects whereby the intensity and duration of exposure to unfavorable environments adversely affects health status, according to a dose–response relationship.[3–7]

The essence of the latency model is that specific biological factors (e.g., low birth weight) or developmental opportunities (e.g., adequate exposure to spoken language) at critical/sensitive periods in (early) life have a lifelong impact on health and well-being, regardless of subsequent life circumstances. The fact that crucial elements of emotional control, peer social skills, language development, and the understanding relative quantity all have critical periods in the first five years of human life adds biological plausibility to the latency model.[8]

Biological plausibility is reinforced by evidence, such as the studies of Romanian orphans who spent more than eight months of their first few years of life in Romanian orphanages during the Soviet era. These studies show that putting adequately nourished children in unstimulating emotional and intellectual environments can retard cognitive and behavioral development in a manner that is not entirely reversible.[9] It has also been argued that the association between low birth weight and cardiovascular disease in adulthood is evidence of a latent effect.[10] Similarly, the results from early childhood stimulation programs for disadvantaged children are consistent with a latent effect, given their effectiveness in improving adult well-being and competence through enrichment programs that are confined to the early years, and do not involve ongoing elements from school age to adulthood.[11,12]

In practice, latent effects can be difficult to disentangle from pathway effects. This is because the pathways model acknowledges that differences in early life environment may direct children onto different life courses. To illustrate, stimulation, stability, and security in early childhood affect a child's cognitive readiness for schooling in terms of both quantitative skills[13] and receptive language.[14,15] Also, the prevalence of aggressive behavior in childhood does not peak in the teenage years as is commonly thought, but rather by 24 months of age.[16] The principal opportunity for socializing nonaggressive behavior falls between age two and five. In turn, lack of school readiness leads to an increased risk of failure to adjust to school[17] as well as academic failure. Behavioral problems and failure in school lead to low levels of mental well-being in early adulthood.[18] Meanwhile, the status of one's parents helps to determine the community where one grows up, which, by the early school years, starts to influence the child's life chances through the social networks, community values, and opportunities that present themselves.[19–21]

The third process linking early life environment and adult health recognizes the importance of cumulative effects, wherein the focus is on the accumulation of advantage or disadvantage over time, based on the duration and intensity of exposure to factor(s) that have the potential to confer advantage or disadvantage. For instance, a cumulative effect of income is suggested by the stronger association with mortality found for earnings over several years than for single-year earnings.[22] With respect to socioeconomic circumstances, it was shown that mortality risk in a prospective study of Scottish men was graded by cumulative social class, comprising class of origin, at labor market entry, and in later adulthood.[23]

Life course influences on health status have been established, in the greatest detail, in the 1958 British Birth Cohort.[24,25] Cumulative and pathway effects were confirmed: socioeconomic conditions from birth to age 33 were shown to have a cumulative effect on self-rated health, over and above the independent effect of level of education achieved (a pathway effect). Latent effects were also confirmed.[26] The variable "parents read to child at age 7" predicted self-rated health at age 33 even after subsequent educational attainment had been considered. The rate of growth in early childhood, as indexed by the "percent of adult height at age 7" is also a predictor of adult self-rated health. Finally, early behavioral adjustment is an important predictor of adult self-rated health, even when subsequent behavioral state is taken into account.

When this perspective is considered, then the most valid explanatory model for the socioeconomic gradient would appear to be one that simultaneously considers life course factors, contemporary circumstances, and the interactions between them (FIG. 1). Life course factors (latent, pathway, and cumulative) would be seen to interact with contemporary circumstances at various levels of social aggregation on a moment-by-moment basis and over time, with differential health status emerging as a function of these interactions. This approach brings together the hitherto disparate

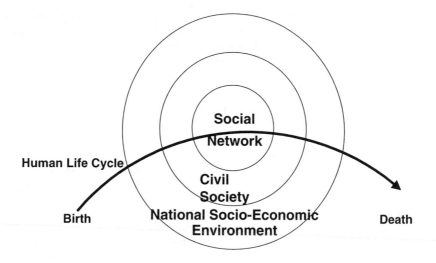

FIGURE 1. Framework for human development and the determinants of health.

approaches of previous studies that tend to focus exclusively on life course explanations for adult health outcomes[27–30] or, exclusively, on contemporary circumstances.

CONTEMPORARY CIRCUMSTANCES

A key element of the explanatory model described above is the notion that contemporary circumstances should be grouped according to different levels of social aggregation. At the most "macro" or broadest level of social aggregation, there is the socioeconomic environment of a society as a whole. The principal determinants of health at this level are its income per capita and how equitably it is distributed.[31,32] Among countries with per capita incomes below $11,000 US, increasing national income strongly correlates with increasing health status[33]; above this level, equity of income distribution appears to matter more than variations in income *per se.*

At the "meso" or civil society level, there are a series of factors that include voluntarism; social affiliation, trust, and cohesion; discrimination and social exclusion; and the capacity of important social institutions to respond to current and changing human needs. These factors can be seen as elements of organized society that may either buffer or exacerbate the stresses of daily living. Thus, variables as diverse as psychosocial work characteristics and the level of membership in service organizations can be regarded as aspects of civil society. By emphasizing both the voluntary and the structural, this construct includes the full range of characteristics studied separately by other investigators.[34–37]

Finally, at the most "micro" level, there are the determinants of health associated with private life.[38] In practice, this comprises the nature and quality of personal social support: intimate relationships, friendship, and the availability of personal help when needed.

In Canada, the National Longitudinal Study of Children and Youth has shown that the life course of young children interacts with factors at these three levels of social aggregation to produce gradients in cognitive and behavioral readiness for school by age five.[39–41] At the micro level, there is a socioeconomic gradient in the prevalence of low-functioning families, whose function negatively affects children's development.[42] At the meso level, high levels of neighborhood cohesion and safety are positively associated with children's development, whereas uniformly low neighborhood income (as opposed to low average neighborhood income with a small proportion of middle income residents) and frequent residential moves are negatively associated with children's development.[43] At the societal level, low income *per se,* and lack of affordable access to organized child care are negatively associated with children's development.[44,45]

BIOLOGIC EMBEDDING

How do life course factors, interacting with contemporary circumstances, create systematic differences in host resilience? It is possible to offer a hypothesis that systematic differences in the quality of early environments, in terms of stimulation and emotional and physical support, will affect the sculpting and neurochemistry of the central nervous system in ways that will adversely affect cognitive, social, and behavioral development. Because the central nervous system, which interprets the environment, interacts closely with the immune, hormone, and clotting systems, systematic differences in life experiences and circumstances will ultimately affect three things: physiological patterns of "host response"; the "objective" stressfulness of the experiences and circumstances to which the host must respond; and, also, the biological interpretation of these experiences and circumstances. These differences have the potential to change the long-term function of organ systems and create socioeconomic differentials in morbidity and mortality that cut across a wide variety of disease processes. The process whereby differential human experiences systematically affect the healthfulness of life across the life cycle has been termed "biological embedding."[46]

The first place to look for evidence of biological embedding is in the "life of the hypothalamo–pituitary–adrenal (HPA) axis in society." This axis is central because of its role in host perception of, and response to, stressful circumstances. One end product of HPA stimulation, cortisol secretion, has widespread metabolic effects on organ systems in the human body. These effects are adaptive in the acute phase, but may be damaging to end-organs with chronic overexposure.

Animal studies provide a preliminary model of the role the HPA axis may play in general vulnerability and resistance to disease. Three lines of evidence are particularly pertinent here. First, Meaney[47,48] has shown that, in rats, an intervention ("handling") in early life can permanently condition the way the HPA axis responds to living conditions over the life course. This conditioning only takes place during a discrete time in early life, which suggests that it depends on appropriate stimulation during a highly circumscribed window of opportunity in brain development (i.e., a critical period). Most important, once the HPA axis has been conditioned, the effects may be lifelong. In this study, handling reduced total lifetime exposure of corticosterone to the brain. Chronic overexposure to corticosterone endangers selected neurons in the hippocampus of the brain, such that the rate of loss of hippocampal neurons was reduced in the handled rats over their life span. Cognitive functions are sensitive to relatively small degrees of hippocampal damage, and so by twenty-four months of age, elderly by rat standards, the handled rats had been spared some of the cognitive deterioration typical of aging. The significance of this was demonstrated by performance on a learning task wherein rats had to find a submerged platform in a pool of opaque water, relying entirely upon visuospatial cues from the surrounding room. Nonhandled rats had a progressive deterioration in their performance with age; in contrast, no deterioration occurred in aged handled rats.

Second, the relationship has been demonstrated,[49] in rhesus monkeys, between nature, nurture, social mobility, and the life of the HPA across the life course. Suomi has shown that a minority of rhesus monkeys (approximately 15%) are born predisposed to a high reactivity state, which involves both behavioral and metabolic dimensions.[49] The behaviors are not adaptive, in that they involve avoidance of novel stimuli, as well as anxious and depressive reactions to maternal separation. On the metabolic level, the HPA axis is overstimulated, with exaggerated cortisol responses to daily stresses. In adulthood, highly reactive males are usually low status, and highly reactive females are at increased risk of neglecting their offspring. However, Suomi has shown that arranging to have highly reactive rhesus monkeys raised by exemplary parents can transform all three tendencies: reactive behavior is transformed into vigilance on behalf of the troop; the HPA axis is stabilized; adult males tend towards high status; and adult females adopt the parenting styles of their foster parents.

The final line of evidence comes from Sapolsky's studies of free-ranging baboon populations of the Serengeti.[50] With a knowledge of the life circumstances of each baboon, Sapolsky defined four factors that lead to variation in basal cortisol levels in the wild. In terms of the life of the HPA axis, lower basal cortisol can be thought of as the superior state, in terms of well-being. These four factors are:

1. *Rank*—When all other factors are held constant, higher rank in the baboon community means lower basal cortisol.

2. *Social stability and its enforcement*—When baboon societies are stable, those in dominant positions have lower basal cortisols than they do during periods of instability. When stability is imposed by high levels of violence and coercion, the nondominant baboons have higher basal cortisols than when it is maintained with low levels of violence and coercion.

3. *The experience of rank, stability, and enforcement*—When social instability occurs, some nondominant baboons will actually experience decreases in basal cortisol. This is because their relationships with those higher in the hierarchy are traditionally stressful. These relationships may be interrupted by the preoccupations the more dominant baboons have with each other during fights for supremacy. Other low-ranked baboons, however, will do worse if they become the victims of displaced aggression from the losers in the fight for social dominance.

4. *Personality and coping styles*—Individual characteristics matter, too. The ability to distinguish seriously threatening situations from ruses; to distinguish winning from losing a fight; to relieve stress by displacing aggression; and to be able to develop friendships and strategic alliances all lead to increased well-being. Each of

these characteristics has a component that is related to circumstances of upbringing and mentorship.

Taken together, these studies of different species suggest that the life of the HPA axis parallels the determinants of health in human societies. Hierarchy and social stability are, fundamentally, characteristics of whole societies, although they may be encrypted either within society as a whole (social stability) or in the individual (place in hierarchy). There is a parallel between the pattern of lower average basal cortisol in baboon communities with low levels of violence and coercion, and findings in human populations that show that relative income equality[51,52] and shallow social class gradients in health[53] are determinants of longevity in human societies. The experience of hierarchy, stability, and enforcement (e.g., the day-to-day stresses of good times, such as a positive workplace and home life, and bad times, for example, loss of control at work, layoffs, or long-term unemployment, are in the terminology used here "civil society" functions that reside in an intermediate zone between the individual and the state. Personality and coping styles are embedded in the individual, but have both a social network aspect and a life course aspect. The importance of the latter is reinforced by the work of both Meaney and Suomi.

Does the HPA axis have the same life in human society that it seems to in animals? Evidence here has been much slower to accumulate. However, there are at least four lines of inquiry that converge with the evidence presented above.

- It has been shown[54] that the quality of maternal–child attachment affects the HPA axis and behavior, such that poorly attached toddlers have both more reactive HPA axes and less adaptive behavioral responses in social conflict situations.

- Long-term Romanian orphans tend to be high cortisol reactors.[b]

- Systematic social class differences in basal cortisol levels among both primary and secondary school children have been shown.[b]

- Systematic differences have been demonstrated[55] in cortisol responses of 50-year-old Swedish and Lithuanian men to standardized challenges that are specific to cortisol. By analogy to Saplosky's baboons, the Swedish men show a pattern of higher well-being than the Lithuanian men. This is of tremendous interest because the life circumstances of men who have lived through the experience of the Soviet era and the period of political and social transformation that followed it are systematically different from those of affluent Western countries such as Sweden. Moreover, mortality among men in Central and Eastern Europe used to be similar to the West, but has become much higher over the past 30 years.

- Finally, it has been shown[56] that high levels of cortisol reactivity in the elderly are associated with more rapid rates of cognitive decline. This is analogous to Meaney's experiments with handled rats.

---

[b]The comments marked by the superscript b are from a workshop on biological pathways and reflect presentations by various investigators, including Gunnar, Lupien, Lundberg, and Tarlov, which are not yet available in published form.

The preceding discussion is not meant to suggest that the HPA axis is the only route to socioeconomic gradients in health status. Other pathways operating through perceptual mechanisms, such as the sympatho-adrenal medullary axis certainly exist.[b] Moreover, life circumstances may help create gradients through mechanisms that have no perceptual element at all. Chemical exposures in the environment would be an example here. However, it is principally the mechanisms that operate through perception, memory, and learned response that have the capacity to link the life course to contemporary circumstances and, in turn, to the socioeconomic gradient in health.

DOES IT MATTER?

The questions, why the socioeconomic gradient in health emerges and how it emerges, come together when considering international comparisons of socioeconomic gradients in children's and young adults' performance on tests of literacy.[57] In general, the average level of achievement of those countries that show relatively shallow socioeconomic gradients (by parental socioeconomic status) in literacy is higher than those countries whose gradients are steep (FIG. 2). The suggestion here is that gradients in cognitive development, like gradients in health, may "flatten up." If so, the social conditions that flatten gradients ought to be of great interest to researchers and policy makers alike. Perhaps the best example to cite is Sweden, which has a relatively flat socioeconomic gradient in mortality,[58] accompanied by high life

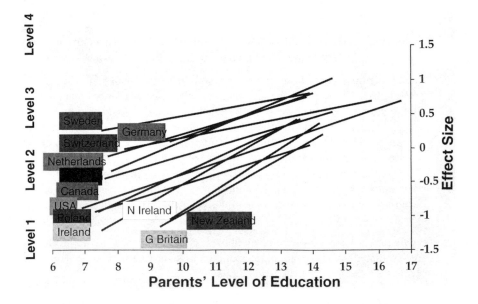

FIGURE 2. Quantitative literacy scores for youth aged 16–25. International Adult Literacy Study, 1994

expectancy, as well as high levels of literacy among young adults, with a similarly flat socioeconomic gradient. In a world that demands increasing sophistication in the cognitive realm, this would seem to be the most desirable state for a modern society.

REFERENCES

1. HERTZMAN, C., S. KELLY & M. BOBAK, Eds. 1996. East–West Life Expectancy Gap in Europe: Environmental and Non-environmental Determinants. Kluwer Academic Publishers, Dordrecht.
2. RAMEY, C.T. & S.L. RAMEY. 1998. Prevention of intellectual disabilities: early interventions to improve cognitive development. Prev. Med. **27:** 224–232.
3. KUH, D.L. & Y. BEN-SHLOMO. 1997. A Life Course Approach to Chronic Disease Epidemiology: Tracing the Origins of Ill Health from Early to Adult Life. Oxford University Press, Oxford.
4. MARMOT, M. & M. WADSWORTH, Eds. 1997. Fetal and early childhood environment: long term health implications. Br. Med. Bull. **53:** 1.
5. POWER, C. & C. HERTZMAN. 1997. Social and biological pathways linking early life and adult disease. Br. Med. Bull. **53**(1): 210–221.
6. DAVEY SMITH, G., C. HART, D. BLANE, C. GILLIS & V. HAWTHORNE. 1997. Lifetime socioeconomic position and mortality: prospective observational study. Br. Med. J. **314:** 547–552.
7. LYNCH, J.W., G.A. KAPLAN & S.J. SHEMA. 1997. Cumulative impact of sustained economic hardship on physical, cognitive, psychological, and social functioning. N. Engl. J. Med. **337**(26): 1889–1895.
8. DOHERTY, G. 1997. Zero to six: the basis for school readiness. Research Paper R-97-8E. Applied Research Branch. Human Resources Development Canada. Ottawa, ON.
9. RUTTER, M. & THE ENGLISH AND ROMANIAN ADOPTEES (ERA) STUDY TEAM. 1998. Developmental catch-up, and deficit, following adoption after severe global early privation. J. Child Psychol. Psychiatry **39:** 465–476.
10. BARKER, D.J.P., Ed. 1992. Fetal and Infant Origins of Adult Disease. 1st edit. British Medical Journal. London.
11. PALMER F.H. 1979. Long-term gains from early intervention: findings from longitudinal studies. *In* Project Head Start: A Legacy of the war on poverty. E. Zigler & J. Valentine, Eds. The Free Press, New York.
12. SCHWEINHART, L.J., H.V. BARNES & D.P. WEIKART. 1993. Significant benefits: the High/Scope Perry preschool study through age 27. Monog. High/Scope Educ. Res. Foundat. **10.**
13. CASE, R. & S. GRIFFIN. 1991. Rightstart: an early intervention program for insuring that children's first formal learning of arithmetic is grounded in their intuitive knowledge of numbers. Report to the James S. McDonnell Foundation.
14. KOHEN, D.E, C. HERTZMAN & J. BROOKS-GUNN. 1998. Neighbourhood influences on children's school readiness. Working Paper W-98-15E. Human Resources Development Canada, Ottawa, ON.
15. ROSS, D.P. & P. ROBERTS. 1999. Income and child well-being: a new perspective on the poverty debate. Canadian Council on Social Development, Ottawa, ON.
16. TREMBLAY, R.E., C. JAPEL, D. PERUSSE, M. BOIVIN, M. ZOCCOLILLO, J. MONTPLAISIR & P. McDUFF. 1999. The search for the age of "onset" of physical aggression: Rousseau and Bandura revisited. *In* Criminal Behavior and Mental Health. In press.
17. PULKKINEN, L. & R.E. TREMBLAY. 1992. Patterns of boys' social adjustment in two cultures and at different ages: a longitudinal perspective. Int. J. Behav. Dev. **15:** 527–553.
18. POWER, C., O. MANOR & J. FOX. 1991. Health and Class: The Early Years. Chapman & Hall, London.
19. KOHEN, D.E., C. HERTZMAN & J. BROOKS-GUNN. 1998. Neighbourhood influences on children's school readiness. Working Paper W-98-15E. Human Resources Development Canada. Ottawa, ON.

20. KOHEN, D.E., C. HERTZMAN & M. WIENS. 1998. Environmental changes and children's competencies. Working Paper W-98-25E. Human Resources Development Canada. Ottawa, ON.
21. KLEBANOV, P.K., J. BROOKS-GUNN, C. MCCARTON, M.C. MCCORMICK. 1998. The contribution of neighborhood and family income to developmental test scores over the first three years of life. Child Dev. **69:** 1420–1436.
22. MCDONOUGH, P., G.J. DUNCAN, D. WILLIAMS & J. HOUSE. 1997. Income dynamics and adult mortality in the United States, 1972 through 1989. Am. J. Pub. Health **87:** 1476–1483.
23. DAVEY SMITH, G., C. HART, D. BLANE, C. GILLIS & V. HAWTHORNE. 1997. Lifetime socioeconomic position and mortality: prospective observational study. Br. Med. J. **314:** 547–552.
24. POWER, C. & C. HERTZMAN. 1997. Social and biological pathways linking early life and adult disease. Br. Med. Bull. **53**(1): 210–221.
25. POWER, C. & S. MATTHEWS. 1998. Accumulation of health risks across social groups in a national longitudinal study. *In* Human Biology and Social Inequality. S.S. Strickland & P.S. Shetty, Eds.: 36–57. Cambridge University Press, Cambridge.
26. HERTZMAN, C, C. POWER & S. MATTHEWS. 1999. Using an interactive framework of society and lifecourse to explain self-rated health in early adulthood. Soc. Sci. Med. Submitted.
27. WANNAMETHEE, G., P. WHINCUP, G. SHAPER & M. WALKER. 1996. Influence of father's social class on cardiovascular disease in middle-aged men. Lancet **348:** 1259–1263.
28. GLIKSMAN, M.D., I. KAWACHI, D. HUNTER, G.A. COLDITZ, J.E. MANSON, M.J. STAMPFER, F.E. SPEIZER, W.C. WILLETT & C.H. HENNEKENS. 1995. Childhood socioeconomic status and risk of cardiovascular disease in middle aged US women: a prospective study. J. Epidemiol. Commun. Health. **49:** 10–15.
29. VAGERO, D. & D. LEON. 1994. Effect of social class in childhood and adulthood on adult mortality. Lancet **343:** 1224–1225.
30. MARE, R.D. 1990 Socio-economic careers and differential mortality among older men in the United States. *In* Measurement and Mortality: New Approaches. J. Vallin, S. de Souza & A. Polloni, Eds.: 362–387. Oxford University Press. New York.
31. WILKINSON, R.G. 1997. Health inequalities: relative or absolute material standards? Br. Med. J. **314:** 591–595.
32. KAPLAN, G.A., E.R. PAMUK, J.W. LYNCH, R.D. COHEN & J.L. BALFOUR. 1996. Inequality in income and mortality in the United States: analysis of mortality and potential pathways. Br. Med. J. **312:** 999–1003.
33. WORLD BANK. 1993. World Development Report. Investing in Health. World Development Indicators. Oxford University Press. New York.
34. PUTNAM, R.D. 1993. Making Democracy Work: Civic Traditions in Modern Italy. Princeton University Press, Princeton.
35. ROSE, R. 1995. Russia as an hour-glass society: a constitution without citizens. East Eur. Constitut. Rev. **4:** 34–42.
36. KAPLAN, G.A., E.R. PAMUK, J.W. LYNCH, R.D. COHEN & J.L. BALFOUR. 1996. Inequality in income and mortality in the United States: analysis of mortality and potential pathways. Br. Med. J. **312:** 999–1003.
37. KAWACHI, I., B.P. KENNEDY, K. LOCHNER & D. PROTHROW-STITH. 1997. Social capital, income inequality, and mortality. Am. J. Pub. Health **87:** 1491–1498.
38. BERKMAN, L.F. 1995. The role of social relations in health promotion. Psychosom. Med. **57:** 245–254.
39. ROSS, D.P. & P. ROBERTS. 1999. Income and child well-being: a new perspective on the poverty debate. Canadian Council on Social Development. Ottawa, ON.
40. KOHEN, D.E., C. HERTZMAN & J. BROOKS-GUNN. 1998. Neighbourhood influences on children's school readiness. Working Paper W-98-15E. Human Resources Development Canada. Ottawa, ON.
41. KOHEN, D.E., C. HERTZMAN & M. WIENS. 1998. Environmental changes and children's competencies. Working Paper W-98-25E. Human Resources Development Canada. Ottawa, ON.

42. Ross, D.P. & P. Roberts. 1999. Income and child well-being: a new perspective on the poverty debate. Canadian Council on Social Development. Ottawa, ON.
43. Kohen, D.E, C. Hertzman & M. Wiens. 1998. Environmental changes and children's competencies. Working Paper W-98-25E. Human Resources Development Canada. Ottawa, ON.
44. Ross, D.P. & P. Roberts. 1999. Income and child well-being: a new perspective on the poverty debate. Canadian Council on Social Development, Ottawa, ON.
45. Kohen, D. & C. Hertzman. 1999. The importance of quality child care. Chapter 15. *In* Vulnerable Children in Canada. D. Willms, Ed.: In press.
46. Hertzman, C. & M. Wiens. 1996. Child development and long-term outcomes: a population health perspective and summary of successful interventions. Soc. Sci. Med. **43**(7): 1083–1095.
47. Meany, M.J. 1999. Stress, maternal care, and infant brain development. Ann. N.Y. Acad, Sci. **896:** this volume.
48. Sapolsky, R.M. 1992. Stress, the Aging Brain, and the Mechanisms of Neuron Death. The MIT Press, Cambridge.
49. Suomi, S.J. 1999. Developmental trajectories, early experiences, and community consequences: lessons from studies with rhesus monkeys. *In* Developmental Health and the Wealth of Nations. D.P. Keating & C. Hertzman, Eds.: The Guildford Press, New York.
50. Sapolsky, R.M. 1995. Social subordinance as a marker of hypercortisolism: some unexpected subtleties. Ann. N.Y. Acad. Sci. **771:** 626–639.
51. Wilkinson, R.G. 1992. Income distribution and life expectancy. Br. Med. J. **304:** 165–168.
52. Wilkinson, R.G. 1997. Health inequalities: relative or absolute material standards? Br. Med. J. **314:** 591–595.
53. Vagero, D. & O. Lundberg. 1989. Health inequalities in Britain and Sweden. Lancet **ii:** 35–36.
54. Gunnar, M.R. & C.A. Nelson. 1994. Event-related potentials in year-old infants: relations with emotionality and cortisol. Child Dev. **65:** 80–94.
55. Kristenson, M. 1998. The LiVicordia study: possible causes for the differences in coronary heart disease mortality between Lithuania and Sweden. Linkoping University Medical Dissertations #547. Linkoping University, Sweden.
56. Lupien, S.J., M. de Leon, S. de Santi, A. Convit, C. Tarshish, N.P.V. Nair, M. Thakur, B.S. McEwan, R.L. Hauger & M.J. Meaney. 1998. Cortisol levels during human aging predict hippocampal atrophy and memory deficits. Nature Neurosci. **1:** 69–73.
57. Willms, J.D. 1997. Literacy skills of Canadian youth. Statistics Canada and Human Resources Development Canada. #89-552-MPE, Statistics Canada. Ottawa, ON.
58. Vagero, D & O. Lundberg. 1989. Health inequalities in Britain and Sweden, Lancet **ii:** 35–36.

Hierarchies of Life Histories and Associated Health Risks

BURTON SINGER[a,b] AND CAROL D. RYFF[c]

[b]Office of Population Research, Princeton University, Princeton, New Jersey 08544, USA

[c]Department of Psychology, University of Wisconsin, Madison, Wisconsin 53706, USA

ABSTRACT: Widely documented inverse associations between socioeconomic standing and incident chronic disease and mortality invite explanation in terms of pathways to these outcomes. Empirical identification of pathways, or histories, requires measures that assess cumulative wear and tear on physiological systems following from psychosocial adversity and genetic predispositions. Such an assessment, allostatic load, has been shown to predict later life mortality, incident cardiovascular disease, and decline in physical and cognitive functioning. Using data from the Wisconsin Longitudinal Study (WLS), we seek precursors to allostatic load via ordered categories of cumulative adversity relative to advantage over the life course. We operationalize these histories via unfolding economic circumstances and social relationship experiences (e.g., parent–child interactions, quality of spousal ties). Findings reveal a strong direct association between the extent of adversity relative to advantage in an ordering of these histories and likelihood of high allostatic load. Importantly, resilient individuals with economic disadvantage, but compensating positive social relationship histories also show low prevalence of high allostatic load.

INTRODUCTION

The provision of defensible explanations for the inverse associations between position in socioeconomic hierarchies and later-life morbidity and mortality requires integrated investigation of psychosocial and physiological interrelationships over the life course. Most extant studies do not incorporate long-term processes, or cumulative experience, when attempting to identify features of life histories that predict later-life chronic disease and mortality or disability-free well-being into old age. Nevertheless, there is suggestive evidence indicating that cumulative processes across multiple life domains are of central importance for understanding how socioeconomic status (SES)/health associations come about.[1–10]

At the level of income dynamics and its connection to health over the life course, there has been emphasis on economic inequality resulting from cumulative processes, particularly permanent income.[11–13] Deaton,[12] for example, shows that elevated permanent income, rather than contemporary cross-sectional income, has a strong protective effect on mortality. The cumulative negative impact of persistent poverty on health has also received considerable attention.[14,15] In an insightful review, em-

[a]Address for correspondence: Burton Singer, Office of Population Research, Princeton University, 21 Prospect Ave., Princeton, NJ 08544. 609-258-5938 (voice); 609-258-1039 (fax).

e-mail: singer@opr.princeton.edu

phasizing the bidirectional relationships between health and both income and wealth, Smith[11] emphasized the need for more extensive investigation of the role of permanent and transitory changes in income and unemployment on health risks. Despite this literature, cumulative economic processes have received limited attention in prior analyses of socioeconomic differences in income and wealth.[13,16–19]

The import of cumulative effects also pertains to psychosocial experiences. It has long been argued that early life conditions, including the fetal environment, are linked with later life expectancy and disease risks.[2] However, there is great plasticity in factors influencing later-life health and length of life, and cumulative adversity and advantage are consequential. A distant awareness of this point is exemplified by Greenwood's[20] valedictory address for Karl Pearson to the Royal Statistical Society in 1936: "I do not think persons over the age of 40 need abandon hope that social and hygienic betterments introduced after their school days may increase their expectations of life." In more contemporary reviews, we find further support for cumulative effects. Ben-Shlomo and Davey-Smith[21,22] note that "the strong correlations seen between early environment and adult mortality may simply be an effect of continued deprivation leading to an accumulation of detrimental health effects."

Studies of social stress and its consequences for mental health frequently also evaluate childhood and lifetime traumas as well as track chronic, enduring difficulties.[23] The importance of cumulation is illustrated by results showing that the presence of a single stressor (or no stressor at all) produced a 1% increment in psychiatric disorder in children.[24,25] Two stressors in the family complex provide a 5% rise in the disorder rate; three stressors, a 6% increment; and four or more stressors a 21% increment in the rate of childhood psychiatric disorders. Cumulatively, the presence of stressors accounted for a 33% rise in the disorder rate, with multiple stressors accounting for the largest proportion of the disorders.

Because we are also interested in understanding recovery from and resistance to adversity, it is important to give equal consideration to positive aspects of people's lives and particularly to cumulation of advantage. The components of cumulative advantage may come in the form of starting resources (e.g., growing up in an intact family), personal capacities and abilities (e.g., IQ), the realization of expected life transitions (e.g., job promotions, marriage), or having positive evaluations of one's life (e.g., job satisfaction, marital quality). The idea of cumulation of advantage is not new, having been invoked to explain inequalities in scientific productivity[26,27] or health in the context of educational attainment.[28]

Simultaneous consideration of cumulative adversity and advantage as they pertain to understanding health outcomes, including resilience, has been the theme of several recent investigations.[29–31] In understanding pathways into, and recovery from, episodes of depression, it is important to identify the cumulative processes of both negative and positive valence.[23] The basic point is that pathways to diverse health outcomes depend on an interplay of both positive and negative experience across multiple life domains.

At the level of physiology *per se*, a recently introduced[32–34] indicator of the long-term physiological response to stress, called allostatic load, provides an important bridge between measures of cumulative psychosocial adversity relative to advantage and their biological signature. The basic idea derives from the notion of allostasis[35]—the ability to adapt to change while maintaining physiological systems within normal operating ranges. Through allostasis, the autonomic nervous system, the hypothalamic–pituitary–adrenal (HPA) axis, and the cardiovascular, metabolic, and immune systems protect the body by responding to internal and external stress. The price of this accommodation to stress is referred to as allostatic load, meaning the wear and tear that results from chronic overactivity or underactivity of allostatic systems. An operationalization of allostatic load[36,37] has been shown to predict later-life incident cardiovascular disease, decline in physical and cognitive functioning, and mortality. An important feature of the present paper is the empirical demonstration that allostatic load represents a physiological signature of cumulative adversity relative to advantage in the domains of economic resources and social relationships.

Revisiting the idea of hierarchy, the central question is how to incorporate cumulative processes in multiple life domains in the specification of an ordered family of histories. In most of the literature dealing with SES–health associations, the relevant hierarchies are simply orderings of individuals on the basis of years of education, income based on a cross-sectional ascertainment, or occupational prestige. When taking a life course perspective, an ordering of histories can be based on degrees of cumulative adversity alone, the degree of cumulative adversity relative to advantage, or some other measure that quantifies cumulative experience across one or more life domains and that is associated with health outcomes. The primary goal is then to demonstrate an association between position in a hierarchy of life histories, based on assessments of cumulation in multiple life domains, and the probability of a health or disease outcome. Specifically, the greater the degree of cumulative adversity relative to advantage in the life history specification, the higher the probability of later-life chronic disease, disability, or mortality. Conversely, low cumulative adversity relative to advantage should be associated with high well-being and low probability of incident chronic disease into old age. The advantage of studying SES–health associations in terms of hierarchies of life histories is that the cumulative adversity and advantage specifications provide the ingredients for explanations of *how* the cruder cross-sectional associations come about.

A related and important point is the observation that there is considerable variation in health outcomes at all levels of the cross-sectional hierarchies used in the SES–health literature. Moreover, the variance in outcomes is larger at the bottom of these hierarchies—that is, for low levels of education and income—than at the upper end. For persons at low levels in these hierarchies who nevertheless have positive health outcomes, the question arises of how this resilience in the face of adversity comes about.

Life history representations can facilitate answering this question. Because resilient people do not conform to normative expectations, their life histories should also not be a part of a hierarchy of histories that represent the normative pathways to either disease/disability or good health into late life. Thus, their histories represent pathways to positive outcomes, but where there is also a high degree of cumulative adversity. The details of the pathway specification represent a step toward explanation of the processes that underlie the phenomenon of resilience.

A fundamental feature of pathways of resilience is the demonstration that early-life disadvantage and adversity need not lead to later-life negative outcomes, provided there are compensating positive experiences in the intervening years. Dramatic evidence that risks for negative health consequences can be altered by changing postnatal and later-life social environments can be seen in recent animal (rat) studies. There are beneficial health effects in later life derived from maternal licking and grooming of rat pups.[38,39] However, rats reared in emotionally impoverished environments react to stress more radically throughout their lives than rats reared in enriched environments. This effect, however, is *reversible*. Rats exposed to inadequate nurturing in early life can, if subsequently reared by a high licking and grooming foster mother, have normal functioning and healthy adult lives.[40]

With these observations in mind, the purposes of this paper are to (i) illustrate the process of creating hierarchies of life history pathways using information from two life domains, cumulative economic standing and cumulative relationship profiles; (ii) investigate whether degree of adversity relative to advantage in a hierarchy of pathways is linked to the probability of exhibiting multiple physiological indicators (i.e., allostatic load) that predict later-life incident cardiovascular disease and decline in physical and cognitive functioning; and (iii) determine whether there is a subpopulation of persons from economically disadvantaged backgrounds but who have experienced positive relationship histories that show low allostatic load at ages 59–60.

Social relationships are a central feature of our pathway specifications because of the substantial literature linking the interpersonal realm to mortality outcomes and, when positive, to protective factors.[41–46] The subpopulation identified under objective (iii) defies the expected trend that persons from low-SES backgrounds will have higher allostatic load in mid- to later life, thereby underscoring variability in trajectories of SES to health. These individuals also illustrate pathways of resilience and thus routes from low SES in childhood to good health in later life.

In the next section, we first describe our empirical data base. Attention is then focused on measuring instruments at both the psychosocial and physiological levels. An operationalization of the predisease physiological indicator of cumulative wear and tear, allostatic load, is described in detail. This is accompanied by a brief overview of the scales used to assess parent–child interactions and relations with a significant other in adulthood. Household income of parents while the respondents were in high school and of the respondents themselves at age 50 was derived directly from the WLS survey responses. Finally, we specify the combined cumulative economic and social relationship pathways, accompanied by a rationale for them.

The third section, RESULTS, demonstrates the associations between pathway specifications and allostatic load. We conclude with a discussion of the implications of these results for understanding how cross-sectional associations between SES and morbidity/mortality rates come about. We also emphasize the importance of studying pathways of resilient persons—those who do well in the face of persistent SES-related adversity—as part of a larger program of understanding positive human health[47–52] and the routes to it, particularly under challenging life circumstances.

DATA AND METHODS

Our study population is a subsample ($n = 84$) of persons from the much larger Wisconsin Longitudinal Study (WLS)—with $n = 10,317$—but for whom a range of biomarker assessments and survey responses focused on intimacy in social relationships have been obtained. The primary WLS is a survey of a random sample of

10,317 men and women who graduated from Wisconsin high schools in 1957. Data were collected on the original respondents in 1957, 1975, and 1992/93. For a comprehensive overview of WLS and many of the findings from it, see Hauser *et al.*[53]

The subsample of WLS respondents used in the investigations presented here was selected (in 1997) to match income distributions of respondents' family household income in 1957 and own household income in 1992–1993 for the full WLS population. In 1997, each person completed a social relationship questionnaire, described in detail below. They also participated in a physical health examination and contributed blood and urine samples, from which laboratory assays provided the requisite biomarker measurements. The social relationship measures focus on the key emotional features of social ties, viewed from a life history perspective. That is, the aim was to evaluate early relationship experiences with parents[54] as well as multiple aspects of intimacy with spouse or significant other in adulthood. Together, such assessments allowed for the creation of positive and negative relationship pathways.

Relationship Measures

Caring, supportive, and affectionate relationships between parents and children are hypothesized to be important components of cumulative advantage pathways that ultimately are linked with good physical and mental health in later life. Conversely, the experience of uncaring and even abusive interactions with one or both parents is anticipated to be a defining feature of a negative social relationship pathway that would be associated with physiological indicators operating outside normal ranges in later life. TABLE 1 lists the twelve "caring" items in the Parental Bonding Scale[55] that are the basis for discriminating between genuine caring and warmth in the parent–child bond, as opposed to indifference and rejection. The WLS respondents were asked about their relationship with their mother and father separately—specifically, "When you were growing up, how much did she (he)

TABLE 1. The parental bonding scale

(+)	1.	She (he) spoke to me with a warm and friendly voice.
(+)	2.	She (he) was affectionate to me.
(−)	3.	She (he) seemed emotionally cold to me.
(+)	4.	She (he) appeared to understand my problems and worries.
(+)	5.	She (he) helped me as much as I needed.
(+)	6.	She (he) enjoyed talking things over with me.
(+)	7.	She (he) frequently smiled at me.
(+)	8.	She (he) seemed to understand what I needed or wanted.
(−)	9.	She (he) made me feel I wasn't wanted.
(+)	10.	She (he) could make me feel better when I was upset.
(+)	11.	She (he) communicated with me very much.
(+)	12.	She (he) took an active interest in my habits and school activities.

NOTE: (+) Positively scored item, (−) negatively scored item. Mother caring $\alpha = 0.95$; father caring $\alpha = 0.75$.

behave in each of the following ways?" Response options were "Never," "Some," "A Lot." With the exception of possibly two items (#5 and #12), these questions probe explicitly emotional, affectual, caring features of one's relationship to mother and father.

Shifting attention to mid-life relationships, four aspects of connection to a spouse or significant other are hypothesized to contribute to cumulative relationship pathways that should, in turn, be associated with later life physiological indicators of wear and tear on the body. We assessed different aspects of intimacy by using four subscales of the PAIR (personal assessment of intimacy relationships) inventory.[56] The *emotional* and *sexual* subscales were included because of their focus on the most intimate forms of connection between two people. The *intellectual* and *recreational* subscales emphasize mutually enjoyed experience, companionship, and the scope of shared communication. We did not use the social subscale of the PAIR because it concentrates on the mutual friends of the couple. Similarly, the conventionality subscale was deleted in our pathway constructions because it focused on efforts to create a good impression. Neither of these latter subscales are explicitly tapping feelings and connections between marital partners.

The PAIR seeks to (a) identify the degree to which each partner presently feels intimate in each relational area considered and (b) identify the degree to which each partner would like to be intimate. The items comprising the emotional, sexual, intellectual, and recreational subscales are listed in TABLE 2. For each statement the respondent answers on a five-point scale from strongly agree to strongly disagree.

Biological Measures

Allostasis, meaning "stability through change"[35] is a concept that emphasizes the dynamism of internal physiology and the fact that healthy functioning requires ongoing adjustments and adaptations of the internal physiologic milieu. Normally functioning physiological systems exhibit fluctuating levels of activity as they respond and adapt to environmental demands. Through allostasis, the autonomic nervous system, the hypothalamic–pituitary–adrenal (HPA) axis, and the cardiovascular, metabolic, and immune systems protect the body by responding to internal and external stress.

The long-term, or cumulative, effect of physiological accommodations to stress represent a price paid by the body to maintain systems within normal operating ranges. We conceptualize this price with the term *allostatic load*. It is a measure of the wear and tear that results from chronic overactivity and underactivity of the stabilizing allostatic systems.[32–34] The first operationalization of allostatic load was designed to summarize levels of physiologic activity across a range of regulatory systems pertinent to disease risks.[36,37] Allostatic load for an individual was defined as the number of indicators from the list in TABLE 3 for which an individual's assessed value satisfies the stated inequality.

Cortisol, the catecholamines norepinephrine and epinephrine, and DHEA are mediators of physiological responses to adverse challenge. In particular, 12-hour urinary cortisol excretion is an integrated measure of HPA axis activity, while DHEA-S is a functional HPA axis antagonist serving to reset elevated cortisol levels to basal conditions following stressful challenge. Twelve-hour urinary norepinephrine and epinephrine are integrated measures of sympathetic nervous system activity. Blood pressure, waist–hip ratio, total and HDL cholesterol and glycosylated hemoglobin are viewed as reflecting secondary consequences of stressful challenge. Systolic and diastolic blood pressure are indices of cardiovascular activity. Waist–hip ratio is an index of long-term levels of metabolism and adipose tissue deposition, thought to be influenced by glucocorticoid activity.[37] Serum high-density lipoprotein (HDL) and total cholesterol levels are indices of cardiovascular risk. Total

TABLE 2. Personal assessment of intimacy in relationships (PAIR) subscale statements

Emotional ($\alpha = 0.89$)

(−)	I often feel distant from my partner.
(+)	My partner can really understand my hurts and joys.
(−)	I feel neglected at times by my partner.
(+)	My partner listens to me when I need someone to talk to.
(+)	I can state my feelings without him/her getting defensive.
(−)	I sometimes feel lonely when we're together.

Sexual ($\alpha = 0.85$)

(+)	I am satisfied with our sex life.
(−)	I feel our sexual activity is just routine.
(+)	I am able to tell my partner when I want sexual intercourse.
(−)	I "hold back" my sexual interest because my partner makes me feel uncomfortable.
(+)	Sexual expression is an essential part of our relationship.
(−)	My partner seems disinterested in sex.

Intellectual ($\alpha = 0.87$)

(+)	My partner helps me clarify my thoughts.
(−)	When it comes to having a serious discussion it seems that we have little in common.
(−)	I feel "put down" in a serious conversation with my partner.
(−)	I feel it is useless to discuss some things with my partner.
(+)	We have an endless number of things to talk about.
(−)	My partner frequently tries to change my ideas.

Recreational ($\alpha = 0.85$)

(+)	I think that we share some of the same interests.
(−)	I share in very few of my partner's interests.
(−)	We seldom find time to do fun things together.
(+)	We enjoy the same recreational activities.
(+)	We enjoy the out-of-doors together.
(+)	We like playing together.

NOTE: (+) Positively scored item, (−) negatively scored item.

TABLE 3. Allostatic load parameterization

Systolic BP	≥ 148 mmHg
Diastolic BP	≥ 83 mmHg
Waist–hip ratio	≥ 0.94
Ratio total cholesterol/HDL	≥ 5.9
Glycosylated hemoglobin	$\geq 7.1\%$
Urinary cortisol 9	≥ 25.7 µg/g creatinine
Urinary norepinephrine	≥ 48 µg/g creatinine
Urinary epinephrine	≥ 5 µg/g creatinine
HDL cholesterol	≤ 37 mg/dl
DHEA-S	≤ 350 ng/ml

glycosylated hemoglobin is an integrated measure of glucose metabolism over a period of several days.

The allostatic load measure, based on counting the number of indices in TABLE 3 for which a person's assessed value satisfies the stated inequality, has been shown to be predictive of incident cardiovascular disease and later life decline in physical functioning and memory loss.[36,37] The same protocol used to operationalize allostatic load in this initial work was also employed with the WLS biological subsample. We view the full array of biomarkers, and their summary via allostatic load scores, as *intermediate outcomes* in a cohort study.[57] That is, they are measurements assessed after exposure to cumulative adversity and advantage but before clinical appearance of disease. They therefore quantify early biological and/or altered structure/physiological function before pronounced declines in physical and cognitive functioning and incident chronic disease.

Economic Indicators

We use household income assessments at two points in the life course as the basis for linking our pathway constructions to more conventional measures of socioeconomic status. Household income in 1957 for WLS respondents is an indicator of the economic circumstances of the parents of each individual. These figures were assembled at the first wave of WLS data collection and are derived from Wisconsin state tax records. Because parents' income plays a major role in shaping the childhood environment, we will use it in conjunction with the parental bonding scale parent–child relationship assessments as part of pathway constructions that use both kinds of information. We also utilize respondents household income, assessed in 1992–1993, when they were 52–53 years of age. This allows for a set of pathways to be specified that are based on changes in economic circumstances alone or in combination with cumulative social relationship histories.

PATHWAY SPECIFICATIONS

Relationship Pathways

We define an individual as positive (+) or negative (−) on the mother caring (respectively, father caring) component of the Parental Bonding Scale according to whether she/he has a score that is above or below the median. Thus there are four categories of parent–child relationships based on both mother caring (MC) and father caring (FC). These are, for the pairs (MC category, FC category), given by (+,+), (+,−), (−,+), and (−,−).

From the PAIR inventory, we viewed emotional (E) and sexual (S) items as probes of the most personal and intimate aspects of spousal ties and thus combined these subscales in the concatenation, E+S. Intellectual (I) and recreational (R) items were viewed as probing more companionate and cognitive forms of spousal connection and were combined in the concatenation of subscales I+R. We classified persons as positive (+) or negative (−) on each of E+S and I+R according as their scores were above or below the median on the respective concatenation of subscales. Then the possible (E+S category, I+R category) responses become (+,+), (+,−), (−,+), and (−,−).

Putting the early parental ties and adult spousal connection classifications together, we define an individual to be on the *negative pathway* if s/he scores (−,−) on the parental bonding classification and/or (−,−) on the concatenated subscales of the PAIR inventory. Thus, these individuals experienced negative relationships with *both* parents and/or negative interaction with a spouse on both combined aspects of intimacy described above. We define an individual to be on a *positive pathway* if s/he has at least one + on (MC category, FC category)—that is, (+,−), (−,+), or (+,+)—and at least one + on (E+S category, I+R category). Thus, the positive path requires some positive relational experience with one or both parents in childhood and at least one of the two combined forms of intimacy in adulthood. This pathway underscores the cumulative nature of positive emotional experiences with significant others in childhood and adulthood.

Economic Change

We define an individual to have been in a positive childhood economic environment (+) if the household income of the parents in 1957—when the respondents were 18 years of age—was at or above the median household income for the state of Wisconsin in that year. An individual will be regarded as having been in a negative childhood economic environment (−) if the parents' household income in 1957 is below the statewide median. Analogously, a respondent at ages 52–53 (i.e., in 1992–1993) will be defined to be in positive (+) (respectively, negative [−]) economic circumstances if s/he has household income at or above (respectively, below) the median household income for the state of Wisconsin in 1992–1993. Because these categories are defined in terms of ranked observations, they are insensitive to inflationary factors and do not require any adjustments to constant dollars.

With these ingredients at hand, we define four possible economic pathways in terms of the vector (1957 income, 1992–1993 income). The possible realized vectors are (−,−), (−,+), (+,−), and (+,+). Although more refined income categories (e.g., tertiles, quartiles, and quintiles) of household income can clearly be created, the relatively small number of observations in the biological sample, ($n = 84$) would render comparisons across distinct pathways to be quite unstable. Splitting the income distributions at the median for the childhood and adult responses represents the limiting resolution of the present data set.

Composite Pathways

Household income categories will be combined with relationship pathways in two ways, depending on the kinds of questions being addressed. First, we are interested in how the childhood economic environment concatenated with each of the relationship pathways relates to allostatic load in later life—that is, age 60. To this end, we introduce the composite pathways defined by the vector (1957 household income, relationship pathway). The possible vectors are (–, negative), (–, positive), (+, negative), and (+, positive). It will be useful for subsequent discussion to single out the hierarchy of pathways—ordered from most to least adversity—defined by the sequence: (–, negative); (+, negative); and (+, positive). *A priori*, we hypothesize that the decreasing adversity implied in these pathways is also associated with decreasing proportions of individuals at high allostatic load. The distinguished pathway (–, positive) is viewed *a priori* to be associated with resilient individuals. In particular, this pathway represents persons who grew up in economically disadvantaged environments but who, nevertheless, have positive relationship pathways. We also expect that this population will exhibit physiological resilience in the sense that they should have a substantially smaller proportion of individuals at high allostatic load than those persons on, for example, the (–, negative) pathway.

A second family of combined pathways that are interesting in their own right, and are the building blocks for coarser levels of income history/relationship history combinations, are those defined by pairing each economic pathway with each social relationship pathway. Several hierarchies of composite pathways based on these pairings are displayed in the next section in conjunction with their relationship to allostatic load scores. Interpretations of these hierarchies and a comparison with the more conventional socioeconomic stratification systems are given in the discussion section.

RESULTS

Analogous to much of the literature documenting an inverse association between SES and morbidity and mortality rates,[16–19] we first exhibit the inverse association between household income category and allostatic load. TABLE 4 shows these associations for parents' household income in 1957 and, separately, for respondents' household income in 1992–1993 vs. the percentage of individuals in each stratum at high allostatic load.

The ordering of income categories from high to low disadvantage shows the expected association with allostatic load. The high disadvantage categories exhibit higher percentages of individuals at high allostatic load. There is a greater difference (10%) in percentages at high load for respondents' own household income at age 52–53 than for parents income (5%). This is not surprising, since—as indicated below—

TABLE 4. Household income and allostatic load

Household income category	Percentage with allostatic load at or above 3
1957	
(−)	0.44 (*n* = 41)
(+)	0.39 (*n* = 43)
1992–1993	
(−)	0.47 (*n* = 43)
(+)	0.37 (*n* = 41)

there is a considerable diversity of pathways evolving from each of the 1957 economic environments, with an accompanying diversity of later life (age 60) physiological status as assessed by allostatic load scores.

Greater variation in allostatic load scores across economic strata is anticipated when the strata are defined by pathways representing economic environments at different ages in the life course. We operationalize the economic pathway categories by the vectors (1957 income category, 1992–1993 income category), the possible responses being (−,−), (−,+), (+,−), and (+,+). In TABLE 5 these pathways are arrayed in an order of decreasing adversity. Each path is associated with a percentage of persons on it who are at high allostatic load at age 59–60. We interpret downward mobility (+,−) to be more adverse than upward mobility (−,+). A decrease in economic resources relative to peers is not only negative in terms of real income but also instills an obvious negative social comparison. This interpretation is supported by the corresponding ordering of high allostatic load percentages—0.43 on (+,−) and 0.37 on (−,+).

Across the full hierarchy from (−,−) to (+,+), the corresponding allostatic load percentages are, as one would anticipate *a priori,* strictly decreasing. The association between these rudimentary pathways and the predisease marker, allostatic load, provides a first glimpse of the substantial variation that is hidden behind the usual single-point-in-time SES measure, as in TABLE 4, cross-classified with a health or illness/disease indicator (e.g., mortality, incident cardiovascular disease). The increased spread between the top and bottom of this hierarchy (14%) as compared with the maximum spread in TABLE 4 (10%) is admittedly modest. However, as more refined life history information and, correlatively, nuance of experience, is added to the

TABLE 5. Economic change pathways and allostatic load

Pathway	Percentage with allostatic load at or above 3
(−,−)	0.50 (*n* = 22)
(+,−)	0.43 (*n* = 21)
(−,+)	0.37 (*n* = 19)
(+,+)	0.36 (*n* = 19)

pathway representations, we expect greater differentiation of population subgroups to emerge.

Some insight in this direction derives from examining the association between a relationship pathway hierarchy and allostatic load in TABLE 6. These pathways, of course, do not incorporate any of the economic indicators.

There is a statistically significant difference ($p < 0.01$) between these percentages. A comparison of TABLES 5 and 6 indicates that relationship pathways alone have more discriminatory power than economic pathways, at least in terms of identifying population subgroups at high versus low allostatic load.

TABLE 6 is consistent with a substantial literature indicating that persistent negative relationships are associated with impaired immune function, elevated blood pressure, and later-life illness and chronic disease propensity.[48,58-61] It is also consistent with evidence documenting the role of positive and supportive relationships with parents during childhood and lower incidence of later-life diagnosed diseases. For example, in the 35-year follow-up of the Harvard Mastery of Stress study population,[48] 91% of participants who did not perceive themselves to have had a warm relationship with their mothers—as on the negative pathway (N)—had diagnosed diseases in mid-life including coronary artery disease, hypertension, duodenal ulcer, and alcoholism. This is to be compared with 45% of the people who had a warm positive relationship with their mother but who exhibit the same set of diagnosed diseases.

TABLE 6 suggests that one would anticipate that cumulative positive relationships might ameliorate the negative effects of economic adversity. To assess this hypothesis, we augment the relationship pathways with the indicator of childhood economic environment, that is, 1957 household income. This yields the associations with allostatic load displayed in TABLE 7.

Despite the modest subgroup sizes, the difference between the first two percentages and between the first and last percentages are both statistically significant ($p < 0.05$). Three interpretive points are in order. First, if we think in terms of the economic hierarchy—that is, the categories (−) and (+) for 1957 income—there is

TABLE 6. Relationship pathways and allostatic load

Pathway	Percentage with allostatic load at or above 3
Negative (N)	0.56 ($n = 41$)
Positive (P)	0.28 ($n = 43$)

TABLE 7. {1957 Household income vs. relationship pathway} × allostatic load

{Income − relationship} pathway	Percentage with allostatic load at or above 3
(−, N)	0.64 ($n = 22$)
(−, P)	0.21 ($n = 19$)
(+, N)	0.47 ($n = 19$)
(+, P)	0.33 ($n = 24$)

decidedly greater spread in allostatic load percentages among relationship pathways at the lower end of the hierarchy (i.e., 0.64 to 0.21) than at the upper end (i.e., 0.47 to 0.33). This seems to be a generic situation for a variety of health measures. It is indicative of an important feature of SES–health associations that is masked by the emphasis in the extant literature given to gradients based on average scores on health measures within strata.

A second feature of this table is the allostatic load score (0.21) for the pathway (–, P). This suggests a group of resilient individuals who started out relatively disadvantaged economically but for whom cumulative positive relationships served as a protective factor against breakdown of allostasis across multiple physiological systems.[33,34] Third, there are two hierarchies of pathways to consider. They are ordered from highest to lowest adversity and are specified as follows: (i) (–, N), (+, N), and (+, P) and (ii) (–, N), {(–, P) or (+, N)}, (+, P). The first set of pathways deletes the resilient group and describes an ordering of histories with a corresponding ordering of allostatic load percentages, namely, 0.64, 0.47, and 0.33, respectively. The second hierarchy has an intermediate category with either economic disadvantage and positive relationships or economic advantage and negative relationships. The associated allostatic load percentages are, respectively, 0.64, 0.34, and 0.33. The second hierarchy, of course, masks the resilient group. This serves to emphasize the importance, in general, of exploring multiple forms of hierarchy en route to developing explanations for the very coarse level but widely documented SES–health gradients.

The most fine-grained set of pathways that can be constructed with the economic and social relationship components are formed by concatenation of all possible pairs of economic pathway and social relationship pathway. These are summarized with corresponding allostatic load percentages in TABLE 8. Because the total population for which we have biomarker data is of modest size ($n = 84$), each of the individual concatenated pathways is identified with a small number of individuals. Nevertheless, the pattern of "pathway × allostatic load" relationships is very suggestive of what one should look for in future investigations with larger data sets. Specifically, we would now hypothesize that cumulative positive social relationship pathways have a strong ameliorating effect on allostatic load for persons with any economic adversity (lines 5, 6, and 7 of TABLE 8). Conversely, being on a negative relationship

TABLE 8. [Economic pathway vs. relationship pathway] × allostatic load

(Economic, relationship) pathway	Percentage with allostatic load at or above 3
(–,–); N	0.69 ($n = 13$)
(+,–); N	0.65 ($n = 8$)
(–,+); N	0.55 ($n = 9$)
(+,+); N	0.36 ($n = 11$)
(–,–); P	0.22 ($n = 9$)
(+,–); P	0.31 ($n = 13$)
(–,+); P	0.20 ($n = 10$)
(+,+); P	0.36 ($n = 11$)

pathway enhances the negative impact of any economic adversity (lines 1, 2, and 3 of TABLE 8). Finally, having persistent economic advantage (+,+) overrides the impact of the negative relationship pathway (line 4 of TABLE 8). In fact, lines 4 and 8 indicate that the relationship pathways do not influence allostatic load at the top of the income trajectory hierarchy.

There is a useful hierarchy based on an aggregate of these pathways, where the subgroup sizes are larger and where strong differentiation on the basis of allostatic load is apparent. Such a hierarchy is exhibited in TABLE 9. What this hierarchy implies is that persistent economic advantage is protective against physiological wear and tear, regardless of relationship history. Alternatively, having at least one episode of economic adversity combined with negative relational experience is conducive to high allostatic load.

TABLE 9. Aggregate pathways and allostatic load

Pathway	Percentage with allostatic load at or above 3
At least one economic (−), N	0.63 ($n = 30$)
(+,+)	0.36 ($n = 22$)

There is also an aggregate resilience pathway [at least one economic (−); P} with corresponding percentage at high allostatic load of 0.25 ($n = 32$). This is a refinement of the prior finding on resilience (i.e. TABLE 7), which was restricted only to childhood economic adversity combined with a positive relationship pathway. From the more elaborated hierarchies, we see a pattern of resilience that pertains to any period of economic adversity combined with positive relational experience and low allostatic load.

Without relationship pathways there is far less capacity to discriminate those at high versus low allostatic load. TABLE 10, illustrates this point; that is, with only economic information, positive and negative, from both childhood and adulthood, we see limited distinguishability in the percentage of persons at high allostatic load as a function of economic stratum.

TABLE 10. Hierarchy of economic pathways and allostatic load

Economic Pathway	Percentage with allostatic load at or above 3
At least one economic (−)	0.44 ($n = 62$)
(+,+)	0.36 ($n = 22$)

DISCUSSION

Most of the literature relating SES to health measures focuses on mortality and chronic disease outcomes.[1–10,16–19,62] Our focus here is on a predisease indicator—an early warning signal—allostatic load. The same qualitative association that holds between SES and incident disease and mortality—that is, the higher the position in the SES hierarchy, the lower the disease and mortality rates—has been shown to hold for SES, operationalized as household income, and allostatic load. Specifically, the higher the position in the household income hierarchy, the smaller the percentage of persons with high allostatic load.

Any attempt to explain how these associations come about must bring in additional life history information that is linked to SES indicators—household income in the present study—and also to biomarkers of physiological functioning. The primary objective is the specification of a taxonomy of pathways that relate one or more forms of psychosocial experience, emphasizing cumulative adversity and advantage, to predisease indicators and ultimately, to chronic disease and mortality. We have operationalized this idea by constructing income histories and social relationship pathways. The income histories are specified in terms of household income of the respondent's parents in 1957 and their own household income when they are 52–53 years of age (i.e., in 1992–1993). The relationship histories are based on parent–child interactions when the respondents were growing up and on the character of intimate interactions with a spouse or significant other in adulthood. Both sets of pathways were ordered in terms of degree of adversity relative to advantage. The conventional cross-sectional hierarchies based on SES indicators are replaced by longitudinally defined hierarchies that provide the basis for explanations of the cross-sectional associations and, more importantly, provide characterizations of pathways to elevated risk of disease or to the absence of it into older ages.

Another central feature of the longitudinal pathways is that they facilitate exposure of sources of substantial variation in outcomes that exist within cross-sectional strata. This was illustrated in the present analyses by the fact that the combined economic–social relationship pathways differentiate low versus high allostatic load subpopulations to a greater extent than either of the cross-sectional economic indicators. Furthermore, pathways of resilience are exposed. This provides the basis for formulating primary prevention programs targeted at increasing the proportion of individuals from disadvantaged early life circumstances who, nevertheless, have as good or better physiological functioning at older ages as persons with advantageous childhood circumstances. The substantial difference in proportion of persons at high allostatic load between positive and negative relationship pathways—among those persons starting out in disadvantageous economic circumstances (0.64 on the negative pathway vs. 0.21 on the positive pathway [TABLE 7])—suggests that the science of interpersonal flourishing and interventions such as emotion coaching[63,64] could have significant influence in maintaining allostasis in mid- and later life.

The relative importance, for later-life health, of economic status over time versus other forms of cumulative psychosocial experience is of considerable interest. We have shown in Table 8 that for any income history that involves some episode of disadvantage, a positive relationship history has a compensating influence in the sense that the individuals with such a history are decidedly less likely to have high allostatic load than individuals with a negative relationship history. On the other hand, individuals with a persistently advantageous income history—the category (+,+) in TABLE 8—have the same probability of being at high allostatic load (0.36), regardless of which relationship pathway they are on. It will be useful to explore this issue on a larger subsample of the WLS population, where the income distribution can be split into quartiles or quintiles while maintaining counts of 40 or more persons in each stratum. In particular, it is conceivable that some mobility among the upper two income quartiles only—or among the upper two quintiles—would define pathways for which the probability of having high allostatic load is still insensitive to the relationship history.

Future research will also have to take account of the fact that what is salient for some individuals may not be their position in an SES hierarchy defined by conventional indicators such as income, years of education, or occupational status. The strong influence of cumulative social relationship histories on allostatic load exemplifies this point. Thus, an important next step in the program of characterizing pathways to predisease indicators, or sustained allostasis, is the specification of more elaborate histories that incorporate information about experience across a greater multiplicity of life domains than household income dynamics and intimate social relationships with parents and a significant other.

More nuanced psychosocial pathways should, in the future, be accompanied by repeated biomarker assessments over time on the same individuals. This would facilitate identification of integrated physiological/psychosocial pathways to both predisease endpoints and, subsequently, to the onset of a broad range of chronic diseases. For pathways where cumulative advantage dominates adversity and where allostasis is maintained into later life, we would have a more sharply focused picture of the factors that promote health and are protective against illness.

The compelling nature of the above program has been pointed out on several occasions in the past by a diverse group of investigators, albeit with some variation in emphases about what does or does not belong in the pathway specifications.[65–67] The limiting factor in advancing the subject has been the dearth of longitudinal birth cohort studies on humans that follow individuals into middle and older ages. Exceptions to this general rule are two birth cohort studies in England[68,69] that have been increasingly utilized to study pathways to diverse health outcomes. However, both data sets are limited by a lack of direct physiological assessments. This situation is changing rapidly with current and future planned assessments designed to remedy the imbalance between an abundance of psychosocial and self-reported health measures and the virtual absence of such important physiological indicators as cortisol and the catecholamines epinephrine and norepinephrine.

In the United States, the Wisconsin Longitudinal Study—utilized here—follows the birth cohort of 1939. However, it was initiated as a random sample of the high school graduating class of 1957 in the state of Wisconsin. Thus, it lacks very early childhood information while remaining an invaluable resource for studying cumulative effects from adolescence through, at the present time, age 60. Our allostatic load analyses were derived from a subsample of this population on whom biomarker assessments were carried out when the respondents were 59 years old.

Returning to the global question of providing explanations for SES–health gradients, it is our position that more elaborate hierarchies of histories should be constructed with birth cohort data including prenatal information at a psychosocial and physiological level. This would form an empirical basis for integrating evidence about the role of the fetal environment on later-life health[2] with data on impact of cumulative adversity and advantage across the life course. In addition, the growing literature on resilience—particularly at older ages[29]—prompts more extensive studies than heretofore with a focus on plasticity and improved functioning with increasing age. Investigations of this kind can serve to identify multiple pathways to disease and disability as well as, in complementary fashion, pathways to flourishing and resilience even in the face of cumulative adversity.

ACKNOWLEDGMENTS

This research was funded by the John D. and Catherine T. MacArthur Foundation Networks on Socioeconomic Status and Health (BS) and Successful Midlife Development (CDR) and National Institute on Aging (NIA) Grant AG13613-01. We have benefited from discussions with Teresa Seeman, based on an earlier draft. Special thanks are due to Robert M. Hauser and Taissa Hauser for facilitating the data collection on which this study is based and for insightful comments on a myriad of design issues. Gayle Love provided invaluable technical assistance.

REFERENCES

1. ARNESON, E. & A. FOREDAHL. 1985. The Tromso Heart Study: coronary risk factors and their association with living conditions during childhood. J. Epidemiol. Commun. Health **39:** 210–214.
2. BARKER, D.J.P. & C. OSMOND. 1986. Infant mortality, childhood nutrition, and ischaemic heart disease in England and Wales. Lancet **I:** 1077–1081.
3. COHEN, S., J.R. KAPLAN & S.B. MANUCK. 1994. Social support and coronary heart disease: underlying psychological and biological mechanisms. *In* Social Support and Cardiovascular Disease. S.A. Shumaker & S.M. Czajkowski, Eds.: 195–221. Plenum Press, New York.
4. HARRIS, J.E. 1989. Social and Economic Causes of Cancer. *In* Pathways to Health. J.P. Bunker, D.S. Gomby & B.H. Kehrer, Eds.: 165–216. The Henry J. Kaiser Family Foundation, Menlo Park, CA.
5. MARMOT, M.G., H. BOSMA, H. HEMINGWAY, E. BRUNNER & S. STANSFIELD. 1997. Contribution of job control and other risk factors to social variations in coronary heart disease incidence. Lancet **350:** 235–239.
6. POWER, C. & S. MATTHEWS. 1998. Accumulation of health risks across social groups in a national longitudinal study. *In* Human Biology and Social Inequality. S.S. Strickland & P.S. Shetty, Eds.: 36–57. Cambridge University Press, Cambridge.
7. SAPOLSKY, R.M. 1994. Why Zebras Don't Get Ulcers: A Guide to Stress, Stress-Related Diseases, and Coping. W.H. Freeman, New York.
8. SEEMAN, T.E. & S.L. SYME. 1987. Social networks and coronary artery disease: a comparative analysis of network structural and support characteristics. Psychosom. Med. **49:** 341–354.
9. SEEMAN, T.E. & B.S. MCEWEN. 1996 Impact of social environment characteristics on neuroendocrine regulation. Psychosom. Med. **58:** 459–471.
10. WILLIAMS, D. & C. COLLINS. 1995. U.S. socioeconomic and racial differences in health: patterns and explanations. Annu. Rev. Sociol. **21:** 349–386.
11. SMITH, J.P. 1999. Healthy bodies and thick wallets: the dual relation between health and economic status. J. Econ. Perspect. **13**(2): 145–166.
12. DEATON, A. 1999. Inequalities in income and inequalities in health. NBER Working Paper 7141. National Bureau of Economic Research, Cambridge, MA.
13. MELLOR, J.M. & J. MILYO. 1999. Income inequality and health status in the United States: evidence from the current population survey. National Bureau of Economic Research, Cambridge, MA.

14. KORENMAN, S. & J.E. MILLER. 1997. Effects of long-term poverty on physical health of children in the National Longitudinal Survey of Youth. *In* Consequences of Growing Up Poor. G.J. Duncan & J. Brooks-Gunn, Eds.: 70–99. Russell Sage Foundation, New York.

15. STARFIELD, B., S. SHAPIRO, J. WEISS, K.Y. LIANG, D. RA, D. PAIGE & X. WANG. 1991. Race, family income, and low birth weight. Am. J. Epidemiol. **134**(10): 1167–1174.

16. MARMOT, M.G., G. DAVEY-SMITH, S. STANSFIELD, C. PATEL, F. NORTH, J. HEAD, I. WHITE, E. BRUNNER & A. FEENEY. 1991. Health inequalities among British civil servants: The Whitehall II Study. Lancet (June 8) **337**: 1387–1393.

17. ECOB, R. & G. DAVEY-SMITH. 1999. Income and health: what is the nature of the relationship? Soc. Sci. Med. **48**: 693–705.

18. MACINTYRE, S. 1997. The black report and beyond: what are the issues? Soc. Sci. Med. **44**(6): 723–746.

19. MACINTYRE, S. 1998. Social inequalities and health in the contemporary world: comparative overview. *In* Human Biology and Social Inequality. S.S. Stricland & P.S. Shetty, Eds.: 20–35. Cambridge University Press, Cambridge.

20. GREENWOOD, M. 1936. English death-rates, past, present and future. A valedictory address. J. R. Stat. Soc. **99**: 674–713.

21. BEN-SHLOMO, Y. & G. DAVEY-SMITH. 1991. Deprivation in infancy or adult life: which is more important for mortality risk? Lancet **337**: 530–534.

22. KUH, D. & G. DAVEY-SMITH. 1993. When is mortality risk determined? Historical insights into a current debate. J. Soc. Hist. Med. 101–123.

23. SINGER, B., C.D. RYFF, D. CARR & W. MAGEE. 1998. Linking life histories and mental health: a person-centered strategy. *In* Sociological Methodology, 1998. A. Raftery, Ed.: 1–51. American Sociological Association, Washington.

24. GARMEZY, N. 1993. Children in poverty: resilience despite risk. Psychiatry **56**: 127–136.

25. GARMEZY, N. 1993. Vulnerability and resilience. *In* Studying Lives Through Time: Personality and Development. D.C. Funder, R.D. Parke, C. Tomlinson-Keaset & K. Widaman, Eds.: 377–399. American Psychological Association, Washington.

26. COLE, J.R. & B. SINGER. 1991. A theory of limited differences: explaining the productivity puzzle in science. *In* The Outer Circle: Women in the Scientific Community. H. Zuckerman, J.R. Cole & J. Bruer, Eds.: 277–340. Norton, New York.

27. MERTON, R.K. 1968. The Matthew effect in science. Science **159**: 59–63.

28. ROSS, C.E. & C.L. WU. 1996. Education, age, and the cumulative advantage in health. J. Health Soc. Behav. **37**: 104–120.

29. RYFF, C.D., B. SINGER, G.D. LOVE & M.J. ESSEX. 1998. Resilience in adulthood and later life. *In* Handbook of Aging and Mental Health: An Integrative Approach. J. Lomranz, Ed.: 69–96. Plenum Press, New York.

30. SINGER, B. & C.D. RYFF. 1997. Racial and ethnic inequalities in health: environmental, psychosocial, and physiological pathways. *In* Intelligence, Genes, and Success: Scientists Respond to the Bell Curve. B. Devlin, S.E. Fienberg, D. Resnick & K. Roeder, Eds.: 89–122. Springer-Verlag, New York.

31. ELDER, G.H., L.K. GEORGE & M.J. SHANAHAN. 1996. Psychosocial stress over the life course. *In* Psychosocial Stress: Perspectives on Structure, Theory, Life Course, and Methods. H. Kaplan, Ed.: 247–291. Academic Press, Orlando.

32. MCEWEN, B.S. & E. STELLAR. 1993. Stress and the individual: mechanisms leading to disease. Arch. Intern. Med. **153**: 2093–2101.

33. MCEWEN, B.S. 1998. Protective and damaging effects of stress mediators. N. Engl. J. Med. **338**(3): 171–179.

34. MCEWEN, B.S. & T. SEEMAN. 1999. Protective and damaging effects of mediators of stress: elaborating and testing the concepts of allostasis and allostatic load. Ann. N.Y. Acad. Sci. **896**: this volume.

35. STERLING, P. & J. EYER. 1988. Allostasis: a new paradigm to explain arousal pathology. *In* Handbook of Life Stress, Cognition, and Health. J. Fisher & J. Reason, Eds.: 629–649. John Wiley and Sons, New York.

36. SEEMAN, T., B. SINGER, B. MCEWEN, R. HORWITZ & J. ROWE. 1997. The price of adaptation: allostatic load and its health consequences—MacArthur studies of successful aging. Arch. Intern. Med. **157:** 2259–2268.
37. SEEMAN, T., B. SINGER, C. WILKINSON & B. MCEWEN. 1999. Exploring a new concept of cumulative biological risk—allostatic load and its health consequences: MacArthur studies of successful aging. In review.
38. CALDJI, C., B. TANNENBAUM, S. SHARMA, D. FRANCIS, P. PLOTSKY & M. MEANEY. 1998. Maternal care during infancy regulates the development of neural systems mediating the expression of fearfulness in the rat. Proc. Nat. Acad. Sci. USA **95:** 5335–5340.
39. CENTER FOR THE ADVANCEMENT OF HEALTH. 1999. To learn about people, ask the animals. facts of life: an issue briefing for health reporters. **4**(6): 1–6.
40. CENTER FOR THE ADVANCEMENT OF HEALTH. 1999. Facts of life: an issue briefing for health reporters **4**(4): 1–6.
41. RYFF, C.D. & B. SINGER. 1999. Interpersonal flourishing: a positive health agenda for the new millennium. Perspect. Soc. Sci. Rev. In press.
42. RUBERMAN, W., E. WEINBLATT & J.D. GOLDBERG. 1984 Psychosocial Influences on mortality after myocardial infarction. N. Engl. J. Med. **311:** 552–559.
43. SPIEGEL, D., J.R. BLOOM & I. YALOM. 1981. Group support for patients with metastatic cancer: A randomized outcome study. Arch. Gen. Psychiatry **38:** 527–533.
44. TAYLOR, S.E., R.L. REPETTI & T. SEEMAN. 1997. Health psychology: what is an unhealthy environment and how does it get under the skin? Annu. Rev. Psychol. **48:** 411–447.
45. SEEMAN, T.E., L.F. BERKMAN, F. KOHOUT, A. LACROIX, R. GLYNN & D. BLAZER. 1993. Intercommunity variation in the association between social ties and mortality in the elderly: a comparative analysis of three communities. Ann. Epidemiol. **3:** 325–335.
46. BURMAN, B. & G. MARGOLIN. 1992. Analysis of the association between marital relationships and health problems: an interactional perspective. Psychol. Bull. **112:** 39–63.
47. RYFF, C.D. & B. SINGER. 1998. The contours of positive human health. psychological inquiry. **9**(1): 1–28.
48. CARTER, C.S. 1998. Neuroendocrine perspectives on social attachment and love. Psychoneuroendocrinology **23**(8): 779–818.
49. KNOX, S.S. & K. UVNAS-MOBERG. 1998. Social isolation and cardiovascular disease: an atherosclerotic pathway? Psychoneuroendocrinology **23**(8): 877–890.
50. MCEWEN, B.S. 1997. Meeting Report—is there a neurobiology of love? Mol. Psychiatry **2:** 15–16.
51. UVNAS-MOBERG, K. 1997. Physiological and endocrine effects of social contact with special reference to oxytocin. In The Integrative Neurobiology of Affiliation. C.S. Carter, I. Lederhendler & B. Kirkpatrick, Eds. Ann. N.Y. Acad. Sci. **807:** 146–163.
52. UVNAS–MOBERG, K. 1998. Oxytocin may mediate the benefits of positive social interaction and emotions. Psychoneuroendocrinology **23**(8): 819–835.
53. HAUSER, R.M., D. CARR, T. HAUSER, J. HAYES, M. KRECKER, D.K. HSIANG-HUI, W. MAGEE, D. PRESTI, D. SHINBERG, M. SWEENEY, T. THOMPSON-COLON, S.C.N. UHRIG & J.R. WARREN. 1993. The class of 1957 after 35 years: overview and preliminary findings. Center for Demography and Ecology Working Paper No. 93-17. University of Wisconsin—Madison.
54. RUSSEK, L.G. & G.E. SCHWARZ. 1997. Feelings of parental caring predict health status in midlife: A 35-year follow-up of the Harvard Mastery of Stress Study. J. Behav. Med. **20**(1): 1–13.
55. PARKER, G., H. TUPLING & L.B. BROWN. 1979. A parental bonding instrument. Br. J. Med. Psychol. **52:** 1–10.
56. SCHAEFER, M.T. & D.H. OLSON. 1981. Assessing intimacy: the PAIR inventory. J. Marital Family Ther. **7:** 47–60.
57. MUNOZ, A. & S.J. GANGE. 1998. Methodological issues for biomarkers and intermediate outcomes in cohort studies. Am. J. Epidemiol. **20**(1): 29–42.

58. COHEN, S. 1988. Psychosocial models of the role of social support in the etiology of physical disease. Health Psychol. **7:** 269–297.
59. COE, C.L. & G.R. LUBACH. 1999. Social context and psychological influences on the development of immunity. *In* Emotion, Social Relationships and Health. C.D. Ryff & B. Singer, Eds.: Oxford University Press, New York. In press.
60. KIECOLT-GLASER, J.K., R. GLASER, J.T. CACIOPPO, R.C. MACCALLUM, M. SNYDER-SMITH, K. CHEONGTAG & W.B. MALARKEY. 1997. Marital conflict in older adults: endocrinological and immunological correlates. Psychosom. Med. **59:** 339–349.
61. KIECOLT-GLASER, J.K., R. GLASER, S. GRAVENSTEIN, W.B. MALARKEY & J. SHERIDAN. 1996. Chronic stress alters the immune response to influenza virus vaccine in older adults. Proc. Nat. Acad. Sci. **93:** 3043–3047.
62. KUNST, A. & J. MACHENBACH. 1994. International variations in the size of mortality differences associated with occupational status. Int. J. Epidemiol. **23:** 742–750.
63. GOTTMAN, J., L.F. KATZ & C. HOOVEN. 1996. Parental meta-emotion philosophy and the emotional life of families: theoretical models and preliminary data. J. Family Psychol. **10:** 243–268.
64. GOTTMAN, J.M. 1999. Meta-emotion, children's emotional intelligence, and buffering children from marital conflict. *In* Emotion, Social Relationships and Health. C.D. Ryff & B. Singer, Eds.: Oxford University Press, New York.
65. KELLY, S., C. HERTZMAN & M. DANIELS. 1997. Searching for the biological pathways between stress and health. 1997. Annu. Rev. Pub. Health **18:** 437–462.
66. REPETTI, R., S.E. TAYLOR & T.E. SEEMAN. 1999. Risky Families: Family Social Environments and the Mental and Physical Health of Offspring. University of California, Los Angeles. In review.
67. ROBERT, S. 1999. Socioeconomic position and health: The independent contribution of community socioeconomic context. Annu. Rev. Sociol. **25:** 489–516.
68. WADSWORTH, M.E.J. & D.J.L. KUH. 1997. Childhood influences on adult health: a review of recent work from the British 1946 National Birth Cohort Study, the MRC National Survey of Health and Development. Ped. Perinat. Epidemiol. **11:** 2–20.
69. POWER, C., O. MANOR & A.J. FOX. 1991. Health and Class: The Early Years. Chapman Hall, London.

Part III Summary: What is the Role of the Social Environment in Understanding Inequalities in Health?

GEORGE A. KAPLAN[a]

Department of Epidemiology, School of Public Health, University of Michigan, 109 S. Observatory St., Ann Arbor, Michigan 48109-2029, USA

That the social environment is inextricably involved in the health of individuals and populations was recognized long ago, extending back beyond the parallel activities in England, France, and Germany during the mid-1800s that led to the beginnings of the public health movement.[1] Despite the important contributions of early urban sociologists,[2,3] for the next century and a half the discussion of the social environment tended to focus on material living conditions such as housing, sanitation, water quality, and so forth. During the last quarter of a century, the discussion of the social environment broadened with John Cassel's paper "The Contribution of the Social Environment to Host Resistance" being a sentinel marker of this change.[4] In this paper, Cassel called upon evidence that linked poorer health to social disorganization of counties, social instability and poverty level of census tracts, levels of family competence, acculturation, and life stress and poor social support. More recent papers have shown that characteristics of the areas in which people live,[5] patterns of social connections,[6] social and economic policies,[7] organization of work,[8] and other aspects of the social environment are associated with important variations in health status. The papers presented in this part of the symposium show that this explosion of interest is alive, well, and exciting.

But what is the social environment? We can relatively easily define the physical environment, whereas a definition of the social environment is elusive. While it may actually not be important to come up with an exact definition, inspection of FIGURE 1, or other similar representations,[9–12] gives some idea of the magnitude of the terrain that is involved when we speak broadly of the social environment. Thus, we can think of social and economic policies setting the context for the development of particular institutions and regulatory systems related to health care, education, public safety, local and regional development, and working conditions. It is important to remember that these social and economic policies are embedded in history and geography and contain cross-currents related to discrimination and culture. The nature of neighborhoods and communities, living conditions, both material and neomaterial, and patterns of social relationships between individuals and groups set in place processes that facilitate or impede the development of individual risk factors, both behavioral and psychosocial, that may feed back on upstream determinants. Thus, in order to understand the day-to-day experience of individuals and groups and

[a]Address for correspondence: 734-764-5435 (voice); 734-764-3192 (fax).
e-mail: gkaplan@umich.edu

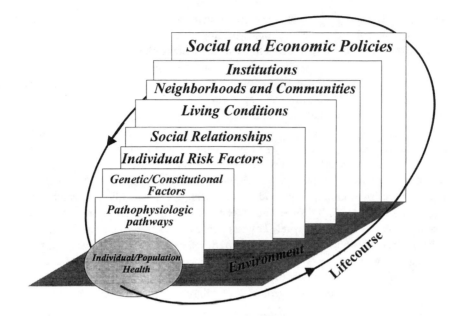

FIGURE 1.

how that translates into better or worse health among the richer and poorer,[13] we will have to consider the social environment from a dynamic, multilevel, and upstream perspective.

How, then, can knowledge concerning the impact of the social environment on health contribute to our understanding of the relationship between socioeconomic status and health? Consideration of FIGURE 1 shows that there will be no easy answers. The contemporary penchant for statistically estimating the "independent" effects of single variables is not likely to be useful when analyzing dynamic, multilevel phenomena with feedback between levels. Furthermore, such techniques may be misleading because they often fall victim to being "prisoners of the proximate."[14–15] That is, they epistemologically privilege causal factors that are more proximate to the disease outcome, whereas consideration of FIGURE 1 would lead to an appreciation of the joint role of multiple factors, across levels—all being potentially involved in the causal explanation of the reasons for socioeconomic gradients in health. It is likely that the most complete understanding of the reasons for socioeconomic gradients in health, the role of the social environment, and what we can do to reduce these gradients will come from efforts to build bridges across the multiple levels shown in FIGURE 1. Such efforts hold the greatest potential for elucidating both the pathways by which economic inequalities in health are generated—the "how"—as well as the determinants of these pathways—the "why."[16]

Within this framework how are we to understand the interesting work presented in this session? First, it is clear that an upstream focus is called for. The authors of the papers examining health outcomes in humans point to the importance of social and economic policies in determining working conditions, the impact of racist ideology and history on the socioeconomic and socioenvironmental disadvantage experienced by African-Americans, and the role of economic forces in eroding social capital and cohesion. Furthermore, in their studies of cynomologus monkeys, Kaplan and Manuck[17] point out an important parallel between nonhuman primates and humans—namely, the contextual nature of the relationship between rank and health. Thus, they posit that the impact of rank, used metaphorically by some as equivalent to social class, will only be felt physiologically where rank is associated with inequities in access to material goods and other resources. Thus, it is not rank *per se* but instead the interaction of rank and the differential distribution of demands and resources by rank that allow individual differences in reactivity to social stress to be expressed physiologically. This expanded view of hierarchy and dominance, which has been way overinterpreted by some researchers studying social inequalities in health, is consistent with a growing recognition among primatologists that social rank may have far less to do with physiology than previously thought. In fact, referring to differences in physiology and stress-related disease, Sapolsky argues "...[how]...little, in fact, rank predicts any of these endpoints" (Ref. 18, p. 39).

Second, we are only beginning to get an understanding of how racial discrimination, high-stress jobs, low social rank, or living in an area with low social capital contributes to differences in the day-to-day experiences of people, and how these experiences influence behavior and biology. As an example—how does income inequality lead to poor health?[19] Is it a marker for underinvestments in human and physical capital? Poorer health care and education? How are they experienced? Does it lead to increased stress or depression with fewer effective coping resources available? Perhaps we need to address the role of the social environment in health inequalities more from the perspectives used by primatologists and anthropologists when they attempt to capture the every-day experience of individuals and groups.

Finally, if aspects of the social environment contribute to socioeconomic gradients in health, we need to ask how the social environment can be changed in order to reduce inequalities. Our lack of knowledge in such areas is variable. In the area of work stress there is a considerable amount known.[20] While the recent Independent Inquiry into Inequalities in Health Report[21] contained many useful suggestions on ways to potentially reduce inequalities in health, detailed suggestions for interventions on the social environment were relatively few. What this underscores is a need for expanded efforts to evaluate the impact on inequalities of health of interventions conducted at all levels shown in FIGURE 1. Some would argue that many of these interventions would be outside the pale of medicine and public health. Surely without such changes it is likely that we may see little reduction in health inequalities. Given the magnitude of the health burden associated with socioeconomic inequalities in health, there is little choice but to mount an interdisciplinary approach, venturing out into an area of intervention where the success is uncertain but the payoff could be dramatic.

REFERENCES

1. ROSEN, G. 1993. A History of Public Health—Expanded Edition. Johns Hopkins University Press, Baltimore.
2. SHAW, C.R. & H.D. MCKAY. 1942. Juvenile Delinquency and Urban Areas: A Study of the Rate of Delinquents in Relation to Differential Characteristics of Local Communities in American Cities. University of Chicago Press, Chicago.
3. FERRIS, R.E.L & H.W. DUNHAM. 1960. Mental Disorders in Urban Areas: An Ecological Study of Schizophrenia and Other Psychoses. 2nd ed. (1st ed., 1939). Hafner Publishing Co., New York.
4. CASSEL, J. 1976. The contribution of the social environment to host resistance: the Fourth Wade Hampton Frost Lecture. Am. J. Epidemiol. **104:** 107–122.
5. KAPLAN, G.A. 1996. People and places: Contrasting perspectives on the association between social class and health. Int. J. Health Serv. **26**(3): 507–519.
6. COHEN, S. & S.L. SYME. 1985. Social Support and Health. Academic Press, New York.
7. KAPLAN, G.A., E. PAMUK, J.W. LYNCH, R.D. COHEN & J.L. BALFOUR. 1996. Inequality in income and mortality in the United States: analysis of mortality and potential pathways. Br. Med. J. **312:** 999–1003.
8. SCHNALL, P.C., P.A. LANDSBERGIS & D. BAKER. 1994. Job strain and cardiovascular disease. Ann. Rev. Pub. Health **15:** 381–411.
9. EVANS, R.G. & G.L. STODDART. 1994. Producing health, consuming health care. *In* Why Are Some People Healthy and Others Not: The Determinants of Health of Populations. R.G. Evans, M.L. Barer & T.R. Marmor, Eds. Aldine de Gruyter, New York.
10. BEAGLEHOLE, R. 1995. Conceptual frameworks for the investigation of mortality from major cardio-vascular diseases. *In* Adult Mortality in Developed Countries: From Description to Explanation. A. Lopez, G. Caselli & T. Valkonen, Eds. Clarendon Press, London.
11. PATRICK, D.L. & T.M. WICKIZER. 1995. Community and Health. *In* Society and Health. B.C. Amick, S. Levine, A.R. Tarlov & D.C. Walsh, Eds. Oxford University Press, New York.
12. KAPLAN, G.A. & J.W. LYNCH. 1999. Socioeconomic considerations in the primordial prevention of cardiovascular disease. Prevent. Med. In press.
13. KAPLAN, G.A. 1995. Where do shared pathways lead: some reflections on a research agenda. Psychosom. Med. **57:** 208–212.
14. MCMICHAEL, A.J. 1999. Prisoners of the proximate: loosening the constraints on epidemiology in an age of change. Am. J. Epidemiol. **149**(10): 887–897.
15. KAPLAN, G.A. 1998. The role of epidemiologists in eradicability of poverty. Lancet **352**(9140): 1627.
16. LYNCH, J.W., G.A. KAPLAN, R.D. COHEN, J. TUOMILEHTO & J.T. SALONEN. 1996. Do cardiovascular risk factors explain the relationship between socioeconomic status, risk of all-cause mortality, cardiovascular mortality and acute myocardial infarction? Am. J. Epidemiol. **144**(10): 934-942.
17. KAPLAN, J.R. & S.B. MANUCK. 1999. Social status, stress, and atherosclerosis: the role of environment and individual behavior. Ann. N.Y. Acad. Sci. **896:** this volume.
18. SAPOLSKY, R.M. 1999. Hormonal correlates of personality and social contexts: from nonhuman to human primates. *In* Hormones, Health and Behavior. C. Panter-Brick & C.M. Worthman, Eds.: 18–46. Cambridge University Press, New York.
19. LYNCH, J.W. & G.A. KAPLAN. 1997. Understanding how inequality in the distribution of income affects health. J. Health Psychol. **2**(3): 297–314.
20. KARASEK, R.A., & T. THEORELL. 1990. Health Work: Stress, Productivity, and Reconstruction of Working Life. Basic Books, New York.
21. ACHESON, D. 1998. Independent Inquiry into Inequalities in Health Report. The Stationery Office, London.

Social Capital and Community Effects on Population and Individual Health

ICHIRO KAWACHI[a]

Department of Health and Social Behavior and the
Harvard Center for Society and Health, Harvard School of Public Health,
Harvard University, Boston, Massachusetts 02115, USA

ABSTRACT: Social capital refers to those features of social relationships—such as levels of interpersonal trust and norms of reciprocity and mutual aid—that facilitate collective action for mutual benefit. Social capital is believed to play an important role in the functioning of community life across a variety of domains, ranging from the prevention of juvenile delinquency and crime, the promotion of successful youth development, and the enhancement of schooling and education to the encouragement of political participation. More recently, researchers have begun to apply the concept to explain variations in health status across geographic localities. In preliminary analyses, the higher the stocks of social capital (as indicated by measures of trust and reciprocity in social surveys), the higher appear to be the health achievement of a given area. Strengthening the social capital within communities may provide an important avenue for reducing socioeconomic disparities in health.

THE "BOWLING ALONE" HYPOTHESIS

Social affiliation and sociability are on the wane in American society. Over the past two to three decades, membership has declined by about 25 to 50% across a broad swath of civic organizations including the PTA, the League of Women Voters, labor unions, and the Red Cross.[1] Perhaps no other metaphor for this trend has captured the public imagination as well as the political scientist Robert Putnam's observation that membership in bowling leagues has plummeted during the past decade, even as individual Americans continue to patronize bowling alleys. Between 1980 and 1993, the total number of bowlers in America increased by 10%, while league bowling dropped by 40%.[2] Although Putnam's claims have been contested,[3,4] new data[5] appear to confirm the overall trend: America's stock of "social capital" has been shrinking for more than a quarter of a century. Time budget studies suggest that Americans are spending less and less time on informal socializing with neighbors, friends, and even family. In a related trend, data from the General Social Surveys conducted in a nationally representative sample since 1972 indicate that the degree to which Americans say they trust each other has declined by roughly a third during the past two and a half decades.[1]

[a]Address for correspondence: Dr. I. Kawachi, Department of Health and Social Behavior, Harvard School of Public Health, 677 Huntington Avenue, Boston, MA 02115. 617-432-0235 (voice); 617-432-3123 (fax).
e-mail: Ichiro.Kawachi@channing.harvard.edu

Should Americans worry about these trends? A growing body of research has pointed to the crucial role that social affiliation and "social capital" play in the functioning of community life across a variety of domains, spanning from (in order of micro- to macro-phenomena): (i) the prevention of juvenile delinquency and crime (e.g., Sampson et al.[6]); (ii) the promotion of successful youth development (e.g., Parcel and Menaghan[7]; Furstenburg and Hughes[8]); (iii) the development of norms of labor market attachment (Wacquant and Wilson[9]; Case and Katz[10]); (iv) the enhancement of schooling and education (e.g., Coleman[11] and Goldin and Katz[12]); (v) the smooth functioning of democracy and political governance (e.g., Putnam[13] and Verba et al.[14]); and (vi) the advancement of economic development (e.g., Fukuyama[15]). Given this lengthy list of benefits claimed for "social capital"—many of which have direct or indirect consequences for the opportunity range available to individuals—it should come as no surprise that health researchers have lately turned to this notion to account for socioeconomic disparities in health outcomes across communities.

Before turning to review the evidence linking "social capital" to health status, some definitions are in order. The term "social capital" has been used to refer to features of social relationships—such as levels of interpersonal trust and norms of reciprocity and mutual aid—that facilitate collective action for mutual benefit.[16] The concept originally grew out of sociology and political science to describe the resources available to individuals through their affiliative behaviors and membership in community networks. In contrast to financial capital, which resides in people's bank accounts, or human capital, which is embodied in individuals' investment in education and job training, social capital inheres in the structure and quality of social relationships between individuals.

By definition, social capital can assume several forms. It may take the form of a moral resource such as levels of interpersonal trust or norms of reciprocity, or it may exist in the form of what Coleman[16] termed "appropriable" social organizations. An example of an appropriable social organization cited by Coleman[16] is the case of a resident's association in an urban housing project that formed initially for the purpose of lobbying builders to fix problems such as leaks and crumbling sidewalks. After the problems were fixed, the organization remained as available social capital to improve the quality of life for residents.

From this brief definition, it is not too farfetched to suggest that social capital might play a role in determining the level of health achievement of individuals and communities. Even apparently trivial differences in the willingness of neighbors to help each other (e.g., through cash loans or labor in kind) might conceivably affect the health of individuals living in deprived communities. An extensive literature in social epidemiology attests to the health benefits of social affiliation.[17] It is by now well established that socially isolated individuals are at increased risk of premature mortality, reduced survival after major illness, and poor mental health.[18] The mechanisms underlying the protective effect of social integration appear to be through access to various forms of social support, for example, instrumental support, emotional support, and the provision of information. But whereas epidemiologists have tended to conceptualize and measure social integration at the individual level, the notion of social capital is properly conceived at the collective level, or as a property of the social structure. What, then, is the evidence that social capital is related to health outcomes?

SOCIAL CAPITAL IN RELATION TO
COMMUNITY AND INDIVIDUAL HEALTH

The evidence linking social capital to health outcomes is still quite sparse, reflecting the relatively recent application of this concept to the realm of population health. Kawachi et al.[19] carried out an ecological analysis linking variations in social capital to mortality rates across the states of the United States. Following the definitions adopted by political scientists[2,13] and economists,[12] indicators of social capital were aggregated to the state level from responses to social surveys. Levels of interpersonal trust, norms of reciprocity, and density of associational membership were obtained from residents in 39 states responding to the General Social Surveys conducted by the National Opinions Research Center between 1986 and 1990. Among other questions, the survey asked about membership in a wide range of civic organizations—church groups, sports groups, hobby groups, fraternal organizations, labor unions and so on. Density of organizational membership (a proxy measure of sociability) varied considerably across states, ranging from a low of 1.2 per capita in Arkansas to 3.5 per capita in North Dakota. In turn, per capita group membership in each state was significantly inversely correlated with age-adjusted, all-cause mortality ($r = -0.49$, $p < 0.0001$). In regression analyses adjusted for household poverty rates, a one unit increment in the average per capita group membership was associated with a lower age-adjusted overall mortality rate of 66.8 deaths per 100,000 population (95% confidence interval: 26.0 to 107.5).[19]

Predictably, the extent to which people participated in civic associations was related to the degree of trust between citizens ($r = 0.65$) as well as expectations about reciprocity and mutual aid (0.54). Trust was assessed in the General Social Surveys by asking respondents whether "most people can be trusted—or you can't be too careful in dealing with people"; and reciprocity by asking whether "most of the time people try to be helpful—or are they mostly looking out for themselves." In turn, the level of mistrust (the proportion of residents in each state agreeing that "most people *can't* be trusted") was strikingly correlated with age-adjusted mortality rates ($r = 0.79$, $p < 0.0001$) (FIG. 1; from Kawachi et al.[19]). In regression models, variations in the level of trust explained 58% of the variance in total mortality across states, including statistically significant associations with most major causes of death including heart disease, malignant neoplasms, stroke, homicide, and infant mortality.

More recently, Kawachi et al.[20] carried out a multilevel study of the relationship between state-level social capital and individual self-rated health. Self-rated health—assessed by the question: "Would you say your overall health is excellent, very good, good, fair, or poor?"—has been found in over two dozen studies to predict subsequent mortality, independent of other medical, behavioral, or psychosocial risk factors.[21] The study was carried out among 167,259 individuals residing in 39 U.S. states, sampled by the Centers for Disease Control's Behavioral Risk Factor Surveillance System (BRFSS). Logistic regression was carried out with the SUDAAN procedure to estimate the odds ratios of fair/poor health (as opposed to excellent/good health). A strength of this particular study was the availability of information on individual-level confounds, including health insurance coverage, smoking status, overweight, as well as sociodemographic characteristics including household income level, educational attainment, and whether the person lived alone.

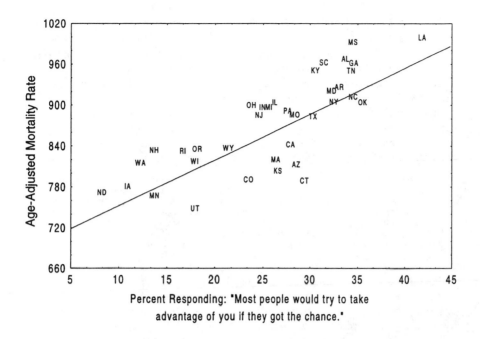

FIGURE 1. Relationship between state-level measure of social trust and age-adjusted total mortality rates (from Kawachi *et al.*[19]; used with permission from the *American Journal of Public Health*).

Predictably, strong associations were found between individual risk factors (e.g., low income, low education, smoking, obesity, lack of access to health care) and poor self-rated health. However, even after adjusting for these proximal variables, individuals residing in states with low social capital were at increased risk of poor self-rated health. For example, the odds ratio for fair/poor health associated with living in areas with the lowest levels of trust was 1.41 (95% confidence interval: 1.33 to 1.50) compared to those living in high-trust states. In other words, the findings were consistent with an apparent contextual effect of state-level social capital on individual well-being, independent of the more proximal predictors of self-rated health.

MECHANISMS LINKING SOCIAL CAPITAL TO HEALTH

Correlation does not prove causation, and the still sparse evidence on the relationship between social capital and health has been limited by the cross-sectional nature of the studies, as well as the lack of adjustment for social integration measured at the individual level. Despite the preliminary nature of the evidence, there are nonetheless sound theoretical reasons to believe that social capital could enhance the health achievement of individuals and communities. The mechanisms underlying this relationship most likely varies according to the level of aggregation at which social capital is conceptualized and measured.

At the *state* level, social capital has been hypothesized to affect health outcomes via political processes.[22] Political scientists have maintained that the degree of political participation by the citizenry depends on the extent to which members are embedded in the institutions of civil society. Social institutions—such as voluntary groups, churches, and labor unions—play a major role in stimulating citizens to take part in politics by cultivating psychological engagement in politics and by serving as the locus of recruitment into political activity. As the political scientist Sidney Verba and colleagues[14] discovered in their path breaking study of political participation:

> Ordinary and routine activity on the job, at church, or in an organization, activity that has nothing to do with politics or public issues, can develop organizational and communications skills that are relevant for politics and thus can facilitate political activity. Organizing a series of meetings at which a new personnel policy is introduced to employees, chairing a large charity benefit, or setting up a food pantry at church are activities that are not in and of themselves political. Yet they foster the development of skills that can be transferred to politics (Verba et al.,[14] p. 17–18).

As citizen participation in voluntary associations wanes, so do the stocks of civic skills that are indispensable for taking part in politics. As corroboration of this hypothesis, the extent of depletion in social capital (measured by levels of mistrust) turn out to be inversely correlated at the state level with measures of political activity, such as voter turnout at elections ($r = -0.46, p < 0.05$).[23]

How does political participation affect health? By mobilizing voters across the socioeconomic spectrum, a higher level of political participation ensures that governments are more responsive in their policies toward taking care of the needs of the most disadvantaged members of society. For example, Hill and Leighley[24] carried out a pooled time series analysis for the 50 U.S. states from 1978 to 1990, examining the relationship between the degree of mobilization of lower class voters at election time and the generosity of welfare benefits provided by state governments. Even after adjusting for other plausible factors that might affect state welfare policy—such as the degree of public liberalism in the state, the federal government's welfare cost-matching rate for individual states, and the state tax effort, the researchers found robust relationships between the extent of political participation by lower class voters and the degree of generosity of state welfare payments. Indeed, policy indicators such as the generosity of welfare benefits have been shown to vary systematically with the stocks of social capital in a state (FIG. 2, from Kawachi and Kennedy[25]). The lower the levels of trust between citizens, the more hostile the social policies geared toward the poor. In other words, who participates in politics matters for political outcomes, and in turn the resulting policies have an important influence on the opportunities available to the poor to lead a healthy life.

Turning to the *neighborhood* level, social capital plausibly affects health outcomes via processes of informal social control, maintenance of healthy norms, and the provision of access to various forms of social support. Evidence from criminology suggests that neighborhoods enriched with stocks of social capital are better able to exert informal control over juvenile delinquency and crime. The mechanism seems to operate through neighbors being willing to monitor activities on street corners and intervene in situations where youths appear to be "up to no good."[26] Extending the argument to the health realm, it is not too much of a leap to suggest that

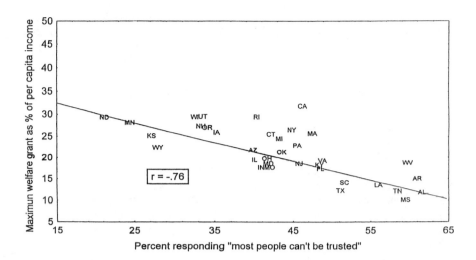

FIGURE 2. Relationship between state-level measure of social trust and maximum welfare grant as a percentage of state per capita income (from Kawachi and Kennedy[25]; used with permission from *Health Services Research*).

neighbors who are willing to help one another might intervene to report instances of "deviant" youth behavior such as drug taking, alcohol abuse, or underage smoking. A recent study of American college campuses suggests that levels of social capital (assessed by the average hours of student voluntarism in the past month) is a powerful protective force against binge drinking and alcohol abuse among students.[27] Where norms of health consciousness exist in the community—such as local action to restrict smoking in restaurants through ordinances—neighborhood social capital might also serve to reinforce healthy behaviors (like refraining from lighting up even in public places that are not covered by such ordinances).

Finally, social capital increases the likelihood of access to various forms of social support during times of need. For example, the ability to borrow money from a neighbor to purchase prescription medicines or to borrow a car to get to the doctor or to arrange child care at short notice depends on (a) levels of trust between neighbors and (b) the expectation that a good deed will be repaid or reciprocated in the future. Such seemingly trivial favors could conceivably make the difference in terms of access to preventive and medical services, especially in deprived neighborhoods. Ultimately, differences in access to social support must translate into individual physiological differences. Research in the fields of psychoneuroimmunology and neuroendocrinology have begun to map out the mediators and mechanisms by which the availability of social support and other environmental conditions might influence individual health (see chapter by McEwen and Seeman[12a] in these proceedings).

Unfortunately, economic disadvantage and lack of social capital often run together.[13] For instance, it is much more difficult for neighbors to trust and provide support for one another when the chances of having a loan repaid are low and the consequences of default are potentially disastrous to the lender. That said, much of the burgeoning interest in social capital lies in the observation that there are substantial variations in the stocks of trust across impoverished communities and the possibility that something can be done to build social capital even in deprived neighborhoods.

SOCIAL CAPITAL AND WIDENING SOCIOECONOMIC DISPARITIES

We return to the mystery posed at the beginning of this article: Why is social capital on the wane in American society? Various suspects have been named including residential mobility and surbubanization, the movement of women into the paid labor force and the time pressures associated with dual-career families, the disruption of marriage and family ties, period effects associated with historical events (Watergate, Vietnam), the growth of the welfare state leading to the "crowding out" of voluntarism and private initiative, and technological changes including the rise of television watching and Internet surfing.[1]

One distal feature of American society that seems to tie together several of these disparate trends is the surge in income inequality that has occurred over the past two decades. Beginning in about 1973, the affluent sections of American society have been pulling sharply away from the middle-class and poor.[28] Between 1977 and 1992, the average after-tax incomes of the top fifth of American families rose by 28%. By contrast, the average incomes of the middle fifth of families remained stagnant over the same 15-year period, ticking up by just 1%. At the bottom, the incomes of poor families actually fell by 17%. Forty percent of American families have lower real income today than in 1977. More recent Census data indicate that the rich have continued to get richer, and the poor poorer, while the middle class is getting squeezed in between. Between 1995 and 1996, the average inflation-adjusted family incomes of the poorest fifth of American families dropped by $210, while those of the top 5% rose by $6,443.[29]

These trends in inequality have forced Americans to spend longer hours at work and to send more family members into the work-force, just to keep from slipping back down the economic ladder. According to one calculation, production and non-supervisory employees, who make up 80% of the American labor force, must now work an extra 245 hours, or 6 extra weeks per year, just in order to keep up with their 1973 standard of living.[30] Spending more time at work translates into less time to devote to socializing and volunteer activities. According to the economist Robert Frank,[31] widening economic disparities have resulted in a growing imbalance in consumption practices. As inequalities widen, and the top earners begin to set new standards in the pattern of conspicuous consumption (e.g., in the form of bigger houses and bigger cars), it forces the rest of society to engage in "defensive spending" to maintain relative status. Earning the extra income to be able to keep up with the rising levels of conspicuous consumption has come at the expense of what Frank calls "inconspicuous" forms of consumption—namely, the forms of consumption that do not raise our relative standing in the social hierarchy, but nonetheless really make a difference to our well-being, such as spending more time with family and friends, or volunteering in community activities.

To give a concrete example, income inequality is a major reason why the average size of the American home has gotten much bigger. The process begins when sharply rising incomes prompt the rich to build bigger homes, contributing to residential mobility and suburban sprawl. In 1970, the average size of a new home was 1,500 square feet, but by 1997, it was 2,150 square feet, even though the average household size in America declined from 3.14 to 2.64 persons over the same period.[32] The affluent have been steadily abandoning metropolitan areas to retreat to suburbs where they have been able to assure decent public schooling for their children, financed out of property taxes, which are in turn linked to real estate prices. Even if those lower on the economic ladder didn't care about living in "trophy" homes, they may be forced nonetheless to work harder and longer hours if their goal is to afford a house in a neighborhood where their children can also get the best education. Unfortunately, if everyone else does the same, at best their relative positions will remain unaffected (since there are only a limited number of positions in the best schools), and at worst they merely succeed in driving up housing prices in that neighborhood. We each end up with a worse bargain than was reckoned with before the transaction was undertaken. Meanwhile, the time that parents spend at work ends up displacing the hours that could have been invested in strengthening social and domestic bonds, whereas residential mobility contributes independently to the erosion of the sense of community. Society as a whole suffers as a result of the neglect of "inconspicuous" consumption.

A growing literature points to the deleterious health consequences of income inequality: the greater the disparity in incomes between the top and bottom, the worse the level of health achievement of that society.[22] Although this effect has been attributed to the harmful social comparisons and psychological perceptions triggered by relative deprivation, at least part of the causal chain linking income inequality to poor health is likely to be mediated by the erosion of sociability, trust, and reciprocity. Indicators of social capital have been declining roughly during the same period that America experienced a sharp rise in income inequality. Looking cross-sectionally across the U.S. states, variations in the stocks of social capital (as measured, for example, by levels of trust) are strikingly correlated with levels of household income inequality ($r = 0.71$, $p = 0.001$).[19]

SOCIAL CAPITAL AND THE REVITALIZATION OF CIVIL SOCIETY

The apparent connection between growing economic inequality and the erosion of social capital hints at the possibility of revitalizing civil society through fixing the "upstream" problem of income maldistribution. The subject is intensely debated, however. A valid criticism of the growing enthusiasm for social capital is that the concept has been used to justify contradictory policy prescriptions.[33] In one view, state–society relations are zero-sum, that is, as the state waxes, civil institutions wane. It has been argued that the welfare state, through the paternalistic provision of a variety of social services, tends to "crowd out" civic voluntarism and norms of mutual care.[15,34] Opposing views regard state–society relations as positive-sum, that is, the state can actively nurture civil society. Skocpol,[35] for one, argues that many of the existing civic associations in America came about as a result of deliberate government intervention and support.

Several commentators[33,36,37] have cautioned against the tendency to portray social capital as an unqualified social good. Without doubt, there are important downsides of social capital, which include the exclusion of "out" groups, the occasionally excessive claims made on members of "in" groups, as well as restrictions on individual liberty and freedom of expression. To the extent that social capital is made available only to members of a closed system, such as residents within "gated" communities, encouraging such forms of capital formation may actually end up reinforcing disparities in health along the dimensions of class and race/ethnicity.

Within economically distressed communities, social capital may paradoxically act as a source of role strain. Contrary to the usual beneficial effects ascribed to social integration, under certain circumstances, social ties may actually impose stressful obligations. LeClere et al.[38] have hypothesized that a high proportion of single female-headed households within a neighborhood may imply a high burden of demands for financial assistance, care giving, and other types of support from surrounding networks of kin and acquaintances. When the material resources of everyone within a neighborhood are taxed to the limit, such obligations may lead to a diminishment of health status on the part of those to whom others turn for support. Minority women in disadvantaged communities may be especially vulnerable to this form of stress, for example, through neglect of self-care and preventive activities. Although we alluded earlier to the role of social capital in promoting norms of healthy behavior, it is also possible that within close-knit neighborhoods, social affiliation might enhance the diffusion of *unhealthy* behaviors, such as cigarette smoking and excessive drinking. Finally, some forms of social capital, such as that provided by membership of criminal gangs, impose negative externalities on the rest of society; that is, they confer the benefits of social affiliation to individual members but contribute little to social cohesion.

Based on the foregoing caveats, it is clear that social capital is not a panacea for addressing social disparities in health. Nevertheless, the concept provides a useful framework for identifying the potential resources available within a community to improve the health of its members. Research on area variations in health have tended to focus exclusively on community stressors, typically measured in terms of the extent of material deprivation (e.g., percent households receiving public assistance, percent unemployment, the proportion of overcrowded housing, and so on). However, the health status of individuals most likely reflects the *balance* of stressors and resources within a given locality. Attention to social capital therefore provides a much needed redirection of focus toward strengthening the assets and resources that already exist even within disadvantaged communities.

Exactly how we should go about building or strengthening social capital still remains to be charted. Few would realistically advocate turning back the clock and exhorting communities to return to an overly idealized Tocquevillian past. Instead, the new sources of social capital are likely to be found in settings where people now spend most of their time, for example, at work. Creative solutions to revitalize Americans' civic commitment will likely involve partnerships with the private sector to encourage more flexible work arrangements, more generous family leave policies, and affordable child care, as well as incentives to enable employees to invest more on the "inconspicuous" forms of consumption that really make a difference to the well-being of our families and communities.

REFERENCES

1. PUTNAM, R.D. 1996. The strange disappearance of civic America. Am. Prospect **24**(Winter): 34–48.
2. PUTNAM, R.D. 1995. Bowling alone. America's declining social capital. J. Democr. **6:** 65–78.
3. WUTHNOW, R. 1998. Loose Connections. Harvard University Press, Cambridge, MA.
4. HALL, J.A. & C. LINDHOLM. 1999. Is America Breaking Apart? Princeton University Press, Princeton.
5. PUTNAM, R.D. 2000. Bowling Alone. Simon & Schuster, New York. In press.
6. SAMPSON, R.J., S.W. RAUDENBUSH & F. EARLS. 1997. Neighborhoods and violent crime: a multilevel study of collective efficacy. Science **277:** 918–924.
7. PARCEL, T. & E. MENAGHAN. 1993. Family social capital and children's behavior problems. Soc. Psychol. Q. **56:** 120–135.
8. FURSTENBURG, F.F. & M.E. HUGHES. 1995. Social capital and successful development among at-risk youth. J. Marriage Family **57:** 580–592.
9. WACQUANT, L.J.D. & W.J. WILSON. 1989. The cost of racial and class exclusion in the inner city. Ann. Am. Acad. Polit. Soc. Sci. **501:** 8–25.
10. CASE, A.C. & L.F. KATZ. 1991. The company you keep: the effects of family and neighborhood on disadvantaged youths. NBER Working Paper No. W3705. National Bureau of Economic Research, Cambridge, MA.
11. COLEMAN, J.S. 1988. Social capital in the creation of human capital. Am. J. Sociol. **94**(Suppl): S95–S120.
12. GOLDIN, C. & L.F. KATZ. 1998. Human capital and social capital: the rise of secondary schooling in American 1910 to 1940. NBER Working Paper No. W6439. National Bureau of Economic Research, Cambridge, MA.
12a. MCEWEN, B.S. & T. SEEMAN. 1999. Protective and damaging effects of mediators of stress: elaborating and testing the concepts of allostasis and allostatic load. Ann. N.Y. Acad. Sci. **896:** this volume.
13. PUTNAM, R.D. 1993. Making Democracy Work. Civic Traditions in Modern Italy. Princeton University Press, Princeton.
14. VERBA, S., K. LEHMAN SCHLOZMAN & H.E. BRADY. 1995. Voice and Equality. Civic Voluntarism in American Politics. Harvard University Press, Cambridge, MA.
15. FUKUYAMA, F. 1995. Trust: The Social Virtues and the Creation of Prosperity. The Free Press, New York.
16. COLEMAN, J.S. 1990. Foundations of Social Theory. Harvard University Press, Cambridge, MA.
17. HOUSE, J.S., K.R. LANDIS & D. UMBERSON. 1988. Social relationships and health. Science **214:** 540–545.
18. BERKMAN, L.F. 1995. The role of social relations in health promotion. Psychosom. Med. **57:** 245–254.
19. KAWACHI, I., B.P. KENNEDY, K. LOCHNER & D. PROTHROW-STITH. 1997. Social capital, income inequality, and mortality. Am. J. Pub. Health **87:** 1491–1498.
20. KAWACHI, I., B.P. KENNEDY & R. GLASS. 1999. Social capital and self-rated health: a contextual analysis. Am. J. Pub. Health. **89:** 1187–1193.
21. IDLER, E.L. & Y. BENYAMINI. 1997. Self-rated health and mortality: a review of twenty-seven community studies. J. Health Soc. Behav. **38:** 21–37.
22. KAWACHI, I., B.P. KENNEDY & R.G. WILKINSON. 1999. Income Inequality and Health: A Reader. The New Press, New York.
23. KAWACHI, I. & B.P. KENNEDY. 1997. Health and social cohesion: why care about income inequality? Br. Med. J. **314:** 1037–1040.
24. HILL, K.Q. & J.E. LEIGHLEY. 1992. The policy consequences of class bias in state electorates. Am. J. Polit. Sci. **36:** 351–363.
25. KAWACHI, I. & B.P. KENNEDY. 1999. Income inequality and health: pathways and mechanisms. Health Serv. Res. **34:** 215–227.
26. SAMPSON, R.J. 1995. The community. In Crime. J.Q. Wilson & J. Petersilia, Eds.: 193–216. Institute for Contemporary Studies, San Francisco.

27. WEITZMAN, E.R. 1999. Giving Is Receiving. The Protective Effect of Social Capital on Binge Drinking on College Campuses. Ph.D. Thesis, Harvard University, Boston.
28. SHAPIRO, I. 1995. Unequal shares: recent income trends among the wealthy. November, 1995. Center on Budget and Policy Priorities, Washington, DC.
29. CENTER ON BUDGET AND POLICY PRIORITIES. 1997. Poverty rate fails to decline as income growth in 1996 favors the affluent. Center on Budget and Policy Priorities, Washington, DC.
30. SCHOR, J.B. 1991. The Overworked American. The Unexpected Decline of Leisure. Basic Books, New York.
31. FRANK, R.H. 1999. Luxury Fever. Why Money Fails to Satisfy in an Era of Excess. The Free Press, New York.
32. COX, W.M. & R. ALM. 1999. Myths of Rich & Poor. Why we're better off than we think. Basic Books, New York.
33. WOOLCOCK, M. 1998. Social capital and economic development: toward a theoretical synthesis and policy framework. Theory Soc. 27: 151–208.
34. MCKNIGHT, J. 1995. The Careless Society. Basic Books, New York.
35. SKOCPOL, T. 1996. Unravelling from above. Am. Prospect 25: 20–25.
36. KAPLAN, G.A. & J.W. LYNCH. 1997. Whither studies on the socioeconomic foundations of population health? Am. J. Pub. Health 87: 1409–1411.
37. PORTES, A. 1998. Social capital: its origins and applications in modern sociology. Annu. Rev. Sociol. 24: 1–24.
38. LeCLERE, F.B., R.G. ROGERS & K. PETERS. 1998. Neighborhood social context and racial differences in women's heart disease mortality. J. Health Soc. Behav. 39: 91–107.

Socioeconomic Status and Chronic Stress

Does Stress Account for SES Effects on Health?

ANDREW BAUM,[a] J.P. GAROFALO, AND ANN MARIE YALI

University of Pittsburgh Cancer Institute, Suite 405,
Iroquois Building, Pittsburgh, Pennsylvania 15213, USA

ABSTRACT: Socioeconomic status (SES) is an important predictor of a range of health and illness outcomes. Research seeking to identify the extent to which this often-reported effect is due to protective benefits of higher SES or to toxic elements of lower social status has not yielded consistent or conclusive findings. A relatively novel hypothesis is that these effects are due to chronic stress that is associated with SES; lower SES is reliably associated with a number of important social and environmental conditions that contribute to chronic stress burden, including crowding, crime, noise pollution, discrimination, and other hazards or stressors. In other words, chronic stress may capture much of the variance in health and social outcomes associated with harmful aspects of lower social status. Low SES is generally associated with distress, prevalence of mental health problems, and with health-impairing behaviors that are also related to stress. Research targeting this hypothesis is needed to determine the extent to which stress is a pathway linking SES and health.

INTRODUCTION

Interest in the effects of socioeconomic status (SES) on health and well-being has waxed and waned over the past several decades, in part because of changing socio-political climates and emphases in behavioral and social sciences. More recently, SES has been cast as a public health factor and its links to disease, health, and life quality have received increasing attention. This research has reaffirmed the importance of this multidimensional variable and has convincingly shown that SES is associated with a variety of health outcomes.[1–9] More broadly, SES appears to influence well-being as well, suggesting possible mechanisms underlying these effects.[10] However, explanations of SES influence have not been comprehensive enough or have otherwise failed to account for the range of observed relationships. Inherent in the construct is the assumption that higher social status affords protective health benefits that are not available to people of lower status. At the same time it can be argued that toxic ingredients of lower SES, that is, the greater danger and stress of lower social status, underlie SES–health relationships. One can concentrate either on hazards associated with lower social status or on special protection afforded upper strata. However, many of the toxic ingredients in the mix of variables that contribute to or are associated with lower SES have not been identified, and the lessons of this important relationship have not been fully learned.

[a]Address for correspondence: 412-624-4800 (voice); 412-647-1936 (fax).
e-mail: baum@pcicirs.pci.pitt.edu

One possible explanation for the health-modulating effects of SES lie in its relationship with chronic stress. Although definitions and operational translations of chronic stress have been variable, chronic stress generally refers to stress that persists "abnormally" or that lasts for a long time, either because it occurs repeatedly or episodically, continuously, or because it poses severe threats that are not easily adapted or overcome. It refers to background or ambient stress due to more-or-less constant stressors embedded in living or working environments and to acute-incident stressors that have effects that persist well beyond the initiating event. Data strongly suggest that this persistent stress is associated with poorer health outcomes. Vulnerability to infectious illness, the extent and intensity of inflammatory and healing processes, and reactivation of latent viruses such as herpes simplex or Esptein-Barr are affected by stress as are heart disease, cancer, and HIV disease.[11–21] Higher chronic stress levels are generally associated with more chronic social and nonsocial burdens or hazards, and one could argue that SES also correlates with the prevalence of these sources of stress. If true, this would suggest that one pathway by which SES affects health and happiness is by establishing a chronic level of burden or stress.

Related to chronic stress, the concept of allostatic load specifies the wear and tear associated with repeated or prolonged activation of stress "systems" in the body, such as the hypothalamic–pituitary–adrenal (HPA) axis or the sympathetic nervous system. Consequently, allostasis and allostatic load refer to physiological activity that initiates and terminates adaptation to a range of threatening stimuli. It is relevant or likely to increase when stressors occur frequently, when inactivation is ineffective, when adaptation cannot be achieved, or when the elasticity of these systems results in slower cessation of response.[22] Chronic stress parallels these constructs to the extent that it is associated with episodic stress or repeated impact of multiple stressors, to persistent stress or ineffective adaptation, or to constitutional barriers to recovery.[23] However, chronic stress extends well beyond the activity of allostatic systems, and the reasons for or effects of chronic activation of these and other bodily systems are not yet clear. Allostasis is a useful representation of an important component of persistent stress and its contribution to the etiology of chronic or acute disease, and it can be considered to be a component of chronic stress representing the cumulative burden posed by activation of neural, neuroendocrine, and immune systems that achieve homeostasis in the face of stressors. It reflects that part of chronic stress associated with dysfunction or wear and tear on the body due to frequent or prolonged activation.[22]

This paper considers the possibility that a substantial portion of SES effects on health and well-being are due to the fact that SES is inversely related to chronic stress and allostatic load. That is, low SES, often together with ethnic background, places people in particular settings that are potentially more stressful or hazardous than the settings that higher SES fosters or promotes. Space does not permit lengthy reviews of the literatures on SES or chronic stress, so we will assume that each is associated with health outcomes. First, we consider some potential mechanisms by which SES may affect these outcomes and then turn our attention to the manner in which they might be associated with stress.

SES AND HEALTH

Research on the pathways linking SES with health and well-being has been hindered by the lack of clear, coherent conceptualizations and operationalizations. Several demographic markers have been used to measure SES and definitions centering on social class, income, education, and other constructs have been proposed. Although these different markers are correlated with one another, they represent only partially overlapping conditions or circumstances and can imply different mechanisms (see TABLE 1). Income-based measures of SES often concentrate on more instrumental advantages of higher SES and may yield different findings than approaches that focus on education, social class, or relative deprivation. For example, people from lower SES groups may experience more distress and poorer health outcomes because they lack the ability to purchase goods or services that reduce stress, minimize sources of stress, or that can be used to prevent or treat illnesses.[24] This kind of effect may be different from effects of SES due to powerlessness, helplessness, or poorer coping skills.[25–27] Further clouding the issue are the mixed results of studies of these various constituents of SES. For example, some studies suggest that occupational social class is the strongest correlate of illness or health, but other studies indicate that income variables are more closely linked to health outcomes.[28–30] Occupational status is also correlated with SES and with stress. Higher income was associated with more happiness and self-confidence, and lower income was linked with greater perceived vulnerability.[31] Another study suggested that occupational status was associated with psychological and physiological symptoms of stress.[32] Job characteristics also appear to mediate SES effects on depression,[33] supporting the argument that stress or its sources and constrained coping are central. Research has also affirmed that education variables predict health outcomes, and these effects have been found to extend beyond those associated with access to higher social status or income.[34] The only conclusion one can reach is that all of these variables are associated with health and that together they explain SES effects on health. Alternatively, these conditions cause people to live in more stressful, hazardous environments and subject them to social and fiscal privations. This leaves the SES construct as a general variable that includes loosely associated conditions that individually affect health and well-being or that are correlated with other conditions that are stressful.

TABLE 1. Factors that may account for SES effects on health[a]

Factors	Presumed Mechanisms
Sociodemographic	Relative deprivation, instrumental benefits, privation
Ethnicity	Discrimination, relative deprivation, access to health care
Access to medical care	Quality of health care
Environment (residential)	Exposure to hazards, limited coping
Diet and nutrition	Quality of nutrition
Occupational status	Role mismatches, underemployment

[a]All of these factors are associated independently with SES and health and well-being.

Ethnicity

Ethnicity or minority status is closely related to these sociodemographic variables that constitute common measures of SES, and one can argue that social conditions such as discrimination and prejudice typically linked to minority status may come to be associated with lower SES groups as well. Minorities in this country are more likely to be lower SES than are whites.[35] At the same time, minorities have higher morbidity and mortality than do whites.[36] Higher Mexican-American, Native American, and African-American mortality rates have been attributed to the socioeconomic disadvantages these populations typically encounter.[35] However, differences between whites and African-Americans are present across SES levels and mortality rates remain higher among African-Americans even after controlling for education.[36] Data also suggest that the disparity between minorities and whites may be magnified by SES; differences in mortality are greater at lower SES levels.[36]

Access to Medical Care

Another mechanism hypothesized to account for the disparity in morbidity and mortality among social classes is access to medical care. People who do not have health insurance are not receiving the care they may require, because they generally report fewer ambulatory care visits each year compared to those with health insurance.[11] Inadequate access is also associated with the use of emergency rooms rather than establishing a relationship with an outpatient clinic, thereby resulting in a lack of continuity and inadequate care.[38] It is possible that the accessibility and frequency of medical visits to outpatient clinics accounts for delayed detection/diagnosis of diseases and the higher incidence of advanced stage detection among lower SES groups. People with adequate health care coverage may routinely engage in appropriate surveillance activities, whereas those with health coverage may neglect these activities. There are data that suggest that the inadequate access to health care reported by lower social classes is an important risk factor for poor health, but that like education, income, or social class, access to health care does not fully account for these disparities across SES gradients. Even when health insurance is present, people with lower incomes tend to report poorer health outcomes. For example, Adler *et al.*[3] found that differences in health by social position or SES hold up in countries with universal health coverage.

Residential Environment

An important but understudied aspect of SES is the residential environment and the extent to which it exposes people to hazards such as crime, drug use, or access to health care. Generally, lower SES is associated with greater limits on choices about where one will live, leading to overrepresentation of lower SES people in these more impoverished settings.[4] At the same time, environments in which lower SES groups live are associated with greater mortality, independent of effects of SES.[7] Several studies show correlations between SES and the frequency of environmental exposures to social or nonsocial hazards.[6,37] The association of residential environment with all-cause mortality was significant even after controlling for age, race, sex, initial health status, SES, and other variables often tied to SES.[6] A study of community-level SES and individual-level health found that individual participants' health was related to the SES characteristics of the community, controlling for income and educational level.[38]

Health Behaviors

Another approach has been to look at health behaviors. There are a number of behaviors, like tobacco use, diet, exercise, and alcohol use, that appear to have large effects on health and illness. Research suggests that many of these behaviors vary across social strata. For example, studies found that those who attend college are more likely to avoid smoking, report less obesity, are more likely to use seat belts, and exercise more than those who have not graduated from high school.[41,42] Taira *et al.*[43] found a similar pattern across income level for the aforementioned variables. Ford *et al.*[44] observed qualitative and quantitative differences in physical activity among men and women that appeared to be moderated by the SES of the individual. Higher SES women spent more time in leisure-time physical activity, job-related physical activity, and household physical activity than did lower SES women, and higher SES men reported more leisure physical activity than did lower SES men. These differences in activities and behaviors that have clear effects on health may also account for the effects of SES.

Diet and nutrition also vary by SES and appear to contribute to health and well-being.[45] First, low income may restrict households from buying essential foods that meet daily nutritional needs. Lack of access to private transportation may also interfere with access to groceries, particularly in areas where local markets have moved away or closed. Inadequate nutrition poses a risk factor for many health problems across the life span that also account for some of the health effects of SES.

Researchers have also examined alcohol and drug use across SES. For example, less educated and poorer families consumed alcohol more frequently than more advantaged families.[46] Higher alcohol consumption has also been observed among men in lower educational groups.[47] In terms of meeting actual clinical substance disorder criteria, Dohrenwend *et al.*[48] found a negative association between SES and substance use disorders where more disorders were found in low social gradients. Recent studies have reported contradictory results. For example, Wohlfarth and Van Den Brink[49] found a positive association between SES and substance abuse disorders in which people in higher social gradients report greater abuse.

Psychological Factors

Several psychological aspects of SES have been proposed as mechanisms underlying SES effects on health, and several appear to be important parts of this relationship. However, many of these factors are products of environmental exposures associated with lower or higher SES, such as learned helplessness, a sense of powerlessness, or an orientation towards mastery and efficacy,[23,50,51] or are related to opportunities for coping or stressful exposure.[54,55] Data suggest, for example, that lower SES is related to more frequent life events and more reported distress.[55,56] Because these variables do not explain the effects of SES alone, it is possible that the greater exposure to stressors associated with lower SES causes people to experience greater vulnerability to individual stressors.[4] For the most part research has considered other psychological variables (such as depression) that are typically considered to be outcomes but that could predispose or mediate some SES–health relationships.

Summary

These data suggest that a number of variables moderate the relationships between SES and health outcomes, including the enabling effects of higher SES, ethnicity, access to medical care, residential environments, health behaviors, and psychological processes. None of these variables appears to explain all of the variance in health outcomes, and one could argue that the direction of this effect is actually the reverse of the common view, that health determines social position and that the disparities in mortality and disparity among social classes is a product of drift down the social hierarchy.[57,58] In other words, poor health causes people to earn less, complete less education, or otherwise achieve lower social status. This downward drift would be perpetuated by illnesses, lost productivity, and social mobility. Despite the support found for this argument in studies of schizophrenia, it does not account for the disparities in overall health among different SES populations.[10] Despite the evolutionary appeal of this perspective, data do not bear it out, and we are left continuing to search for the protective elements of privileged life and the toxic effect of privation.

STRESS AND SES

The finding that community-level SES predicted individual health above and beyond the effects of education and income suggests a broader environmental context for SES effects on health and well-being. Does varying SES correlate with environmental variation such that lower SES groups find themselves living in harsher environments? Environmental conditions and the opportunities they afford are powerful determinants of behavior and likely influenced the evolution of our species.[59] One way in which environments affect people is the extent to which they engender and support chronic stress. Just as the environments that our ancestors occupied posed certain hazards and threats while affording specific opportunities for survival, our environments pose sources of stress and permit only some solutions or coping. As suggested earlier, a strong connection between SES and the nature of one's neighborhood or community is likely. Lower SES is likely to be correlated with settings with higher population density, noise, crime, pollution, discrimination, poor access to resources, and with hazards or privations. Limited income, education, and/or lower social class may cause people to live in poorer, stressful settings or may perpetuate their living in such areas. Higher SES communities appear to have fewer hazards or privations, more support, and to be able to afford more options for coping with problems that do occur.

This notion is similar to the theory proposed by Anderson, McNeily, and Myers[5] to explain the relationship between stress reactivity and hypertension in African-Americans. The environmental context in which many or most African-Americans lived was disproportionately likely to be characterized by lower SES and by more of the hazards we have already described. The basis of the model reflected the belief that ethnic minorities are more frequently exposed to life stressors than are others. These stressors would include prejudice, racism, discrimination, unemployment, low income, underemployment, and environments marked by higher crime rates, residential crowding, and poorer living conditions.[35,60] These socioecological stressors appear to correlate strongly with some health outcomes, suggesting that as characteristics of one's environment worsen, so does one's health. For example, Harburg *et al.*[61] observed high blood pressure among African-Americans living in low-SES neighborhoods characterized by high crime and divorce rates compared to blacks living in low-SES but more stable environments. Interestingly, socioecological stressors were not significantly related to blood pressure among whites, suggesting that African-Americans encounter more stressors than whites and may consequently be more susceptible to the health-impairing effects of these social and environmental stressors.

Although minority status is not exclusively related to lower SES, the largest groups of minority citizens in the United States are found in lower SES brackets: about half of African-Americans are classified as lower SES, while membership in upper SES brackets is much smaller (10%).[62] The brackets for poverty include a lower percentage of whites (25%) and a larger percentage is in the upper brackets.[62] Poverty among African-Americans is approximately 32% compared to 11% for other Americans.[63] Older African-American women are also disproportionately represented among underinsured Americans, thereby, hindering their access to important health-promoting services (e.g., screening, diagnosis, and treatment).[64] Kessler and Neighbors[65] found that African-Americans with low SES reported more stress in their lives than did whites with low SES. They also had more stress than upper income blacks. Although they had a higher incidence of negative life events (e.g., marital difficulty, deaths in family, and divorce) and were more likely to compose the lower class group, African-Americans were not more depressed than whites.[64] As income increased in a sample of 661 white and 114 black adults, psychological distress decreased, and this was especially true for African-Americans. However, there was no significant difference in distress between whites and blacks among the lower social classes.[67]

The hazard or sources of stress that are posed by the environments in which low-SES groups typically live and the constraint of coping and adjustment these settings impose derive from several conditions. Features of the home environment are an important source of stressors and constraint. Residential density and crowding, inadequate housing, poor sanitation, noise, and fear of crime are all more characteristic of lower SES environments and are potential stressors. Data suggest that more impoverished communities were perceived as the most hazardous (more drive-by shootings, violent crime, property damage, gangs, drug use, graffiti, and police brutality) and threatening.[68] Further, the more threatening a neighborhood was perceived to be the more common the symptoms of depression, anxiety, and conduct disorder.[69] The quality of one's home life can also be affected; financial problems or economic stress can affect marital quality and distress among children,[70] and there is some evidence that domestic violence is more common in lower than in middle or upper SES brackets.[71–73]

The point of this discussion is that SES may exert some of its effects by increasing the likelihood of exposure to stressors that are due to minority status or to living in more hazardous environments. In other words, SES is correlated with exposure to stressful environments and conditions that contribute to chronic stress, which in turn affects health. Low-SES environments may augment the likelihood of encountering stressors that tax the individual in the absence of an adequate support system that would optimally alleviate this stress burden; health consequences may be extensive.[74] At the same time, SES and the environmental conditions associated with SES may limit the range of options that are feasible or likely to address the stressor successfully. This model would suggest that SES effects on health are mediated by stress (see FIG. 1), but is there any evidence that low SES is associated with more stress or high SES with less stress or fewer burdens?

The evidence for this hypothesis is circumstantial, and what direct evidence there is suggests that stress does not account for SES effects. However, these studies are limited in their approaches to operationalizing and/or defining stress. There are reasons to suspect that stress may be involved in more complex relationships. Lower

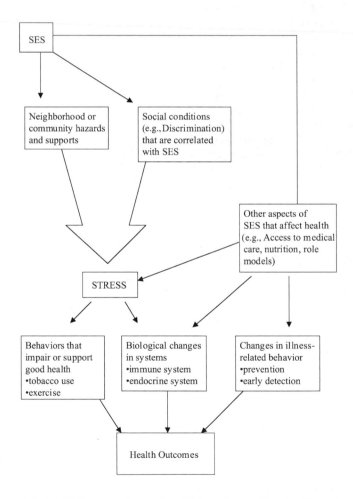

FIGURE 1. Model for the pathways by which SES may affect health.

family income has been associated with more difficult experiences and psychological distress, including feelings of hopelessness, depression, and life dissatisfaction.[75] Social status is associated with the frequency of stressful life events and with emotional responses during stress.[55,76–78] Depression, mental health problems, and other indices of distress are more common in lower SES groups than in middle or upper SES groups.[66,79–81] It is possible that poorer mental health is responsible for lower SES, but data suggest that SES is more likely to be antecedent to distress. A longitudinal study spanning 17 years indicated that incomes below the poverty level were associated with an increased likelihood of difficulties with activities of daily living, even after controlling for age, sex, and health behaviors.[82] In addition, those who had three episodes of economic hardship over the course of the study were at greater risk for depression and were more likely to be cynically hostile, lack optimism about their future, and report more cognitive difficulties.[82]

Similar findings were reported from a study of 877 depressed patients in Italy. In this sample, the diagnosis of bipolarity was more frequent in lower social classes than in higher classes.[83] Diagnoses of anxiety/somatization, loss of weight, impairment at work, somatic anxiety, and hypochondriasis were more common in lower SES groups while "feelings of guilt," depersonalization, and obsessional/compulsive symptoms and cognitive disturbance were more common among higher SES groups. Cumulative exposure to chronic stress should be higher in an environment characterized by more hazards and fewer resources, suggesting that lower SES and minority populations in this country experience more stress.

The similarity of stress effects on health behaviors and health outcomes to those associated with SES also suggest that a significant portion of SES effects may be due to chronic stress levels. Constrained diet and nutrition, increased tobacco use, alcohol use, drug use, and violence are behavioral components of the stress–health relationship,[84] and these factors appear to show similar patterns when stress is high or SES is low. Lower SES populations and African Americans appear to be affected by chronic stress derived from several sources including residential settings, racial discrimination, poverty, and economic constraints.[85]

There are no data that definitively indicate whether lower SES environments are more stressful than higher SES settings or whether differences in chronic stress or vulnerability to chronic stress are responsible for SES effects.[75] However, the associations implied or directly inferred in this model are consistent with prevailing stress theory, and circumstantial evidence suggests that most or all of the effects or proposed mechanisms of SES influence on health and well-being are potentially attributable to stress. The characteristic features of lower SES, including lower social class, income, education, or occupational status are widely thought to be associated with more stress; and one reason for this may be that the conditions associated with lower SES environments are stressful. In addition, stress affects behaviors or conditions hypothesized as mechanisms for SES—health behaviors, including tobacco, alcohol, and drug use, poorer diet, less exercise, and poorer utilization/adherence regarding health care are all affected by stress. Whether these relationships hold up over time and the extent to which these associations explain SES effects on health and well-being must await further research.

Another source of circumstantial evidence of chronic stress mediation of SES–health relationships is the literature on physiological changes that are associated with stress and SES independently. Most of these data are for hypertension and blood pressure, and the many factors governing these outcomes make it difficult to draw firm conclusions. Higher SES is associated with lower blood pressure and less hypertension, and lower SES is associated with higher blood pressure and more hypertension.[86,87] Lower levels of education were linked with higher blood pressure and poorer lipid profiles in a study of risk factors for heart disease in women.[88] Other studies have found evidence of SES modulation of biological risk for illness, and in most cases, the outcomes associated with lower SES are also associated with stress.[4] The complexity of the processes underlying these bodily states places strong limits on appropriate interpretation of these findings, and more work on such linkages is needed.

CONCLUSIONS

We are proposing that the sum total of stressors experienced contribute to persistent, background stress that characterizes people's daily lives and affects how people respond to new stressors or how quickly adaptation is achieved. In other words, all of the stressors that are routinely experienced, including things like commuting to work, problems with a difficult neighbor, discrimination, crime, noise, persistent occupational stressors, and other stressors add to this background and form the context for experiencing and responding to less common life events or changes. Many of the conditions associated with lower SES probably contribute directly to this background stress, suggesting that low SES is associated with greater chronic stress. Because chronic stress has a number of direct and indirect effects on health and well-being, stress associated with life circumstances characteristic of residents of lower SES environments may account for some of its consequences and determine how these residents respond to changes in health (e.g., seeking medical care). Chronic stress appears greater among those in a lower social position, and response to stressors also seems to be different than among people with higher social status. The relationships among the many stressors associated with low SES and health outcomes suggest that excess chronic stress burden may interfere with health maintenance, affect response to acute stressors, and influence survival and well being.

We have noted that this model is speculative and supported by covariation more than anything else. The association between SES and stress is intuitively appealing, is supported by available data, and could logically account for many of the outcomes associated with SES. The likelihood that chronic stress affects reactions to new stressors is also appealing but is very complex and requires further study. The extent to which chronic stress is ongoing, resolved, episodic, or similar to new stressors appears to affect its impact on stress reactivity.[89,90] Further, the likelihood that chronic stress affects psychophysiological vulnerability to new stressors has been suggested but remains key to understanding the role played by stress in SES–health relationships. More work, particularly prospective assessments on ongoing and more isolated stressors as well as reactions to them, is needed.

REFERENCES

1. ADLER, N.E. 1995. Socioeconomic status and health: do we know what explains the association? Advances **11**(3): 6–9.
2. ADLER, N.E. *et al.* 1993. Socioeconomic inequities in health: no easy solution. JAMA **269:** 3140–3145.
3. ADLER, N.E. *et al.* 1994. Socioeconomic status and health: the challenge of the gradient. Am. Psychol. **49**(1): 15–24.
4. ANDERSON, N.B. & C.A. ARMSTEAD. 1995. Toward understanding the association of socioeconomic status and health: a new challenge for the biopsychosocial approach. Psychosom. Med. **57**(3): 213–225.
5. ANDERSON, N.B., M. MCNEILLY & H.F. MYERS. 1993. A biopsychosocial model of race differences in vascular reactivity. *In* Cardiovascular Reactivity to Psychological Stress and Disease. APA Science Volumes. J.J. Blascovich, E.S. Katkin, *et al.*, Eds.: 83–108. American Psychological Association, Washington, DC.
6. HAAN, M., G.A. KAPLAN & T. CAMACHO. 1987. Poverty and health. Prospective evidence from the Alameda County Study. Am. J. Epidemiol. **125**(6): 989–998.
7. HAAN, M., G.A. KAPLAN & S.L. SYME. 1989. Socioeconomic status and health: old observations and new thoughts. *In* Pathways to Health: The Role of Social Factors. J. Bunker, D. Gomby & B. Kehrer, Eds. Henry H. Kaiser Family Foundation, Menlo Park.
8. KOCHANEK, K.D., J.D. MAURER & H.M. ROSENBERG. 1994. Why did black life expectancy decline from 1984 through 1989 in the United States? Am. J. Pub. Health **84:** 938–944.
9. MARMOT, M.G. *et al.* 1998. Contribution of psychosocial factors to socioeconomic differences in health. Milbank Q. **76**(3): 403–448.
10. MARMOT, M.G. *et al.* 1997. Social inequalities in health: next questions and converging evidence. Soc. Sci. Med. **44**(6): 901–910.
11. KAPLAN, G.A. & J.E. KEIL. 1993. Special report: socioeconomic factors and cardiovascular disease: a review of the literature. Circulation **88**(4): 1973–1998.
12. ANDERSEN, B.L., J.K. KIECOLT-GLASER & R. GLASER. 1994. A biobehavioral model of cancer stress and disease course. Am. Psychol. **49**(5): 389–404.
13. BAUM, A. 1990. Stress, intrusive imagery, and chronic distress. Health Psychol. **9:** 653–675.
14. COHEN, S. *et al.* 1998. Types of stressors that increase susceptibility to the common cold in healthy adults. Health Psychol. **17:** 214–233.
15. COHEN, S., D.A. TYRRELL & A.P. SMITH. 1991. Psychological stress and susceptibility to the common cold. N. Engl. J. Med. **325**(9): 606–612.
16. COHEN, S. & G.M. WILLIAMSON. 1991. Stress and infectious disease in humans. Psychol. Bul. **109:** 5–24.
17. GLASER, R. *et al.* 1994. Plasma cortisol levels and reactivation of latent Epstein-Barr virus in response to examination stress. Psychoneuroendocrinology **19**(8): 765–772.
18. KIECOLT-GLASER, J.K. *et al.* 1998. Psychological influences on surgical recovery: perspectives from psychoneuroimmunology. Am. Psychol. **53:** 1209–1218.
19. MARUCHA, P.T., J.K. KIECOLT-GLASER & M. FAVAGEHI. 1998. Mucosal wound healing is impaired by examination stress. Psychosom. Med. **60:** 362–365.
20. MCKINNON, W. *et al.* 1989. Chronic stress, leukocyte subpopulations, and humoral response to latent viruses. Health Psychol. **8:** 389–402.
21. O'LEARY, A. 1990. Stress, emotion, and human immune function. Psychol. Bul. **108**(3): 363–382.
22. LAZARUS, R.S. & S. FOLKMAN. 1984. Stress, Appraisal, and Coping. Springer, New York.
23. BRESNAHAN, J.L. & W.L. BLUM. 1971. Chaotic reinforcement: a socioeconomic leveler. Dev. Psychol. **4**(1): 89–92.
24. RAHKONEN, O., E. LAHELMA & M. HUUHKA. 1997. Past or present? Childhood living conditions and current socioeconomic status as determinants of adult health. Soc. Sci. Med. **44:** 327–336.

25. VAN DE MHEEN, H. *et al.* 1997. The contribution of childhood environment to the exploration of socioeconomic inequalities in health in adult life. Soc. Sci. Med. **44:** 12–24.

26. HAY, D.I. 1988. Socioeconomic status and health status: a study of males in the Canada Health Survey. Soc. Sci. Med. **27**(12): 1317–1325.

27. LANTZ, P.M. *et al.* 1998. Socioeconomic factors, health behaviors, and mortality: results from a nationally representative prospective study of U.S. adults. JAMA **279**(21): 1703–1708.

28. SMITH, G.D. & C. HART. 1998. Socioeconmic factors, health behaviors, and mortality: results from a nationally representative prospective study of US adults. JAMA **280**(20): 1744–1745.

29. ADELMANN, P.K. 1987. Occupational complexity, control, and personal income: their relationship to psychological well-being in men and women. J. Appl. Soc. Psychol. **72:** 529–537.

30. ULBRICH, P.M., G.J. WARHEIT & R.S. ZIMMERMAN. 1989. Race, socioeconomic status, and psychological distress: an examination of differential vulnerability. J. Health Soc. Behav. **30**(1): 131–146.

31. LINK, B.G., M.C. LENNON & B.P. DOHRENWEND. 1993. Socioeconomic status and depression: the role of occupations involving direction, control, and planning. Am. J. Sociol. **98:** 1351–1387.

32. REYNOLDS, J.R. & C.E. ROSS. 1998. Social stratification and health: education's benefit beyond economic status and social origins. Soc. Problems **45**(2): 221–247.

33. JAYNES, G.D. & R.M. WILLIAMS. 1989. A Common Destiny: Blacks and American society. National Academy Press, Washington, DC.

34. PAPPAS, G. *et al.* 1993. The increasing disparity in mortality between socioeconomic groups in the United States, 1960 and 1986. N. Engl. J. Med. **329**(2): 103–109.

35. ROGERS, R.G. *et al.* 1996. Demographic, socioeconomic, and behavioral factors affecting ethnic mortality by cause. Soc. Forces **74**(4): 1419–1438.

36. FLACK, J.M. *et al.* 1995. Panel I: epidemiology of minority health. Health Psychol. **14**(7): 592–600.

37. KRIEGER, N. 1991. Racial and gender discrimination: risk factors for high blood pressure? Soc. Sci. Med. **7:** 1273–1281.

38. ROBERTS, S.A. 1998. Community-level socioeconomic status effects on adult health. J. Health Soc. Behav. **39**(1): 18–37.

39. HOFER, T.P. & S.J. KATZ. 1996. Health behaviors among women in the United States and Ontario: the use of preventive care. Am. J. Pub. Health **86:** 1755–1759.

40. ROSS, C.E. & C. WU. 1995. The links between education and health. Am. Soc. Rev. **60**(5): 719–745.

41. TAIRA, D.A. *et al.* 1997. The relationship between patient income and physician discussion of health risk. JAMA **278:** 1412–1417.

42. FORD, E.S. *et al.* 1991. Physical activity behaviors in lower and higher socioeconomic status populations. Am. J. Epidemiol. **133**(12): 1246–1256.

43. PHILIP, W. *et al.* 1997. Socioeconomic determinants of health: the contribution of nutrition to inequalities in health. Br. Med. J. **314**(7093): 1545–1549.

44. DUNCAN, T.E., S.C. DUNCAN & H. HOPS. 1998. Latent variable modeling of longitudinal and multilevel alcohol use data. J. Stud. Alcohol **59**(4): 399–408.

45. VAN OERS, J.A.M. *et al.* 1999. Alcohol consumption, alcohol-related problems, problem- drinking, and socioeconomic status. Alcohol Alcoholism **34**(1): 78–88.

46. DOHRENWEND, B.P. & B.S. DOHRENWEND. 1974. Social and cultural influences on psychopathology. Annu. Rev. Psychol. **25:** 417–452.

47. WOHLFARTH, T. & W. VAN DEN BRINK. 1998. Social class and substance use disorders: the value of social class as distinct from socioeconomic status. Soc. Sci. Med. **47**(1): 51–58.

48. SELIGMAN, M.E.P. 1975. Helplessness: On Depression, Development, and Death. W.H. Freeman & Co. San Francisco.

49. UMBERSON, D. 1993. Sociodemographic position, world views, and psychological distress. Soc. Sci. Q. **74:** 575–589.

50. BILLINGS, A. & R.H. MOOS. 1981. The role of coping responses and social resources in attenuating the stress of life events. J. Behav. Med. **4:** 157–189.
51. MCGOWN, A. & G. FRASER. 1995. The effect of sociodemographic variables on the use of active and avoidance coping strategies. Psychol. Stud. **40:** 157–169.
52. SCHUSSLER, G. 1992. Coping strategies and individual meanings of illness. Soc. Sci. Med. **34:** 427–432.
53. MCLEOD, J.D. & R.C. KESSLER. 1990. Socioeconomic status differences in vulnerability to undesirable life events. J. Health Soc. Behav. **31:** 162–172.
54. KESSLER, R.C. 1979. Stress, social status and psychological distress. J. Health Soc. Behav. **20:** 259–273.
55. FREEMAN, H. 1994. Schizophrenia and city residence. Br. J. Psychiatry **164**(Suppl. 23): 39–50.
56. MUNK-JORGENSEN, P. & P.B. MORTENSEN. 1992. Soc. Psychiat. Epidem. **27**(3): 129–134.
57. DIAMOND, J.M. 1998. Guns, Germs, and Steel: The Fates of Human Societies. W.W. Norton & Co. New York.
58. WILSON, W. 1993. The Ghetto Underclass: Social Science Perspectives. Sage Publications, Newbury Park, CA.
59. HARBURG, E. *et al.* 1973. Socioecological stress, suppressed hostility, skin color and black–white male blood pressure: Detroit. Psychosom. Med. **35:** 276–296.
60. DANA, R.H. 1993. Multicultural Assessment Perspectives for Professional Psychology. Simon & Schuster, Boston.
61. NATIONAL CENTER FOR HEALTH STATISTICS. 1993. Health, United States, 1992. Public Health Service, Hyattsville, MD.
62. FORTE, D.A. 1995. Community-based breast cancer intervention program for older African American women in beauty salons. Pub. Health Rep. **110**(2): 179–183.
63. KESSLER, R.C. & H.W. NEIGHBORS. 1986. A new perspective on the relationships among race, social class, and psychological distress. J. Health Soc. Behav. **27:** 107–115.
64. STEELE, R.E. 1978. Relationship of race, sex, social class, and social mobility to depression in normal adults. J. Soc. Psychol. **104:** 37–47.
65. COCKERHAM, W.C. 1990. A test of the relationship between race, socioeconomic status, and psychological distress. Soc. Sci. Med. **31:** 1321–1326.
66. HOUSLEY, K. *et al.* 1987. Self-esteem of adolescent females as related to race, economic status, and area of residence. Percept. Motor Skills **64:** 559–566.
67. ANESHENSEL, C.S. & C.A. SUCOFF. 1996. The neighborhood context of adolescent mental health. J. Health Soc. Behav. **37:** 293–310.
68. GE, X. *et al.* 1992. Linking family economic hardship to adolescent distress. J. Res. Adol. **2:** 351–378.
69. KANTOR, G.K. & M.A. STRAUS. 1990. The drunken bum theory of wife beating. *In* Physical Violence in American Families. M.A. Straus & R.J. Gelles, Eds. Transaction, New Brunswick, NJ.
70. TRICKETT, P.K. *et al.* 1991. Relationship of socioeconomic status to the etiology and developmental sequelae of physical child abuse. Dev. Psychol. **27:** 148–158.
71. MCCLOSKEY, L.A. 1996. Socioeconomic and coercive power within the family. Gender Soc. **10:** 449–463.
72. PINCUS, T. & L. CALLAHAN. 1995. What explains the association between socioeconomic status and health: primarily access to medical care or mind–body variables? Advances **11**(1): 4–36.
73. FISCELLA, K. & P. FRANKS. 1997. Does psychological distress contribute to racial and socioeconomic disparities in mortality. Soc. Sci. Med. **45**(12): 1805–1809.
74. KESSLER, R.C. & P.D. CLEARY. 1980. Social class and psychological distress. Am. Soc. Rev. **45:** 463–478.
75. TURNER, R.J. & S. NOH. 1988. Physical disability and depression: a longitudinal analysis. J. Health Soc. Behav. **27:** 78–89.
76. STRONKS, K. *et al.* 1998. The importance of psychosocial stressors for socioeconomic inequalities in perceived health. Soc. Sci. Med. **46**(4–5): 611–623.

77. MURPHY, J.M. *et al.* 1991. Depression and anxiety in relation to social status: a prospective epidemiologic study. Arch. Gen. Psychiatry **48:** 223–229.
78. DOHRENWEND, B.P. *et al.* 1992. Socioeconomic status and psychiatric disorders: the causation–selection issue. Science **255:** 946–952.
79. KESSLER, R.C., R.H. PRICE & C.B. WORTMAN. 1985. Social factors in psychopathology: stress, social support, and coping processes. *In* Annual Review of Psychology. M.R. Rosenzweig & L.W. Porter, Eds.: 531–572. Annual Reviews, Stanford, CA.
80. LYNCH, J.W., G.A. KAPLAN & M.S. SHEMA. 1997. Cumulative impact of sustained economic hardship on physical, cognitive, psychological, and social functioning. N. Engl. J. Med. **337:** 1889–1895.
81. LENZI, A. *et al.* 1993. Social class and mood disorders: clinical features. Soc. Psychiat. Epidemiol. **28:** 56–59.
82. BAUM, A. & D. POSLUSZNY. 1999. Health psychology: mapping biobehavioral contributions to health and illness. Annu. Rev. Psychol. **50:** 137–163.
83. JOHNSON, K.W. *et al.* 1995. Panel II: Macrosocial and environmental influences on minority health. Health Psychol. **14**(7): 601–612.
84. DYER, A.R. *et al.* 1976. The relationship of education to blood pressure: findings on 40,000 employed Chicagoans. Circulation **54**(6): 987–992.
85. SYME, S.L. *et al.* 1974. Social class and racial differences in blood pressure. Am. J. Pub. Health **64:** 619–620.
86. MATTHEWS, K.A. *et al.* 1989. Educational attainment and behavioral and biologic risk factors for coronary heart disease in middle-aged women. Am. J. Epidemiol. **129**(6): 1132–1144.
87. GUMP, B.B. & K.A. MATTHEWS. 1999. Do background stressors influence reactivity to and recovery from acute stressors. J. Appl. Soc. Psychol. **29**(3): 469–494.
88. DOUGALL, A.L., K.J. CRAIG & A. BAUM. 1999. Assessment of characteristics of intrusive thoughts and their impact on distress among victims of traumatic events. Psychosom. Med. **61:** 38–69.

Status, Stress, and Atherosclerosis: The Role of Environment and Individual Behavior

JAY R. KAPLAN[a,b] AND STEPHEN B. MANUCK[c]

[b]Department of Pathology (Comparative Medicine),
Wake Forest University School of Medicine, Medical Center Boulevard,
Winston-Salem, North Carolina 27157-1040, USA

[c]Department of Psychology, Behavioral Physiology Laboratory,
506 Engineering Hall, 4015 O'Hara Street, University of Pittsburgh,
Pittsburgh, Pennsylvania 15260, USA

ABSTRACT: Atherosclerosis induced by moderate hyperlipoproteinemia in group-housed cynomolgus monkeys differs significantly between animals of dominant and subordinate social status. The nature of this association also varies by sex, and in males, by stability of the social environment. Dominant males develop more extensive atherosclerosis than subordinates when housed in unstable, but not stable, social groups; in contrast, subordinate females develop greater atherosclerosis than dominants, and do so irrespective of the conditions of social housing. Experimental investigations reveal that the first of these associations (males) is mediated by concomitant sympathoadrenal activation and the second (females) by ovarian impairment associated with the stress of social subordination. We believe our findings offer clues to the neuroendocrine mediation of behavioral influences on coronary artery disease in humans. This is particularly true where these influences reflect asymmetries in the power or status relationships among individuals within similar social environments, or when dimensions of temperament or disposition give rise to such relationships. We propose that these data also may be informative regarding the pathophysiological sequelae of social stratification (in which disease incidence varies by class membership within populations), but only where social environments engendered by class inequalities exacerbate status-dependent behavioral differences among individuals within communities of associates.

INTRODUCTION

Recent decades have provided abundant evidence of an inverse association between socioeconomic status (SES) and both total and disease-specific mortality.[1,2] To some extent, this association reflects variation in access to health care and in the distribution of health-related behaviors, such as smoking, alcohol consumption, dietary and exercise patterns, and hygienic practices.[3] However, much of the variance in disease incidence associated with the SES gradient remains unexplained even after adjustment for these factors.[3,4] An alternative hypothesis is that a "low" position in the SES gradient is associated with certain behavioral or psychological factors (e.g., stress and "demoralization") that in turn predispose to disease and premature

[a]Address for communication: 336-716-1522 (voice).
e-mail: jkaplan@wfubmc.edu

mortality.[3,4] Presumably, such behavioral conditions would potentiate disease through associated perturbations of the body's principal axes of neuroendocrine response, such as the hypothalamic–pituitary–adrenocortical and sympathetic-adrenomedullary systems.[5–8] These systems normally coordinate an organism's physiological response to environmental challenge and hence are routinely activated as a part of daily existence. Although such routine reactions are not thought to be pathogenic, it is widely hypothesized that prolonged or excessive activation of these systems—as might occur under chronic stress, for instance—could adversely affect immunologic, cardiovascular, and central nervous system function, which may in turn augment risk for disease (e.g., Refs. 5 and 9).

The hypothesis that neuroendocrine factors mediate behavioral influences on disease (including those associated with the SES gradient) is of long standing, but is yet supported by little direct evidence.[5] However, we believe that recent research in cynomolgus monkeys (*Macaca fascicularis*) helps elucidate the relationship between behavioral factors and one prominent disease process, atherosclerosis. In this paper we review a series of studies conducted in socially housed male and female animals of this species, in which atherosclerosis is linked to both behavior and neuroendocrine activation. In addition to demonstrating that neuroendocrine factors contribute to vascular pathology, the outcomes of these studies implicate the relative social status of individuals as a major behavioral factor predicting susceptibility to disease. The ways in which the relationship between social status and cardiovascular disease, as observed in male and female monkeys, may be informative with respect to the SES gradient as a predictor of disease and mortality within human populations is discussed in the final sections.

APPLYING ANIMAL MODELS TO THE STUDY OF ATHEROSCLEROSIS

Atherosclerosis refers to the development of fibrofatty plaques (atheromas) within the inner lining or intima of arteries. It can be characterized as an inflammatory process that generally proceeds for decades before the appearance of clinical manifestations, the most prominent of which is coronary heart disease (CHD). Atherosclerotic lesions begin developing when the endothelial cells lining the artery wall undergo functional changes provoked by risk factors such as elevated plasma concentrations of low density lipoprotein cholesterol (LDLC), hypertension, and perhaps psychosocial stress.[10,11] In turn, functionally altered endothelial cells allow the infiltration of lipid particles and blood monocytes (macrophages) and lymphocytes into the artery wall. Smooth muscle cells from the arterial media also migrate to the nascent lesion. Together, the constituent cells of the emerging lesion release growth factors that further stimulate plaque development and encourage the accumulation of lipid and the proliferation of an extracellular matrix.[10,12] Over time, the progressing lesion often becomes complicated by calcification, necrosis, and internal hemorrhage, and is subject to rupture and subsequent thrombus formation. These processes eventually culminate in the various clinical expressions of CHD, including transient ischemia and infarction, and increased susceptibility to cardiac arrhythmias and sudden cardiac death.

Clinical and epidemiologic investigation provide increasing evidence that psychosocial factors contribute both to the development of coronary artery atherosclerosis and to its acute clinical expression as CHD.[13,14] Detailed study of the origins and mechanisms of behavioral influences on CHD is limited, however, both by the protracted nature of atherogenesis and by ethical considerations that preclude human experimentation and invasive diagnostic procedures in asymptomatic individuals. It is thus difficult to investigate satisfactorily, in human beings, factors that affect progression of coronary artery atherosclerosis in advance of the usual clinical manifestations of CHD.

The use of animal models addresses some of these limitations by permitting experimental control of pertinent environmental and dietary factors and an earlier and more precise quantification of lesion characteristics than is generally possible in studies involving human subjects.[15] Macaque monkeys (*Macaca*) are particularly appropriate for the investigation of atherogenesis because, when consuming diets that induce a moderate increase in plasma lipids, they develop lesions that are similar in morphological characteristics and location to those seen in human beings.[15] Moreover, lesion development progresses in macaques through the same stages and occurs in the same pattern as in humans. In cynomolgus macaques (*M. fascicularis*), for example, males develop more extensive atherosclerosis than do reproductively intact (i.e., premenopausal) females.[16] and males experience myocardial infarction at a rate similar to that seen in their human counterparts.[17]

THE BEHAVIOR OF CYNOMOLGUS MACAQUES

Cynomolgus monkeys not only resemble people in the pathobiology of atherosclerosis, but also exhibit social behaviors reminiscent of those thought to confer increased risk for CHD in humans (e.g. aggressiveness).[15,18] These group-living animals are characterized by elaborate patterns of positive social interaction, including generation-spanning networks of affiliation, alliance, and mutual support, as well as well-defined social status ("dominance") relationships and hierarchies.[15] In the latter regard, both wild and captive macaques form hierarchies of social status in which some animals (*dominants*) reliably defeat others (*subordinates*) in competitive interactions.[19] Once such hierarchies are formed, fights among individuals are generally unambiguous in outcome, with dominant monkeys exhibiting only attack gestures and subordinates only those gestures associated with flight.[20] The predilection of monkeys to form status hierarchies allows the categorization of animals within groups as either winners (dominants) or losers (subordinates) in response to conspecific challenge and stimulation. Dominant monkeys are usually, but not always, more aggressive (in frequency and intensity) than subordinates.[15] Although long-term genealogical and peer associations contribute to dominance ranking in naturally constituted groups, the ranks animals habitually achieve in small, unisexual groups (such as those incorporated in the experiments described here) probably reflect underlying traits of temperament.[21]

In addition to their propensity to establish well-delineated dominance relationships, cynomolgus macaques respond antagonistically to new animals attempting to join their social groupings. This behavioral phenomenon is well suited to experimental manipulation, as by recurrent reorganization of social group membership. The appearance of unfamiliar monkeys intensifies confrontations among animals as monkeys attempt to reestablish hierarchic relationships and affiliative coalitions.[22] Such encounters with unfamiliar conspecifics are not uncommon in the natural history of macaque males; these animals typically disperse from their natal groups at adolescence and thereafter tend to be socially transient.[23] The repeated exposure of males to unfamiliar conspecifics thus represents an ethologically salient stressor, since it mimics the typical adult male experience of moving from one social group to another. In contrast, females typically remain with their group of birth throughout their lives, and therefore encounter strangers (i.e., unfamiliar females) only on rare occasions.

In the following sections we first review the results of two investigations showing that psychosocial factors (specifically, dominant social status and social group instability) predispose male cynomolgus monkeys to the development of coronary atherosclerosis, and do so via activation of the sympathoadrenal system. Next, we describe evidence that subordinate social status potentiates coronary artery atherosclerosis in females of the same species, and does so through a mechanism involving stress-induced ovarian impairment.

THE BEHAVIORAL EXACERBATION OF ATHEROSCLEROSIS IN MALES

In an initial study,[18] 30 male cynomolgus monkeys fed a moderately atherogenic diet (similar to that consumed in industrialized countries) were housed in five-member social groups and assigned in equal numbers to one of two experimental conditions. In one of these conditions, termed "unstable," animals were redistributed among groups on a regular basis to model the social instability typically experienced by macaque males. Furthermore, an estrogen-implanted female was placed into each of these groups in the latter half of each reorganization period to provide an additional stimulus for intermale competition. The remainder of the animals constituted a "stable" condition, in which initial group memberships were maintained without disruption (and without females) throughout the 22-month experiment. Repeated behavioral observations also permitted identification of individuals as relatively more "dominant" or "subordinate" in their social groups. In this and other experiments, dominant animals, in both unstable and stable groups, tended to retain their high rankings; similarly, subordinate individuals tended to remain subordinate irrespective of their social condition. For analytic purposes, animals that on average ranked above the median rank of all animals were considered dominant; the remainder were labeled subordinate.

Subsequent quantitative evaluation of the coronary arteries of these animals (males only) revealed that animals housed in reorganized social groups developed about twice the coronary atherosclerosis seen among animals in the stable environment, but *only* if they were of high social rank (i.e., dominant) (FIGURE 1). Subordinate animals, irrespective of social environment, showed an amount of atherosclerosis approximately equivalent to that of dominant monkeys housed in a stable social setting. These results suggest that the behavioral demands of retaining

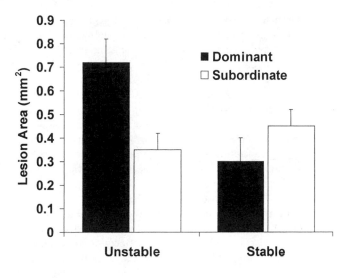

FIGURE 1. Atherosclerosis extent in the coronary arteries of dominant and subordinate monkeys housed in stable or unstable (periodically reorganized) social groups. Dominant monkeys in unstable groups had more atherosclerosis than dominant monkeys in stable groups, and more than subordinates in either condition ($p < 0.05$) (adapted from Ref. 18).

preeminence in an unstable social environment potentiate atherogenesis, at least in males of this species. Consistent with this suggestion is the observation that the dominant monkeys living in unstable social groups initiated significantly more episodes of nonritualized, contact aggression (grabbing, chasing) than did their counterparts assigned to the stable condition in this experiment. Moreover, other forms of social behavior were also disrupted by the periodic reorganization of group memberships, as reflected in a marked alteration of ordinary grooming relationships and in changes in the frequency of passive affiliation among animals assigned to the unstable social condition.

The outcome of this experiment may seem surprising in view of the generally prevailing belief that subordinates are under greater social stress than dominants. Furthermore, the mechanism underlying the behavioral exacerbation of atherosclerosis in dominants is unclear in this experiment, as the preceding results were independent of variation in other risk factors, such as serum lipid concentrations (that is, total plasma cholesterol [TPC] and high density lipoprotein cholesterol [HDLC]) and blood pressure. A similar outcome—that is, the exacerbation of disease in high-status animals—has been observed among colony-housed male mice; specifically, dominant mice exhibited pronounced sympathoadrenal activation when actively suppressing the behavior of subdominants and, upon termination of the experiment, were found to have larger aortic lesions (characterized by dissolution and fragmentation of smooth muscle cell layers).[24] On the basis in part of this result and observations relating excessive sympathetic drive to atherosclerosis in rabbits,[25] we speculated that dominant monkeys assigned to unstable groups in our initial experiment (and therefore forced to cope with repeated challenges to their social status) experienced recurrent sympathetic arousal with accompanying increases in heart rate, blood pressure, and catecholamine release (e.g., Ref. 6). These hemodynamic and metabolic responses, in turn, may have altered endothelial function (and thus provoked the initiation of lesion formation), or they may have resulted in the further exacerbation of diet-induced lesions.[26]

On the hypothesis that socially induced sympathetic activation might promote atherogenesis in predisposed (i.e. dominant) animals, 30 monkeys in a subsequent study (again, males) were *all* housed in periodically reorganized social groups and fed a cholesterol-containing diet for 26 months. Estrogen-implanted females were again placed in the social groups midway through each reorganization to prolong the social disruption. One-half of the study males also received a β-adrenoreceptor antagonist, propranolol, throughout the study period.[27] While β-adrenergic blockade did not alter either the social behavior or the serum lipid concentrations (TPC, HDLC) of these animals,[27] it did modulate the effects of social status on coronary atherosclerosis (FIG. 2). Untreated dominant monkeys again had twice the coronary atherosclerosis of their subordinate counterparts, replicating the results from the unstable condition of the first experiment. Dominant monkeys administered propra-

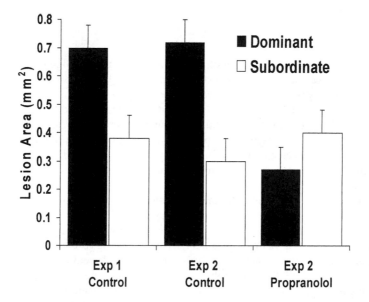

FIGURE 2. Atherosclerosis extent in the coronary arteries of dominant and subordinate monkeys housed in unstable groups (both from experiment 1 and the present experiment) and either treated or not with a beta-blocker (propranolol). Atherosclerosis was pronounced in untreated dominant animals from both experiments; treatment with propranolol markedly inhibited atherosclerosis in dominant animals but did not affect subordinates ($p < 0.05$) (adapted from Ref. 27).

nolol, on the other hand, developed less than half the coronary atherosclerosis of untreated dominants and had roughly the same extent of lesion as both treated and untreated subordinate animals. Hence, the more pronounced atherosclerosis characteristic of untreated (i.e., autonomically intact), dominant monkeys—when housed in groups of rotating membership and fed a cholesterol-containing diet—can be prevented by the long-term administration of an adrenergic inhibitor and is therefore mediated by concomitant sympathoadrenal activation.

The generalized effects of propranolol on blood pressure and heart rate, which occurred irrespective of social status, cannot account for the selective protection accorded dominant monkeys in the treated condition. However, the atherogenicity of psychosocial factors may result from the hemodynamic and/or metabolic adjustments experienced by susceptible animals during naturally occurring periods of social challenge or stress. Such responses are likely to be transient, and therefore elude detection in measurements recorded under usual laboratory conditions. This latter speculation is supported by an additional observation, namely that naturally occurring social interactions occasion substantial changes in heart rate in these animals and that during periods of active social reorganization such changes are more pronounced in *dominant* than subordinate monkeys; these status-dependent cardiac effects are also mitigated by propranolol. Thus, β-receptor blockade may have exerted an antiatherogenic effect in the above study by ameliorating the physiological manifestations of sympathoadrenal reactions experienced most appreciably by dominant monkeys during episodes of social challenge.

The studies with male cynomolgus monkeys suggest two major conclusions: (1) atherosclerosis is exacerbated among individuals that are habitually successful in their aggressive encounters with social strangers, thereby retaining dominant social status in an unstable environment; and (2) the increased risk of atherosclerosis experienced by such animals is related, in part, to the sympathoadrenal activation occasioned by the demands of retaining dominant status in an unstable environment. As shown below, female monkeys respond differently than males to the challenges of group formation, and in a way that puts subordinate, rather than dominant, monkeys at risk.

THE BEHAVIORAL EXACERBATION OF ATHEROSCLEROSIS IN FEMALES

The relative sparing of premenopausal women in relation to similarly aged men is a prominent feature of CHD, ischemic stroke, and atherosclerosis.[28] Although this phenomenon is sometimes referred to as "female protection," it is more accurately characterized as a delay in disease onset, with the incidence curve for women lagging behind that of men by about 10 years.[29] Inasmuch as atherosclerosis progresses over decades, we hypothesized that the clinical events occurring in postmenopausal women would have their beginnings in the premenopausal years. A series of studies in female cynomolgus macaques (which have 28-day menstrual cycles that are similar hormonally to those of women) allowed evaluation of this hypothesis and revealed that relative "protection" against coronary atherosclerosis is a benefit experienced by some, but not all, premenopausal monkeys; specifically, outcome varies significantly as a function of animals' social status.

In the first study,[30] 30 premenopausal females were housed in social groups of five animals, each containing a single, vasectomized male. Two of these groups were stable in composition while three were unstable, with females switched between groups approximately monthly. Ten additional males were housed in two groups of five animals each, and all monkeys consumed a moderately atherogenic diet. As before, repeated behavioral observations allowed identification of individuals as more dominant or subordinate in their social groups over the course of the experiment. In addition to behavioral assessment, all females were subjected to daily vaginal swabbing to monitor menses. Furthermore, we collected blood samples for the determination of plasma estradiol and progesterone concentrations across the menstrual cycle. Measurement of coronary lesions on completion of the study indicated that female protection from atherosclerosis extended only to *dominant* animals; subordinates, approximately half of the animals in each social group, could not be distinguished from males in extent of lesion development (FIG. 3). Social instability did not influence this outcome.

As in the previous studies involving males, status-dependent effects on atherosclerosis among females were statistically independent of variation in plasma lipid concentrations and blood pressure. However, we did observe that subordinate females had five times as many anovulatory menstrual cycles and three times as many menstrual cycles characterized by luteal phase progesterone deficiencies (peak plasma progesterone concentrations between 2.0 and 4.0 ng/dl) as their dominant coun-

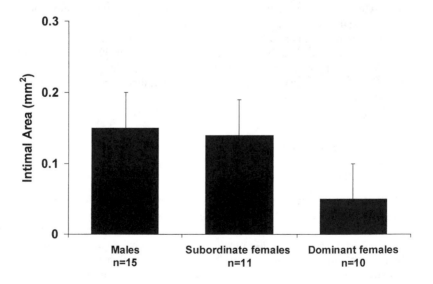

FIGURE 3. Atherosclerosis extent in the coronary arteries of socially housed male and female monkeys. Females are reproductively intact. Dominant females have less atherosclerosis than either males or subordinate females ($p < 0.05$); subordinate females do not differ from males (adapted from Ref. 30).

TABLE 1. Ovarian and adrenal indices (median values) in dominant and subordinate monkeys[a]

	Dominant	Subordinate	p Value[b]
Luteal-phase peak plasma progesterone (mg/ml)	8.9	4.0	< 0.01
Percent anovulatory cycles	3.5	16.5	< 0.01
Percent cycles with luteal-phase deficiencies	8.9	24.3	< 0.01
Adrenal weight (mg/kg body weight)	168	201	< 0.05

[a]Data from Reference 30.
[b]By Mann-Whitney test.

terparts (TABLE 1).[30,31] Other studies indicate that subordinate monkeys typically have plasma estradiol concentrations of about 60 pg/ml, whereas estradiol levels of dominants average around 130 pg/ml.[32] Thus, in comparison to dominant females, subordinate monkeys experience ovulatory impairment and relative estrogen deficiency. Additionally, subordinate females in the foregoing study also experienced significant adrenal enlargement and hypersensitivity (TABLE 1), which suggests that these animals were under substantial stress. This association between stress and ovarian dysfunction, in turn, is one of the most reliable observations in mammalian socioendocrinology.[33,34]

We hypothesized that estrogen deficiency was predominantly responsible for the worsened atherosclerosis of the subordinate monkeys. In women, for example, a history of menstrual irregularity is linked to a significantly increased risk for acute myocardial infarction, a thickened arterial lining, and elevated plasma fibrinogen concentrations (a risk factor for atherosclerosis).[35,36] Also, premenopausal women with angiographically confirmed CHD have significantly lower plasma estradiol concentrations than do controls.[37] Hence, estradiol concentrations of "at risk" women are approximately 80 pg/ml, compared to 120 pg/ml for controls. These values, in turn, are comparable to those described above for subordinate and dominant female monkeys, respectively, animals that differ in atherosclerosis extent.[30,32]

A subsequent experiment was designed to explore the mechanism mediating the association among social status, ovarian impairment, and atherosclerosis. Specifically, if estrogen deficiency potentiates atherosclerosis, it follows that treatment with exogenous estrogen should be inhibitory, especially in those animals at highest risk for such deficiency by virtue of their subordinate social status. We tested this hypothesis in a study involving approximately 190 premenopausal monkeys, all housed in social groups of five or six animals each and consuming a moderately atherogenic diet.[38] Additionally, half of the monkeys were given in their diet the triphasic oral contraceptive (OC) Triphasil™, containing ethinyl estradiol (an estrogen) and levonorgestrel (a progestin). At the end of 26 months, we measured atherosclerosis extent in an iliac artery biopsy (as a surrogate for the coronary arteries) from each animal. Animals were again ranked either dominant or subordinate over the course of the experiment.

As in previous studies of females, untreated subordinates showed more extensive lesion than untreated dominants. However, treatment with the OC inhibited lesion development in subordinates, rendering them indistinguishable from dominants,

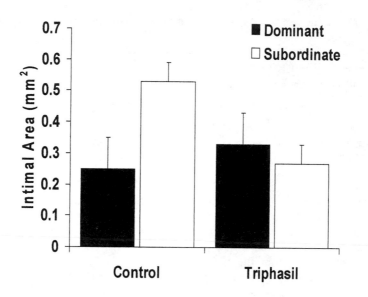

FIGURE 4. Atherosclerosis extent in the iliac arteries of dominant and subordinate females either treated or not with an oral contraceptive (Triphasil). Untreated subordinate animals had more atherosclerosis than untreated dominants and more atherosclerosis than treated animals, irrespective of status (adapted from Ref. 38).

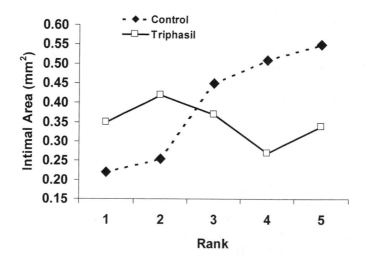

FIGURE 5. Atherosclerosis extent in the iliac arteries of females plotted against average social rank from high (*1*) to low (*5*). Oral contraceptive treatment eliminated the inverse association between rank and atherosclerosis (adapted from Ref. 38). In all cases $SE < 0.10$.

treated or untreated (FIG. 4). Parallel evaluation of plasma lipid concentrations indicated that HDLC concentrations were suppressed in treated compared with untreated animals, and in subordinates compared to dominants ($p < 0.05$ in all cases). Nonetheless, the protective effect of OC treatment on subordinate monkeys persisted even after statistical adjustment for changes in plasma lipids. Hence, plaque development was inhibited in treated monkeys despite the reduction in HDLC that accompanied OC exposure. Finally, owing to the substantial number of animals in this experiment, it was possible to plot atherosclerosis extent against average social status grouped into five categories (from high to low) (FIG. 5). This plot suggests the presence of an inverse, linear association (i.e., a "dose-response" relationship) between social status and atherosclerosis among the control animals, an association that was eliminated by OC treatment.

The results of this experiment confirmed that the effects of social status on atherosclerosis in female monkeys are mediated by concomitant ovarian impairment in subordinate animals. Hence, subordinate social status was associated with worsened atherosclerosis among untreated monkeys, whereas treatment with an OC inhibited the development of atherosclerosis in subordinates and, in fact, entirely eliminated the difference in lesion extent between dominant and subordinate monkeys. To the extent that these results reflect analogous processes in women—for example the presence of stress-induced ovarian impairment[34,39-41]—the studies conducted in female monkeys highlight the potential importance of behavioral stressors in the development of atherosclerosis during the premenopausal period (e.g., Refs. 35 and 36). They also illuminate the possible antiatherogenic effects of contraceptive steroids among premenopausal women with estrogen deficiency.

THE PATHOGENICITY OF SOCIAL STATUS IN MALE AND FEMALE MONKEYS

Why should low status be pathogenic in female monkeys, irrespective of social stability, while *high* status is pathogenic in males, but only under conditions of social instability? The answer, we believe, relates to differences in the social biology and natural history of male and female monkeys, which in turn caused similar experimental manipulations to have different costs and benefits for animals of the two sexes and to activate different neuroendocrine mechanisms.

As stated previously, male macaques disperse from their groups at adolescence and tend to switch groups frequently during adulthood. As a result, males must often decide when to challenge and break into an existing hierarchy and when to avoid such situations. By inclination or temperament, some males are probably more aggressive and thus successful in these encounters (although at greater risk of injury), while others are more passive (and at less risk of injury). Our experimental instability manipulation forced males to confront social strangers repeatedly, and each animal responded in its habitual way to this challenge—either engaging and winning such contests (i.e., the eventual dominants) or engaging but losing competitive interactions (i.e., the eventual subordinates). Such repeated challenges were absent in the stable social groups, where status was decided on a single occasion at the beginning of the experiment. On the basis of experimentation with mice, Henry suggested that attempts to maintain social control are accompanied by preferential sympathoadrenal activation (and increased risk of cardiovascular disease), whereas behavioral conservation and withdrawal are associated with pituitary–adrenocortical activation.[6] Our data on the males support Henry's suggestions. Not only did we observe exacerbation of atherosclerosis among unstable dominants and the subsequent inhibition of disease in such animals following β-adrenergic blockade, we also observed enlarged adrenal glands in all subordinate males, irrespective of housing conditions.[42]

The females present a different picture than the males, behaviorally as well as biologically. Female monkeys almost never leave the groups into which they are born, but structure all of their social interactions around their relatives and lifelong peers.[43] As a result, females tend to be more intolerant of same-sex social strangers than males. Upon introduction to strangers, the more aggressive and competitive female monkeys (the dominants) engage in prolonged harassment of the animals destined to be subordinate. This harassment tends to continue undiminished over long periods of time, even if the social group is subsequently kept stable in composition. Hence, irrespective of social stability, the pituitary–adrenocortical activation and ovarian impairment experienced by subordinates in response to harassment by dominants comprise the major physiologic outcomes in groups of adult females initially put together as social strangers. As a result, subordinate females are always at risk of accelerated atherogenesis. Biologically, stress-associated ovarian impairment is possibly adaptive, because it allows a female mammal to delay an energetically expensive pregnancy until safer, more propitious circumstances prevail. No such analogous feature need apply to male mammals, for whom reproduction is usually inexpensive, at least energetically.

More generally, social status distinctions, like most behavioral adaptations, entail elements of benefit and elements of cost. For dominant animals, the benefits are preferential access to resources, be they food, space, or mates, and the costs are those associated with the behavioral demands of achieving and retaining preeminence against competitors in a social group. For subordinate animals, the costs are limited access to the same resources and ritualized or overt subjugation in encounters with more dominant animals. The benefits are less clear, but acquiescence to subordinate status probably reduces injury, ameliorates conflict until a time more advantageous for achieving higher status, and (in natural environments) may involve alternative (e.g. surreptitious) behavioral strategies for resource acquisition. As a result, either dominant or subordinate status may have pathophysiologic consequences, depending on the balance of cost to benefit and the nature of accompanying neuroendocrine reactions. Importantly, salient aspects of the social and physical environment modulate the costs and benefits associated with different levels of social status. In the unstable social environment of our experiments in males, for example, re-establishment of high status represents a net cost and is accompanied by sympathoadrenal activation. Following initial status determinations, as for example in a stable social group, dominant and subordinate males tolerate each other well despite being social strangers. Conceivably, if the same animals housed in stable groups were exposed to a more resource-poor environment (less space, fewer perches, a limited food supply, etc.), subordinate males might suffer disproportionately instead, due the necessity of directly competing with animals dominant to them.

In contrast to males, within groups of females that have not been reared together, the constraints of space and social demands reify and exacerbate status-dependent interactions between individuals, with subordinates the focus of recurrent harassment. However, heightened competition for status (as through daily, as opposed to monthly, introduction of new animals) might reduce the usual status–atherosclerosis gradient described for females by placing increased behavioral demands on dominant monkeys; analogously, the exacerbation of lesion development in subordinates might be reduced by "softening" the conditions of housing (e.g., by providing abundant space, avenues for social escape), thus reducing contact between monkeys of different status. Hence, for both males and females, it may be possible to create environmental conditions or demands under which either dominants or subordinates would suffer pathophysiological consequences selectively.

THE CHALLENGE OF THE GRADIENT

Insofar as the data reported here were derived from phylogenetically close relatives to man, it may be asked whether they are relevant to understanding the SES–disease relationship in humans or the mediation of this relationship. There are two conceptual issues that block an easy translation of results from monkeys to people, at least with respect to the SES gradient: (1) as suggested in the previous paragraphs, there is nothing inherently pathogenic in either dominant or subordinate social status in monkeys—in contrast, low SES is uniformly associated with increased disease risk in humans; and (2) social status in monkeys and social class or SES in people are not equivalent constructs in definition or implication. Regarding the first point, as we have seen, the relationship between status and disease in monkeys is variable, depending on sex and conditions of the social environment. Thus, while there is an inverse association between social status and atherosclerosis extent in premenopausal monkeys, an opposite association is obtained in males of the same species when such animals are exposed to repeated reorganization of group membership. Further complicating the picture of status–disease relationships, we also have reported that subordinate male monkeys have significantly greater susceptibility to upper respiratory infections than do dominants, an effect that is independent of the conditions of social housing.[44]

The second problem identified above is the lack of conceptual concordance between social status as described in monkeys and the SES gradient in people. In monkeys, status distinctions reflect behavioral asymmetries among individuals associated by common group membership. In contrast, SES in humans is generally defined in terms of demographic attributes that delineate strata of society and may thereby be taken to imply classes of individuals or groups effectively anonymous to each other. If human status is conceived in this latter sense, the relationship to monkeys with respect to patterns of disease is not clear, except insofar as class differences (between anonymous strata) might evoke similar patterns of neuroendocrine response and similar disease sequelae. Here, the effects on health might share the same pathogenic mechanism as that seen in relation to primate social status, but not reflect the same behavioral construct—even though going by the same name (i.e., the "demoralization" of low SES, where such individuals are largely anonymous with respect to persons of higher "class" membership, versus low status derived from asymmetries of outcomes in competitive encounters among members of a primate social group).

However, an alternative conceptualization of environment in monkeys and of social class and status in people may allow interpretations of human disease patterns in terms of the primate data. Suppose, for example, we envision the environmental conditions or demands imposed on the monkeys (i.e., stability of groups, resource distribution) as analogous to different levels of social class. Stable and unstable monkeys would then be seen as comprising different classes of animals, made distinct by their environmental conditions (harsher in the unstable than in the stable). Within a class, individuals are differentiated by their social status, which emerges from behavioral interactions. Depending on the specific demands imposed at a class level, either dominants or subordinates may be at a relative health advantage. With regard to humans, suppose that social class retains its meaning as pertaining to the various strata of society, each characterized by a particular level of constraints and demands (or lack thereof). Then, the term "social status," in reference to humans, might be taken to imply objective or perceived social ranking within a community of associates at a particular societal stratum. Under this model—which now resembles the monkey situation—we would expect that the effects of "social class" would not equally affect all individuals in a class, but would confer disproportionate risk as a function of individual differences in status (where status refers to behavioral outcomes, attributes, or perceptions, rather than economic condition *per se*).

The foregoing conceptualization leads to a number of predictions for both monkeys and people. First, it might be expected that, in monkeys, levels of increasing environmental demand (i.e., going from higher to lower "class") would be accompanied by generally increasing levels of disease. Such increases would occur despite any differential in disease that might be observed between animals of different status *within* a class. Male monkeys provide some evidence in this regard, as there is somewhat more atherosclerosis overall among animals living in unstable social groups than among those in stable groups.[18,45] In a general sense, then, the monkeys would be expected to show a health gradient across classes (i.e., across levels of environmental demand and constraints) similar to that observed with respect to the SES gradient. A second prediction in monkeys would be that, within any "class" (i.e., degree of constraint), susceptibility to disease should be a function of the relative costs and benefits associated with dominant and subordinate status. In our previous experiments, we have burdened dominant males by forcing them to reassert their preeminence in groups of changing composition. Reversing the burden might alter the relative risks between subordinate and dominant males.

Applied to humans, the monkey model predicts that at any SES level (i.e., class level), there will be significant variation in health outcomes related to individual differences in social status or associated behavior. Such differences with respect to infectious disease are, in fact, reported in another chapter of this volume.[46] The monkey model also allows predictions with respect to the neuroendocrine mediation of status-induced differences in disease. Heart disease in males, for example, might be driven by the sympathoadrenal activation that accompanies aggressive and competitive behavior. This effect might be especially prominent in the middle and lower SES strata, where the opportunities for such interactions (in the workplace) might be most prevalent. Although the human analogue for subordinate female monkeys is not clear, there is a stress-associated syndrome (functional hypothalamic amenorrhea, also called "psychogenic" amenorrhea) involving the same triad of ovarian dysfunction, adrenal hyperactivity, and behavioral withdrawal or depression that characterizes subordinate monkeys.[39–41] It is tempting to relate the substantial amount of atherosclerosis now known to occur in one-third of premenopausal women[47] to periodic and perhaps subclinical, stress-induced ovarian dysfunction (e.g., Refs. 48 and 49). This effect would seem most pronounced at the lower strata of the SES gradient, where resources are most constrained and social and economic demands are the greatest.

CONCLUSION

The conceptualization presented in the foregoing paragraphs suggests that results of studies such as ours are potentially relevant to an understanding of the pathophysiological sequelae of social stratification among people. This is particularly true where the social environment engendered by class inequities (as observed *between* SES strata) exacerbates status-dependent behavioral differences among regularly interacting individuals (as observed *within* a stratum). Here, it is not a struggle between classes that potentiates pathogenesis, but rather a struggle within a community of associates, with such contests more intense at lower SES strata. This conceptual framework may offer a way to bridge human and nonhuman primate studies. As yet, however, the translation of results between human and monkey studies with respect to the SES gradient remains more a promise than a reality.

REFERENCES

1. ADLER, N.E., T. BOYCE, M.A. CHESNEY, S. COHEN, S. FOLKMAN, R.L. KAHN, & S.L. SYME. 1994. Socioeconomic status and health: the challenge of the gradient. Am. Psychol. **49:** 15–24.
2. DUTTON, D.B. & S. LEVINE. 1989. Overview: methodological critique, and reformulation. *In* Pathways to Health. J.P. Bunker, D.S. Gomby & B.H. Kehrer, Eds.: 29–69. The Henry J. Kaiser Family Foundation, Menlo Park.
3. ADLER, N.E. & K. MATTHEWS. 1993. Health psychology: Why do some people get sick and some stay well? Ann. Rev. Psychol. **45:** 229–259.
4. MARMOT, M.G., M.J. SHIPLEY & G. ROSE. 1984. Inequalities in death: specific explanations of a general pattern? Lancet **1:** 1003–1006.
5. MANUCK, S.B., A.L. MARSLAND, J.R. KAPLAN & J.K. WILLIAMS. 1995. The pathogenicity of behavior and its neuroendocrine mediation: An example from coronary artery disease. Psychosom. Med. **57:** 275–283.
6. HENRY, J.P. & P.M. STEPHENS. 1977. Stress, health and the social environment. *In* A Sociobiological Approach to Medicine. Springer-Verlag, New York.
7. HERD, J.A. 1977. Physiological basis of behavioral influences in atherosclerosis. *In* Coronary Prone Behavior. T.M. Dembroski, S.M. Weiss, S.L. Shields, *et al.*, Eds. Springer-Verlag, New York.
8. SCHNEIDERMAN, N. 1987. Psychophysiologic factors in atherosclerosis and coronary heart disease. Circulation **76**(Suppl. I): 141–147.
9. MCEWEN, B.S. 1998. Protective and damaging effects of stress mediators. N. Engl. J. Med. **338:** 171–179.
10. HENDERSON, A. 1996. Coronary heart disease: overview. Lancet **348:** S1–S4.

11. SKANTZE, H.B., J. KAPLAN, K. PETTERSSON, S. MANUCK, N. BLOMQVIST, R. KYES, K. WILLIAMS & G. BONDJERS. 1998. Psychosocial stress causes endothelial injury in cynomologus monkeys via β,1-adrenoceptor activation. Atherosclerosis 136: 153–161.

12. LIBBY, P. 1996. Atheroma: more than mush. Lancet 348: S4–S7.

13. ROZANSKI, A., J.A. BLUMENTHAL & J. KAPLAN. 1999. Impact of psychological factors on the pathogenesis of cardiovascular disease and implications for therapy. Circulation 99: 2192–2217.

14. MANUCK, S.B., J.R. KAPLAN & K.A. MATTHEWS. 1986. Behavioral antecedents of coronary heart disease and atherosclerosis. Arteriosclerosis 6: 2–14.

15. KAPLAN, J.R., S.B. MANUCK, T.B. CLARKSON & R.W. PRICHARD. 1985. Animal models of behavioral influences on atherosclerosis. Adv. Behav. Med. 1: 115–163.

16. HAMM, T.E., JR., J.R. KAPLAN, T.B. CLARKSON & B.C. BULLOCK. 1983. Effects of gender and social behavior on the development of coronary artery atherosclerosis in cynomolgus macaques. Atherosclerosis 48: 221–233.

17. BOND, M.D., B.C. BULLOCK, D.A. BELLINGER & T.E. HAMM. 1980. Myocardial infarction in a large colony of nonhuman primates with coronary artery atherosclerosis. Am. J. Pathol. 101: 675–692.

18. KAPLAN, J.R., S.B. MANUCK, T.B. CLARKSON, F.M. LUSSO & D.M. TAUB. 1982. Social status, environment and atherosclerosis in cynomolgus monkeys. Arteriosclerosis 2: 359–368.

19. KAPLAN, J.R. & S.B. MANUCK. 1998. Monkeys, aggression, and the pathobiology of atherosclerosis. Aggres. Behav. 24: 323–334.

20. BERNSTEIN, I.S. 1981. Dominance: the baby and the bathwater. Behav. Brain Sci. 4: 419–457.

21. KAPLAN, J.R., T.B. CLARKSON, M.R. ADAMS, S.B. MANUCK & C.A. SHIVELY. 1991. Social behavior and gender in biomedical investigations using monkeys: studies in atherogenesis. Lab. Anim. Sci. 41: 334–342.

22. BERNSTEIN, I.S., T.P. GORDON & R.M. ROSE. 1974. Aggression and social controls in rhesus monkey (Macaca mulatta) groups revealed in group formation studies. Folia Primatol. 21: 81–107.

23. BERARD, J.D. 1989. Life histories of male Cayo Santiago macaques. P.R. Health Sci. J. 8: 61–64.

24. ELY, D.L. 1981. Hypertension, social rank, and aortic atherosclerosis in CBA/j mice. Physiol. Behav. 26: 655–661.

25. SPENCE, J.D., D.G. PERKINS, R.L. KLEIN, M.A. ADAMS & M.D. HAUST. 1984. Hemodynamic modifications of aortic atherosclerosis: Effects of propranolol versus hydralazine in hypertensive hyperlipidemic rabbits. Atherosclerosis 50: 325–333.

26. KAPLAN, J.R., K. PETTERSSON, S.B. MANUCK & G. OLSSON. 1991. Role of sympathoadrenal medullary activation in the initiation and progression of atherosclerosis. Circulation 84(Suppl. VI): VI-23–VI-32.

27. KAPLAN, J.R., S.B. MANUCK, M.R. ADAMS, K.W. WEINGAND & T.B. CLARKSON. 1987. Inhibition of coronary atherosclerosis by propranolol in behaviorally predisposed monkeys fed an atherogenic diet. Circulation 76: 1364–1372.

28. MCGILL, H.C. & N.P. STERN. 1979. Sex and atherosclerosis. Atheroscler. Rev. 4: 157–242.

29. HIGGINS, M. & T. THOM. 1993. Cardiovascular disease in women as a public health problem. In Cardiovascular Health and Disease in Women. N.K. Wenger, L. Speroff & B. Packard, Eds.: 15–19. LeJacq Communications, Inc., Greenwich.

30. KAPLAN, J.R., M.R. ADAMS, T.B. CLARKSON & D.R. KORITNIK. 1984. Psychosocial influences on female "protection" among cynomolgus macaques. Atherosclerosis 53: 283–295.

31. ADAMS, M.R., J.R. KAPLAN & D.R. KORITNIK. 1985. Psychosocial influences on ovarian endocrine and ovulatory function in Macaca fascicularis. Physiol. Behav. 35: 935–940.

32. WILLIAMS, J.K., C.A. SHIVELY & T.B. CLARKSON. 1994. Determinants of coronary artery reactivity in premenopausal female cynomolgus monkeys with diet-induced atherosclerosis. Circulation 90: 983–987.

33. CHRISTIAN, J.J. 1980. Endocrine factors in population regulation. *In* Biosocial Mechanisms of Population Regulation. N.N. Cohen, R.S. Malpass & H.G. Klein, Eds.: 55–116. Yale University Press, New Haven.

34. CAMERON, J.L. 1997. Stress and behaviorally induced reproductive dysfunction in primates. Sem. Reprod. Endocrinol. **15:** 37–45.

35. LaVECCHIA, C., A. DECARDI, S. FRANCESCHI, A. GENTILE, E. NEGRI & F. PARAZZINI. 1987. Menstrual and reproductive factors and the risk of myocardial infarction in women under fifty-five years of age. Am. J. Obstet. Gynecol. **157:** 1108–1112.

36. PUNNONEN, R., H. JOKELA, R. AINE, K. TEISALA, A. SALOMAKI & H. UPPA. 1997. Impaired ovarian function and risk factors for atherosclerosis in premenopausal women. Maturitas **27:** 231–238.

37. HANKE, H., S. HANKE, O. ICKRATH, K. LANGE, B. BRUCK, A.O. MUCK, H. SEEGER, M. ZWIRNER, R. VOISARD, R. HAASIS & V. HOMBACH. 1997. Estradiol concentrations in premenopausal women with coronary heart disease. Coron. Artery Dis. **8:** 511–515.

38. KAPLAN, J.R., M.R. ADAMS, M.S. ANTHONY, T.M. MORGAN, S.B. MANUCK & T.B. CLARKSON. 1995. Dominant social status and contraceptive hormone treatment inhibit atherogenesis in premenopausal monkeys. Atheroscler. Thromb. Vasc. Biol. **15:** 2094–2100.

39. REINDOLLAR, R.H., M. NOVAK, S.P. THO & P.G. McDONOUGH. 1986. Adult-onset amenorrhea: a study of 262 patients. Am. J. Obstet. Gynecol. **155:** 531–543.

40. BERGA, S.L., T.L. DANIELS & D.E. GILES. 1997. Women with functional hypothalamic amenorrhea but not other forms of anovulation display amplified cortisol concentrations. Fertil. Steril. **67:** 1024–1030.

41. JUDD, S.J., J. WONG, S. SALONIKLIS, M. MAIDEN, B. YEAP, S. FILMER & L. MICHAILOV. 1995. The effect of alprazolam on serum cortisol and luteinizing hormone pulsatility in normal women and in women with stress-related anovulation. J. Clin. Endocrinol. Metab. **80:** 818–823.

42. KAPLAN, J.R. & S.B. MANUCK. 1997. Using ethological principles to study psychosocial influences on coronary atherosclerosis in monkeys. Acta Physiol. Scand. **161**(Suppl. 640): 96–99.

43. SADE, D.S. 1972. A longitudinal study of social behavior of rhesus monkeys. *In* The Functional and Evolutionary Biology of Primates. R. Tuttle, Ed.: 378–398. Aldine-Atherton, Inc., Chicago.

44. COHEN, S., S. LINE, S.B. MANUCK, E. HEISE & J.R. KAPLAN. 1997. Chronic social stress, social dominance and susceptibility to upper respiratory infections in nonhuman primates. Psychosom. Med. **59:** 213–221.

45. KAPLAN, J.R., S.B. MANUCK, T.B. CLARKSON, F.M. LUSSO, D.M. TAUB & E.W. MILLER. 1983. Social stress and atherosclerosis in normocholesterolemic monkeys. Science **220:** 733–735.

46. COHEN, S. 1999. Social status and susceptibility to respiratory infections. Ann. N.Y. Acad. Sci. **896:** this volume.

47. STRONG, J.P., G.T. MALCOM, C.A. McMAHAN, R.E. TRACY, W.P. NEWMAN III, E.E. HERDERICK & J.F. CORNHILL. 1999. Prevalence and extent of atherosclerosis in adolescents and young adults. Implications for prevention from the Pathobiological Determinants of Atherosclerosis in Youth Study. JAMA **281:** 727–735.

48. PRIOR, J.C., Y.M. VIGNA, M.T. SCHECHTER & A.E. BURGESS. 1990. Spinal bone loss and ovulatory disturbances. New Engl. J. Med. **323:** 1221–1227.

49. PRIOR, J.C., Y.M. VIGNA, S.I. BARR, S. KENNEDY, M. SCHULZER & D.K.B. LI. 1996. Ovulatory premenopausal women lose cancellous spinal bone: a five year prospective study. Bone **18:** 261–267.

Stress Responses in Low-Status Jobs and Their Relationship to Health Risks: Musculoskeletal Disorders

ULF LUNDBERG[a]

Department of Psychology, Stockholm University, S-106 91 Stockholm, Sweden

ABSTRACT: Conditions typical of many low-status jobs are known to induce elevated stress. In keeping with this, blue-collar workers show elevated psychophysiological stress levels both during and after work compared with workers in more stimulating and flexible jobs. Health-related behaviors, such as cigarette smoking and drug abuse, that are known to contribute to the social gradient in health, can be seen as ways of coping with a stressful work situation in order to get short-term relief. Negative emotional states associated with low-status jobs, combined with a lack of economic resources, are also likely to reduce the individual's motivation to seek proper medical treatment and, thus, increase the risk that transient symptoms develop into chronic illness. With regard to musculoskeletal disorders, it is well documented that physically monotonous or repetitive work is associated with an increase in neck, shoulder, and low back pain problems. However, recent studies also report an association between psychosocial factors and muscle pain syndromes. Possible mechanisms explaining these findings involve the assumption that psychological stress may induce sustained activation of small, low-threshold motor units that may lead to degenerative processes, damage, and pain. Analysis of short periods of very low muscular electrical activity (EMG gaps) shows that female workers with a high frequency of EMG gaps seem to have less risk of developing myalgia problems than do workers with fewer gaps. Stress induced by psychosocial conditions at work, which is usually more lasting than that resulting from physical demands, may prevent the individual from shutting off their physiological activation and reduces the time for rest and recovery. In the modern work environment, with strong emphasis on a high work pace, competitiveness, and efficiency, it is possible that lack of relaxation is an even more important health problem than is the absolute level of contraction or the frequency of muscular activation.

SOCIAL CONDITIONS, STRESS, AND HEALTH

The social gradient in health is well documented and, in many countries, there are indications that inequalities in health have increased during the last decade. This pattern can only partly be explained by differences in exposure to adverse physical conditions, such as poor housing, pollution, chemicals, noise, and crowding. Health-related behaviors, such as cigarette smoking, alcohol abuse, poor eating habits, and

[a]Address for correspondence: Ulf Lundberg, Ph.D., Department of Psychology, Stockholm University, S-106 91 Stockholm, Sweden. 46-8-163874 (voice); 46-8-167847 (fax).
e-mail: ul@psychology.su.se

lack of exercise, are also known to contribute to health differentials. However, relative socioeconomic status seems more relevant to health than the absolute standard of living,[1] and the differences in life style between different social groups can, to a large extent, be considered consequences of environmental conditions. Under the influence of economic stress, low job satisfaction, unemployment or the threat of unemployment, and lack of influence and control over one's life, the individual is more likely to adopt a passive and emotional coping style, involving denial, escapism, overeating, use of tobacco, alcohol, and other drugs. These may give short-term relief in a stressful situation, but contribute to long-term health risks. A passive emotional coping style, combined with lack of economic resources, is also likely to influence the individual's motivation to seek proper medical treatment and, thus, increase the risk that minor symptoms develop into chronic illness.

In addition to the direct effects of the external environment on health (e.g., the influence from noise, vibration, heat, and cold), many health risks are knowledge-based, without direct sensory information (e.g., exposure to UV radiation, radioactive fallout, water and air pollution). In such cases, it is often unclear to what extent the harmful effects are caused by actual exposure or by the fear and anxiety associated with the exposure. In addition, a considerable number of people report symptoms that they tend to attribute to environmental conditions not (yet) known to induce health problems. These include exposure to electromagnetic fields from video display units (VDUs), cellular telephones, or other electrical equipment, amalgam fillings in teeth, and new foods and products. Although many people are convinced that their symptoms are caused by specific environmental factors, so far no scientific evidence exists for these relationships and no mechanisms have been described that can convincingly explain them. Psychological and social factors and media influences on the experience of such symptoms are likely to be great.[2,3]

Most people experience somatic symptoms from time to time for which the professionals cannot provide a medical diagnosis.[4] As humans try to find the environment understandable, predictable, and meaningful,[5] it seems natural for the individual to seek alternative explanations for his or her symptoms. With regard to, for example, lower back pain, most people believe that their symptoms are caused by a physical injury, although this is seldom the case. This could start a vicious circle, where they will avoid exposure to physical demands that they think will create more pain. Through learning mechanisms, this avoidance behavior will be reinforced by reducing anxiety, and the individual will thus avoid exposure to biomechanical demands more and more frequently. Successively, he or she will become weaker and more isolated, eventually ending up with a serious physical and social handicap.[6] Interaction with environmental conditions and personality characteristics will make these relationships even more complex and difficult to analyze. Similar multifactorial phenomena are likely to explain the development of symptoms attributed to, for example, electromagnetic fields.

Social and economic status is largely determined by type of employment, which is closely associated with education. Conditions typical of many low status jobs, such as time pressure, lack of influence over one's work, and constant involvement in repetitive tasks of short duration, are known to cause work stress or strain as described by the Demand–Control Model.[7] High work strain, combined with lack of social support, has been associated with elevated risk of, for example, coronary heart disease.[8]

RESPONSES TO STRESS

Several psychobiological studies[9,10] show that the impact of psychosocial conditions on the individual can be measured in terms of elevated psychophysiological arousal, such as cardiovascular activity and stress hormone levels. Physiological recordings may serve as objective indicators of the stress that an individual is exposed to but, at the same time, these bodily reactions are assumed to link psychosocial factors to somatic symptoms. The various biological functions, such as the autonomic nervous, hypothalamic–pituitary–adrenal cortical (HPA), cardiovascular, metabolic, and immune systems, serve an important role in the organism's adaptation to the environment by protecting and restoring the body. However, under certain conditions, they may also have health-damaging consequences.

Henry[11] integrated findings from animal and human research into a model describing the biological effects and health risks associated with different coping styles. In response to acute stress or threat, the individual's earlier experiences, personality characteristics, and genetic makeup determine his or her way of coping. Two different types of coping strategies can be distinguished: the active defense reaction associated with sympathetic arousal and increased levels of catecholamines, sex hormones, blood lipids, glucose, and so on, and the passive withdrawal or defeat reaction associated with elevated activity of the HPA-axis and cortisol (corticosterone) secretion.

Henry's model[11] is strongly supported by animal research.[12] For example, dominant male baboons on top of the social hierarchy and in control of the group have elevated testosterone levels and low cortisol secretion, whereas subordinate animals show the opposite hormonal pattern with increased activity of the HPA system due to disturbed feedback mechanisms on a central level.[13] Dominant tree shrews (*Tupaia belangeri*) increase their catecholamine output, whereas submissive animals increase their cortisol levels.[14] Similar findings are reported by Kaplan for cynomolgus monkeys in this volume. Although the studies on humans are less conclusive, a similar pattern of responses has been noticed[15] with, for example, elevated cortisol levels associated with anxiety and depressive symptoms,[16] and markedly reduced testosterone levels in male tennis players after losing a match.[17]

As described by McEwen and Seeman in this volume, a new stress model, the allostatic load model,[18,19] refers to the ability to achieve stability through change. Activation of the allostatic systems is necessary for successful coping and survival, whereas over- or underactivity of the allostatic systems may add to the wear-and-tear of the organism. Examples include frequent and intensive activation of physiological systems (cardiovascular, hormonal, metabolic, immune function) without enough time for rest and recovery, or an inability to shut off the allostatic response after the stress exposure, which may cause overactivity and exhaustion of the systems. Lasting high levels of stress hormones increase the risk of cardiovascular illness and immune deficiency, as well as cognitive impairment. Lack of adequate response in one system due to exhaustion may cause compensatory overactivation of other systems.[18]

Health problems are consistently more common among blue-collar workers with low education and income, lack of influence in their work situation, and work that involves monotonous and repetitive tasks than among white-collar workers with more stimulating and varying types of work tasks and more influence over the content and pace of their work. In keeping with this, studies of repetitive and monotonous blue-collar jobs generally show that these workers have more elevated psychophysiological stress levels compared with those in more stimulating and flexible jobs. A review of catecholamine responses to work shows that, whereas white-collar workers increase their epinephrine but not their norepinephrine output at work, manual workers increase both their epinephrine and norepinephrine levels.[20] Thus, blue-collar workers seem to be exposed to greater allostatic loads at work and, in addition, to more elevated stress levels after work.[21] Women seem to be at particular risk,[10] because of the extra burden from unpaid work at home and because they, more often than men, are employed in low-status jobs. This may be relevant for women's greater health problems.[22]

The health risks associated with certain life styles and physical conditions are fairly well documented, whereas less is known about the psychobiological factors linking psychosocial stress to somatic illness. However, as indicated above and in the other chapters of this book, recent research has provided new information on possible mechanisms. In view of the important role played by pain syndromes in the neck, shoulder, and lower back in industrialized countries today, this chapter will focus on the possible pathways between psychosocial factors and musculoskeletal disorders.

MUSCULOSKELETAL DISORDERS

In industrialized countries, large parts of the population suffer from pain syndromes in the neck, shoulders, and lower back; and the costs associated with musculoskeletal disorders (absenteeism, early retirement, medical treatment, and rehabilitation) are considerable. For example, in the Nordic countries, the costs have been estimated to be between 3 and 5% percent of the gross national product and about 30% of these costs can be attributed to work-related factors. Such pain syndromes are more often reported by workers at lower occupational levels, even when the physical work conditions are very similar. Aronsson et al.[23] found that the prevalence of neck and shoulder symptoms was twice as high among workers involved in monotonous VDU work (data entry) compared with that of programmers and system operators.

Musculoskeletal disorders differ from many other major health problems, such as cardiovascular disease and cancer, in that symptoms often appear very early in life and after a relatively short exposure to adverse environmental conditions. In repetitive work, pain syndromes are often reported after only 6–12 months on the job.[24] Thus, people may suffer over very long time periods, and interventions at the workplace aimed at reducing symptoms have, so far, not been very successful.[25–27]

Attempts have been made to establish threshold limit values for static load (e.g., thresholds of 2–5% of maximal voluntary contraction have been suggested for shoulder muscles[28]). However, Westgaard[29] concluded that even very low levels of activation might contribute to the development of chronic pain syndromes.

It is well known that physically monotonous or repetitive work is associated with increased risk of shoulder and neck pain,[30] but recent studies also report an association between psychosocial factors at the workplace and musculoskeletal disorders.

Conditions typical of many low status jobs often characterize jobs associated with a high risk for muscular problems.[31–36] The high prevalence of musculoskeletal disorders in psychologically stressful but light physical work, such as assembly work and data entry, indicate that mental stress plays an important role. In keeping with this, experimental studies show that mental stress, also in the absence of physical demands, increases muscle tension.[37–39]

Thus, several studies indicate that not only physical demands but also psychosocially induced stress may be of significant importance for the development of musculoskeletal disorders. Psychosocial and psychological factors may prevent the individual from shutting off his or her physiological activation and returning to baseline during breaks at work and after the work shift.

Complementing traditional theories, which explain musculoskeletal disorders in terms of insufficient blood circulation due to the high intramuscular pressure during contraction,[40] new theories have been proposed to explain the development of musculoskeletal disorder symptoms in psychologically stressful jobs with a moderate or low physical load.[41–43] The model proposed by Hägg,[41] "The Cinderella Hypothesis" (referring to Cinderella of the fairy tale; who was first to rise and last to go to bed), is based on earlier findings by Henneman et al.,[44] who showed that the motor units of a given muscle are recruited in a fixed order. Small, low-threshold motor units are recruited at low levels of contraction before larger ones, and kept activated until complete relaxation of the muscle. Not only physical demands but also ongoing psychological stress may keep low-threshold motor units active more or less continuously. Wærsted et al.[45] demonstrated continuous activation of low-threshold motor units during a 10-min exposure to cognitive demands in the laboratory. Although these small motor units are assumed to be fatigue resistant, there is likely to be an upper limit for continuous activation.[39] Long-lasting activation of these units may cause degenerative processes, damage, and pain.[39,46]

According to a theory proposed by Schleifer and Ley,[43] stress-induced hyperventilation decreases peak CO_2 levels and increases the blood pH level (which beyond 7.45 becomes alkalosis). Under such conditions, migration of CO_2 molecules from intra- to extracellullar fluid contributes to heightened neuronal excitability, elevated muscular tension, and a suppression of parasympathetic activity. The sympathetic dominance may amplify the responses to catecholamines.

Pain and tension syndromes are often located in the neck–shoulder region, where the density of muscle spindles is very high.[42] The muscle spindles play an important role in the regulation of muscle stiffness and are influenced by mental stress.[47] Inflammatory metabolites from muscle contractions, such as arachidon acid, bradykinin, and serotonin, have strong effects on muscle spindle activity and, at the same time, increase pain sensitivity. This may start a vicious circle,[42] where reduced blood flow in the contracted muscle increases the concentration of the metabolites, which affects the muscle spindles, which increases muscle stiffness and so on. Through nerve signals, increased muscle stiffness and activity of the muscle spindles may spread to other muscles, including muscles located far from the primary one.

A possible pathogenic mechanism for muscle pain is that nociceptors are sensitized as a result of local metabolic changes in fatigued low-threshold (Type I) muscle fibers.[48] The hypothesis of overload of certain motor units is supported by the observation of an increased number of "ragged red" Type I muscle fibers in the trapezius muscle of workers exposed to monotonous shoulder load.[49–51] This is not conclusive evidence, however, because such changes have also been reported in normal muscles.[52]

These models are not contradictory, but all involve the assumption that mental stress may cause muscle tension. Thus, it is likely that stressful jobs may create elevated risk for musculoskeletal disorders through muscular tension induced by psychological stress, which usually is more lasting than physical stress. In addition, there are studies indicating that mental and physical demands may interact and further increase muscle tension and the risk of musculoskeletal disorders.[37]

In an interesting prospective study, Veiersted et al.[24] measured electromyographic (EMG) activity in 21 female packing workers (mean age 25 years) during work and involuntary breaks at work every 10th week from the start of employment. Thirteen women contracted clinically diagnosed trapezius myalgia within the first year, half of them after just six months. EMG data shows that women developing trapezius myalgia problems had higher muscle activity during breaks at work but not during actual work. It was concluded that "sustained low-level muscle activity seems to be a risk factor for muscular pain" (Ref. 24, p.18).

Additional information may be obtained from analysis of the short periods of very low muscular electrical activity (i.e., "EMG gaps"). Female workers with a high frequency of EMG gaps seem to have a reduced risk of developing myalgia problems compared with subjects with a lower level.[53] Similar findings have been reported by Hägg and Åström for female medical secretaries.[54] Recently, we found that female cashiers with trapezius myalgia problems had less EMG rest (20%) in trapezius during work, compared with cashiers without symptoms (30%), although the difference was not statistically significant.[35]

According to a large body of evidence, repetitive and monotonous blue-collar jobs with a high prevalence of back pain problems are associated with elevated psychophysiological stress levels[55–58] and slower physiological unwinding after work, compared with more flexible jobs.[21, 59–62] It is possible that a negative psychosocial work environment will induce health problems independently of the physical situation or, perhaps, even enhance the effects of exposure to adverse physical conditions.

In a recent real-life study of 72 female cashiers working in the supermarket (mean age 37 years), it was found that only 22 women were free of neck–shoulder symptoms.[35] Psychophysiological arousal measured by self reports, blood pressure, heart rate, urinary catecholamines, and EMG activity of the trapezius muscle increased significantly during work. The increase in EMG activity was most pronounced among cashiers with neck and shoulder symptoms, who also reported more tension during and after work and had higher systolic and diastolic blood pressure. Examples of EMG patterns from single individual cashiers showed a successive increase in EMG activity and a decrease in the amount of rest in the trapezius muscle during a two-hour work period. A very unfavorable work–rest pattern in the muscle was already observed after one hour of work.

Unfavorable work–rest patterns may be of significant importance for the development of musculoskeletal disorders. Muscle pain associated with psychological factors at the workplace could be explained by a blocking of pauses in muscle activity unrelated to the actual biomechanical work being performed.[63] This will reduce restitution and contribute to a sustained activity in low-threshold motor units.

CONCLUSIONS

There is evidence that both the temporal pattern and the level of upper trapezius activity are relevant risk indicators for neck and shoulder disorders. Any factor that provokes sustained muscle activity may increase the risk for contracting work-related muscle pain. Thus, it is relevant to explore to what extent mental aspects of low-status jobs contribute to sustained muscle activity in sedentary work with low physical demands, as well as in physically more demanding jobs. In summary, workers involved in repetitive work tasks with lack of influence and control seem to be exposed to higher chronic stress levels and, consequently, more lasting muscle tension than workers in more flexible and stimulating jobs.

In the modern work environment, with its emphasis on time pressure, effectiveness, competitiveness, lean production, and downsizing, it is possible that lack of relaxation is an even more important health risk than is the absolute level of contraction or the frequency of muscular activation because of the way it prevents rest and recovery of the allostatic systems.

A tentative model[64] for the development of musculoskeletal disorders is presented in FIGURE 1. According to this model, mental as well as physical load contributes to elevated muscle tension and physiological stress levels at work. However, conditions at work, such as monotonous and repetitive tasks, lack of influence and control, and a high work pace may influence conditions after work and cause sustained stress levels and muscle tension. Unpaid workload from household chores and children may further contribute to keeping stress levels and muscle tension elevated after work, particularly in women and, thus, contribute to overactivity of the allostatic systems.

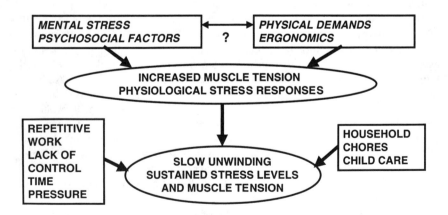

FIGURE 1. A tentative model of musculoskeletal disorders (based on Melin and Lundberg[64]).

CONCLUDING REMARKS

Inequalities in health in the industrialized countries cannot be explained only in terms of differences in exposure to adverse physical conditions and/or health-related behaviors associated with socioeconomic status. Numerous studies suggest an important role for psychosocial factors in the major health problems today, and several plausible psychobiological mechanisms have been proposed for how low social status translates into ill health. Even relative inequality, such as not being able to give your children the same material level as that of your neighbors' children or not being able to travel as often as other people, may create feelings of unfairness and marginalization and induces a passive and emotional coping strategy and an unhealthy life style. In addition, psychobiological stress reactions associated with such conditions as overactivity of the HPA axis, have been demonstrated to increase the risk for a number of health problems, including cardiovascular illness, diabetes, compromised immune function, and cognitive impairment.[18,65] In view of the important role played by neck, shoulder, and back pain problems in the modern work environment, the possible psychobiological mechanisms linking psychosocial work conditions to musculoskeletal disorders are of particular interest.

Information on the psychobiological pathways between psychosocial factors, symptoms, and illness is of great importance for the possibility of preventing and treating environmentally induced ill health. Such knowledge could also help individuals better understand their own health problems and find ways of breaking vicious circles between behavior and symptoms. It may also help to create a more understanding attitude in general toward people who, under negative psychosocial conditions, have developed somatic symptoms. However, most important is that knowledge about these mechanisms is a strong incentive for implementing structural and organizational changes in society in order to prevent people from ending up in socioeconomic conditions contributing to mental and physical disorders. The psychobiological parameters may be used as "warning signals." They may also offer new opportunities for evaluating changes aimed at contributing to better socioeconomic conditions before these are reflected in somatic illness patterns, which usually—but not always—takes a long time. With regard to the enormous costs and suffering associated with, for example, the musculoskeletal disorders, actions leading to even a moderate or small reduction of these health problems would be extremely cost efficient.

ACKNOWLEDGMENT

Financial support has been obtained from the Swedish Council for Work Life Research, the Swedish Council for Research in the Humanities and Social Sciences, and the Bank of Sweden Tercentenary Foundation.

REFERENCES

1. MARMOT, M.G. 1994. Social differentials in health within and between populations. Health Wealth J. Am. Acad. Arts Sci. **123:** 197–216.
2. URSIN, H. 1997. Sensitization, somatization and subjective health complaints. Int. J. Behav. Med. **4:** 105–116.

3. WESSELY, S. 1995. The epidemiology of chronic fatigue syndrome. Epidemiol. Rev. **17:** 139–151.
4. TELLNES, G. 1989. Days lost by sickness certification. Scand. J. Prim. Health Care **7:** 245–251.
5. ANTONOVSKY, A. 1990. The salutogenic model of health. *In* The Healing Brain: A Scientific Reader. R. E. Ornstein & C. Swencioni, Eds.: 231–243. Guilford Press, New York.
6. LINTON, S.J. 1994. The role of psychological factors in back pain and its remediation. Pain Rev. **1:** 231–243.
7. KARASEK, R.A. 1979. Job demands, job decision latitude and mental strain: implications for job redesign. Admin. Sci. Q. **24:** 285–307.
8. JOHNSON, J.V., E. HALL & T. THEORELL. 1989. The combined effects of job strain and social isolation on the prevalence of cardiovascular disease and death in a random sample of the Swedish working male. Scand. J. Work Environ. Health **15:** 271–279.
9. FRANKENHAEUSER, M. 1983. The sympathetic–adrenal and pituitary–adrenal response to challenge: comparison between the sexes. *In* Biobehavioral Bases of Coronary Heart Disease. T.M. Dembroski, T.H. Schmidt & G. Blümchen, Eds.: 91–105. Karger, New York.
10. LUNDBERG, U. 1996. The influence of paid and unpaid work on psychophysiological stress responses of men and women. J. Occup. Health Psychol. **1:** 117–130.
11. HENRY, J.P. 1992. Biological basis of the stress response. Integr. Physiol. Behav. Sci. **1:** 66–83.
12. FOLKOW, B. 1993. Physiological organization of neurohormonal responses to psychosocial stimuli: Implications for health and disease. Ann. Behav. Med. **15:** 236–244.
13. SAPOLSKY, R.M. 1990. Stress in the wild. Studies of free-ranging baboons in an African reserve are helping to explain why human beings can differ in their vulnerability to stress-related disease. Science **262:** 106–113.
14. HOLST, V.D., E. FUCHS & W. STÖHR. 1983. Physiological changes in male *Typaia belangeri* under different types of social stress. *In* Biobehavioral Bases of Coronary Heart Disease. T.M. Dembroski, T.H. Schmidt & G. Blümchen, Eds. Karger, Basel/New York.
15. HENRY, J.P. & P.M. STEPHENS. 1977. Stress, health, and the social environment. A sociobiological approach to medicine. Springer Verlag, New York.
16. SACHAR, E.J. 1970. Psychological factors related to activation and inhibition of the adrenal cortical stress response in man: a review. *In* Progress in Brain Research. Vol. 32. D. de Wied & J.A.M.W. Weijnen, Eds. Elsevier, Amsterdam.
17. MAZUR, A. & A. BOOTH. 1999. Testosterone and dominance in men. Behav. Brain Sci. **21:** 353–363.
18. MCEWEN, B.S. 1998. Protective and damaging effects of stress mediators. N. Engl. J. Med. **238:** 171–179.
19. MCEWEN, B.S. & E. STELLAR. 1993. Stress and the individual: mechanisms leading to disease. Arch. Int. Med. **153:** 2093–2101.
20. LUNDBERG, U. & G. JOHANSSON. 1999. Stress and health risks in repetitive work and supervisory monitoring work. *In* Engineering Psychophysiology: Issues and Applications. R. Backs & W. Boucsein, Eds. Lawrence Erlbaum, New Jersey.
21. MELIN, B., U. LUNDBERG, J. SÖDERLUND & M. GRANQVIST. 1999. Psychophysiological stress reactions of male and female assembly workers: a comparison between two different forms of work organizations. J. Org. Behav. **20:** 47–61.
22. FRANKENHAEUSER, M., U. LUNDBERG & M. CHESNEY. 1991. Women, Work and Health. Stress and Opportunities. Plenum Press, New York.
23. ARONSSON, G., M. DALLNER & C. ÅBORG. 1994. Winners and losers from computerization: a study of the psychosocial work conditions and health of Swedish state employees. Int. J. Hum. Comp. Inter. **6:** 17–35.
24. VEIERSTED, K.B., R.H. WESTGAARD & P. ANDERSEN. 1993. Electromyographic evaluation of muscular work pattern as a predictor of traplezius myalgia. Scand. J. Work Environ. Health **19:** 284–290.
25. EKBERG, K. 1994. An Epidemiological Approach to Disorders in the Neck and Shoulders. Ph.D. Thesis, Linköping University, Sweden.

26. JOSEPHSON, M. 1998. Work Factors and Musculoskeletal Disorders. An Epidemiological Approach Focusing on Female Nursing Personnel. Ph.D. Thesis, Karolinska Institute and National Institute for Working Life, Stockholm, Sweden.
27. LAGERSTRÖM, M. & M. HAGBERG. 1997. Evaluation of a 3 year education and training program for nursing personnel at a Swedish hospital. A. Å. O. H. N. J. **45:** 83–92.
28. JONSSON, B. 1982. Measurement and evaluation of local muscular strain in the shoulder during constrained work. J. Hum. Ergol. **11:** 73–88.
29. WESTGAARD, R. 1988. Measurement and evaluation of postural load in occupational work situations. Eur. J. Appl. Physiol. **5:** 291–304.
30. BERNARD, B.P. 1997. Musculoskeletal disorders and workplace factors. A critical review of epidemiologic evidence for work-related musculoskeletal disorders of the neck, upper extremity, and low back. U.S Department of Health and Human Services, Public Health Service, CDC, and NIOSH, Washington, DC.
31. BAMMER, G. 1990. Review of current knowledge—musculoskeletal problems. *In* Work with Display Units 89. L. Berlinguet & D. Berthelette, Eds.: 113–120. Elsevier Science Publishers B.V., North-Holland.
32. BONGERS, P.M., C.R. DE WINTER, M.A.J. KOMPIER & V.H. HILDEBRANDT. 1993. Psychosocial factors at work and musculoskeletal disease. Scand. J. Work Environm. Health **19:** 297–312.
33. HALDEMAN, S. 1991. Presidential address, North American Spine Society: failure of the pathology model to predict back pain. Spine **15:** 718–724.
34. JOHANSSON, J. 1994. Psychosocial Factors at Work and Their Relation to Musculoskeletal Symptoms. Ph.D. Thesis, Göteborg University, Sweden.
35. LUNDBERG, U., I. ELFSBERG DOHNS, B. MELIN, L. SANDSJÖ, G. PALMERUD, R. KADEFORS, M. EKSTRÖM & D. PARR. 1999. Psychophysiological stress responses, muscle tension and neck and shoulder pain among supermarket cashiers. J. Occup. Health Psychol. **4:** 245–255.
36. MOON, S.D. & S.L. SAUTER, Eds. 1996. Psychosocial Aspects of Musculoskeletal Disorders in Office Work. Taylor & Francis, London.
37. LUNDBERG, U., R. KADEFORS, B. MELIN, G. PALMERUD, P. HASSMÉN, M. ENGSTRÖM & I. ELFSBERG DOHNS. 1994. Psychophysiological stress and EMG activity of the trapezius muscle. Int. J. Behav. Med. **1:** 354–370.
38. SVEBAK, S., R. ANJIA & S.I. KÅRSTAD. 1993. Task-induced electromyographic activation in fibromyalgia subjects and controls. Scand. J. Rheumatol. **22:** 124–130.
39. WÆRSTED, M. 1997. Attention-Related Muscle Activity—a Contributor to Stustained Occupational Muscle Load. Ph.D Thesis, Department of Physiology, National Institute of Occupational Health, Oslo, Norway.
40. MAEDA, K. 1977. Occupational cervicobrachial disorder and its causative factors. J. Hum. Ergol. **6:** 193–202.
41. HÄGG, G. 1991. Static work loads and occupational myalgia—a new explanation model. *In* Electromyographical Kinesiology. P.A. Anderson, D.J. Hobart & J.V. Danhoff, Eds: 141–144. Elsevier Science, Amsterdam.
42. JOHANSSON, H. & P. SOJKA. 1991. Pathophysiological mechanisms involved in genesis and spread of muscular tension in occupational muscle pain and in chronic musculoskeletal pain syndromes: a hypothesis. Med. Hypot. **35:** 196–203.
43. SCHLEIFER, L.M. & R. LEY. 1996. Macroergonomics, breathing, and musculoskeletal problems in computer work. *In* Human Factors in Organizational Design and Management. O. Brown, Jr. & H.W. Hendrick, Eds.: 261–266. Elsevier Science, Amsterdam.
44. HENNEMAN, E., G. SOMJEN & D.O. CARPENTER. 1965. Excitability and inhibitibility of motoneurons of different sizes. J. Neurophys. **28:** 599–620.
45. WÆRSTED, M., T. EKEN & R.H. WESTGAARD. 1996. Activity of single motor units in attention-demanding tasks: firing pattern in the human trapezius muscle. Eur. J. Appl. Physiol. **72:** 323–329.
46. KADEFORS, R., M. FORSMAN, B. ZOÉGA & P. HERBERTS. 1999. Recruitment of low threshold motor units in the trapezius muscle in different arm positions. Ergonomics **42:** 359–375.

47. PEDERSEN, J. 1997. Effects Exerted by Chemosensitive Muscle Afferents and Muscle Fatigue on the g-Muscle-Spindle System and on Proprioception. Ph.D Thesis, Department of Physiology and Technology, National Institute for Working Life, Umeå, and Department of Orthopedics, University of Umeå, Umeå, Sweden.
48. SEJERSTED, O.M. & N.K. VØLLESTAD. 1993. Physiology of muscle fatigue and associated pain. In Progress in Fibromyalgia and Myofascial Pain. H. Værøy & H. Merskey, Eds.: 41–51. Elsevier Science, Amsterdam.
49. LARSSON, S.E., A. BENGTSSON, L. BODEGÅRD, K.G. HENRIKSSON & J. LARSSON. 1988. Muscle changes in work related chronic myalgia. Acta Orthop. Scand. 59: 552–556.
50. LARSSON, B., R. LIBELIUS & K. OHLSSON. 1992. Trapezius muscle changes unrelated to static work load. Chemical and morphologic controlled studies of 22 women with an without neck pain. Acta Orthop. Scand. 63: 203–206.
51. LINDMAN, R., M. HAGBERG, K.-A. ÄNGQVIST, K. SÖDERLUND, E. HULTMAN & L.E. THORNELL. 1991. Changes in muscle morphology in chronic trapezius myalgia. Scand. J. Work Environ. Health 17: 347–355.
52. LINDMAN, R. 1992. Chronic Trapezius Myalgia—a Morphological Study. M.D. Thesis, University of Umeå, Umeå, Sweden.
53. VEIERSTED, B. 1995. Stereotyped Light Manual Work, Individual Factors and Trapezius Myalgia. M.D. Thesis, University of Oslo, Oslo, Norway.
54. HÄGG, G. & A. ÅSTRÖM. 1997. Load pattern and pressure pain threshold in the upper trapezius muscle and psychosocial factors in medical secretaries with and without shoulder/neck disorders. Int. Arch. Occ. Environ. Health 69: 423–432.
55. LUNDBERG, U., M. GRANQVIST, T. HANSSON, M. MAGNUSSON & L. WALLIN. 1989. Psychological and physiological stress responses during work at an assembly line. Work Stress 3: 143–153.
56. COX, S., T. COX, M. THIRLAWAY & C. MACKAY. 1982. Effects of simulated repetitive work on urinary catecholamine excretion. Ergonomics 25: 1129–1141.
57. JOHANSSON, G. 1981. Psychoneuroendocrine correlated of unpaced and paced performance. In Machine Pacing and Occupational Stress. G. Salvendy & M.J. Smith, Eds.: 277–286. Taylor & Francis, London.
58. WEBER, A., C. FUSSLER, J.F. O'HANLON, R. GIERER & E. GRANDJEAN. 1980. Psychophysiological effects of repetitive tasks. Ergonomics 23: 1033–1046.
59. FREUDE, G., P. ULLSBERGER & M. MÖLLE. 1995. Application of Bereitschaftspotentials for evaluation of effort expenditure in the course of repetitive display work. J. Psychophysiol. 9: 65–75.
60. JOHANSSON, G. & G. ARONSSON. 1984. Stress reactions in computerized administrative work. J. Occup. Behav. 5: 159–181.
61. JOHANSSON, G., G. ARONSSON & B.O. LINDSTRÖM. 1978. Social psychological and neuroendocrine stress reactions in highly mechanized work. Ergonomics 21: 583–599.
62. LUNDBERG, U., B. MELIN, G.W. EVANS & L. HOLMBERG. 1993. Physiological deactivation after two contrasting tasks at a video display terminal: learning vs. repetitive data entry. Ergonomics 36: 601–611.
63. ELERT, J.E., S.B. RANTAPÄÄ-DAHLQVIST, K. HENRIKSSON-LARSÉN, R. LORENTZON & B.U.C. GERDLÉ. 1992. Muscle performance, electromyography and fibre type composition in fibromyalgia and work-related myalgia. Scand. J. Rheumatol. 21: 28–34.
64. MELIN, B. & U. LUNDBERG. 1997. A biopsychosocial approach to work-stress and musculoskeletal disorder. J. Psychophysiol. 11: 238–247.
65. BJÖRNTORP, P. 1996. Behavior and metabolic disease. Int. J. Behav. Med. 3: 285–302.

Race, Socioeconomic Status, and Health

The Added Effects of Racism and Discrimination

DAVID R. WILLIAMS[a]

University of Michigan, Department of Sociology and Survey Research Center,
Institute for Social Research, P.O. Box 1248, Ann Arbor, Michigan 48106, USA

ABSTRACT: Higher disease rates for blacks (or African Americans) compared to whites are pervasive and persistent over time, with the racial gap in mortality widening in recent years for multiple causes of death. Other racial/ethnic minority populations also have elevated disease risk for some health conditions. This paper considers the complex ways in which race and socioeconomic status (SES) combine to affect health. SES accounts for much of the observed racial disparities in health. Nonetheless, racial differences often persist even at "equivalent" levels of SES. Racism is an added burden for nondominant populations. Individual and institutional discrimination, along with the stigma of inferiority, can adversely affect health by restricting socioeconomic opportunities and mobility. Racism can also directly affect health in multiple ways. Residence in poor neighborhoods, racial bias in medical care, the stress of experiences of discrimination and the acceptance of the societal stigma of inferiority can have deleterious consequences for health.

This paper provides an overview of the ways in which race and socioeconomic status (SES) combine to affect health status. It first considers patterns of racial differences in health and the role that SES plays in accounting for these disparities. It then describes the nature of racism—the ways in which policies linked to the historic legacy and the persistence of racism have created adverse living conditions that are pathogenic for minority populations. Residential segregation has restricted African-Americans' access to desirable educational and employment opportunities. In combination with other racist mechanisms, it has created the concentrated disadvantage characteristic of many minority communities. The stability of these societal processes has led to remarkable stability in racial economic inequality and in the nonequivalence of SES indicators across race. Finally, the paper considers the ways in which economic discrimination, discrimination in medicine, perceptions of racial bias, and the stigma of inferiority can have pathogenic consequences.

RACE, SES, AND HEALTH

In the United States, race and ethnicity predict variations in health. TABLE 1 illustrates these associations by comparing the mortality rates for all of the major racial/ethnic minority groups to those of the white population.[1] National mortality

[a]Address for correspondence: 734-936-0649 (voice); 734-647-4575 (fax).
e-mail: wildavid@umich.edu

data reveal that the overall death rate for American Indians is similar to that of whites. However, compared to whites, American Indians have lower death rates for cardiovascular disease and cancer but higher rates of death from injuries, the flu and pneumonia, diabetes, suicide, and cirrhosis of the liver. It should be noted that mortality rates for American Indians who live on or near reservations are higher than the national rates for their group.[2] The overall mortality rates for the Hispanic population is lower than that of the white population but Hispanics have higher death rates for diabetes, cirrhosis of the liver, and HIV/AIDS than whites. For all of the leading causes of death in the United States, the Asian Pacific Islander population has mortality rates that are considerably lower than those of whites.

Several factors must be considered to put these data into perspective. First, a nontrivial proportion of nonblack minorities are misclassified as white on the death certificate. This numerator problem leads to an underestimate of the death rates for American Indians, Asian and Pacific Islanders, and Hispanics.[3–4] Second, there is considerable heterogeneity within each of the major racial/ethnic populations that importantly predicts variation in health status within each group. Third, a relatively high proportion of the Hispanic, and especially the Asian-American population, is foreign-born, and their health profile reflects in part the impact of immigration. Immigrants tend to enjoy better health status than the native-born population, even when those immigrants are lower in SES.[5–6] However, with increasing length of stay in the United States and adaptation to mainstream behavior, the health status of immigrants deteriorates.

African Americans (or blacks) have an overall death rate that is 1.6 times higher than that of the white population. Elevated mortality rates for the black compared to the white population exists for eight of the ten leading causes of death. These racial

TABLE 1. Age-adjusted death rates (per 100,000 population) for whites and minority/white ratios for the 10 leading causes of death, United States 1996[a]

Causes	White (W) (Rate)	Black/W Ratio	AmI[b]/W Ratio	API[b]/W Ratio	Hispanic/W Ratio
All causes	**466.8**	**1.58**	**0.98**	**0.59**	**0.78**
1. Heart disease	129.8	1.47	0.78	0.55	0.68
2. Cancer	125.2	1.34	0.68	0.61	0.62
3. Stroke	24.5	1.80	0.86	0.98	0.80
4. Pulmonary disease	21.5	0.83	0.59	0.40	0.41
5. Unintentional injuries	29.9	1.23	1.93	0.54	0.97
6. Flu and pneumonia	12.2	1.45	1.15	0.81	0.80
7. Diabetes	12.0	2.40	2.32	0.73	1.57
8. HIV/AIDS	7.2	5.75	0.58	0.31	2.26
9. Suicide	11.6	0.57	1.12	0.52	0.58
10. Liver cirrhosis	7.3	1.27	2.84	0.36	1.73

[a]Taken from the National Center for Health Statistics.[1]
[b]AmI, American Indian; API, Asian–Pacific Islander.

TABLE 2. Mortality rates for blacks and black/white ratios (age-adjusted death rates per 100,000 for the leading causes of death in 1995)[a]

	1950		1995	
Causes of Death	Black Rate	B/W Ratio	Black Rate	B/W Ratio
All causes	**1236.7**	**1.55**	**765.7**	**1.58**
1. Heart disease	379.6	1.26	198.8	1.49
2. Cancer	129.1	1.04	171.6	1.35
3. Cerebrovascular disease	150.9	1.81	45.0	1.82
4. Pulmonary disease	—	—	17.6	0.83
5. Unintentional injury	70.9	1.27	37.4	1.25
6. Flu and pneumonia	57.0	2.49	17.8	1.44
7. Diabetes	17.2	1.24	28.5	2.44
8. HIV/AIDS	—	—	51.8	4.67
9. Suicide	4.2	0.36	6.9	0.58
10. Cirrhosis	7.2	0.84	9.9	1.34
11. Homicide	30.5	11.73	33.4	6.07

[a]Taken from the National Center for Health Statistics.[1]

disparities have been documented for a long time and have been widening in recent years for multiple indicators of health status. TABLE 2 presents the mortality rates for blacks and the black/white mortality ratios for 1950 and 1995.[1] Although the overall mortality rate for African Americans has declined over time, for several causes of death (cancer, diabetes, suicide, cirrhosis of the liver, and homicide) the mortality rate is higher in 1995 than in 1950. Moreover, the black/white ratio for all-cause mortality in 1995 is virtually identical to that of 1950. Black/white mortality ratios over this 45-year period are virtually unchanged for some causes of death, such as stroke and unintentional injury, and smaller for two causes of death (the flu

TABLE 3. United States life expectancy, at age 45 by family income (1980 dollars)[a]

	Females			Males		
Family Income	White	Black	Difference	White	Black	Difference
All[b]	**36.3**	**32.6**	**3.7**	**31.1**	**26.2**	**4.9**
1. Less than $10,000	35.8	32.7	3.1	27.3	25.2	2.1
2. $10,000–$14,999	37.4	33.5	3.9	30.3	28.1	2.2
3. $15,000–$24,999	37.8	36.3	1.5	32.4	31.3	1.1
4. $25,000 or more	38.5	36.5	2.0	33.9	32.6	1.3

[a]1979–1989; Taken from the National Center for Health Statistics.[1]
[b]1989–1991; Taken from the National Center for Health Statistics.[7]

and pneumonia and homicide). However, the black/white mortality ratios in 1995 are larger than those in 1950 for heart disease, cancer, diabetes, and cirrhosis of the liver.

Socioeconomic status predicts variation in health within minority and white populations and accounts for much of the racial differences in health. TABLE 3 illustrates these data for life expectancy. At age 45, white males have a life expectancy that is almost five years more than their black counterparts.[7] Similarly, white females have a life expectancy at age 45 that is 3.7 years longer than that of their black peers. However, there is considerable variation in life expectancy within both racial groups.[1] Black men in the highest income group live 7.4 years longer than those in the lowest income group. The comparable numbers for whites was 6.6 years. Thus, the SES difference within each racial group is larger than the racial difference across groups. A similar pattern is evident for women, although the SES differences are smaller. At age 45, black women in the highest income group have a life expectancy that is 3.8 years longer than those in the lowest income group. Among whites, the SES difference is 2.7 years. Also evident in the life expectancy data is an independent effect of race even when SES is controlled. At every level of income, for both men and women, African Americans have lower levels of life expectancy than their similarly situated white counterparts. This pattern has been observed across multiple health outcomes and for some indicators of health status, such as infant mortality, the racial gap becomes larger as SES increases.[1]

RACE AND RACISM IN THE UNITED STATES

How do we understand these differences? What is race, and what contribution does racism make to these persisting patterns of racial differences in health? Our current racial categories were created before the development of valid scientific theories of genetics and do not capture biological distinctiveness.[8–10] The American Association of Physical Anthropology[11] recently stated that "Pure races in the sense of genetically homogenous populations do not exist in the human species today, nor is there any evidence that they have ever existed in the past." There is considerable biological variation in human populations, but our racial categories fail to capture it. There is more genetic variation within our existing racial groups than between them. Moreover, genetics is not static but changes over time as human populations interact with their natural and social environment. In the United States, our racial groups importantly capture differences in power, status, and resources. Three of the five official racial/ethnic categories were used in the inaugural census in 1790 and these groups were not regarded as equal. In compliance with the First Article of the United States Constitution, that census enumerated whites, blacks as three-fifths of a person, and civilized Indians (that is, Indians who paid taxes). The Thirteenth Amendment abandoned the three-fifths rule, and over time new racial categories were developed to keep track of new immigrants.[12]

Historically, racial categorization has been rooted in racism, and racial classification schemes have had an implicit or explicit relative ranking of various racial groups. Within the U.S. context, whites have always been at the top, blacks at the bottom, and other groups in between. The construct of racism can enhance our understanding of racial inequalities in health. By racism, I mean an ideology of inferiority that is used to justify unequal treatment (discrimination) of members of groups defined as inferior, by both individuals and societal institutions. This ideology of inferiority may lead to the development of negative attitudes and beliefs towards racial outgroups (prejudice), but racism primarily lies within organized institutional structures and not in individual attitudes or behaviors.[13]

First, is the endorsement of an ideology of inferiority a relic of a bygone era? On the one hand, there have been dramatic improvements in the racial climate in the United States in the last 50 years.[14] For example, national data reveal that in 1942 only 32% of whites with school-aged children believed that white and black children should go to the same schools. Ninety-six percent of white parents supported that view in 1995. Similarly, in 1958 only 37% of whites stated that they would vote for a qualified black man for President of the United States. In 1997, 95% of whites indicated that they would vote for a black person for President. At the same time, other data indicate that racial attitudes are complex. Overwhelming support for the principle of equality coexists with a reluctance to support policies that would reduce racial inequalities.[14]

Moreover, data on stereotypes reveal the persistence of negative images of minority racial/ethnic populations in the United States. National data reveal that 45% of whites believe that most blacks are lazy, 51% indicated that most blacks are prone to violence, 29% that most blacks are unintelligent, and 56% that most blacks prefer to live off welfare.[15] These data also reveal a reluctance to endorse positive stereotypes of African Americans. Only 17% of whites indicated that most blacks are hard-working, 15% that most blacks are not prone to violence, 21% that most blacks are intelligent, and 12% that most blacks prefer to be self-supporting. These data are even more striking when compared with whites' perceptions of themselves and other groups. In general, whites view all minority racial groups more negatively than themselves, with blacks being viewed more negatively than any other group. Hispanics tend to be viewed twice as negatively as Asians. Jews tend to be viewed more positively, and southern whites more negatively, than whites in general.

RACISM AND SES

How does racism affect health? First, and most importantly, racism has restricted socioeconomic attainment for members of minority groups. By determining access to educational and employment opportunities, segregation has been a key mechanism by which racial inequality has been created and reinforced.[16] It is generally recognized that there are large racial differences in SES, and health researchers routinely adjust for SES when examining the race–health association. However, SES is not just a confounder of racial differences in health but part of the causal pathway by which race affects health. Race is an antecedent and determinant of SES, and racial differences in SES reflect, in part, the successful implementation of discriminatory policies premised on the inferiority of certain racial groups.

Arguably, the single most important policy of this type that continues to have pervasive adverse effects on the socioeconomic circumstances and the health of African Americans is residential segregation. Beliefs about black inferiority and an explicit desire to avoid social contact with this out-group led to the development of policies in the early 20th century that aimed at ensuring the physical separation of blacks from whites in residential areas.[17] This physical separation was possible through co-operative efforts of major societal institutions.[18] Between 1900 and the 1940s, fed-eral housing policies, the lending practices of banks, restrictive covenants, and discrimination by the real estate industry, individuals and vigilant neighborhood organizations, ensured that housing options for blacks were restricted to the least desirable residential areas. Audit studies reveal that explicit discrimination in hous-ing persists,[19] but most of the institutional discrimination that created segregation is now illegal. However, the structure of segregation and its consequences have re-mained relatively intact over time.

TABLE 4 shows the average levels of segregation in the 30 metropolitan areas with the largest black populations between 1970 and 1990.[20] Data are provided for two of the most commonly used measures of segregation. The index of dissimilarity, a measure of unevenness, captures the percent of blacks who would have to change neighborhood residence to achieve complete integration. The isolation index indi-cates the percent of blacks in the census tract where the average black person resides. Segregation is slightly higher in the North than in the South but in both regions the levels of segregation are very high. In 1990, for example, 78% of blacks in northern metropolitan areas would have to move in order to achieve a random distribution of blacks and whites. In the South, 67% of blacks would have to move. Similarly, in 1990 the average African American living in the North resided in a census tract that was 69% black. In the South, the average black lived in a neighborhood that was 65% black. There has been little change in these levels of segregation in the last 20 years. While other groups have experienced residential segregation in the United States, no immigrant population has ever lived under the high levels of segregation that current-ly characterize the living circumstances of African Americans.[16] Moreover, the high level of segregation of the black population is not self-imposed because blacks re-flect the highest support for residence in integrated neighborhoods.[21]

Residential segregation has led to racial differences in the quality of elementary and high school education. Because the funding of education is at the local level, community resources importantly determine the quality of the neighborhood school.

TABLE 4. Average segregation in 30 metropolitan areas with largest black populations[a]

Area[b]	1970	1980	1990
Non-South			
1. Unevenness	84.5	80.1	77.8
2. Isolation	68.7	66.1	68.9
South			
1. Unevenness	75.3	68.3	66.5
2. Isolation	69.3	63.5	64.9

[a]Taken from Massey.[20]

[b]Unevennes, percent of blacks who would have to change residence to achieve an even spatial distribution; isolation, percent of blacks in the census tract where the average black person resides.

Residential segregation had led to the concentration of poverty in residential areas and thus the concentration of poverty in the classroom. Not withstanding a unanimous Supreme Court ruling in *Board vs. Board of Education,* elementary and high school public education in the United States today is still highly segregated and decidedly unequal.[22] Moreover, even in integrated schools, black students are disproportionately allocated or tracked into low-ability and non–college preparatory classes that are characterized by a less demanding curriculum and lower teacher expectations.[18]

Two-thirds of African-American students and three-fourths of Hispanic students attend schools where more than half the students are black or Latino.[23] The proportion of black and especially Hispanic students in predominantly minority schools has been increasing in recent years. There is nothing inherently negative with having most of one's fellow classmates being members of minority groups. The problem is the very strong relationship between racial composition of schools and concentrated poverty. In the United States a student in an intensely segregated African-American and/or Latino school is 14 times more likely to be in a high-poverty school than a student in a school where less than 10% of the students are black and Latino.[22] Nationally, the correlation between minority percentage and poverty is 0.66.[23] In metropolitan Chicago this percentage is 0.90 for elementary schools.[22] There are millions of poor whites in the United States, but most poor white families do not live in areas of concentrated poverty and thus have access to better options in terms of educational opportunities. In 96% of predominantly white schools in the United States the majority of the students come from middle class backgrounds,

Residential segregation also adversely affects SES by having a profound negative impact on employment. Several mechanisms appear to be at work. William Julius Wilson[24–25] has documented that the selective out-migration of whites and some middle class blacks from the core areas of cities (where most blacks reside) to the suburbs over the last several decades has been accompanied by the movement of high-pay, low-skill jobs to the suburbs. This movement of jobs is related to larger processes of urbanization and industrialization, but some evidence suggests that considerations of race have explicitly played a role. African Americans have had significantly higher rates of industrial job losses than whites in recent decades, and research reveals that both U.S.-based and foreign companies explicitly use the racial composition of areas in their decision-making process regarding where to locate new plants.[26] This is true both for the placement of new plants and for the relocation of other plants to more rural and suburban areas. Consistent with this evidence, a *Wall Street Journal* analysis of over 35,000 U.S. companies that report to the Equal Employment Opportunity Commission found that blacks were the only racial group that experienced a net job loss during the 1990–1991 economic downturn.[27] African Americans had a net job loss of 59,000 jobs, compared with net gains of 71,100 for whites, 55,100 for Asians, and 60,000 for Latinos. These job losses did not reflect individual discrimination but rather were the result of restructuring, relocation, and downsizing. In many cases, they reflected the movement of employment facilities to suburban, rural, and southern areas where the proportion of blacks in the labor force was low.

Discrimination at the individual level also plays a role in reducing employment opportunities for minority group members. Studies of white employers reveal that they consciously and deliberately use negative racial stereotypes to deny employment opportunities to black applicants.[28–29] Some of the best evidence of the persistence of discrimination in employment comes from audit studies conducted by the Urban Institute. In these studies, white applicants were favored over black applicants with identical qualifications 20% of the time.[19] Thus, negative racial stereotypes of African Americans appear to play a role both when individual employers evaluate potential applicants, as well as when corporate decision makers deliberate about the location of employment facilities.

Impoverished segregated areas have multiple adversities that may combine in additive and interactive ways to adversely affect SES. Lack of access to jobs produces high rates of male unemployment. There is a strong relationship, for both blacks and whites, between rates of marriage and rates of male unemployment and average male earnings. Thus, the concentration of economic disadvantage in impoverished segregated areas is a major force underlying high rates of out-of-wedlock births and female-headed households and the consequent feminization of poverty that occurs in many urban areas.[30–31] The resulting concentration of poverty isolates youth in segregated communities from both role models of stable employment and social networks that can provide linkages to employment opportunities.[24] Long-term exposure to these conditions can undermine a strong work ethic and devalue academic success.

Racism can also affect SES attainment through the impact of negative racial stereotypes on educational outcomes. Steele[32] has reviewed the evidence that suggests that the negative cultural images of blacks may adversely affect academic performance. He indicates that there is little racial difference between blacks and whites on standardized tests in the first grade. However, a racial gap widens with each year in school and is two full grade levels by the sixth grade. This pattern is not explained by either SES or group differences in skills. Moreover, achievement gaps between blacks, as well as non-Asian minorities, are evident at all levels of SES and sometimes widen with increasing SES. Further, at every skill level, non-Asian minorities receive lower grades than whites. A similar pattern exists for women relative to men but only in those areas of academic performance where women are sterotypically viewed as deficient (such as in the physical sciences and in advanced math courses). Research from the U.K., Israel, Japan, India, and other countries reveal that groups viewed as lower in social status consistently have lower academic achievement.[33] Steele[32] suggests that among lower SES blacks the internalization of negative societal stereotypes may become a self-fulfilling prophecy leading to low performance. In contrast, among high SES, self-confident blacks, the threat of poor performance in a stereotype-relevant domain may lead to anxieties that adversely affect academic performance.

STABILITY OF RACIAL INEQUALITY

Institutional policies have played a major role in creating large racial differences in SES. Because of the persistence of the institutional mechanisms underlying racial inequality, there has been remarkable stability in the racial gap in SES over time. The President's Council of Economic Advisors' recent review of trends in racial econom-

TABLE 5. Median income and poverty rates for whites and blacks, United States 1978–1996[a]

Year	Median Income			Poverty Rate		
	Whites	Blacks	B/W Ratio	Whites	Blacks	B/W Ratio
1978	42,695	25,288	0.59	8.7	30.6	3.52
1980	41,759	24,162	0.58	10.2	32.5	3.19
1982	40,379	22,317	0.55	12.0	35.6	2.97
1984	41,809	23,302	0.56	11.5	33.8	2.94
1986	44,105	25,201	0.57	11.0	31.1	2.83
1988	44,981	25,636	0.57	10.1	31.3	3.10
1990	44,315	25,717	0.58	10.7	31.9	2.98
1992	43,245	23,600	0.55	11.9	33.4	2.81
1994	43,284	26,148	0.60	11.7	30.6	2.62
1996	44,756	26,522	0.59	11.2	28.4	2.54

[a]Taken from the Economic Report of the President.[34]

ic inequalities documented that the expansion of the black middle class and the convergence toward equality between blacks and whites was greatest in the 1960s.[34] In spite of current efforts to dismantle affirmative action policies, the data clearly show that the economic progress of blacks relative to whites stalled in the mid-1970s, and there has been 20 years of stagnation since then. Moreover, income inequality has increased since 1970 overall and within both racial groups.

TABLE 5 shows that in 1978, the median family income of blacks ($25,288) was 59 cents for every dollar earned by whites in median family income ($42,695). In 1996, the black/white ratio of median family income was identical to that of 1978, and there had been little change during the intervening 23 years. Similarly, the poverty levels for both blacks and whites have been relatively stable over time.[34] The poverty rate of blacks (30.6%) was 3.5 times higher than that of whites (8.7%) in 1978. The black poverty rate declined to 28.4 in 1996, and the poverty rate of whites increased somewhat to 11.2 in 1996. Thus, the black/white ratio fell slightly, with blacks being 2.5 times more likely to live in poverty in 1996, compared to whites. Longer trend data tell the same story. TABLE 6 presents the unemployment rates for blacks and whites from 1950 to 1995.[34] Since 1950, African Americans have had unemployment rates that have been about twice as high as that of whites. Over time, the unemployment of both blacks and whites have moved up and down with the business cycle, but the changes for African Americans have been at about twice the rate for whites. There have been modest gains in unemployment in the last few years, but in 1995 blacks still had an unemployment rate that was twice that of whites. These data provide striking evidence of persistent racial inequality in the United States.

Because of the operation of these large-scale societal processes, indicators of SES are not equivalent across racial groups. That is true at the level of the community, the household, and the individual. Because of residential segregation, black and white

TABLE 6. Unemployment rates for blacks and whites, 1950–1995[a]

Year	Black	White	B/W Ratio
1950	9.0	4.9	1.84
1955	8.7	3.9	2.23
1960	10.2	5.0	2.04
1965	8.1	4.1	1.98
1970	8.2	4.5	1.82
1975	14.8	7.8	1.90
1980	14.3	6.3	2.27
1985	13.7	6.2	2.21
1990	11.4	4.8	2.38
1995	9.6	4.9	1.96

[a]Taken from the Economic Report of the President.

neighborhoods differ dramatically in the availability of jobs, family structure, opportunities for marriage, educational quality, and exposure to conventional role models. They also differ in the quality of life and access to resources and amenities that sustain health. For example, Sampson and Wilson[35] found that in the 171 largest cities in the United States, there is not even one city where whites live in ecological equality to blacks in terms of poverty rates and rates of single-parent households. In fact, Sampson and Wilson concluded that, "The worst urban context in which whites reside is considerably better than the average context of black communities."[35]

TABLE 7 presents racial differences in the income return from education for blacks, whites, and Hispanics in 1996.[36] These national data reveal that at every level of education blacks and Hispanics have lower levels of income than whites. Although part of this difference may be due to differences in educational performance and quality, some evidence suggests that other factors are at work. For example, a recent study documented that even after taking racial differences in test scores into account, young black males earned 7.5% less than their white counterparts.[37] Other

TABLE 7. Median income by educational attainment for whites, blacks, and hispanics aged 18 years and older, United States 1996[a]

Education Level	White	Black	Hispanic
Not a high school graduate	$9,762	$7,365	$9,486
High school graduate	$16,331	$13,294	$13,408
Some college or associate degree	$23,480	$20,249	$20,225
Bachelor's degree or more	$30,121	$26,160	$25,302
Professional degree	$56,436	$42,237	—

[a]Taken from the U.S. Bureau of the Census.[36]

data reveal that blacks have higher costs for goods and services than whites due to higher prices on average for a broad range of services such as housing, food, and insurance in the central city areas where blacks live than in suburban areas where most whites reside.[38]

Moreover, racial differences in income understate the true magnitude of the racial differences in economic resources. National data reveal that at every level of income there are large racial differences in wealth. For example, white households have a median net worth that is 10 times that of African-American households.[39] Whites in the lowest quintile of income have a median net worth of $10,257 compared to $1 for comparable blacks. Because much of the wealth of most American families exists in the form of home equity, a substantial part of this racial difference is linked to housing policies and institutional discrimination experienced in the past.[40] These racial differences in economic circumstances are consequential to the day-to-day struggle for survival for minority group members. In the early 1990s, the Census Bureau's Survey of Income and Program Participation collected data on the economic hardship experienced by American households. These data reveal that after adjustment for SES (income, education, transfer payments, home ownership, employment status, disability, and health insurance) and demographic factors (age, gender, marital status, the presence of children, and residential mobility), African Americans were more likely than whites to experience six of nine hardships examined: unable to meet essential expenses, unable to pay for rent or mortgage, unable to pay full utility bill, had utilities shut off, had telephone service shut off, and evicted from apartment or home.[41] There were no racial differences on lacking visits to a doctor and not having enough food. Blacks were less likely than whites to have no visit to a dentist.

RACISM AND HEALTH: DIRECT EFFECTS

A growing body of research also suggests that in addition to its effects on health indirectly through socioeconomic position, exposure to racism and discrimination can also more directly adversely affect health. First, residential segregation can create pathogenic housing and living conditions. Segregation is often a key determinant of quality of life in neighborhoods. Residents of highly segregated neighborhoods have less access to a broad range of services provided by municipal authorities.[42] Reductions in spending and the delivery of services leads to the neglect and deterioration of the physical environment in poor neighborhoods. The redlining by banks can result in the disproportionate representation of undesirable land uses, such as deserted factories, warehouses, and landfills in segregated areas. Persons who reside in segregated neighborhoods may also be disproportionately exposed to environmental toxins and poor-quality housing. The largest black–white difference in mortality noted earlier was for homicide. Research reveals that the combination of concentrated poverty, male joblessness, and residential instability leads to high rates of single parent households and these factors together account for variation in the levels of violent crime.[35] Importantly, the association between these factors and violent crime for whites was virtually identical in magnitude with the association for African Americans.

Several studies have found a positive association between both adult and infant mortality and residence in segregated areas. One recent study has documented elevated mortality rates for both blacks and whites in cities high on two indices of segregation compared to cities with lower levels of segregation.[43] This pattern suggests that beyond some threshold of segregation, the adverse conditions linked to highly segregated cities may negatively affect the health of all persons who reside there.

Another mechanism by which discrimination can affect health status is through access to medical care. The stigma of racial inferiority appears to affect the way that minority group members are treated in the health care system. A large body of evidence indicates that even after adjustment for SES, health insurance, and clinical status whites are more likely than blacks to receive a broad range of specific medical procedures.[44] Especially striking is data from the Veterans Administration Hospital System[45] and from analyses of the receipt of diagnostic and treatment procedures among black and white inpatients covered by Medicare.[46] Among Medicare inpatients, blacks were less likely than whites to receive all of the 16 most common procedures. Further examination revealed that there were only four procedures that blacks were more likely to receive than whites. Blacks were more likely than whites to have the amputation of a lower limb, the removal of both testes, the removal of tissue related to decubitus ulcers and the implantation of shunts for renal dialysis.[46] These procedures all reflected delayed diagnosis or initial treatment, poor or infrequent medical care and the failure in the management of chronic disease.

A recent study by Hannan et al.[47] demonstrated that African Americans were less likely than whites to receive bypass surgery when rigorous criteria demonstrated that the procedure was appropriate, as well as when rigorous criteria indicated that it was necessary. Similarly, a study by Peterson et al.[48] documented that blacks were less likely than whites with comparable disease to receive bypass surgery even among those patients with the most severe disease and with the greatest predictive benefit of survival. Moreover, this study found that the five-year survival rate was significantly lower for blacks. Other recent research indicates that patient preferences and patient refusals play little role in racial differences in the receipt of medical procedures.[47] Taken together, these studies suggest that consciously or unconsciously, a nontrivial proportion of the health care workforce discriminates against African Americans.

Some research also suggests that the subjective experience of discrimination may be an important type of stress that can adversely affect health. A review of these studies reveals that exposure to stress in a laboratory setting can lead to cardiovascular and psychological reactivity among blacks, as well as for a broad range of other groups.[49] In addition, population-based epidemiologic studies also reveal that experiences of discrimination are adversely related to both physical and mental health. One recent study of a major metropolitan area characterized exposure to a broad range of unfair treatment experiences.[50] This study documented that compared to whites, African Americans experienced higher levels of both chronic and acute measures of discrimination and markedly higher levels of discrimination based on race or ethnicity. Importantly, analyses of these data documented that most of the racial difference in physical health was accounted for by SES. However, the consideration of experiences of discrimination made an incremental contribution in accounting for racial differences in self-reported measures of physical health. Studies of the health consequences of experiences of discrimination are still in their infancy, and there is an urgent need for prospective studies that would identify the temporal ordering of the relationship between discrimination and health.

What does it mean for a child to grow up in a society where he or she is viewed as being inferior and where those messages are routinely communicated in multiple ways? A small body of research suggests that the prevalence of negative stereotypes and cultural images of stigmatized groups can adversely affect health status. Researchers have long identified that one response of minority populations would be to accept the dominant society's ideology of their inferiority as accurate. Several studies have operationalized the extent to which African Americans internalize or endorse these negative cultural images. These studies have found that internalized racism is positively related to psychological distress, depressive symptoms, substance use, and chronic physical health problems.[51-53]

CONCLUSION

Striking racial differences in health and their persistence over time are not acts of God. Neither can they be understood as simply reflecting racial differences in individual behavior or biology. Instead, considerable evidence suggests that they reflect, in large part, the successful implementation of specific policies. Racism has been responsible for the development of an organized system of policies and practices designed to create racial inequality. Research is needed that would identify how large societal forces shape individual beliefs and behavior and combine with preexisting resources and vulnerabilities to affect health status. Social factors ultimately affect health through specific physiological mechanisms and processes. The concept of allostatic load provides a useful framework for tracing the pathways from environmental exposure to adverse changes in health status via explicit physiological processes.[54] Racial differences in health importantly reflect the impact of the social environment and the cumulation of adversity across multiple domains. Efforts to improve the health of racial minority group members and reduce racial disparities in health may have to be equally comprehensive in the implementation of strategies that address the fundamental underlying causes of these disparities.

ACKNOWLEDGMENTS

Preparation of this paper was supported by Grant 1 RO1 MH59575 from NIMH and the John D. and Catherine T. MacArthur Foundation Research Network on Socieoeconomic Status and Health. I wish to thank Scott Wyatt and Colwick Wilson for research assistance and Car Nosel for preparing the manuscript.

REFERENCES

1. NATIONAL CENTER FOR HEALTH STATISTICS. 1998. Health, United States, 1998 with Socioeconomic Status and Health Chartbook. USDHHS. Hyattsville, MD.
2. DEPARTMENT OF HEALTH AND HUMAN SERVICES-INDIAN HEALTH SERVICE. 1997. Regional Differences in Indian Health. DHHS. Rockville, MD.

3. SORLIE, P.D., E. ROGOT & N.J. JOHNSON. 1993. Validity of demographic characteristics on the death certificate. Epidemiology **3:** 181–184.
4. HAHN, J.A. 1992. The state of federal health statistics on racial and ethnic groups. JAMA **267:** 268–271.
5. SINGH, G.K. & S.M. YU. 1996. Adverse pregnancy outcomes: differences between U.S.- and foreign-born women in major U.S. racial and ethnic groups. Am. J. Public Health **86:** 837–843.
6. HUMMER, R.A., R.G. ROGERS, C.B. NAM & F.B. LeCLERE. 1999. Race/ethnicity, nativity, and U.S. adult mortality. Soc. Sci. Q. **80:** 136–153.
7. NATIONAL CENTER FOR HEALTH STATISTICS. 1997. U.S. Decennial Life Tables for 1989–91. Hyattsville, MD. U.S. Life Tables **1**(1): 12–29.
8. MONGATU, A. 1964. The Concept of Race. New York Press, Glenco.
9. GOULD, S.J. 1977. Why we should not name human races: a biological view. *In* Ever Since Darwin. S.J. Gould, Ed.: 231–236. W.W. Norton, New York.
10. LEWONTIN, R.C. 1972. The apportionment of human diversity. *In* Evolutionary Biology. Vol. 6. T. Dobzhansky, M.K. Hecht & W.C. Steere, Eds.: 381–386. Appleton-Century-Crofts, New York.
11. AMERICAN ASSOCIATION OF PHYSICAL ANTHROPOLOGY. 1996. AAPA statement on biological aspects of race. Am. J. Phys. Anthropol. **101:** 569–570.
12. ANDERSON, M. & S.E. FEINBERG. 1995. Black, white, and shades of gray (and brown and yellow). Chance **8:** 15–18.
13. BONILLA-SILVA, E. 1996. Rethinking racism: toward a structural interpretation. Am. Sociol. Rev. **62:** 465–480.
14. SCHUMAN, H., CH. STEEH, L. BOBO & M. KRYSAN. 1997. Racial Attitudes in America: Trends and Interpretations. Rev. edit. Harvard University Press, Cambridge.
15. DAVIS, J.A. & T.W. SMITH. 1990. General Social Surveys, 1972–1990 NORC edit. National Opinion Research Center, Chicago.
16. MASSEY, D.S. & N.A. DENTON. 1993. American Apartheid: Segregation and the Making of the Underclass. Harvard University Press, Cambridge.
17. CELL, J. 1982. The Highest Stage of White Supremacy: The Origin of Segregation in South Africa and the American South. Cambridge University Press, New York.
18. JAYNES, G.D. & R.M. WILLIAMS. 1987. A Common Destiny: Blacks and American Society. National Academy Press, Washington, D.C.
19. FIX, M. & R.J. STRUYK. 1993. Clear and Convincing Evidence: Measurement of Discrimination in America. Urban Institute Press, Washington, D.C.
20. MASSEY, D. 1999. Residential segregation and neighborhood conditions in U.S. metropolitan areas. *In* America Becoming: Racial Trends and Their Consequences. William Julius Wilson & Faith Mitchel, Eds. National Research Council Commission on Behavioral and Social Sciences and Education. National Academy of Sciences Press, Washington, DC. In press.
21. BOBO, L. & C.L. ZUBRINSKY. 1996. Attitudes on residential integration: perceived status differences, mere in-group preference, or racial prejudice? Soc. Forces **74:** 883–909.
22. ORFIELD, G. & S.E. EATON. 1996. Dismantling desegregation: The Quiet Reversal of *Brown v. Board of Education.* The New Press, New York.
23. ORFIELD, G. 1993. The growth of segregation in American schools: changing patterns of separation and poverty since 1968. A report of the Harvard Project on School Desegregation to the National School Boards Association.
24. WILSON, W.J. 1987. The Truly Disadvantaged. University of Chicago Press, Chicago.
25. WILSON, W.J. 1996. When Work Disappears: The World of the New Urban Poor. Alfred A. Knopf, New York.
26. COLE, R.E. & D.R. DESKINS, JR. 1988. Racial factors in site location and employment patterns of Japanese auto firms in America. Calif. Manage. Rev. **31:** 9–22.
27. SHARPE, R. 1993. In latest recession, only blacks suffered net employment loss. Wall St. J. **LXXIV:** no. 233.
28. KIRSCHENMAN, J. & K.M. NECKERMAN. 1991. "We'd love to hire them, but...": the meaning of race for employers. *In* The Urban Underclass. C. Jencks & P.E. Peterson, Eds.: 203–232. The Brookings Institution, Washington, D.C.

29. NECKERMAN, K.M. & J. KIRSCHENMAN. 1991. Hiring strategies, racial bias, and inner-city workers. Soc. Problems **38:** 433–447.
30. TESTA, M., N.M. ASTONE, M. KROGH & K.M. NECKERMAN. 1993. Employment and marriage among inner-city fathers. *In* The Ghetto Underclass. W.J. Wilson, Ed.: 96–108. Sage, Newberry Park.
31. WILSON, W. & K.M. NECKERMAN. 1986. Poverty and family structure: the widening gap between evidence and public policy issues. *In* Fighting Poverty. S.H. Danziger and D.H. Weinberg, Eds.: 232–259. Harvard University Press, Cambridge.
32. STEELE, C.M. 1997. A threat in the air: how stereotypes shape intellectual identity and performance. Am. Psychol. **52:** 613–629.
33. FISCHER, C.S., M. HOUT, M.S. JANKOWSKI, S.R. LUCAS, A. SWIDLER & K. VOSS. 1996. Race, ethnicity and intelligence. *In* Inequality by Design: Cracking the Bell Curve Myth. C.S. Fischer, M. Hout, M.S. Jankowski, S.R. Lucas, A. Swidler & K. Voss, Eds. Princeton University Press, Princeton.
34. ECONOMIC REPORT OF THE PRESIDENT. 1998. U.S. Government Printing Office, Washington, DC.
35. SAMPSON, R.J. & W.J. WILSON. 1995. Toward a theory of race, crime, and urban inequality. *In* Crime and Inequality. J. Hagan & R.D. Peterson, Eds.: 37–54. Stanford University Press, Stanford.
36. U.S. BUREAU OF THE CENSUS. 1997. Income by educational attainment for persons 18 years old and over, by age, sex, race, and Hispanic origin: March 1996, Current Population Report. U.S. Government Printing Office, Washington, D.C.
37. NEAL, D.A. & W.R. JOHNSON. 1996. The role of premarket factors in black–white wage differences. J. Polit. Econ. **104:** 869–895.
38. WILLIAMS, D.R. & C. COLLINS. 1995. U.S. socioeconomic and racial differences in health. Ann. Rev. Sociol. **21:** 349–386.
39. ELLER, T.J. 1994. Household Wealth and Asset Ownership: 1991. U.S. Bureau of the Census, Current Population Reports, P70–34. US Government Printing Office (USGPO), Washington, D.C.
40. OLIVER, M.L. & T.M. SHAPIRO. 1997. Black Wealth/White Wealth: A New Perspective on Racial Inequality. Routledge, New York.
41. BAUMAN, K. 1998. Direct measures of poverty as indicators of economic need: Evidence from the survey of income and program participation. U.S. Census Bureau Population Division Technical Working Paper No. 30.
42. ALBA, R.D. & J.R. LOGAN. 1993. Minority proximity to whites in suburbs: an individual-level analysis of segregation. Am. J. Sociol. **98:** 1388–1427.
43. COLLINS, C. & D.R. WILLIAMS. 1999. Segregation and mortality: the deadly effects of racism? Sociol. Forum **14**(3): 493–521.
44. COUNCIL ON ETHICAL AND JUDICIAL AFFAIRS. 1990. Black–white disparities in health care. JAMA **263:** 2344–2346.
45. WHITTLE, J., J. CONIGLIARO, C.B. GOOD & R.P. LOFGREN. 1993. Racial differences in the use of invasive cardiovasular procedures in the Department of Veterans Affairs. N. Engl. J. Med. **329:** 621–626.
46. MCBEAN, A.M & M. GORNICK. 1994. Differences by race in the rates of procedures performed in hospitals for Medicare beneficiaries. Health Care Finan. Rev. **15:** 77–90.
47. HANNAN, E.L., M. VAN RYNE, J. BURKE, D. STONE, D. KUMAR, D. ARANI, W. PIERCE, S. RAFII, T.A. SANBORN, S. SHARMA, J. SLATER & B.A. DEBUONO. 1999. Access to coronary artery bypass surgery by race/ethnicity and gender among patients who are appropriate for surgery. Med. Care **37:** 68–77.
48. PETERSON, E.D., L.K. SHAW, E.R. DELONG, D.B. PRYOR, R.M. CALIFF & D.B. MARK. 1997. Racial variation in the use of coronary-revascularization procedures—Are the differences real? Do they matter? N. Engl. J. Med. **337**(7): 480–486.
49. WILLIAMS, D.R., M. SPENCER & J.S. JACKSON. 1999. Race-related stress and physical health: is group identity a vulnerability factor or a resource? *In* Self, Social Identity, and Physical Health: Interdisciplinary Explorations. R.J. Contrada & R.D. Ashmore, Eds.: 71–100. Oxford University Press, New York. In Press.

50. WILLIAMS, D.R., Y. YU, J. JACKSON & N. ANDERSON. 1997. Racial differences in physical and mental health: socioeconomic status, stress, and discrimination. J. Health Psychol. **2:** 335–351.
51. TAYLOR, J. & B. JACKSON. 1990. Factors affecting alcohol consumption in black women, part II. Int. J. Addict. **25:** 1415–1427.
52. WILLIAMS, D.R. & A-M. CHUNG. 1999. Racism and Health. *In* Health in Black America. R. Gibson & J.S. Jackson, Eds. Sage Publications, Thousand Oaks. In press.
53. TAYLOR, J., D. HENDERSON & B.B. JACKSON. 1991. A holistic model for understanding and predicting depression in African American women. J. Commun. Psychol. **19:** 306–320.
54. MCEWEN, B.S. & T. SEEMAN. 1999. Protective and damaging effects of mediators of stress: elaborating and testing the concepts of allostasis and allostatic load. Ann. N.Y. Acad. Sci. **896:** this volume.

Part IV Summary: Psychobiological and Psychosocial Pathways and Mechanisms to Disease

MARK R. CULLEN[a]

Occupational and Environmental Medicine Program, Yale University School of Medicine, New Haven, Connecticut 06510, USA

In the previous session we reviewed the emerging concept of social environment—family, neighborhood, community, workplace—and explored the potential contributions such environments may make to the socioeconomic status (SES) and health gradients. Although less directly discussed, each speaker also acknowledged the crucial role of physical environment—air quality, diet, habitual behaviors, workplace hazards, noise, and so forth. Although the precise contributions of each of these factors remains uncertain, there is substantial evidence that these factors are deleterious to health and heavily determined by SES.

In this session we turned our attention to the next link in the chain, how these environmental factors get internalized. Whatever else we may believe about the societal and social causes of health and disease, it remains axiomatic that health itself is very much an individual characteristic, and at the end of the day, it is individual health that is the target of our research. So we must come to understand not only how the external social and physical environments impact us, but how they "get under our skin," forming the basis for biologic deterioration, or resilience.

In this session several different approaches are discussed. Three speakers addressed current psychological and psychosocial theories that attempt to link external experience with psychologic reaction. Of course, in each case the psychological mechanisms that translate the external to the internal are themselves heavily influenced by SES, yet another level at which the gradient may be explained. Another speaker addressed the complex set of behavioral factors that may modulate the relationships between classic risk factors for heart disease, such as smoking, and subjects in different parts of the SES spectrum, with special attention to the role of longitudinal data for investigation. Yet another intriguing theory, discussed below, is that sleep may serve as an important vehicle by which the experiences of the environment, social and physical, get translated into biologic phenomena. Finally, the session closed with a review of what fraction of currently understood risk factors for cardiovascular disease actually explain of the SES gradient—not much—reminding us of the magnitude of the challenge before us.

[a]Address for correspondence: Mark R. Cullen, M.D., Occupational and Environmental Medicine Program, Yale University School of Medicine, 135 College Street, Room 366, New Haven, CT 06510, USA. 203-785-6434 (voice); 203-785-7391 (fax).
    e-mail: mark.cullen@yale.edu

DISCUSSION

A series of eight questions and comments were posed to the speakers: The first was a general comment exhorting the assembly to ask the deeper "why" question when confronting data about the adverse health behaviors of lower SES groups. To paraphrase, could much of this be explained by social and political policies that reinforce such differential behaviors, rather than by blaming the victims themselves?

A second questioner raised the important issue of the underlying theoretical framework, or lack thereof, that has motivated the psychosocial and behavioral research presented. The relative important of theoretical constructs, as opposed to empirically driven hypotheses divorced from such theory, was briefly discussed, without resolution.

Given the largely still-unexplained role of education, the next questioner asked whether compliance with prescribed medical regimens could be an important pathway. While there is some evidence that this could explain differences in health among comparably insured groups, panel members felt it is unlikely to be the major discriminating reason, even for the differential outcomes in the treatment for established diseases, let alone for differences in disease rates themselves. The importance of relative, as opposed to absolute, differences in social status and wealth was underscored by the next comment, citing the very divergent health indices for heart disease among African Americans, when comparing families of Northern (high CHD mortality), Southern (intermediate), or Caribbean (low CHD mortality) origin.

The next speaker reiterated the concern, raised in several sessions of the conference, about the relative de-emphasis on discrimination and racism as determinants of poor health. Panel members responded in support of this framework, but also cited the strong evidence that SES, more than discrimination experience per se, was predictive of adverse health.

The question was posed to the psychologists on the panel how subconscious emotions and attitudes might be better accounted for in study design. Each of the panelists described the challenges for doing this, while recognizing that self-report is limited in this obvious way. The next question raised the issue of self-esteem, which has not proven a remarkably strong predictor of health, nor is it strongly associated with SES in recent studies. There was speculation from the panel about why it may not be an informative construct, possibly because of some difficulties in effectively measuring self-esteem relative to some of the other emotion-based constructs such as negative affect.

The session closed with a very provocative question about why increased rates of smoking appeared to be having relatively little adverse impact on the health of Japanese in Japan, and indeed what aspect of Japanese society might be responsible for its robust health. The responses included recognition of the very high investment in human and social capital in Japan and the very low levels of inequality, relative to the US, between richest and poorest in society. Though not an excuse for increased smoking, there was consensus that these features of Japanese society were likely protective in terms of human health.

Pathways by Which SES and Ethnicity Influence Cardiovascular Disease Risk Factors

MARILYN A. WINKLEBY,[a] CATHERINE CUBBIN,
DAVID K. AHN, AND HELENA C. KRAEMER

Stanford Center for Research in Disease Prevention, Stanford University School of Medicine, 1000 Welch Road, Palo Alto, California 94304-1825, USA

ABSTRACT: Little is known about pathways by which socioeconomic status (SES) translates into individual differences in cardiovascular disease (CVD) risk factors. Because the socioeconomic structure is not the same for all ethnic subgroups, the pathways that lead to the development of CVD risk factors may vary by both SES and ethnicity. We used data from a large national survey to examine the independent associations of two indicators of SES (education and income) and ethnicity with six primary CVD risk factors. We then used data on smoking that reflected a temporal sequence to examine the extent to which SES and ethnicity influenced smoking at three different time points, from smoking onset, to a serious quit attempt, to successful quitting. These analyses provide an understanding of the relationships between SES, ethnicity, and CVD risk factors and suggest that if the timing, focus, and content of intervention programs take pathways into account they will result in more successful outcomes.

INTRODUCTION

One mechanism through which socioeconomic status (SES) influences cardiovascular disease (CVD) is by its association with more proximal causes, such as recognized risk factors for CVD. Following the concept that SES is a fundamental cause of disease,[1,2] persons of higher SES are more able to avoid CVD risk factors, and thus less likely to develop or to die from the disease than their lower SES counterparts. Avoiding risk factors is possible because persons higher in the socioeconomic hierarchy command greater access to resources, such as health information, high-quality health care, social capital, and healthy social environments; and are more able to take advantage of those resources, compared to those lower in the hierarchy.[1,3] Over time, new information, products, and technology become available to promote heart-healthy behaviors and to prevent and treat CVD, creating a dynamic relationship between SES and CVD. Understanding this dynamic relationship is essential to gain insight about effective intervention strategies to combat CVD, the leading cause of death for women and men in the United States, and a major cause of premature morbidity and mortality.[4]

The epidemiological relationship between SES and CVD risk factors and events persists across gender, age groups, and ethnic groups.[5–7] SES, whether measured by

[a]Address for correspondence: 650-723-7055 (voice); 650-725-6906 (fax).
e-mail: mwinkleby@SCRDP.Stanford.edu

education, income, occupation, or other factors (e.g., neighborhood quality, home ownership, occupational prestige), is strongly associated with heart disease and stroke as well as with CVD risk factors. In studies that have used education as a marker for SES, a strong inverse relationship has been shown between educational attainment and mortality, with the lowest educated group usually experiencing about twice the CVD mortality of the highest educated group.[5,8] Adding strength to these findings are studies that show that the effect of SES is evident early in the natural history of atherosclerotic vascular disease,[9] suggesting that SES is associated with clinical CVD.[10] The relationship between SES and CVD mortality extends to CVD risk factors where highly significant relationships have been documented between several different indicators of SES and blood pressure, total blood cholesterol, physical activity, smoking, and body mass index.[11-14]

Although many studies have examined the association between SES and CVD, few have examined the interrelated effects of both SES and ethnicity with CVD outcomes.[15,16] A recent literature search identified only 19 studies that focused on both SES and ethnicity from hundreds that have been published on CVD in the U.S. in the last 20 years.[17] Many investigators have examined the separate relationships of SES or ethnicity with CVD risk factors and events.[18-21] However, the considerable overlap between SES and ethnicity suggests that to better understand their independent roles in CVD, they should be examined simultaneously using appropriate statistical methods.[22] This is especially important because both SES and ethnicity show strong, independent associations with CVD outcomes.[23]

It is likely that lower SES leads to greater CVD mortality via complex pathways linking behavioral, social, economic, and biological causes. In addition, differences in CVD risk factors among lower SES groups may be cumulative and reflect a lifelong impact of economic and social stressors.[24] Unfortunately, there is little understanding of the pathways through which SES and ethnicity are related to CVD risk factors because the majority of past studies lack data that reflect temporal associations.[25] In addition, past studies commonly use linear models that are sensitive to collinearity among predictor variables, making make them difficult for use in examining pathways that involve multiple factors.[26] Furthermore, linear models often exclude higher order interaction terms that can lend particular insight into high- and low-risk subgroups. Therefore, new methods may be useful in understanding pathways that underlie the relationships between SES, ethnicity, and CVD risk factors which may, in turn, provide insight about the timing, focus, and content of primary, secondary, and tertiary interventions.

In this paper, we use data from a large national survey to address two issues that contribute to our understanding of SES and ethnic differences in CVD risk factors. As background, we examine the associations between two separate indicators of SES (educational attainment—an individual marker, and family income—a household marker) and ethnicity with six primary CVD risk factors for women and men from three of the largest ethnic groups in the United States. Because data are available for smoking that reflect a temporal sequence (from smoking onset, to a serious quit attempt, to successful quitting), we use smoking as an example to explore pathways by which SES, ethnicity, and other risk factors influence critical time-points in the process of smoking. This analysis recognizes that different dimensions of SES and/ or ethnicity may vary in their predictiveness and interact differently at each time point, and that different time points may require different types of intervention programs for the most effective results.

METHODS

We present data from the Third National Health and Nutrition Examination Survey (NHANES III), a large survey conducted from 1988 to 1994 to assess the health and nutrition status of the U.S. population.[27] This survey is noteworthy because it included an oversampling of African-American, Mexican-American, and white women and men who represent both the upper and lower levels of SES. This sampling strategy allowed samples of each ethnic group to be representative of their respective U.S. populations and for superior generalizability.

NHANES III was conducted at 89 sites, from 1988 to 1994. Data were collected via standardized questionnaires and medical examinations at participants' homes and mobile examination centers. The questionnaires included demographic, socioeconomic, dietary, and health history questions; the medical examinations included measurements of blood pressure, lipids, and diabetic status. The questionnaires were translated into Spanish and administered by bilingual, bicultural interviewers to Spanish-speaking participants.

NHANES III included a total sample of 33,994 persons ages 2 months and older. Response rates were high; 78% completed both the home questionnaire and medical examination. The sample for this analysis includes 10,029 black, Mexican-American, and white women and men, ages 25–64, who completed both the home questionnaire and medical examination. We used the lower age cutpoint of 25 to assure that most individuals had completed their highest level of education and the upper age cutpoint of 64 to avoid problems of selection effects due to non-CVD caused morbidity and mortality.[28] We excluded data for women who were pregnant ($n = 168$), those from other ethnic groups ($n = 469$), those whose surveys were coded as unreliable ($n = 19$), and those who completed the home questionnaire but not the medical examination ($n = 921$). The 921 adults who completed only the home questionnaire were similar to the 10,029 adults who completed both the home questionnaire and medical examination on a number of sociodemographic variables including mean age (42.4 vs. 41.5 years, respectively) and mean education (13.0 vs. 12.7 years, respectively). Fewer than 5% of data were missing for the variables we analyzed, except for family income (8% missing).

Definitions of SES and Race/Ethnicity

We recognize that SES is a multidimensional construct and choose educational attainment and family income divided by family size as our measures of SES. Education is an indicator of prestige or status, and income is an indicator of economic resources, two dimensions of social class under Weber's framework.[29] The advantages of using education in epidemiologic research are that it is unlikely to be influenced by CVD morbidity, remains valid throughout adulthood, tends to have few missing data, and is available for retired persons and those who are not employed outside of the home. In addition, previous research has found education to be a strong predictor of heart disease.[5,8] It is important to realize, however, especially when examining health outcomes for different race and ethnic groups, that a given level of education does not confer the same financial returns for all persons.[16,30] For this reason, and because we wanted to measure more than one domain of SES, we choose to use both education and income in our analyses. We also recognize that education and income are correlated[31] and therefore subject to problems of collinearity when entered into the same regression model. To allow for a valid entry of both education and income into the same model, we adjusted income for education before it was entered into our models. We did this by calculating the residuals from regressing family income divided by family size on education, per $1,000. Thus, the effects of income in the regression models represent the additional variance explained after removing the effects of education.

Throughout this paper, we employ the term ethnicity to characterize the three demographic groups in our sample: black, Mexican-American, and white respondents. The ethnic differences in the outcomes, however, do not necessarily imply that ethnicity (customs, common traits, language, beliefs, etc.) is the underlying mechanism. For example, many ethnicities are included within and between the categories of white and black. Because we agree that race is a social construct, we believe that ethnic differences in health and disease are due primarily to the social environment[32,33] rather than ethnicity or biology.

Our two SES measures and race/ethnicity were defined as follows:

- *Education*: Highest grade or year of regular public or private school completed.

- *Family income*: Annual family income divided by family size.

- *Race/ethnicity*: Self-reported race/ethnicity as black, Mexican or Mexican-American, or white (not Hispanic).

Definitions of CVD Risk Factors

The six CVD risk factors we analyzed were defined as follows:

- *Current cigarette smoker*: Defined as smoking at least 100 cigarettes during a respondent's lifetime and currently smoking cigarettes. Serum cotinine levels (>13 nanograms per milliliter) were used to validate self-reported smoking.[34]

- *Hypertension*: Systolic and diastolic blood pressure, measured on the right arm while the participant was seated during the medical examination; the mean of the second and third of three blood pressure readings was used to calculate hypertension which was defined as systolic blood pressure ≥ 140 and/or diastolic blood pressure ≥ 90 and/or current use of antihypertensive medications.

- *Obesity*: Body mass index (BMI) ≥ 30 units, calculated as weight in Kg/height in m^2.

- *Leisure-time inactivity*: Questions adapted from the 1985 National Health Interview Survey,[27] which asked participants whether they had engaged in any leisure time physical activity in the past month, including exercises, sports, or physically active hobbies. Respondents who reported no leisure time activities were considered physically inactive.

- *Hypercholesterolemia*: Measurements came from serum specimens, were derived from nonfasting samples, and were analyzed by standardized protocols. Hypercholesterolemia was defined as total serum cholesterol of ≥240 mg/dl.

- *Non-insulin-dependent diabetes mellitus (NIDDM)*: Fasting plasma glucose levels, available on the entire NHANES III sample, were determined using a microadaptation of the national glucose oxidase reference method.[35] NIDDM was defined as having an ≥8-hour fast and plasma glucose levels ≥126 mg/dl and/or a medical history of diabetes (other than during pregnancy) with an age of onset >25 years.

Smoking Pathway Variables

The three variables we used in the smoking pathway analysis that reflect different time points in the process of smoking were:

- *Smoking onset*: Age first started smoking cigarettes fairly regularly.

- *Serious quit attempt*: Quit smoking for a period of one year or longer.

- *Successful quit attempt*: A quit attempt leading to current nonsmoker status (smoking cessation).

Analytic Approach

We first examined the association between the two measures of SES as well as ethnicity with the six CVD risk factors described above, using multiple logistic regression models. For this analysis we used SUDAAN, version 7.11 (Research Triangle Institute, Research Triangle Park, NC), a software program that adjusts for complex sampling designs and incorporates sampling weights that adjust for unequal sampling probabilities.[36] The independent variables were years of education (continuous and centered at 12 years to aid in the interpretation of the regression coefficients), family income divided by family size (adjusted for education before entry into the model), age (in years, centered at the sample mean), and ethnicity (black, Mexican-American, white). The analysis adjusted for all factors simultaneously. Models were run separately for women and men because of the strong gender differences in CVD risk factors and outcomes shown by past studies.[37] All *p* values are two-tailed.

We then examined the role of SES, ethnicity, and other factors at three time points in the process of smoking, from smoking onset, to a serious quit attempt, to successful quitting. For this analysis we used the signal detection method, a method of recursive partitioning (classification trees) to identify distinct subgroups at each time point, based on SES, ethnicity, and other risk factors that preceded the time point.[38,39] This method is particularly well suited for analyzing and interpreting multiple complex pathways to illnesses and disease. Signal detection models sequentially partition the data to identify subgroups that are mutually exclusive and maximally discriminated from each other, based on the probability of the outcome variable. The predictor variables are entered, and the algorithm then selects a variable and cutpoint based on a combined optimal measure of sensitivity and specificity with regard to the outcome variable. After choosing and splitting on the first optimally efficient variable, the signal detection program separately searches each subgroup or "branch" of the first split for the next most efficient variable and cutpoint, using all initial predictor variables as candidates. This procedure is repeated separately in each subgroup with all the remaining predictor variables, and ends when (1) there are inadequate subjects in a subgroup for further analysis, (2) no further significant discriminating variables ($p < 0.001$) are found, or (3) no further predictor variables remain. The results are displayed as classification trees.

We ran three signal detection analyses, each having a binary outcome that reflected a different time point in the process of smoking: age of smoking onset before 25 years (yes/no), serious quit attempt equal to or longer than one year (yes/no), and successful quitting (yes/no). Age 25 was used as the cut-point for smoking onset because it was the lower bound age for our sample. Each signal detection analysis included only predictor variables that preceded each time point. The first signal detection analysis used gender, birthyear, and ethnicity as predictor variables. The second analysis added two additional variables that preceded the second time point (education and age of smoking onset in addition to gender, birthyear, and ethnicity), and the third analysis added two more variables that preceded the third time point (family income and urban/rural status). Family income was included with and without an adjustment for family size in order to evaluate two dimensions of income. Although the data are from NHANES III, which is cross-sectional in design, these variables represent a temporal sequence, thus allowing us to conduct an exploratory analysis for understanding factors that predict different outcomes in the process of smoking.

RESULTS

Compared with white women and men, Mexican-American women and men had substantially lower levels of education, and both Mexican-American and black women and men had lower levels of income (TABLE 1). Approximately one-half of the Mexican-American sample was born in the U.S., and approximately 40% was Spanish-speaking.

The results of the multiple logistic analysis, which examined the association between the two indicators of SES and ethnicity with the six CVD risk factors, are shown in TABLE 2. The odds ratios, 95% confidence intervals, and p values are presented. Both indicators of SES as well as ethnicity were independently associated with CVD risk factors. For women, higher education and, to a lesser degree, higher income were significantly associated with lower odds of CVD risk factors. For example, the odds ratio of 0.85 for smoking indicates an approximate 15% lower odds of smoking for every additional one year of education. Furthermore, after adjustment for education and income, black and Mexican-American ethnicity were associated with higher odds of risk factors, especially for black women. The results were less consistent and of lower magnitude for men. When the analysis was stratified by the three ethnic groups (data not shown), results were similar but slightly more variable, possibly because of the smaller sample sizes.

TABLE 1. Sociodemographic profile of study population by gender and ethnicity, ages 25–64, NHANES III, 1988–1994

	Women			Men		
	Black	Mexican-American	White	Black	Mexican-American	White
U.S. population	7.7	3.0	47.9	6.4	3.5	47.3
Analytic sample	1769	1489	2031	1460	1536	1744
Education (%)						
< 12 years	30.3	60.2	17.8	34.0	61.8	19.5
12 years	40.5	23.8	41.0	37.1	19.7	32.9
> 12 years	29.2	15.9	41.3	28.9	18.4	47.6
Family income, divided by family size (in dollars)	9,300	7,700	16,900	11,800	8,700	18,000
Age (mean)	40.6	39.6	42.4	39.9	37.9	41.5
Married (%)	43.3	71.7	73.4	57.0	80.4	78.7
Living in urban area (%)	59.5	59.0	43.4	58.5	62.9	45.5
Born in the U.S. (%)	94.0	52.9	95.4	92.5	47.1	95.8
English speaking (%)	98.3	42.1	98.5	97.0	41.2	97.8
No health insurance (%)	16.6	39.4	11.7	21.3	43.7	12.3

TABLE 2. Multiple logistic analyses of SES indicators and ethnicity with six CVD risk factor outcomes, ages 25–64, NHANES III, 1988–1994[a]

Variables in Model	Odds Ratios 95% Confidence Intervals	Smoking	Hypertension	Obesity	Leisure-time Inactivity	Hypercholesterolemia	Diabetes
Women							
Education[b]	OR	0.85***	0.94**	0.93***	0.84***	0.95*	0.93***
	CI	(0.81–0.88)	(0.90–0.98)	(0.90–0.96)	(0.80–0.88)	(0.91–0.99)	(0.89–0.97)
Family income divided by family size[c]	OR	0.98***	0.99	0.99	0.98*	1.00	0.97**
	CI	(0.96–0.99)	(0.98–1.00)	(0.98–1.00)	(0.97–0.99)	(0.99–1.02)	(0.96–0.99)
Black compared with white	OR	0.88	2.86***	1.92***	2.26***	0.87	2.09***
	CI	(0.69–1.13)	(2.26–3.61)	(1.52–2.43)	(1.81–2.81)	(0.68–1.11)	(1.44–3.02)
Mexican-American compared with white	OR	0.19***	0.82	1.48**	1.63**	0.68*	1.48
	CI	(0.14–0.27)	(0.61–1.09)	(1.12–1.94)	(1.23–2.15)	(0.50–0.92)	(0.97–2.26)
Age	OR	0.97***	1.10***	1.02***	1.02***	1.08***	1.06***
	CI	(0.96–0.98)	(1.09–1.11)	(1.02–1.03)	(1.01–1.03)	(1.07–1.09)	(1.04–1.07)
Men							
Education[b]	OR	0.83***	0.98	0.95**	0.83***	1.01	0.92***
	CI	(0.79–0.86)	(0.95–1.01)	(0.92–0.98)	(0.80–0.85)	(0.96–1.06)	(0.88–0.96)
Income adjusted for education[c]	OR	1.00	0.99	0.99	0.98**	1.00	1.00
	CI	(0.99–1.01)	(0.98–1.00)	(0.98–1.00)	(0.96–0.99)	(0.99–1.01)	(0.99–1.02)
Black compared with white	OR	1.27*	1.90***	0.97	1.40*	0.83	1.90***
	CI	(1.06–1.54)	(1.53–2.36)	(0.79–1.18)	(1.08–1.80)	(0.64–1.08)	(1.47–2.46)
Mexican-American compared with white	OR	0.37***	0.92	0.97	1.35	1.10	1.26
	CI	(0.27–0.51)	(0.66–1.29)	(0.74–1.27)	(0.99–1.81)	(0.83–1.44)	(0.87–1.83)
Age	OR	0.98***	1.07***	1.03***	1.02**	1.04***	1.06***
	CI	(0.97–0.99)	(1.06–1.08)	(1.02–1.04)	(1.01–1.03)	(1.03–1.06)	(1.04–1.07)

[a] ***, $p < 0.001$; **, $p < 0.01$; *, $p < 0.05$.
[b] OR reflects every additional one year of education.
[c] OR reflects every additional $1,000 family income, adjusted for education to avoid problems of collinearity.

Process of Smoking

Although the odds ratios provide information about the strength and consistency of the associations between SES and ethnicity with CVD risk factors, they provide little information about the pathways by which SES and ethnicity translate into individual differences in CVD risk factors. As noted, since data were available for smoking that reflected a temporal sequence, we were able to explore the process of smoking at three different time points, from early smoking onset, to a serious quit attempt, to a successful quit attempt (FIG. 1). Thirty-two percent of the sample were current smokers. The first time point in the process of smoking that we examined was smoking onset before age 25. Fifty-two percent of respondents began smoking before the age of 25 and 48% began smoking after the age of 25 or never began smoking. Among these two groups 57% and 5% were current smokers, respectively. Theoretically, if smoking could be prevented or delayed until age 25 or later, smoking rates could be lowered from 32% to 5%. The second time point in the process of smoking was having a serious quit attempt (≥1 year). Among those who began smoking before the age of 25, 58% reported a serious quit attempt and 42% did not. Only 25% of those with a serious quit attempt were current smokers compared with 100% of those with no serious quit attempt. Thus, if a serious quit attempt could be achieved among this latter group, smoking rates could potentially be lowered from 57% to 25%. The last time point in the process of smoking was successful quitting. Among those who began smoking before the age of 25 and who had at least one serious quit attempt, 75% successfully quit smoking and 25% did not.

The signal detection analyses used these three time points to examine the role of SES, ethnicity, and other factors in the process of smoking (FIGS. 2–4). The first signal detection analysis examined factors that predicted smoking onset before the age

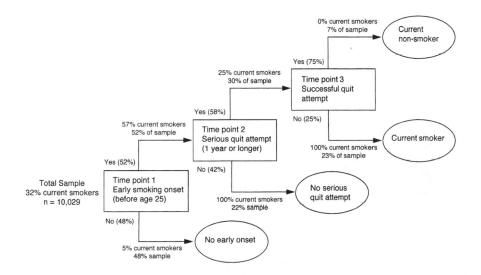

FIGURE 1. Time points in the process of smoking.

of 25. Seven distinct subgroups were identified, all with various rates of smoking (FIG. 2). Overall, 52% of the total sample began smoking before age 25. The first variable that distinguished smoking rates before the age of 25 was gender. Among men, birthyear further distinguished respondents. The group most likely to report smoking before the age of 25 was men born before 1949 (69%, group 1). Smoking rates decreased as a gradient across birth cohorts, with men born after 1958 reporting the lowest rates (49%, group 4). Among women, ethnicity further distinguished respondents, with Mexican-American women reporting the lowest rates of smoking of all groups (23%, group 7).

The second signal detection analyzed data at the second time point in the process of smoking and examined factors that predicted a serious quit attempt (≥1 year) among those who began smoking before the age of 25. Fifty-eight percent of this group reported a serious quit attempt. The signal detection identified eight distinct subgroups (FIG. 3). Birthyear, ethnicity, and education were all significant predictors of quit attempts. The group with the highest rate of serious quit attempts was older Mexican-American and white respondents with higher educational attainment (75%, group 4). This group was more than twice as likely to achieve a serious quit attempt than the group with the lowest rate of quit attempts: younger, lower educated black and white respondents (36%, group 5).

The last signal detection analyzed data at the final time point and examined factors that predicted a successful quit attempt among those who began smoking before the age of 25 and who had a serious quit attempt (≥1 year). This is a select group who already had a successful quit attempt that lasted one year or longer and therefore

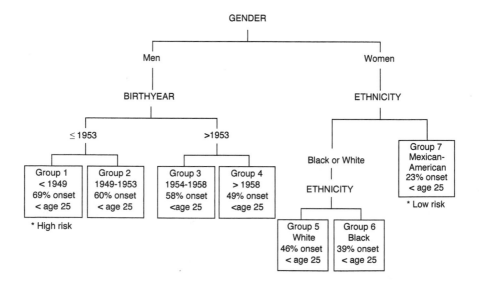

FIGURE 2. Time point 1: Predictors of early smoking onset (less than age 25)—52% overall rate, $n = 10,029$. (Variables in model that preceded outcome: gender, birthyear, ethnicity.)

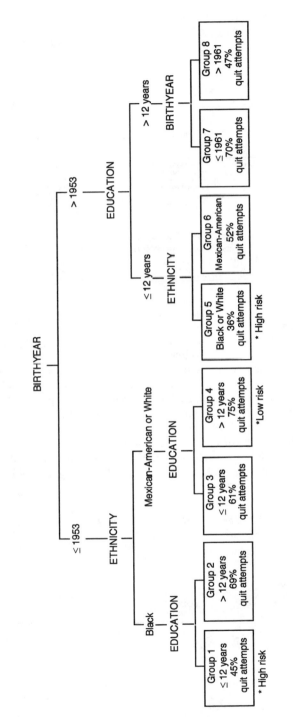
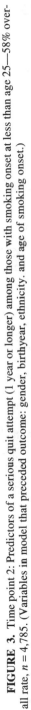

FIGURE 3. Time point 2: Predictors of a serious quit attempt (1 year or longer) among those with smoking onset at less than age 25—58% over-all rate, *n* = 4,785. (Variables in model that preceded outcome: gender, birthyear, ethnicity. and age of smoking onset.)

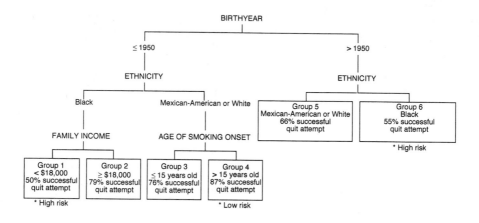

FIGURE 4. Time point 3: Predictors of a successful quit attempt among those with smoking onset at less than age 25 and one or more serious quit attempts—75% overall rate, $n = 2,479$. (Variables in model that preceded outcome: gender, birthyear, ethnicity, education, age of smoking onset, family income, family income divided by family size, and urban/rural status.)

had a high probability of successful quitting. Overall, 75% of this group reported a successful quit attempt (FIG. 4). Birthyear, ethnicity, family income, and age of smoking onset were all significant predictors. Of the six distinct subgroups identified, two groups had particularly low rates of successful quit attempts: older black respondents with lower family incomes (50% successful, group 1) and younger black respondents (55% successful, group 6). The group with the highest rate of successful quit attempts was older Mexican-American and white respondents with a later age of smoking onset (87% successful, group 4).

The results of the three signal detection analyses showed that SES and ethnicity were key predictors at each time point in the process of smoking, except in the case

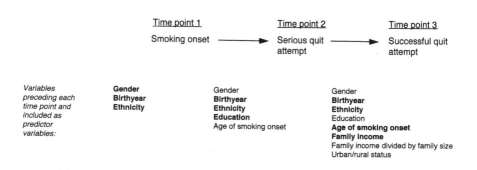

FIGURE 5. Summary of predictive variables in signal detection analyses at each of the time points in the process of smoking. *Bold* indicates variables that were significant predictors at each time point in the signal detection analysis.

of smoking onset where SES during childhood was not available for inclusion in the model (FIG. 5). Furthermore, SES, ethnicity, and other factors varied in their predictiveness at each time point in the process of smoking. For example, while gender was a significant predictor at the first time point, it was not at the latter two time points. Similarly, different dimensions of SES were important at different time points; while education was a predictor of a serious quit attempt, family income was a predictor of a successful quit attempt.

DISCUSSION

In this paper we examined the influence of SES and ethnicity with a set of CVD risk factors using multiple regression models. We then examined the influence of SES, ethnicity, and other factors at different time points in the process of smoking using the signal detection method. In both analyses, SES as well as ethnicity were strongly associated with CVD risk factors and smoking outcomes. The analysis of smoking that used data reflecting a temporal process showed the dynamic nature of SES and ethnicity at various time points, providing insight about effective intervention strategies.

Strengths and Limitations

There are strengths to the data we analyzed as well as the methodologies we used. NHANES III is one of the most comprehensive national surveys to date.[27] Extensive and complete data are available from both the home survey and medical examination. Response rates were high, and there were minimal missing data. Unlike many surveys, NHANES III represents a sample of the U.S. population and therefore results are generalizable to women and men living in the U.S. The multiple regression models we used had the advantage of including two nonoverlapping indicators of SES (education and income adjusted for education before entry into the models) as well as ethnicity, which allowed us to examine the independent associations between education, income, and ethnicity with six primary CVD risk factors. The signal detection model we used to explore smoking pathways had the advantage of examining higher order interactions that are rarely included in traditional regression models. This allowed us to identify groups at particularly high risk for early age of smoking onset, no serious quit attempts, and unsuccessful smoking cessation.

Despite these strengths, there are limitations to our analyses regarding the cross-sectional design of NHANES III and the measurement of several SES and CVD indicators. In our analysis of smoking pathways, we used cross-sectional data that reflect different time points in the process of smoking; however, these data were collected at one point in time and are therefore subject to recall bias (e.g., age of smoking onset). In addition, measures of SES were not available preceding the time of smoking onset, and the income and education questions we used may not have preceded the latter two time points for all respondents. These limitations of cross-sectional data highlight the need for longitudinal studies that collect data at multiple time points in a person's life and allow for a more rigorous testing of causal pathways. The NHANES III question on current smoking status, based on a self-reported question, is also subject to bias. However, NHANES III allowed verification of self-reported smoking, using a biochemical measure, serum cotinine, that was available for most respondents. Among respondents who reported being nonsmokers, the following percentages had positive cotinine values: 9.8%, 4.0%, and 7.6% of black, Mexican-American, and white respondents, respectively, and 9.7%, 6.5%, and 5.1% of respondents completing less than 12, 12, and more than 12 years of education, respectively. These results indicate relatively low levels of underreporting and lend credence to our findings on current smoking status.

Implications for Future Studies

Our findings are exploratory and were undertaken to provide an example of questions that can be asked at critical time points related to CVD risk factors. Our analyses took advantage of cross-sectional data that reflected a temporal sequence. Unfortunately, the temporal sequence of many other CVD risk factors cannot be elucidated using cross-sectional data, and all such data are susceptible to recall bias. Thus, despite the costs and time involved, there remains a critical need for stronger designs, especially longitudinal studies that provide data at multiple time points in a person's life. Longitudinal data, for example, would provide prospective information on other important predictors of CVD risk factors across the lifecourse, such as childhood SES. Such data would also allow for the examination of secular trends (as indicated by birthyear) that we found to be a powerful predictor at all three time points in our signal detection analyses.

Implications for Individually Oriented Interventions

The three time points we examined in the pathway of smoking lend insight to the design of future smoking intervention programs. The goal is to prevent or delay onset of smoking, promote serious quit attempts (especially at early ages before heavy addiction), and achieve smoking cessation without relapse. For example, if interventions could delay smoking onset until age 25 or later, many fewer people would smoke. Similarly, if interventions could promote a serious quit attempt among smokers, most smokers would eventually quit (see FIG. 1).

Our findings suggest that smoking intervention programs should be implemented at different time points in the process of smoking. Certainly, the most important time point is before the onset of smoking. Because some adolescents begin smoking by age 10 and many begin smoking by age 14,[40] intervention programs must begin at early ages, before adolescence. It is important to recognize that many adolescents with the highest rates of smoking do not attend traditional public schools. Therefore, traditional school-based interventions must be broadened to include youth at alternative sites, such as continuation high schools and schools within the foster care and criminal justice system. The timing of programs that address quit attempts and smoking cessation must also occur early, ideally among experimental smokers before they become heavily addicted or have smoked for many years. Because many youth continue smoking into adulthood, and because some people begin smoking during adulthood, programs must also be available that encourage quit attempts and smoking cessation among adults.

Our signal detection results lend insight into the types of smoking intervention programs that may be most effective. In the first signal detection analysis of factors that predict smoking onset before age 25, we observed a strong secular trend for men, with 69% of men born before 1949 reporting smoking before age 25. This decreased as a gradient across four birth cohorts, with 49% of men born after 1958 reporting smoking. This decrease over time suggests that the focus of past smoking intervention programs on community-wide approaches, media campaigns, and public policies[41–43] may have resulted in a higher awareness of the dangers of smoking and less promotion and availability of cigarettes. These broad-based approaches should be continued, with the hope of preventing smoking onset in even larger numbers. Of all groups, early age of smoking onset was lowest among Mexican-American women (23%), a finding that suggests that smoking prevention programs should be developed to reinforce positive cultural beliefs.

The second signal detection analysis of factors that predicted a serious quit attempt identified high-risk groups that may have been missed by past intervention programs and deserve special focus. The two groups with the fewest serious quit attempts were younger black and white respondents with lower educational attainment and older black respondents with lower educational attainment. The identification of these two groups highlights the need for programs that reach women and men with lower educational attainment, in particular black women and men. As noted earlier, these programs should begin during adolescence and continue throughout adulthood. A final group with low quit attempts were younger respondents (born after 1961) with higher educational attainment; however, as this group grows older, their percentage of quit attempts will most likely increase.

The third signal detection analysis identified two additional groups that deserve special attention, based on their low successful quit rates. These groups were older black women and men with lower family incomes, and younger black women and men, regardless of family income. The identification of these groups suggests that interventions need to address both economic and social factors that may influence smoking cessation. This may include providing insurance coverage for smoking cessation programs, free or low-cost nicotine patches or gum, and support groups on stress reduction.

Our findings show the need to design effective CVD intervention programs that reach low SES and ethnic minority populations, especially black Americans.[7,44,45] Many of this group have justifiable reasons to remain distrustful of intervention programs, including those with little or no risk of harm. A history of discrimination has resulted in disenfranchised and segregated low SES and minority populations, both socially and economically, so that the groups with the poorest health outcomes on a number of measures are the most marginalized.[46,47] Public health interventions, designed to promote heart-healthy behaviors, cannot be equally successful in severely disadvantaged communities as in other communities without addressing socioeconomic conditions. For many persons enduring cumulative financial and social stressors, some risk factors, such as smoking or eating foods high in fat, may provide stress relief or comfort, where the long-term health risks seem insignificant in the face of more pressing demands.[24,32,48] This is compounded by the additional barriers to risk factor reduction faced by persons in these communities that include targeted tobacco advertising and limited access to inexpensive, healthy foods.

Unfortunately, it is likely that for the majority of persons in these "high-risk" SES and ethnic minority groups, particularly those who are black and/or of very low SES, substantial barriers will remain to achieving positive lifestyle changes as a result of individually focused interventions. This emphasizes the importance of other means for addressing socioeconomic and ethnic disparities in health, including directly addressing socioeconomic inequalities through social and economic policies and public health policies, such as those that restrict tobacco promotion and availability.[49,50]

Implications for Societal-Oriented Interventions

An individually oriented approach to the prevention of CVD that focuses on modification of lifestyle behaviors or risk factors to the exclusion of the individual's socioeconomic context implies that individuals can and should bear primary responsibility for their health, including changing their behavioral risk factors. This can deflect attention from the issue that individual choices are constrained by the context in which people live and work. As shown by our results, CVD risk factors are not equally distributed along the socioeconomic hierarchy. Indeed, societies dynamically create and shape these patterns of inequality.[3,51] Unfortunately, recent declines in CVD have been shown to be greater for persons with higher SES than for their lower SES counterparts.[52,53] Failure to explicitly take into account the socioeconomic context of health behaviors and other risk factors when designing and implementing health promotion and disease prevention strategies has public policy implications for resource allocation and program development. Many interventions aimed at changing individual CVD risk factors have been shown to be, at best, only moderately effective.[43] Thus, continuing to devote limited resources for interventions that focus solely on providing individuals with information and programs to "enable" them to make lifestyle changes without consideration of their social environment detracts resources from alternative methods that may be more effective.

CONCLUSION

CVD will remain the leading cause of mortality as well as a significant cause of premature morbidity for all SES and ethnic groups in the U.S. over the next decade. Furthermore, CVD is projected to increase dramatically in newly developed and developing countries as their populations experience greater life expectancies and tobacco consumption.[54] Heart disease is projected to be the leader in causes of global disease burden by the year 2020.[54] This increase will be compounded by a concomitant rise in poverty.[30] In order to decrease the burden of CVD, we need a greater understanding of how SES translates into differential risks within and between population groups. We also need a better understanding of the dynamic relationships that underlie the association between SES and CVD in order to design more effective primary and secondary interventions. Our findings suggest that the focus and content of CVD intervention programs should be tailored to different time points in the development of CVD risk factors. Our identification of high-risk populations argues for interventions in collaboration with ethnic minority and socioeconomically disadvantaged communities and for broad public health policies to alleviate social inequalities in health.

ACKNOWLEDGMENTS

This work was done during the tenure of an Established Investigatorship Award to Dr. Winkleby from the American Heart Association, and from an American Heart Association National Grant-in-Aid and a U.S. Public Health Service Grant 1-RO3-HL-57100 from the National Heart, Lung, and Blood Institute to Dr. Winkleby. The authors thank Drs. Rakale Collins, Lori Beth Dixon, Michaela Kiernan, Christopher Gardner, and Jan Sundquist for their insightful comments on an earlier draft, and Alana Koehler for her technical assistance.

REFERENCES

1. LINK, B.G. & J. PHELAN. 1995. Social conditions as fundamental causes of disease. J. Health Soc. Behav. Suppl.: 80–94.
2. SYME, S.L. 1996. Rethinking disease: where do we go from here? Ann. Epidemiol. **6:** 463–468.
3. SUSSER, M., W. WATSON & K. HOPPER. 1985. Sociology in Medicine. Oxford University Press, Oxford.
4. AMERICAN HEART ASSOCIATION. 1993. Heart and Stroke Facts Statistics. 1992. American Heart Association National Center, Dallas.
5. NATIONAL HEART LUNG AND BLOOD INSTITUTE. 1995. Report of the Conference on Socioeconomic Status and Cardiovascular Health and Disease (November 6–7, 1995). Department of Health and Human Services: Public Health Service, Bethesda, MD.
6. KAPLAN, G.A. & J.E. KEIL. 1993. Socioeconomic factors and cardiovascular disease: a review of the literature. Circulation **88:** 1973–1998.
7. WILLIAMS, D.R. & C. COLLINS. 1995. U.S. socioeconomic and racial differences in health: patterns and explanations. Ann. Rev. Sociol. **21:** 349–386.
8. FELDMAN, J.J., D.M. MAKUC, J.C. KLEINMAN & J. CORNONI-HUNTLEY. 1989. National trends in educational differentials in mortality. Am. J. Epidemiol. **129:** 919–933.
9. LYNCH, J., R. COHEN, J. TUOMILEHTO & J. SALONEN. 1996. Do cardiovascular risk factors explain the relation between socioeconomic status, risk of all-cause morality, and acute myocardial infarction? Am. J. Epidemiol. **144:** 934–942.
10. DIEZ-ROUX, A.V., F.J. NIETO, H.A. TYROLER, L.D. CRUM & M. SZKLO. 1995. Social inequalities and atherosclerosis: the Atherosclerosis Risk in Communities Study. Am. J. Epidemiol. **141:** 960–972.
11. WINKLEBY, M.A., S.P. FORTMANN & D.C. BARRETT. 1990. Social class disparities in risk factors for disease: eight-year prevalence patterns by level of education. Prev. Med. **19:** 1–12.
12. SHEA, S., A.D. STEIN, C.E. BASCH, R. LANTIGUA, C. MAYLAHN, D.S. STROGATZ & L. NOVICK. 1991. Independent associations of educational attainment and ethnicity with behavioral risk factors for cardiovascular disease. Am. J. Epidemiol. **134:** 567–582.
13. REYNES, J.F., T.M. LASATER, H. FELDMAN, A.R. ASSAF & R.A. CARLETON. 1993. Education and risk factors for coronary heart disease: results from a New England community. Am. J. Prev. Med. **9:** 365–371.
14. LUEPKER, R.V., W.D. ROSAMOND, R. MURPHY, M.J. SPRAFKA, A.R. FOLSOM, P.G. MCGOVERN & H. BLACKBURN. 1993. Socioeconomic status and coronary heart disease risk factor trends: the Minnesota Heart Survey. Circulation **88**(1): 2172–2179.
15. KINGTON, R.S. & J.P. SMITH. 1997. Socioeconomic status and racial and ethnic differences in functional status associated with chronic diseases. Am. J. Public Health **87:** 805–810.

16. WINKLEBY, M.A., H.C. KRAEMER, D.K. AHN & A.N. VARADY. 1998. Ethnic and socioeconomic differences in cardiovascular disease risk factors: findings for women from the Third National Health and Nutrition Examination Survey, 1988–1994. JAMA **280:** 356–362.

17. MILLS, K.M. & M.A. WINKLEBY. 1999. Race/ethnicity and cardiovascular risk factors: differential across levels of socioeconomic status. Ethnicity Dis. Accepted for publication.

18. GILLUM, R., M. MUSSOLINO & J. MADANS. 1998. Coronary heart disease risk factors and attributable risks in African-American women and men: NHANES I Epidemiologic Follow-Up Study. Am. J. Public Health **88:** 913–917.

19. GOFF, D.C., M.Z. NICHAMAN, W. CHAN, D.J. RAMSEY, D.R. LABARTHE & C. ORTIZ. 1997. Greater incidence of hospitalized myocardial infarction among Mexican-Americans than non-Hispanic whites: the Corpus Christi Heart Project 1988–1992. Circulation **95:** 1433–1440.

20. MARMOT, M. & P. ELLIOT. 1992. Coronary Heart Disease Epidemiology from Aetiology to Public Health. Oxford University Press, New York.

21. WEI, M., B. MITCHELL, S. HAFFNER & M. STERN. 1996. Effects of cigarette smoking, diabetes, high cholesterol, and hypertension on all-cause mortality and cardiovascular disease mortality in Mexican Americans. Am. J. Epidemiol. **144:** 1058–1065.

22. KRAEMER, H.C., A.E. KAZDIN, D.R. OFFORD, R.C. KESSLER, P.S. JENSEN & D.J. KUPFER. 1997. Coming to terms with the terms of risk. Arch. Gen. Psychiatry **54:** 337–343.

23. WINKLEBY, M.A. 1997. Accelerating cardiovascular risk factor change in ethnic minority and low socioeconomic groups. Ann. Epidemiol. **7:** S96–S103.

24. GERONIMUS, A. 1992. The weathering hypothesis and the health of African-American women and infants: evidence and speculations. Ethnicity Dis. **2:** 207–221.

25. KRIEGER, N. 1994. Epidemiology and the web of causation: has anyone seen the spider? Soc. Sci. Med. **39:** 887–903.

26. MARTIN, D.C., P. DIEHR, E.B. PERRIN & T.D. KOEPSELL. 1993. The effect of matching on the power of randomized community intervention studies. Stat. Med. **12:** 329–338.

27. NATIONAL CENTER FOR HEALTH STATISTICS. 1994. Plan and operation of the Third National Health and Nutrition Examination Survey, 1988–1994, series 1: programs and collection procedures. Vital Health Stat. **32:** 1–407.

28. HOUSE, J.S., R.C. KESSLER & A.R. HERZOG. 1990. Age, socioeconomic status, and health. Milbank Q. **68:** 383–411.

29. LIBERATOS, P., B.G. LINK & J.L. KELSEY. 1988. The measurement of social class in epidemiology. Epidemiol. Rev. **10:** 87–121.

30. MASSEY, J.S. 1996. The age of extremes: concentrated affluence and poverty in the twenty-first century. Demography **33:** 395–412.

31. WINKLEBY, M.A., D.E. JATULIS, E. FRANK & S.P. FORTMANN. 1992. Socioeconomic status and health: how education, income, and occupation contribute to risk factors for cardiovascular disease. Am. J. Public Health **82:** 816–820.

32. LILLIE-BLANTON, M. & T. LAVEIST. 1996. Conducting an assessment of health needs and resources in a racial/ethnic minority community. Race/ethnicity, the social environment, and health **43:** 83–91.

33. WILLIAMS, D.R., R. LAVIZZO-MOUREY & R.C. WARREN. 1994. The concept of race and health status in America. Public Health Rep. **109:** 26–41.

34. CUMMINGS, S.R. & R.J. RICHARD. 1988. Optimum cutoff points for biochemical validation of smoking status. Am. J. Public Health **78:** 574–575.

35. REESE, J.W., P. DUNCAN, D. BAYSE, *et al.* 1977. Development and evaluation of a hexokinase-glucose-6-phosphatase dehydrogenase procedure for use as a national glucose reference method. US GPO, Washington, DC.

36. SHAH, B.V., B.G. BARNWELL, P.N. HUNT, P. NILEEN & L.M. LAVANGE. 1991. SUDAAN User's Manual, Release 5.50. Research Triangle Institute, Research Triangle Park, NC.

37. WILLIAMS, E.L., M.A. WINKLEBY & S.P. FORTMANN. 1993. Changes in coronary heart disease risk factors in the 1980s: evidence of a male-female crossover effect with age. Am. J. Epidemiol. **137:** 1056–1067.
38. KRAEMER, H.C. 1992. Evaluating Medical Tests: Objective and Quantitative Guidelines. Sage Publications, Newbury Park.
39. BREIMAN, L., J.H. FRIEDMAN, R.A. OLSHEN & C.J. STONE. 1984. Classification and regression trees. Wadsworth International Group, Belmont.
40. WINKLEBY, M.A., T.N. ROBINSON, J. SUNDQUIST & H.C. KRAEMER. 1999. Ethnic variation in cardiovascular risk factors among children and young adults: findings from the Third National Health and Nutrition Examination, 1988–1994. JAMA **281:** 1006–1013.
41. WINKLEBY, M.A. 1994. The future of community-based cardiovascular disease intervention studies. Am. J. Public Health **84:** 1369–1372.
42. FORTMANN, S.P., J.A. FLORA, M.A. WINKLEBY, C. SCHOOLER, C.B. TAYLOR & J.W. FARQUHAR. 1995. Community intervention trials: reflections on the Stanford Five-City Project Experience. Am. J. Epidemiol. **142:** 576–586.
43. WINKLEBY, M.A., H.A. FELDMAN & D.M. MURRAY. 1997. Joint analysis of three U.S. community intervention trials for reduction of cardiovascular disease risk. J. Clin. Epidemiol. **50:** 148–158.
44. ANDERSON, N.B. 1995. Behavioral and sociocultural perspectives on ethnicity and health. Health Psychol. **14:** 589–591.
45. MOLINA, C., R.E. ZAMBRANA & M. AGUIRRE-MOLINA. 1994. The influence of culture, class, and environment on health care. *In* Latino Health in the US: A Growing Challenge. C. Molina & M. Aguirre-Molina, Eds.: 23–43. American Public Health Association. Washington DC.
46. SCHORR, L.B. 1988. Within Our Reach. Breaking the Cycle of Disadvantage. Anchor Press. New York.
47. BELL, D. 1992. Faces at the Bottom of the Well. The Permanence of Racism. BasicBooks. New York.
48. MEIN, S. & M.A. WINKLEBY. 1998. Concerns and misconceptions about cardiovascular disease risk factors: a focus group evaluation with low income Hispanic women. Hisp. J. Behav. Sci. **20:** 192–211.
49. PIERCE, J.P., W.S. CHOI, E.A. GILPIN, A.J. FARKAS & C.C. BERRY. 1998. Tobacco industry promotion of cigarettes and adolescent smoking. JAMA **279:** 511–515.
50. WALLACK, L. & M. WINKLEBY. 1987. Primary prevention: a new look at basic concepts. Soc. Sci. Med. **25:** 923–930.
51. JOHNSON, K.W., N.B. ANDERSON, E. BASTIDA, J. KRAMER, D. WILLIAMS & M. WONG. 1995. Macrosocial and environmental influences on minority health. Health Psych. **14:** 601–612.
52. MARMOT, M.G. & M.E. MCDOWALL. 1986. Mortality decline and widening social inequalities. Lancet **ii:** 274–276.
53. TYROLER, H.A., S. WING & M.G. KNOWLES. 1993. Increasing inequality in coronary heart disease mortality in relation to educational achievement: profile of places of residence, United States, 1962 to 1987. Ann. Epidemiol. **3**(Suppl.): S51–S54.
54. MURRAY, C.J.L. & A.D. LOPEZ, Eds. 1996. The Global Burden of Disease (Summary). Harvard University Press, Cambridge.

Psychosocial Resources and the SES–Health Relationship

SHELLEY E. TAYLOR[a] AND TERESA E. SEEMAN

Department of Psychology, 1285 Franz Hall, University of California, Los Angeles, P.O. Box 951563, Los Angeles, California 90095-1563, USA

ABSTRACT: Psychosocial resources, which include optimism, coping style, a sense of mastery or personal control, and social support, influence the relationship between SES and health. To varying degrees, these resources appear to be differentially distributed by social class and related to health outcomes. Such resources may partially mediate the impact of SES on health. For example, environments that undermine personal control may have an impact on chronic arousal and the corresponding development of disease, such as CHD. Psychosocial resources may also moderate the impact of SES on health. For example, a large number of positive social relationships and a few conflictual ones may buffer individuals against the adverse effects of SES-related stress. These psychosocial resources are moderately intercorrelated, and so a research strategy that explores their coherence as a psychosocial profile that promotes resilience to stress is tenable and merits empirical examination. The erosion of these resources as one moves lower on the SES scale and specific factors that contribute to such erosion are discussed.

INTRODUCTION

What explains the robust SES gradient with respect to all-cause mortality and health outcomes? How does social class get under the skin so that it adversely affects basic bodily processes and the likelihood of illness? Plausible pathways include the differential practice of health habits, differential availability and use of health services, the cumulative adverse effects of chronic stress, and the inability to meet chronic stress with resources that may help to diffuse its psychological and biological impact.[1] Our analysis focuses on this last pathway, arguing that the availability of psychosocial resources varies by social class, and the effectiveness of those resources for moderating stress may vary by SES as well. We begin by identifying the resources that have been shown to be distributed by SES, to most effectively moderate the effects of stress, to ameliorate the effects of ill health, or all three. Four psychosocial resources meet these criteria: a sense of personal control, optimism, social support, and ways of coping. To varying degrees, these resources seem to be distributed by SES and are associated with health outcomes. As such, they may partially mediate the relation between SES and health; they clearly moderate the SES and health relationship; and, taken together, they present a portrait of the type of person who may best be able to combat the health risks of SES-related chronic stress.

[a]Address for correspondence: e-mail: taylors@psych.ucla.edu

PERSONAL CONTROL

Personal control, also known as a sense of personal mastery, reflects individuals' beliefs regarding the extent to which they are able to control or influence their outcomes. Many theorists have emphasized the importance of perceptions of personal control or mastery and suggested that this desire is a fundamental need of human beings.[2,3] A variety of instruments assess control-related beliefs,[b] with Pearlin and Schooler's[4] "Personal Mastery Scale," the most widely used measure in health research.

Studies have shown a positive association between SES (e.g., higher income and/ or education) and belief in personal control.[5-9] Similar patterns of association are seen for related constructs such as personal mastery[10-12] and self-efficacy,[10] and lower SES has also been associated with greater powerlessness and anomie.[6,13] Social class differences in personal control beliefs may also be importantly influenced by characteristics of the environmental settings that are likely to be inhabited by different social classes. For example, Kohn and Schooler found that work setting characteristics such as environmental complexity and contingency (i.e., control over the process of one's work) can promote the development and persistence of stronger personal agency/control beliefs,[14] and studies of the effects of downward mobility with respect to employment status highlight the negative impact of such experiences on personal control and efficacy beliefs.[10,12]

Evidence linking control beliefs to health is mixed, with evidence for both more positive and more negative health outcomes associated with stronger perceptions of personal control. Some studies show a relation between a higher sense of control and better psychological health,[15] as well as better physical health outcomes, including lower incidence of CHD,[16] better self-rated health and functional status,[17,18] and lower mortality risk.[17,18] However, control beliefs can be associated with poorer health outcomes under certain circumstances,[19,20] especially when expectations for control are high but opportunities to exercise it are constrained.[20-22] Both animal and human studies have found the highest levels of reactivity (that is, increasing cardiovascular or neuroendocrine activity or reduction in immune function) in situations marked by incongruity between expectations for control and situational uncontrollability or difficulty in controlling outcomes.[23-26] The relation between the Type A behavior pattern and increased risk for heart disease may also be an example of such links. Type As have been shown to have a strong need for control,[27] to persist in attempts for control in laboratory situations,[27,28] and to exhibit greater physiologic reactivity in the face of uncontrollable situations.[29] Such persistence, in the face of external realities that limit or prevent actual control over outcomes, along with its accompanying physiological reactivity, may contribute to Type As' increased risk for CHD. Personal control beliefs, however, may also contribute to CHD risk independent of Type A behavior. The presence of stronger personal mastery beliefs, for

[b]These control-related beliefs include: global assessments (e.g., the original Rotter 1-E scale and Pearlin's Personal Mastery scale (see Ref. 115 for details); factorial measures that provide separate measures of beliefs regarding "personal control," "powerful others," and "chance" (e.g., Internality, Powerful Others, and Chance Scales or Spheres of Control; see Ref. 115 for review of measures); domain-specific measures (e.g., "Health Locus of Control"[116]; see Ref. 115 for a more complete review of available scales).

example, has been found to be associated with greater coronary atherosclerosis independent of other known risk factors.[19] To the extent that such strong mastery beliefs promote unrealistic expectations for control, they may be associated with patterns of physiological arousal that promote the development of atherosclerosis.

Socioeconomic status may also moderate the association between control beliefs and health outcomes. Using data from three national samples, Lachman and Weaver[11] found significant interactions of control beliefs with both education and income in relation to health and well-being. Specifically, although beliefs in personal control were associated with more positive health outcomes in all SES groups, the differences in health outcomes associated with stronger versus weaker control beliefs were greater at lower levels of education and income. Among those with less education or income, those with strong control beliefs reported health outcomes comparable to those seen in higher SES groups for self-rated health, acute physical symptoms, depressive symptoms, and life satisfaction. Continued focus on the antecedents of control beliefs, their distribution by SES, and their relation to health outcomes, is clearly justified by the current evidence.

OPTIMISM/PESSIMISM

Optimism refers to outcome expectancies that good things, rather than bad things, will happen. Interest in optimism was fueled initially by a model of behavioral self-regulation derived by Carver and Scheier[30] which assumes that goal-directed behavior is guided by a hierarchy of closed-loop negative feedback systems. Optimism is judged to be a general and stable dispositional resource that influences whether an individual will stay focused on reducing discrepancies between present behavior and a goal or standard selected for pursuit. Both generalized outcome expectancies (dispositional optimism) and specific situational expectancies (situational optimism) are believed to maintain focus and effort.

Dispositional optimism is most commonly measured by the LOT-R,[31] a 10-item scale assessing respondents' agreement with such statements as, "In uncertain times, I usually expect the best." Another approach to assessing dispositional optimism derives from Seligman's[32] theoretical position on learned helplessness. It maintains that, to the extent that generalized expectancies are negative, internal, and global, bad health and mental health consequences will follow. Pessimistic explanatory style, as this response style is called, is measured by content analysis of interview protocols for attributions of negative events to stable, internal, and/or global factors. A third conceptualization of optimism, situational optimism, examines positive outcome expectancies for specific situations. Because specific expectancies are more proximal to specific events than dispositional beliefs, they may be important predictors of psychological and biological responses to specific stressors.[33]

The research literature has not previously addressed the relation of optimistic expectations to SES. To do so, we analyzed four existing datasets with reasonable variability in SES, and an intriguing pattern emerged.[c] In all four data sets, a modest relationship between dispositional optimism and SES was fully explained by pessimism. That is, when the scale items assessing pessimism (negatively worded items) were examined separately from those measuring optimism (the positively worded items), optimism was unrelated to SES, but pessimism was significantly and consistently related at moderately high levels. Thus, SES appears to be related to the development of negative expectations for one's outcomes, though not necessarily positive ones.

A modest amount of evidence has related dispositional optimism/pessimism to health-related outcomes. Schulz et al.[2] found that the pessimism items of the LOT were a significant predictor of early mortality among young patients with recurrent cancer, after controlling for site and symptoms. Conceptually related findings are also reported by Antoni and Goodkin,[34] who found that, among women with atypical neoplastic cervical growth, those who were pessimistic (as assessed by the Millon Inventory) were more likely to have severe disease. In a study of CABG patients, Scheier et al.[35] found that those scoring low in optimism (total LOT score) were significantly more likely to have developed new Q-waves on their electrocardiograms as a result of the surgery and were significantly more likely to have a clinically significant release of the enzyme aspartate aminotransferase. Both are markers for MI, suggesting that the pessimists were significantly more likely than the optimists to have had an infarct during surgery. These relations persisted after controlling for number of grafts, severity of CHD, and a composite index of coronary risk factors. Optimism also significantly predicted rate of recovery, such that optimists were faster to achieve behavioral milestones, such as sitting up in bed and walking, than were pessimists, and were rated by staff members as showing a better physical recovery. At six-month follow-up, optimists continued to have a recovery advantage, reporting that they were more likely to have resumed vigorous physical exercise, to have returned to work, and to have resumed normal activities (see also Ref. 36). In a five-year follow-up, optimists were more likely to be working and, among those experiencing angina, reported less severe chest pain. Optimists were also less likely to be rehospitalized for complications arising from the surgery. Two studies of college students conducted during the last weeks of the academic semester found that optimists reported developing fewer physical symptoms than pessimists over time, taking baseline symptoms into account.[37,38] In addition to its association with disease directly, dispositional optimism has been related to other routes to biological endpoints, including the use of more active and problem-focused coping strategies,[39,40] greater psychological well-being, and better health habits (e.g., Ref. 41; see Ref. 42 for a review). Not all studies show a protective relationship of optimism or a negative effect of pessimism on health. Chesterman et al.[43] found that optimism predicted birth complications in older women, and Cohen et al.[44] found evidence suggesting decreased immunocompetence in optimists in response to stress; however, in another study,[45] pessimism was associated with decreased immunocompetence in response to stress.

Some research has also related situational optimism to health-related outcomes. For example, in the context of HIV infection, negative HIV-specific expectancies

The data sets were a study of Florida residents' recovery from Hurricane Andrew (Gail Ironson, P.I.); the Women and Family Project investigation of women at risk for HIV (Gail Wyatt, P.I.); the MACS Cohort Study, an investigation of the natural history of AIDS in gay men (Roger Detels, P.I.); and an investigation of recovery patterns of 234 coronary artery bypass graft patients (Michael Scheier, P.I.). The authors wish to thank Michael Scheier and Charles Carver for reanalyzing their datasets to reveal these patterns.

predicted immune decline,[46] symptom onset,[47] and survival time for AIDS.[48] In a study on coping with law school,[49] situational optimists had higher NKCC after controlling for the effects of mood. Leedham, Meyerowitz, Muirhead, and Frist[50] found that situationally optimistic expectations were associated with faster recovery following heart transplant.

Studies that have used pessimistic explanatory style as a measure of pessimism have also uncovered relations to health. Pessimistic explanatory style was associated with lower levels of two measures of cell-mediated immunity in a sample of elderly men and women.[51] A study of Harvard University graduates assessing pessimistic explanatory style at age 25 found that these men had significantly poorer health or were more likely to have died when they were assessed 20 to 35 years later.[52]

In conclusion, pessimism appears to be related to SES, and it has shown relationships to important health outcomes. The intriguing asymmetry of positive and negative expectations and their relation to SES merits continued exploration. In particular, research should focus on how these negative expectations develop and whether they partially account for the SES–health relationship.

SOCIAL SUPPORT

Social support refers to the types of help that people receive from others, and it is generally classified into two (sometimes three) major categories: emotional and instrumental (and sometimes informational) support. Emotional support refers to the things that people do that make a person feel loved and cared for and that bolster a sense of self-worth (e.g., talking over a problem, providing encouragement/positive feedback); such support frequently takes the form of nontangible types of assistance. By contrast, instrumental support refers to the various types of tangible help that others may provide (e.g., help with child care/housekeeping, provision of transportation or money). Informational support (sometimes included within the instrumental support category) refers to the help that others may offer through the provision of information.

Investigators have chiefly explored three types of measures of social support. The first is network measures, namely whether people are involved in relationships and groups, and if so, which ones and how many. That is, are people married; do they have children; do they have friends; and are they members of formal and informal community, religious, and interest groups? The second approach assesses social support, that is, people's perceptions that there are others available to them who might provide emotional or instrumental support. The third approach investigates how satisfied people are with the support that they receive from others.

Social support has been found to vary positively with socioeconomic status in studies in the United States,[53–55] England,[8] and Sweden.[56] This pattern is true for both emotional and instrumental support and for both men and women (though the differences appear to be somewhat greater for men.[8] Notably, however, the actual size of the observed variations is relatively small.[8]

The strongest associations between social support (particularly emotional support) and health outcomes are seen in relation to psychological well-being. A large literature documents lower risk for depression and for psychological distress more generally for those who enjoy greater social support (for review see Ref. 57). Relationships to physical health outcomes have also been documented. Much of this research has used measures of social integration, such as network size, rather than social support, and found consistent relations to all-cause mortality and extant disease (e.g., Refs. 58 and 59, for reviews). There is also evidence linking both emotional and instrumental support to less extensive development of coronary atherosclerosis[60,61] and to better survival post-myocardial infarction,[62,63] and post-stroke.[64] More generally, evidence suggests that emotional support is protective with respect to physical function.[65] The effects of instrumental support, however, appear to be more mixed with higher levels of such support associated with greater disability in some cases[66] (for review, see Ref. 67).

Studies also show that emotional support in particular affects both psychological and physical health outcomes in children. Children exposed to deficient nurturing are at increased risk for depression[68,69] and suicidal ideation.[70] Children born to mothers who lacked family support are at increased risk for low birth weight[71] and childhood exposure to less responsive parenting has been related to increased risk for childhood illness[72] and substance abuse among adolescents.[73,74]

A growing body of evidence links social support to physiological regulatory processes. Among children, presence of a supportive caregiver has been shown to lower HPA responses to maternal separation (as indexed by salivary cortisol levels).[75] For adults, social support has likewise been found to predict lower levels of HPA (hypothalamic–pituitary–adrenal) and SNS (sympathetic nervous system) activity in laboratory-based challenge paradigms as well as community settings.[76] Evidence also links social support to lower risk of decline in CD4 T cell counts among HIV-infected men.[77]

To date, social conflict has been a relatively neglected aspect of social relationships in research on SES, social relationships, and health. Social conflict refers to the various types of negative social interaction that may occur within social relationships (e.g., arguments, criticism, hostility, unwanted demands) and may include physical violence. Available data suggest that lower SES is associated with higher levels of social conflict for adults,[78] and evidence also suggests that lower SES is associated with more troubled peer relations among adolescents.[79] Research also suggests that certain social stressors may be more prevalent in lower SES environments (e.g., residential crowding, fear of crime, financial strain); these stressors are associated with lower perceived support[80–83] and may contribute to reductions in reported levels of social support because they foster a distrust of others.[84] However, high levels of support have been found within certain ethnic enclaves (e.g., see Refs. 85–87).

A modest research literature indicates that greater social conflict is associated with greater psychological distress[78,88] (for review, see Ref. 67). Significantly, the impact of social conflict on psychological distress levels is greater among those living in more crowded homes,[83] an effect that appears to be partially mediated by reductions in perceptions of control.[89]

Relationships between social conflict and physical health outcomes have received little research attention to date. However, in both children and adults exposed to social conflict, patterns of heightened physiological reactivity are found, suggesting possible links to poorer health outcomes. Preschoolers exposed to videotapes of angry adult interactions exhibit increases in heart rate and blood pressure.[90] Research also demonstrates relationships between childhood exposure to conflict and/or physical violence and increased risks for depression,[91,92] headaches and stomachaches,[93] and increased risk of mortality.[94] Increased levels of reported stressors in both day-care and family environments (some reflecting social stressors) have also been related to increased incidence of respiratory illness (though specific measures of family conflict were not related to illness).[95] Studies of adults report relationships between social conflict and greater physiologic arousal both with respect to blood pressure[96,97] and neuroendocrine activity.[98]

Unlike control and optimism, for which there are generally preferred measures of the concepts, social support enjoys no preferred measure, and so the lack of a gold standard for assessing social support has impeded progress. Nonetheless, social support, social conflict, and the balance between them may be important moderators of the SES and health relationship.

COPING STRATEGIES

Coping strategies refer to the specific efforts, both behavioral and psychological, that people employ to master, tolerate, reduce, or minimize stressful events. Two general coping strategies have been distinguished: *problem-solving strategies* are efforts to do something active to alleviate stressful circumstances, whereas *emotion-focused strategies* involve efforts to regulate the emotional consequences of stressful or potentially stressful events. Research indicates that people use both types of strategies to combat most stressful events.[99] The predominance of one type of strategy over another is determined, in part, by personal style (e.g., some people cope more actively than others) and also by the type of stressful event. For example, people typically employ problem-focused coping to deal with potentially controllable problems such as work-related problems and family-related problems, whereas stressors perceived as less controllable, such as certain kinds of physical health problems, prompt more emotion-focused coping.

An additional distinction that is often made in the coping literature is between active and avoidant coping strategies. Active coping strategies are either behavioral or psychological responses designed to change the nature of the stressor itself or how one thinks about it, whereas avoidant coping strategies lead people into activities (such as alcohol use) or mental states (such as withdrawal) that keep them from directly addressing stressful events. Generally speaking, active coping strategies, whether behavioral or emotional, are thought to be better ways to deal with stressful events, and avoidant coping strategies appear to be psychological risk factors or markers for adverse responses to stressful life events.[100]

Broad distinctions, such as problem-solving versus emotion-focused, or active versus avoidant, have only limited utility for understanding coping, and so research on coping and its measurement has evolved to address a variety of more specific coping strategies. A variety of idiosyncratic coping measures exist, but in recent years, researchers have typically used one of two instruments: the Ways of Coping measure[99] or the COPE.[39]

In terms of the SES–health relation, coping style may be a psychosocial resource that is farther downstream than those thus far reviewed. That is, coping methods may be, in part, the result of expectations of control, an optimistic or pessimistic way of thinking, and the degree to which one has social support available. This is not to say that coping strategy is unimportant or epiphenomenal in the SES–health relation, but rather that it may be somewhat farther along on the psychosocial chain as a mediator. Consequently, and not surprisingly, the evidence for the relation of coping strategies to SES is rather meager. Only preliminary evidence has found avoidant coping to be higher as SES decreases.[101]

Both the COPE and the Ways of Coping scales have been reliably tied to psychological distress, such that active coping strategies appear reliably to produce better emotional adjustment to chronically stressful events than do avoidant coping strategies. In terms of physical health outcomes, an active versus avoidant coping strategy has been associated with better immune status in HIV-seropositive men,[102,103] in individuals infected with herpes simplex virus,[104] and in men with immunologically-mediated infertility.[105] Use of denial following serostatus notification was associated with more rapid disease progression in HIV-seropositive gay men.[106] Active coping with disease was associated with fewer recurrences and longer survival from melanoma.[107] Avoidance coping was associated with lower numbers of T cells and reduced NK cytotoxity among law school students.[49]

In summary, it appears as if coping strategies may be part of a mediational chain from SES to health risk, but exactly the ways in which they are affected by or reflect SES, and the point at which they affect health, requires further exploration.

OTHER PSYCHOSOCIAL RESOURCES

We reviewed several other psychosocial resources as candidate mediators or moderators of the SES–health gradient. One resource that does not appear to contribute to the SES–health relation is self-esteem. There is little evidence that self-esteem varies by SES or that it is associated reliably with health outcomes.[108] There does seem to be some role for high self-esteem in successful coping with stressful events and in recovery from illnesses (see Ref. 109), but these beneficial outcomes do not appear to be SES-distributed.

Also deserving of consideration are psychosocial resources that may facilitate longevity and good health at the upper ends of the SES–health gradient, which include vitality and vigor and purpose in life. Relative to the resources already discussed, fewer studies have explored the potentially protective effects of these resources, but preliminary research is promising. For example, vitality may be modestly correlated with SES[110] [d] and, on the health side, vitality is associated with fewer chronic physical health conditions,[111] fewer symptoms among people with HIV infection,[112] and fewer symptoms for those with chronic fatigue syndrome.[113] However, measures of vitality do not distinguish between physical and psychological forms, and, therefore, endorsement of exhaustion may represent feelings of physical

[d]We are grateful to Brooks Gump for reanalyzing the Scheier et al.[110] data set to reveal these findings.

exertion in the context of poor health or psychological demands in the context of poor coping.[114] Despite these reservations, the potential protective functions of positive states merits additional consideration.

REACTIVE RESPONDING

To further explore the measurement of psychosocial states that may contribute to the SES and health relationship, the MacArthur SES and Health Psychosocial Working Group has used insights from our understanding of SES and how it might affect health to develop measures to try to get closer to understanding how SES gets under the skin. We began by trying to characterize the attributes of environments that may change as one moves lower on the SES scale and identify what the physiological concomitants of those states might be. The result is a concept, termed "reactive responding," and a set of measures that assesses it.

Reactive responding refers to the self-regulatory patterns believed to develop as a result of exposure to chronically stressful environments that may increase as one is lower on the SES ladder. Development of the concept was guided by the observation that, by virtue of being born into a particular social class, an individual is exposed to a set of environments that differ from those that constitute the experience of individuals in other social classes; these regularities are assumed to produce reliable differences across social classes in the evolution of self-regulatory strategies and skills for dealing with characteristics of SES-related environments. The lower one's social class, the more likely one's environments (that is, family, school, work, neighborhood) may be characterized by a dearth of resources, including time and money, as well as an abundance of chronically stressful conditions, such as crowding, noise, crime, and other risks. In contrast, to the extent that one is higher in social class, one's environments may be more rich in resources, such as money, and lower in chronic stressors, providing opportunities for the development of self-regulatory skills devoted to setting future goals, planning, developing a future temporal orientation, and the like. Regularities across environments within level of social class may produce fairly stable class differences in prevailing modes of responding, such that, through chronic use, such self-regulatory mechanisms become instilled as habits or dispositions, and thus may be employed in new environments where they may not always be maximally useful.

Reactive responding is thought to be characterized by the following:

Chronic vigilance/load: A high level of environmental demands, coupled with danger or urgency, may lead to a state of chronic vigilance, such that individuals chronically monitor the environment for threatening cues.

On-line responding/on-line planning: When individual action is driven by environmental demands rather than an individual's self-generated agenda, there may be little opportunity for anticipatory planning; rather, what planning occurs may be on-line in response to environmental demands.

Emotional action: Responding in demanding environments may be emotionally charged, first due to interruptions from the environment; second, to the extent that risks may be present in the situation; and third, by virtue of an absence of personal control.

Constrained options: When responding occurs as a result of environmental demands rather than self-generated planning, environmental options may be few, and the opportunity for a person to develop alternatives may be low.

Narrow learning and skill development: To the extent that environmental demands drive a person's responses, there may be few opportunities for broad learning. Rather, within the context of constrained options, learning and consequent skills may be quite narrow.

Present orientation: High levels of environmental demands and the need to respond reactively to an environment may foster a present orientation that keeps a person focused on the short-term future.

Simple, short-term goal orientation: A focus on the present, a relative absence of resources, and a relative dearth of opportunities for individual control may lead to the development of relatively simple and short-term goals, as opposed to the creation of long-term goals and opportunities.

We developed a multiscale measure of reactive responding, which attempts to assess these self-regulatory patterns that are believed to develop as a result of exposure to the chronically stressful environments that may increase as one decreases on the SES ladder. In early investigations, three scales have been found to relate to both to SES and to health outcomes: *vigilance,* characterized as the need to chronically monitor the environment for threatening cues (an example of an item is, "I'm on my guard in most situations"); *emotional action*, which measures the extent to which responding in demanding environments is emotionally charged (an example is the reverse-coded item, "I let my emotions cool before I act"); and *goal orientation,* assessing the extent to which people plan where they are going in life and have long-term goals (an example of such an item is, "I have many long-term goals that I work to achieve"). High vigilance, high emotional action, and low goal orientation have been modestly associated with low SES in the samples we have studied thus far, and these same scales appear to be implicated in a variety of health symptoms in several samples. We currently have in place large-scale projects to see if these scales continue to be associated with SES and health in larger and more heterogeneous samples with respect to major health outcomes. What distinguishes our reactive responding scales from the more usual explorations of psychosocial resources and the SES–health relation is, first, the effort to get people to self-rate their behavior in specific and potentially SES-related environments marked by chronic stress and, second, the possible proximity of these experiences to the physiological level, especially vigilance and emotional arousal. Such measures may be helpful in identifying how SES gets under the skin.

CONCLUSIONS

The psychosocial resources reviewed here, although unlikely to be a sufficient explanation for the SES–health relationship, are nonetheless potentially important mediators of SES disparities in health and longevity. Specifically, these are the resources that people bring to stressful encounters that enable them to cope more or less badly with those stressful encounters, both acute and chronic. When we pose the question, "How does SES get under the skin to affect health?" one way in which it may do so is through the psychological mediation or moderation provided by or facilitated by resources such as psychological control, social support, coping style, optimism, and reactive responding.

What remains to be achieved is an integration of psychosocial resources with an understanding of the biobehavioral pathways by which SES affects health. Psychosocial resources influence the perception of events and the degree to which they are experienced as stressful as well as their aftermath and thus, they initiate, exacerbate, or ameliorate the behavioral, physiological, and neuroendocrine responses to stress in ways that ultimately lead to the startling, robust SES gradients in health outcomes that are so commonly observed. Preliminary efforts to develop such models are already under way (see Baum[117]; McEwen and Seeman[118]).

ACKNOWLEDGMENTS

This analysis represents the contributions of the Psychosocial Working Group of the SES and Health MacArthur Foundation Network, and we would like to acknowledge the collaborative role that Nancy Adler, Sheldon Cohen, Karen Matthews, and David Williams have played in the development of this analysis. Preparation of this manuscript was supported by funding from the MacArthur Foundation's SES and Health Network and by a grant from the National Institute of Mental Health (MH 056880) to the first author.

REFERENCES

1. TAYLOR, S.E. et al. 1997. Health psychology: what is an unhealthy environment and how does it get under the skin? Ann. Rev. Psychol. **48:** 411–447.
2. SCHULZ, R. et al. 1994. Pessimism and mortality in young and old recurrent cancer patients. Presented at the Annual Meeting of the American Psychosomatic Society. June. Boston, MA.
3. WHITE, R.W. 1959. Motivation reconsidered: the concept of competence. Psychol. Rev. **66:** 297–335.
4. PEARLIN, L.I. & C. SCHOOLER. 1978. The structure of coping. J. Health Soc. Behav. **19:** 2–21.
5. COHEN, S. et al. 1999. The role of psychological characteristics in the relation between socioeconomic status and perceived health. J. App. Soc. Psychol. **29:** 445–467.
6. MIROWSKY J. & C. ROSS. 1986. Social patterns of distress. Annu. Rev. Sociol. **12:** 23–45.
7. LEVINSON, H. 1981. Differentiating among internality, powerful others, and chance. In Research with the Locus of Control Construct, Vol. 1. H.M. Lefcourt, Ed.: 15–63. Academic Press, New York.
8. MARMOT, M.G. et al. 1997. Contribution of job control and other risk factors to social variations in coronary heart disease incidence. Lancet **350:** 235–239.
9. PINCUS, T. & L.F. CALLAHAN. 1995. What explains the association between socioeconomic status and health: primarily access to medical care or mind-body variables? Advances: J. Mind–Body Health **11:** 4–36.
10. GECAS, V. 1989. The social psychology of self-efficacy. Annu. Rev. Sociol. **15:** 291–316.
11. LACHMAN, M.E. & S.L. WEAVER. 1999. The sense of control as a moderator of social class differences in health and well-being. J. Pers. Soc. Psychol. In press.
12. PEARLIN, L.I. et al. 1981. The stress process. J. Health Soc. Behav. **22:** 337–356.

13. BLAUNER, R. 1964. Alienation and Freedom: The Factory Worker and His Industry. University of Chicago Press, Chicago.
14. KOHN, M.L. & C. SCHOOLER. 1983. Work and Personality: An Inquiry into the Impact of Social Stratification. Ablex Publishing Corp. Stamford, CT.
15. RODIN, J. et al. 1985. The construct of control: biological and psychosocial correlates. Ann. Rev. Gerontol. Geriatr. **5:** 3–55.
16. KARASEK, R.A. et al. 1982. Job, psychological factors and coronary heart disease: Swedish prospective findings and U.S. prevalence findings using a new occupational inference method. Adv. Cardiol. **29:** 62–67.
17. RODIN, J. & E.J. LANGER. 1977. Long-term effects of a control-relevant intervention with the institutionalized aged. J. Pers. Soc. Psychol. **35:** 897–902.
18. SEEMAN, M. & S. LEWIS. 1995. Powerlessness, health and mortality: a longitudinal study of older men and mature women. Soc. Sci. Med. **41:** 517–525.
19. SEEMAN, M. 1991. Alienation and anomie. In Measures of Personality and Social Psychological Attitudes, Vol. 1. J.R. Robinson, et al. Eds.: 291–372. Academic Press, San Diego.
20. THOMPSON, S.C. et al. 1988. The other side of perceived control: disadvantages and negative effects. In The Social Psychology of Health. S. Spacapan & S. Oshkamp, Eds.: 69–93. Sage, Beverly Hills.
21. EVANS, G.W. et al. 1993. Specifying dysfunctional mismatches between different control dimensions. Br. J. Psychol. **84:** 255–273.
22. ROTHBAUM, R. et al. 1982. Changing the world and changing the self: a two-process model of perceived control. J. Pers. Soc. Psych. **42:** 5–37.
23. DEGOOD, D.E. 1975. Cognitive control factors in vascular stress responses. Psychophysiology **12:** 399–401.
24. HOUSTON, B.K. 1972. Control over stress, locus of control, and response to stress. J. Pers. Soc. Psychol. **21:** 249–255.
25. MANUCK, S.B. et al. 1978. Effects of coping on blood pressure responses to threat of aversive stimulation. Psychophysiology **15:** 544–549.
26. SIEBER, W.J. et al. 1992. Modulation of human natural killer cell activity by exposure to uncontrollable stress. Brain Behav. Immunol. **6:** 141–156.
27. MILLER, S.M. et al. 1985. Preference for control and the coronary-prone behavior pattern: "I'd rather do it myself." J. Pers. Soc. Psychol. **49:** 492–499.
28. STRUBE, M.J. & C. WERNER. 1985. Relinquishment of control and the type A behavior pattern. J. Pers. Soc. Psychol. **48:** 688–701.
29. KRANTZ, D.S. et al. 1974. Helplessness, stress level, and the coronary-prone behavior pattern. J. Exp. Soc. Psychol. **10:** 284–300.
30. CARVER, C.S. & M.F. SCHEIER. 1981. Attention and Self-Regulation: A Control-Theory Approach to Human Behavior. Springer, New York.
31. SCHEIER, M.F. et al. 1994. Distinguishing optimism from neuroticism (and trait anxiety, self-mastery, and self-esteem): a reevaluation of the Life Orientation Test. J. Pers. Soc. Psychol. **67:** 1063–1078.
32. SELIGMAN, M.E.P. 1975. Helplessness: On Depression, Development and Death. Freeman, San Francisco.
33. ARMOR, D.A. & S.E. TAYLOR. 1998. Situated optimism: specific outcome expectancies and self-regulation. In Advances in Experimental Social Psychology, Vol. 30. M.P. Zanna, Ed.: 309–379. Academic Press, New York.
34. ANTONI, M.H. & K. GOODKIN. 1988. Host moderator variables in the promotion of cervical neoplasia. I: Personality facets. J. Psychosom. Res. **32:** 327–338.
35. SCHEIER, M.F. et al. 1989. Dispositional optimism and recovery from coronary artery bypass surgery: the beneficial effects on physical and psychological well-being. J. Pers. Soc. Psychol. **57:** 1024–1040.
36. FITZGERALD, T.E. et al. 1993. The relative importance of dispositional optimism and control appraisals in quality of life after coronary bypass surgery. J. Behav. Med. **16:** 25–43.
37. SCHEIER, M.F. & C.S. CARVER. 1991. Dispositional optimism and adjustment to college. Unpublished raw data.

38. TAYLOR, S.E. & L.G. ASPINWALL. 1990. Psychological aspects of chronic illness. *In* Psychological Aspects of Serious Illness. G.R. VandenBos & P.T. Costa, Jr., Eds.: 3–60. American Psychological Association, Washington, DC.
39. CARVER, C.S. *et al.* 1989. Assessing coping strategies: a theoretically based approach. J. Pers. Soc. Psychol. **56:** 267–283.
40. TAYLOR, S.E. *et al.* 1992. Optimism, coping, psychological distress, and high-risk sexual behaviors among men at risk for AIDS. J. Pers. Soc. Psychol. **63:** 460–473.
41. PARK, C.L. *et al.* 1997. The roles of constructive thinking and optimism in psychological and behavioral adjustment during pregnancy. J. Pers. Soc. Psychol. **73:** 584–592.
42. SCHEIER, M.F. & C.S. CARVER. 1992. Effects of optimism on psychological and physical well-being: theoretical overview and empirical update. Cog. Ther. Res. **16:** 201–228.
43. CHESTERMAN, E. *et al.* 1990. Trait optimism as a predictor of pregnancy outcomes. Poster presented at the First International Congress on Behavioral Medicine, Uppsala, Sweden.
44. COHEN, F. *et al.* 1999. Differential immune system changes with acute and persistent stress for optimists vs. pessimists. Brain Behav. Immun. **13:** 155–174.
45. BACHEN, E. *et al.* 1991. Effects of dispositional optimism on immunologic responses to laboratory stress. Unpublished data.
46. TAYLOR, S.E. *et al.* 1999. Psychological resources, positive illusions, and health. Am. Psychol. In press.
47. REED, G.M. *et al.* 1999. Negative HIV-specific expectancies and AIDS-related bereavement as predictors of symptom onset in asymptomatic HIV-positive gay men. Health Psychol. **18:** 1–10.
48. REED, G.M. *et al.* 1994. Realistic acceptance as a predictor of decreased survival time in gay men with AIDS. Health Psychol. **13:** 299–307.
49. SEGERSTROM, S.C. *et al.* 1998. Effects of optimism and coping on stressor-related mood and immune changes. J. Pers. Soc. Psychol. **74:** 1646–1655.
50. LEEDHAM, B. *et al.* 1995. Positive expectations predict health after heart transplantation. Health Psychol. **14:** 74–79.
51. KAMEN-SIEGEL, L. *et al.* 1991. Explanatory style and cell-mediated immunity in elderly men and women. Health Psychol. **10:** 229–235.
52. PETERSON, C. *et al.* 1988. Pessimistic explanatory style is a risk factor for physical illness: a thirty-five-year longitudinal study. J. Pers. Soc. Psychol. **55:** 23–27.
53. MATTHEWS, K.A. *et al.* 1989. Educational attainment and behavioral and biological risk factors for coronary heart disease in middle-aged women. Am. J. Epidemiol. **129:** 132–144.
54. HUANG, G. & M. TAUSIG. 1990. Network range in personal networks. Soc. Networks **12:** 261–268.
55. CAMPBELL, K.E. *et al.* 1986. Social resources and socioeconomic status. Soc. Networks **8:** 97–117.
56. OSTERGREN, P.-O. 1991. Psychosocial Resources and Health. Department of Community Health Sciences, Lund University. Malmo, Sweden.
57. GEORGE, L.K. 1989. Stress, social support, and depression over the life-course. *In* Aging, Stress, Social Support, and Health. K. Markides & C. Cooper, Eds.: 241–267. Wiley, London.
58. HOUSE J.S. *et al.* 1988. Social relationships and health. Science **241:** 540–45.
59. SEEMAN, T.E. 1996. Social ties and health: The benefits of social integration. AEP **6:** 442–451.
60. SEEMAN, T.E. & S.L. SYME. 1987. Social networks and coronary artery disease: a comparative analysis of network structural and support characteristics. Psychosom. Med. **49:** 341–354.
61. BLUMENTHAL, J.A. et al. 1987. Social support, type A behavior, and coronary artery disease. Psychosom. Med. **49:** 331–340.
62. BERKMAN, L.F. *et al.* 1992. Emotional support and survival after myocardial infarction: a prospective, population-based study of the elderly. Psychosom. Med. **58:** 459–471.

63. WILLIAMS, R.B. *et al.* 1992. Prognostic importance of social and economic resources among medically treated patients with angiographically documented coronary artery disease. JAMA **267:** 520–524.
64. GLASS, T. & G.L. MADDOX. 1992. The quality and quantity of social support: stroke recovery as psycho-social transition. Soc. Sci. Med. **34:** 1249–1261.
65. SEEMAN, T.E. *et al.* 1995. Behavioral and psychosocial predictors of physical performance: MacArthur studies of successful aging. J. Gerontol. **50A:** M177–M183.
66. SEEMAN, T.E. *et al.* 1996. Social network characteristics and onset of ADL disability: MacArthur studies of successful aging. J. Gerontol. **51B:** S191–S200.
67. BURG, M.M. & T.E. SEEMAN. 1994. Families and health: the negative side of social ties. Ann. Behav. Med. **16:** 109–115.
68. KASLOW, N.J. *et al.* 1994. Depressed children and their families. Clin. Psychol. Rev. **14:** 39–59.
69. LEWINSOHN, P.M. *et al.* 1994. Adolescent psychopathology. II. Psychosocial risk factors for depression. J. Abnorm. Psychol. **103:** 302–315.
70. ADAMS, D.M. *et al.* 1994. Perceived family functioning and adolescent suicidal behavior. J. Am. Acad. Child Adoles. Psychiatry. **33:** 498–507.
71. COLLINS, N.L. *et al.* 1993. Social support in pregnancy: psychosocial correlates of birth outcomes and postpartum depression. J. Pers. Soc. Psychol. **65:** 1243–1258.
72. GOTTMAN, J.M. & L.F. KATZ. 1989. Effects of marital discord on young children's peer interaction and health. Dev. Psychol. **25:** 373–381.
73. SHEDLER, J. & J. BLOCK. 1990. Adolescent drug use and psychological health: a longitudinal inquiry. Am. Psychol. **45:** 612–630.
74. BAUMRIND, D. 1991. The influence of parenting style on adolescent competence and substance use. J. Early Adoles. **11:** 56–95.
75. GUNNAR M.R. *et al.* 1992. The stressfulness of separation among nine-month-old infants: effects of social context variables and infant temperament. Child Dev. **63:** 290–303.
76. SEEMAN, T.E. & B.S. MCEWEN. 1996. Impact of social environment characteristics on neuroendocrine regulation. Psychosom. Med. **58:** 459–471.
77. THEORELL, T. et al. 1995. Social support and the development of immune function in human immunodeficiency virus infection. Psychosom. Med. **57:** 32–36.
78. SCHUSTER, T.L. *et al.* 1990. Supportive interactions, negative interactions and depressed mood. Am. J. Commun. Psychol. **18:** 423–438.
79. BOLGER, K.E. *et al.* 1995. Psychosocial adjustment among children experiencing persistent and intermittent family economic hardship. Child Dev. **66:** 1107–1129.
80. EVANS G.W. *et al.* 1989. Residential density and psychological health: the mediating effects of social support. J. Pers. Soc. Psychol. **57:** 994–999.
81. LEPORE, S.J. *et al.* 1991. Dynamic role of social support in the link between chronic stress and psychological distress. J. Pers. Soc. Psychol. **61:** 899–909.
82. LEPORE, S.J. *et al.* 1991. Daily hassles and chronic strains: a hierarchy of stressors? Soc. Sci. Med. **33:** 1029–1036.
83. LEPORE, S.J. *et al.* 1991c. Social hassles and psychological health in the context of chronic crowding. J. Health Soc. Behav. **32:** 357–367.
84. KRAUSE, N. 1992. Stress and isolation form close ties in later life. J. Gerontol: Soc. Sci. **46:** S183–S194.
85. GANS, H. 1962. The Urban Villagers: Group and Class in the Life of Italian-Americans. Free Press, New York.
86. STACK, C. 1975. All Our Kin: Strategies for Survival in a Black Community. Harper and Row, New York.
87. MACLEOD, J. 1995. Ain't No Making It. Westview Press, Boulder.
88. ROOK, K.S. 1990. Parallels in the study of social support and social strain. J. Soc. Clin. Psychol. **9:** 118–132.
89. LEPORE, S.J. *et al.* 1992. Role of control and social support in explaining the stress of hassles and crowding. Environ. Behav. **24:** 795–811.
90. EL-SHEIKH, M. *et al.* 1989. Coping with adults' angry behavior: behavioral, physiological, and self-report responding in preschoolers. Dev. Psychol. **325:** 490–498.

91. DOWNEY, G. & E. WALKER. 1992. Distinguishing family-level and child-level influences on the development of depression and aggression in children at risk. Dev. Psychopathol. **4:** 81–95.
92. KOVEROLA, C. *et al.* 1993. Relationship of child sexual abuse to depression. Child Abuse Neglect. **17:** 393–400.
93. MECHANIC, D. & S. HANSELL. 1989. Divorce, family conflict, and adolescents' well-being. J. Health Soc. Behav. **3:** 105–116.
94. SORENSON, S.B. & J.G. PETERSON. 1994. Traumatic child death and documented maltreatment history, Los Angeles. Am. J. Pub. Health **84:** 623–627.
95. BOYCE, W.T. *et al.* 1995. Psychobiological reactivity to stress and childhood respiratory illnesses: results to two prospective studies. Psychosom. Med. **57:** 411–422.
96. EWART, C.K. *et al.* 1991. High blood pressure and marital discord: not being nasty matters more than being nice. Health Psychol. **10:** 155–163.
97. GERIN, W. *et al.* 1992. Social support in social interaction: a moderator of cardiovascular reactivity. Psychosom. Med. **54:** 324–336.
98. KIECOLT-GLASER, J.K. *et al.* 1994. Stressful personal relationships: immune and endocrine function. *In* Handbook of Human Stress and Immunity. R. Glaser & J. Kiecolt-Glaser, Eds.: 321–329. Academic Press, San Diego.
99. FOLKMAN, S. & R.S. LAZARUS. 1980. An analysis of coping in a middle-aged community sample. J. Health Soc. Behav. **21:** 219–239.
100. HOLAHAN, C.J. & R.H. MOOS. 1987. Risk, resistance, and psychological distress: a longitudinal analysis with adults and children. J. Abnorm. Psychol. **96:** 3–13.
101. CARVER, C.S. 1999. Personal communication.
102. GOODKIN, K., N.T. BLANEY, *et al.* 1992. Active coping style is associated with natural killer cell cytotoxicity in asymptomatic HIV-1 seropositive homosexual men. J. Psychosom. Res. **36:** 635–650.
103. GOODKIN, K., I. FUCHS, *et al.* 1992. Life stressors and coping style are associated with immune measures in HIV-1 infection—a preliminary report. Int. J. Psychiatry Med. **22:** 155–172.
104. KEMENY, M.E. 1991. Psychological factors, immune processes, and the course of herpes simplex and human immunodeficiency virus infection. *In* Stress and Immunity. N. Plotnikoff *et al.*, Eds.: 199–210. CRC Press, Boca Raton.
105. KEDEM, P. *et al.* 1992. Psychoneuroimmunology and male infertility: a possible link between stress, coping, and male immunological infertility. Psychol. Health. **6:** 159–173.
106. IRONSON, G. *et al.* 1994. Distress, denial, and low adherence to behavioral intentions predict faster disease progression in gay men infected with human immunodeficiency virus. Int. J. Behav. Med. **1:** 90–105.
107. FAWZY, F.I. *et al.* 1993. Malignant melanoma: effects of an early structured psychiatric intervention, coping, and affective state on recurrence and survival six years later. Arch. Gen. Psychiatry **50:** 681–689.
108. ADLER, N.E. 1998. Self-esteem. *In* Psychosocial Notebook of the MacArthur SES and Health Network. MacArthur Foundation, San Francisco.
109. TAYLOR, S.E. 1999. Health Psychology, 4th edit. McGraw-Hill, New York.
110. SCHEIER, M.F. *et al.* 1999. Optimism and rehospitalization following coronary artery bypass graft surgery. Arch. Int. Med. **159:** 829–835.
111. LERNER, D. *et al.* 1994. Job strain and health-related inequality of life in a national sample. Am. J. Pub. Health **84:** 1580–1585.
112. WU, A.W. *et al.* 1991. A health status questionnaire using 30 items from the Medical Outcomes Study: preliminary validation in persons with early HIV infection. Med. Care **29:** 786–798.
113. BUCHWALD, D. *et al.* 1996. Functional status in patients with chronic fatigue syndrome, other fatiguing illnesses, and healthy individuals. Am. J. Med. **101:** 364–370.
114. GUMP, B. 1998. Vitality and vigor. *In* Psychosocial Notebook of the MacArthur SES and Health Network. MacArthur Foundation, San Francisco.
115. LEFCOURT, H.M. 1991. Locus of control. In Measures of Personality and Social Psychological Attitudes, Vol. 1. J.P. Robinson *et al.*, Eds.: 413–499. Academic Press, San Diego.

116. WALLSTON, K.A. *et al.* 1978. Development of the multidimensional Health Locus of Control Scales. Health Educ. Monogr. **6:** 161–170.
117. BAUM, A. *et al.* 199. Socioeconomic status and chronic stress: does stress account for SES effects on health? Ann. N.Y. Acad. Sci. **896:** this volume.
118. McEWEN, B.S. & T. SEEMAN. 1999. Protective and damaging effects of mediators of stress: elaborating and testing the concepts of allostasis and allostatic load. Ann. N.Y. Acad. Sci. **896:** this volume.

Do Negative Emotions Mediate the Association between Socioeconomic Status and Health?

LINDA C. GALLO AND KAREN A. MATTHEWS[a]

Cardiovascular Behavioral Medicine, The University of Pittsburgh School of Medicine, Pittsburgh, Pennsylvania 15213, USA

ABSTRACT: In this chapter, we examine the possibility that negative emotions contribute to the relationship between socioeconomic status (SES) and health. A model of the associations among SES, emotion, and health is presented first. We then review the evidence for this model, showing associations of SES with depression, hopelessness, anxiety, and hostile affect and cognition, and of these negative emotions with disease. Notably, most of the data supporting the model provide only indirect evidence that negative emotions serve as a key contributor to the proposed associations. We, therefore, conclude with recommendations for longitudinal research, especially in children, that will more directly and comprehensively examine negative emotions as possible mediators of the SES and health relationship.

INTRODUCTION

In this chapter we examine the evidence that negative emotions represent a key link between socioeconomic status and health. We begin by addressing some basic issues regarding the conceptualization of emotion. Next, we describe the model we propose to connect emotional states with SES and health outcomes. We then turn to an overview of research concerning the emotions that may connect SES with health. The issue is whether negative emotions *mediate* the relationship between SES and health. For this model to be plausible, research should show that SES is related to negative emotions, that negative emotions are related to health, and that SES is related to health. Further, when all three constructs are included in a single methodological framework, the relationship between SES and health should be attenuated if negative emotions are controlled for statistically. Here, we assume the connection between SES and health and focus on the other associations in the model. Unfortunately, the majority of the research to date provides only indirect evidence for emotional states as possible mediators—few studies have attempted to integrate SES, emotions, and health. Thus, we conclude with recommendations for future research that will more completely address the proposed model.

[a]Address for correspondence: Karen A. Matthews, Ph.D., Cardiovascular Behavioral Medicine, University of Pittsburgh School of Medicine, 3811 O'Hara St., Pittsburgh, PA 15213, USA. 412-624-2041 (voice); 412-624-0967 (fax).
e-mail: matthewska@msx.upmc.edu

CONCEPTUALIZING EMOTION

The description of emotion has been the focus of considerable attention and disagreement, but many definitions share three components: (1) experienced feelings, based on one's appraisal of the emotion-provoking stimulus; (2) the impulse to behave or act in certain ways; and (3) physiological changes that ready the body for action.[1] Thus, emotions comprise affective, cognitive, behavioral, and physiological correlates. Notably, the terms "emotion" and "mood," though often used interchangeably, denote somewhat distinct affective processes. Parkinson and colleagues[2] suggest that mood can be distinguished from emotion on the basis of its longer duration, more gradual onset, weaker intensity, and less specific precipitants or targets. However, moods and emotions are also likely to be closely and reciprocally related. An individual who is in a "bad mood" has a lower threshold for negative emotions such as anger, anxiety, and sadness. Likewise, an experience that triggers angry emotion may lead to a long-lasting bad mood. Here, we focus on specific emotional states, but we assume that emotions must occur frequently, chronically, or with sufficient intensity to produce significant health effects.

Another commonality across many theories of emotion is the idea that they serve an evolutionary function by signaling a homeostatic imbalance, or need, detected by the individual. Thus, emotions can be considered "transitory adjustment reactions that function to return the organism to a stable, effective relationship with its environment when that relationship is disrupted" (Ref. 3, p.20). By helping the individual regain homeostatic balance, emotions contribute to his or her survival and, ultimately, to species survival. Emotions are therefore adaptive from an evolutionary perspective. Nevertheless, like other potentially adaptive processes such as the physiological stress reaction, emotions have the potential to become maladaptive depending on their appropriateness, frequency, intensity, and duration.[4]

For example, according to the *Diagnostic and Statistical Manual of Mental Disorders* (DSM-IV),[5] a person who has recently lost a loved one may experience great sadness and other symptoms typically associated with major depression (i.e., bereavement). This presentation would not be considered pathological, however, unless it persisted beyond a period of two months and with sufficient intensity to interfere with the individual's functioning. A related issue is the distinction between clinical syndromes, such as depressive or anxiety disorders, and specific emotions. The cardinal feature of clinical depression is sad mood, but it may include other negative emotions, such as guilt, irritability, and anxiety, and nonemotional symptoms such as low appetite, troubled sleep, and poor concentration. Similarly, the fundamental feature of anxiety disorders is fear, but the clinical presentation might include irritability, fatigue, and various behaviors intended to avoid the feared stimuli or reduce the fear itself. Thus, we might conceptualize depression or anxiety disorders as "diseases" of negative emotion. The research we discuss below varies according to whether it focuses primarily on mood and anxiety disorders in their clinically diagnosable forms, or on the quantity of reported symptoms of depression and anxiety. This distinction is important because symptoms of anxiety and depression (i.e., psychological distress) occur relatively frequently in the population, compared with psychiatric disorders. Thus, epidemiological studies demonstrating that diagnosable emotional disorders are not necessary for health effects to occur[6,7] indicate that the effects of negative emotions could have relatively widespread health consequences.

Considerable empirical evidence suggests that the structure of emotion can be captured by two underlying dimensions, which in combination form a circumplex structure.[8-10] The first dimension characterizes the pleasantness (i.e., valence) of the emotion, and the second dimension is variously referred to as activation, arousal, engagement, or attention.[9] Emotions that are more similar in terms of pleasantness, arousal, or both will exhibit higher correlations. This is borne out in research and practice, for example, in the substantial overlap of constructs such as depression and anxiety.[11,12] In a recent empirical investigation of this phenomenon, Feldman[13] demonstrated that individuals weight the pleasantness dimension more heavily than the arousal dimension in describing their moods. Thus, emotions with similar valence are likely to aggregate within an individual.[14] Notably, the literature concerning emotion and SES or health has neglected emotions of positive valence, focusing instead on unpleasant emotions of varying arousal levels. The question of whether positive emotions relate to health and to SES therefore awaits further research.

HOW ARE SES, NEGATIVE EMOTIONS, AND HEALTH RELATED?

FIGURE 1 portrays the model we propose to connect SES, negative emotions, and health. As pictured, individuals who live in low-SES environments are more likely to encounter stimuli associated with threatened or actual harm, and less likely to en-

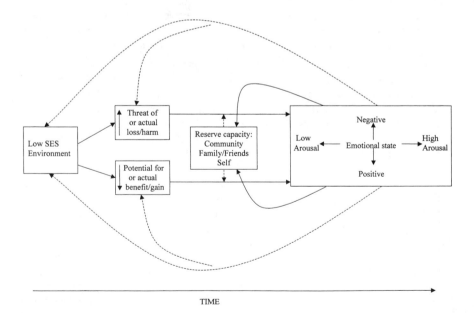

FIGURE 1. The proposed model connecting socioeconomic status, negative emotions, and health.

counter stimuli associated with potential or actual gain. These situational factors are likely to produce congruent emotional responses. Consistent with this model, research shows that lower SES groups do experience more frequent stressful life events.[15,16] At every level of stress exposure, however, they also display higher levels of psychological distress.[17,18] We therefore propose that lower SES individuals are also more *vulnerable* to the negative emotional effects of harmful or threatening stimuli. Their greater vulnerability may reflect a more limited "reserve capacity" of resources with which to manage threatening stimuli (see also Taylor and Seeman, this volume,[19] for discussion of SES and psychosocial resources). Lower SES individuals may have less access to the types of tangible and intangible community resources (e.g., safe neighborhoods, parks, transportation, child care) available to their higher SES counterparts. They may also benefit less from family-provided resources, because lower SES families are more vulnerable to factors that impede familial support, such as domestic violence[20,21] and substance abuse.[22,23] Consistent with this assertion, several studies show that lower SES individuals report fewer and less satisfying social relationships.[24-26] Differential intrapersonal resources may also contribute to the proposed discrepancy in reserve capacity. Lower SES individuals report lower levels of self-efficacy and perceived control,[27] possibly reflecting negative early socialization experiences.[28]

We also propose that because lower SES individuals encounter environmental demands more often, they may be more likely to *deplete* their reserve capacity. In other words, lower SES individuals may be "living on the edge" in terms of their ability to cope with negative stimuli. Because their resources are taxed by the stresses of daily living, lower SES individuals are forced to confront unexpected negative stimuli with an already exhausted system. With no attenuating effect of the reserve capacity, noxious stimuli are likely to persist or escalate, as are negative emotional states. Negative emotions are believed to affect health, in turn, through their associations with health behaviors,[29,30] as well as through alterations in cardiovascular and neuroendocrine responses[29,31,32] and immune functioning.[33] (See also McEwen and Seeman, this volume,[34] for discussion of the physiological sequelae of stress).

As shown, emotional states are likely to feed back on the pathway at several points. Negative emotions may have a direct negative impact on the reserve capacity. For example, a substantial body of literature demonstrates that depression[35,36] and hostility[37,38] are related to poorer marital functioning. Further, negative emotional states such as depression tend to be associated with a poorer self-concept,[39-41] which may interfere with the effective management of harmful or threatening stimuli. Emotional states may also influence appraisals of external stimuli. For example, cognitive theories of depression[42] posit that depression is associated with distorted information processing that tends to reinforce negative mood.[43] Thus, negative emotional states may evoke perceptions that otherwise ambiguous stimuli are threatening or harmful, whereas positive emotional states could lead to more positive appraisals of ambiguous stimuli.

Notably, the path of events we have discussed to this point assumes a *social causation* model of the relationship between SES and physical and emotional health outcomes. From this perspective, one's adult SES plays a causal role in determining health[44] or emotional problems.[45] However, as shown in FIGURE 1, our model also allows for *social drift*, or the causal impact of emotional states on one's social status.

From this perspective, negative emotions—especially in the form of psychiatric disorders—might negatively influence one's ability to complete a higher education program, maintain gainful employment, or secure a high-paying job, thereby causing a decrement in SES. Likewise, positive emotional states might facilitate educational or occupational achievement. The social drift and social causation directional hypotheses have been the subject of considerable research in the literature concerning SES and mental or physical health, and their relative importance is not established.

NEGATIVE EMOTIONS AND HEALTH

In the following sections, we present an overview of the literature concerning the relationships of emotional states with health. We focus on emotions or emotional disorders for which the literature supports an association with documented disease endpoints or other verifiable health outcomes—specifically, depression, hopelessness, and anxiety. We also discuss the literature that has addressed the multidimensional construct of hostility, which includes the emotional component of anger. We emphasize prospective research when possible, because of its ability to demonstrate whether negative emotions predate health outcomes or vice versa. Nevertheless, because prospective studies are correlational, we cannot infer causation from the reported findings. For example, it is possible that negative emotions represent markers of subclinical disease, rather than antecedent causes of disease.

Depression

Depression is an emotion of low arousal and low pleasantness. Clinically diagnosable depressive syndromes are not emotions per se, but reflect a clustering of negative emotions and other symptoms, as noted above. Depressed individuals also frequently report symptoms of anxiety,[46] and this comorbidity makes attempts to determine the individual contribution of each construct difficult and possibly misleading. A variety of measures are used to characterize depression in studies of health and of SES. Some allow the diagnosis of clinical depression, some quantify the level of depressive symptoms, and others address specific symptoms of depression.

Regardless of measure, a growing body of literature indicates that clinical depression or elevated levels of depressive symptoms result in more negative health outcomes. In particular, the literature indicates an effect of depression on cardiovascular health, and recent reviews suggest that depression is associated with the etiology and course of cardiovascular disease.[47,48] Depressive symptoms have been shown to predict stroke in an initially healthy population[49] and stroke and cardiovascular death in patients with essential hypertension.[50] The presence of major depression[51–53] and higher levels of depressive symptoms[53–55] have also been associated with poorer outcomes (e.g., recurrent coronary events, cardiovascular mortality) in patients with established coronary artery disease. Finally, a number of prospective studies have shown that initially healthy persons with a history of clinical depression[56,57] or higher levels of depressive symptoms[6,58] manifest higher rates of cardiovascular morbidity and mortality. However, other studies have reported null findings.[59,60] Positive studies have shown a dose–response relationship between depression and cardiovascular risk.[6,57,58]

In addition to cardiovascular health outcomes, two studies have shown that depressive symptoms and emotional distress predict a poorer immunological course in male HIV-positive patients.[61,62] However, similar studies have not replicated this association.[63,64] Some research also suggests that depressive symptoms increase the risk of cancer mortality,[65] but the majority of studies concerning this association report null findings.[56,66] Finally, research suggests that depressive symptoms[6,55] and major depression[67,68] increase the risk of mortality from all causes. A recent review of the evidence linking depressive symptoms and disorders to mortality emphasizes prevailing methodological problems, but concludes that depression likely increases the risk of mortality from cardiovascular and unnatural causes, but not from cancer.[69]

Hopelessness

Hopelessness is likely to be associated with strong negative emotions, but it is perhaps more accurately described as negative cognition, about the self and the future. Hopelessness is often conceptualized as a symptom of depression,[70] although some researchers consider it a conceptually distinct construct.[71] In one of the first prospective studies to examine the effects of hopelessness, Anda and colleagues[72] found that this construct predicted cardiovascular morbidity and mortality during a 12-year follow-up period. This effect was independent of depression and of other risk factors. Shortly thereafter, Everson and her colleagues[71] reported that hopelessness predicted mortality from all causes and from specific causes including violence and injury, cardiovascular diseases, and cancer. Hopelessness was also associated with incident myocardial infarction (MI) and cancer. Another recent study found that hopelessness predicted faster progression of cardiovascular disease, especially in persons who showed some evidence of disease at baseline.[73]

Anxiety

Anxiety is also an emotion of low pleasantness, but it differs from depression in that it also reflects high arousal. Anxiety may occur in pathological or nonpathological forms, and disordered anxiety seems to be discriminated only by its duration, intensity, or situational appropriateness.[74] Like depression, the research concerning the association of anxiety with health or SES has employed a variety of self-report measures and interviews that address either anxiety symptoms or diagnosable anxiety disorders. The fundamental feature of all anxiety disorders is fear or apprehension about the future, although the corollary symptoms vary.

Consistent with the research concerning depression, most of the anxiety and health research has examined cardiovascular endpoints. Several studies have shown a relationship between anxiety symptoms and incident hypertension,[75,76] but other studies concerning anxiety and hypertension have produced null findings.[77,78] However, this may be at least partially attributable to inadequate sample sizes or assessments of anxiety.[75] Level of anxiety has also been shown to predict complications following MI.[79] Furthermore, several prospective studies have shown anxiety to be an independent predictor of coronary heart disease incidence in men[7,80–82] and women.[83] Two prospective studies of psychiatric patients found that those with panic disorder were more likely to die from coronary causes,[84,85] whereas others have reported null results.[86,87] In a recent review of the research examining the association between anxiety and coronary outcomes, Kubzansky and her colleagues[88] concluded that anxiety contributes to the risk of CHD. She also recommended additional research to address shortcomings of previous studies, including the fact that few studies have included samples of women.

Hostile Attitudes and Affect

Hostility was one of the first psychosocial risk factors studied in relation to health, and the evidence continues to accumulate that hostility is a risk factor for CHD and all-cause mortality.[89] Although this research is generally subsumed under the category of hostility, it more accurately refers to three interrelated but distinct emotional, behavioral, and cognitive constructs,[90] consistent with the definition of emotion outlined above. Anger and related concepts such as contempt and resentment form the primary emotional component. Anger is an emotion of negative valence that is also associated with moderate to high arousal. Verbal and physical aggression form the behavioral component, and hostility most accurately refers to the attitudes and beliefs that comprise the cognitive portion of this multifaceted construct. Studies of hostility have used either interview ratings or questionnaire methods of assessment.[91,92] The different assessment methods tend to be only moderately correlated[93]—a pattern that may reflect the multidimensional structure of this construct.

Several prospective studies have shown that interview ratings of hostility predict incident coronary heart disease.[94–96] Studies using self-report measures of hostility have reported similar findings.[97–99] Hostility scores have also been shown to predict mortality from all causes,[98,99] and to predict the recurrence of coronary problems in persons with established disease.[98] In contrast, several prospective studies using questionnaire measures have reported no relationship between hostility and incident CHD.[100–102] A recent prospective study using a self-report measure of angry affect found that persons with higher scores were more likely to experience any coronary event during a 7-year follow up period.[103] Other studies have examined the association between hostile attitudes or angry affect and the progression of atherosclerotic disease. Julkenen and colleagues[104] found that cynical attitudes and suppression of angry affect were associated with the progression of atherosclerosis in men followed over two years. Matthews and colleagues[105] found that subclinical (i.e., nonsymptomatic) levels of atherosclerosis were associated with scores on measures of hostile attitudes and the tendency to suppress angry affect administered 10 years earlier, even after statistical control for traditional risk factors. Miller and his colleagues[89] recently performed a meta-analysis of studies concerning hostility and health, and they concluded that hostility is a significant risk factor for coronary heart disease and mortality. They also showed that measures of hostile cognition were relatively strong predictors of all-cause mortality. The authors suggested that to some extent, conflicting findings might reflect inconsistencies and limitations of methods, samples, and measurement instruments.

MECHANISMS UNDERLYING THE ASSOCIATIONS
OF NEGATIVE EMOTIONS AND HEALTH

The reviewed research indicates that negative emotions and attitudes are associated with poor health outcomes, including all-cause mortality and cardiovascular disease. In attempting to explain these associations, researchers have examined a number of behavioral and biological pathways. The proposed mediational hypotheses are interesting for their similarity across the different negative emotions and attitudes examined.

Some theories of negative emotions and health posit that these factors are connected through behavioral pathways. For example, research suggests that depressed coronary patients do not adequately adhere to recommended treatment regimens[51,106-107] and that they are more likely to display behavioral risk factors, such as smoking[108-109] and a lack of physical activity.[110] Similarly, anxiety is associated with negative health behaviors,[111,112] as is hostility.[113] However, studies that have controlled for behavioral factors suggest that they do not tell the whole story. Investigators have therefore examined a variety of biological factors associated with negative emotions and with disease outcomes. For example, negative emotions may affect cardiovascular disease mortality through their association with biological risk factors such as hypertension,[75,76,114,115] diabetes,[116] or hyperlipidemia.[117] Similarly, physiological alterations such as hyperactivity of the hypothalamic–pituitary–adrenocortical axis, dysregulation of the sympathoadrenal system, exaggerated platelet reactivity, reduced heart rate variability, and ventricular instability or ischemia in response to stress are hypothesized to relate to negative emotions and attitudes[29,47,88,89,118-120] and may contribute to their relationship with cardiovascular disease. In addition, depression might lead to increased vulnerability to infectious diseases and cancer through its association with suppressed immune functioning.[33] Hostility also appears to be associated with stress-induced changes in immune responses.[121] Thus, a variety of plausible pathways exist and, given that negative emotions and attitudes impact a number of health outcomes, all may be important.

NEGATIVE EMOTIONS AND SES

The reviewed research provides sufficient evidence to connect negative emotions and hostile attitudes with health outcomes, through a number of possible physiological and behavioral mechanisms. Thus, the emotion and health portion of the proposed model appears tenable. Next, we examine the evidence for a connection between negative emotions and SES. We do not present an exhaustive review of this literature. Rather, we focus on studies that are either extensively cited in the literature, provide very recent evidence of SES and emotion associations, or that use especially comprehensive methodological procedures. We also discuss the extent to which gender and ethnicity are associated with vulnerability to each emotional state.

Depression and Hopelessness

A number of studies have examined the associations between SES and scores on dimensional measures of depression or hopelessness.[122-131] This research provides considerable and consistent evidence that SES and depression or hopelessness are inversely related. There is also some evidence relating SES to depressive disorders. In the National Comorbidity Study (NCS), an interview assessment study of psychiatric disorders in the U.S. population, the lowest income group showed higher lifetime and 12-month prevalence rates of affective disorders compared with the highest income group.[23] Education was inversely associated with SES for 12-month, but not lifetime prevalence rates. The Epidemiologic Catchment Area Study (ECA) is another recent study that administered a structured psychiatric diagnostic interview to a large U.S. population. In this study, lifetime prevalence of major depression was not related to occupation, income, or education, although low education was associated with a higher prevalence of bipolar disorder.[133] Rates of affective disorders were higher, however, in persons who were financially dependent on the government (i.e., received welfare or disability payments). Notably, this study used relatively crude distinctions to create socioeconomic groupings, which may have obscured some effects of SES. A six-month follow-up study of the New Haven ECA cohort showed that the group reporting poverty-level income had more new occurrences of major depression.[134] Thus, although the findings regarding SES and depression are somewhat mixed, it appears that groups with very low incomes display higher rates of affective disorders. Notably, given that these data are cross-sectional, this association may reflect the effects of social causation or of social drift.

In both the NCS[23] and the ECA study,[133] prevalence rates of major depression were about twice as high for women as for men. Several studies have also shown that women report higher levels of depressive *symptoms* compared with men.[123,135,136] However, despite women's higher overall vulnerability to depression, sex and SES do not appear to interact in influencing rates of depression.[128,134] Several studies have shown that minority persons experience higher rates of depressive symptoms and hopelessness,[108,123,131,134,135] although some have shown that this difference is attributable to the effects of social class.[131,135] Moreover, the ECA and the NCS both found that black respondents displayed *lower* prevalence rates of affective disorders compared with white respondents.[23,133] In the ECA, Hispanic respondents also showed lower rates, but the NCS found the opposite trend. Thus, there is no clear evidence to suggest that minority status is associated with disproportionate vulnerability to depression, and in fact the opposite may be true.

Anxiety

Two studies that examined scores on self-report measures of anxiety reported inverse relationships with SES.[137,138] Another study found that SES was not associated with prevalent anxiety symptoms at baseline, although SES was marginally inversely associated with anxiety at follow up.[128] Other studies have included measures of "psychophysiologic distress" thought to be indicative of depression and anxiety and have noted an inverse relationship with social class.[28,139] Both the ECA and the NCS studies included assessments of anxiety disorders. In the ECA, education was not associated with prevalence of panic disorder or with prevalence of phobic disorders in women.[140] However, men with lower education tended to have higher rates of phobic disorders. Occupational status did not show a clear relationship with the prevalence of phobic and panic disorders. Men and women who were financially dependent on the government showed higher one-year prevalence rates of panic and phobic disorders. Occupational status and income were inversely associated with one-year prevalence of generalized anxiety disorder (GAD).[141] In addition, persons who were financially dependent on the government were more likely to receive a past-year diagnosis of GAD. Nevertheless, there was no association between education and lifetime or one-year prevalence of GAD. The NCS study found that all groups with income below $70,000 had higher rates of any anxiety disorder, as did all education groups with less than a college degree.[23] Income and education were inversely associated with 30-day prevalence rates of agoraphobia, social phobia, and simple phobia;[142] and lifetime prevalence rates of GAD were found to be higher for the lowest income group compared with the highest income group.[143]

As with depression, several studies have shown that women have higher rates of most anxiety disorders[23] and symptoms[137,138] compared with men. Studies that have examined the effect of minority status on vulnerability to anxiety disorders do not suggest a clear association.[139,140]

Hostility

The studies that have examined the association of hostility and SES show a consistent inverse association between these constructs.[127,144–146] Each of these studies used a self-report measure of hostility, the Cook-Medley, which is primarily associated with cynical hostility or the cognitive aspects of that construct. Scherwitz and his colleagues[146] also reported that SES was inversely associated with item subsets from the Cook-Medley, which assess cynicism, hostile attributions, aggressive responding, and hostile affect. Therefore, SES may be associated with the cognitive, behavioral, and affective components of the hostility construct, although further research is needed to confirm this. Another study showed that women who were lower in education tended to score higher on a measure of anger suppression.[147] Recently, our own laboratory found that for African-American children and adolescents, family and neighborhood SES were inversely associated with a composite hostility factor reflecting the joint influence of hostile attitudes, angry affect, and aggressive behavior.[148] Thus, at least for African-Americans, the association between hostility and SES may begin early in life, although longitudinal research should more specifically address the course of this association. Finally, Mittleman and colleagues[149] showed that persons with lower levels of educational attainment were more likely to experience MIs that were triggered by anger.

In contrast to the findings for depression and anxiety, studies of hostility have shown that men display higher levels than women.[144,146] In addition, Scherwitz and colleagues[146] reported that blacks showed higher hostility scores than whites. This difference was smaller at higher levels of achieved education. Barefoot and colleagues[144] reported a similar association between race and hostility—larger white versus non-white differences in hostility scores were observed at lower SES levels. Similarly, in their recent study of children and adolescents, Gump and colleagues[148] reported that African-American participants scored higher than white participants on a measure of hostile attitudes. These groups did not differ on measures of trait anger or hostile behavior.

SOCIAL CAUSATION VERSUS SOCIAL DRIFT

As shown in our model of SES, negative emotions, and health, SES could have a causal impact on negative emotional states, or negative emotional states could cause changes in SES. The relative impact of these pathways has been the focus of considerable research.[18,45,150,151] We now briefly consider the extent to which the reviewed research provides support for either directional hypothesis. Notably, only those studies that include a longitudinal component can directly evaluate the social drift or causation hypotheses. Moreover, examination of these models requires that the authors report data on the association between SES and changes in negative emotion and between negative emotion and changes in SES.

In their longitudinal research, Murphy and colleagues[128] reported that new cases of depression were more likely to occur in the lower SES groups, supporting a social causation interpretation. However, this study also showed that persons who were depressed at baseline were more likely to show downward social mobility than those who were not depressed, suggesting the effects of social drift. Neither trend was statistically significant, although the causation analysis approached significance. For anxiety, the data did not support a social causation or a social drift effect. The findings of Kaplan and his colleagues[125] are consistent with the social causation hypothesis. Persons who were not depressed at baseline but who reported depression at the nine-year follow-up were more likely to be less educated than those who were not depressed at follow-up. This study did not report the effects of depression on movement within the socioeconomic hierarchy. The data from the New Haven ECA study[134] are also consistent with the social causation hypothesis. New occurrences of major depression and phobia during the six-month follow up were more likely in the poverty group. Again, the authors did not examine the effects of disorder on SES, although little would be expected given the limited follow-up period. No longitudinal studies have addressed the social drift and causation hypotheses in the context of research concerning hostility and SES. However, in an attempt to evaluate the direction of the association between SES and negative emotions and attitudes using a cross-sectional approach, Lynch and colleagues[127] showed that recalled childhood SES was related to adult levels of hostility and hopelessness. Overall, the evidence for either the social drift or causation hypothesis is limited. Consistent with our model, both effects may contribute to the observed associations.

INTEGRATIVE STUDIES OF SES, NEGATIVE EMOTIONS, AND HEALTH—EVIDENCE FOR MEDIATION?

The reviewed literature shows a clear link between negative emotions and health and suggests that an association between SES and negative emotions is likely. SES also appears to be inversely associated with rates of anxiety disorders, and very low income levels appear to be associated with higher rates of depressive disorders. These data provide indirect evidence that negative emotions could mediate the association between SES and health. However, integrative research that directly evaluates the associations among SES, negative emotions, and health is necessary to provide more definitive support for our model. Unfortunately, few studies have attempted this research approach, and those that have report somewhat contradictory findings.

Lynch and colleagues[126] examined the associations between SES and incident MI, cardiovascular mortality, and all-cause mortality across a 4–10-year follow-up period and evaluated the extent to which biological, behavioral, and psychosocial risk factors accounted for these associations. Psychosocial risk factors, including depression, hopelessness, marital status, participation in organizations, and social support, attenuated the excess risk associated with the lowest income group for all three outcomes. Simultaneous inclusion of these factors reduced the relative hazard associated with low income by 35% (from 3.14 to 2.03) for all-cause mortality. For cardiovascular mortality, inclusion of the psychosocial factors reduced the relative hazard estimate by 36%, from 2.66 to 1.71, rendering this association nonsignificant. The relative hazard reflecting the association of SES with nonfatal or fatal MI decreased by only a small amount after controlling for the psychosocial factors, from 4.34 to 4.25. Thus, psychosocial factors accounted for some of the relationship between SES and all-cause or cardiovascular mortality, but not between SES and MI. Notably, when all types of risk factors (e.g., biologic, behavioral, and psychosocial) were controlled, substantial reductions in the associations between SES and all of the health outcomes occurred.

In contrast, another study that examined the associations among SES, depression, and functional status in the 12 months following MI found little evidence for depression as a mediating factor.[124] Both SES and depression were associated with improvements in functional status, and with each other. When the association between SES and functional status was evaluated controlling for depression, stress, and social isolation, only a small reduction in the odds ratio for no improvement occurred. Thus, these psychosocial factors had only a minor role in explaining the association between SES and improvement following MI. Similarly, Fiscella and Franks[123] found little evidence that psychological distress (i.e., depression, hopelessness, life dissatisfaction) accounted for the association between SES and mortality across a 12–16-year follow-up period. Adjustment for psychological factors reduced the relative risks of mortality for the lowest income group by only 3 to 11%. Finally, a recent study showed that SES was associated with cardiovascular reactivity to stressful laboratory tasks, and for African Americans this effect was mediated by individual differences in hostility.[148] Cardiovascular reactivity is one physiological alteration that may underlie the association between psychosocial factors and cardiovascular health outcomes.[152] Thus, this study provides initial evidence that SES could affect cardiovascular outcomes through its relationship with hostility.

CONCLUSIONS AND FUTURE RESEARCH DIRECTIONS

We have presented a model and preliminary evidence suggesting that SES may affect health outcomes, at least in part, through its association with negative emotions and attitudes. SES appears to be inversely associated with levels of negative emotions including depression and anxiety, and negative cognitions such as hopelessness and hostility. Low SES also appears to be associated with higher rates of anxiety disorders and very low income levels may be associated with higher rates of depressive disorders. As suggested by our model, social causation and social drift effects could each be important in connecting SES with negative emotional states, although the evidence for either directional hypothesis is limited at this point. A substantial body of research also shows that negative emotions and attitudes predict worse health outcomes, and a number of behavioral and biological mechanisms could underlie these associations. Woman are especially vulnerable to anxiety and depressive disorders, suggesting that these emotional states may represent especially relevant health risk factors for lower SES women. For lower SES men, hostility may be particularly important. We can draw few conclusions about the relative susceptibility of minority persons to negative emotions, although lower SES African-American men may be especially vulnerable to the health effects of hostility. Unfortunately, there is little direct evidence on which to evaluate our model. Thus, we conclude with recommendations for research that can more directly address this and other possible mediational pathways.

In particular, we suggest that longitudinal research must be undertaken to study the development of negative emotions, negative attitudes, and other behavioral and biological health risk factors. By comparing how these factors develop in low- versus high-SES persons, we can begin to understand the causal nature of the associations we have presented. Notably, evidence suggests that health risk factors tend to aggregate within lower SES persons.[127] Moreover, low SES and other psychosocial risk factors may produce synergistic, negative health effects.[153] Therefore, we may gain a more comprehensive understanding of risk by examining these factors as they occur in natural patterns, rather than by attempting to clarify the independent predictive value of any particular risk factor. This approach also requires that we examine lifecourse trajectories by following children from disparate SES groups from an early age into adulthood. In addition, future research should include assessment of positive as well as negative emotions to examine if positive emotions exert health *protective* effects for higher SES individuals.

In the meantime, our proposed model and review suggest possible intervention strategies for lower SES individuals. The ideal intervention would require amelioration of the SES differential, to eliminate differences in exposure to harmful and beneficial events. However, given that this is not a feasible solution, intervention efforts might be directed toward the reserve capacity we believe moderates the relationship between threatening stimuli and negative emotional states. In particular, lower SES children might benefit from interventions designed to increase skills or sense of efficacy for coping with negative events. Likewise, interventions at the family and community level could bolster these aspects of the reserve capacity. Strategies that improve lower SES persons' ability to effectively manage negative stimuli could have the additional benefit of reducing reliance on negative coping behaviors, such as smoking or alcohol use. Thus, effective interventions could ultimately alter the lifecourse trajectories that we suggest may place lower SES persons at higher risk for health problems.

REFERENCES

1. LAZARUS, R.S. 1991. Emotion and Adaptation. Oxford University Press, New York.
2. PARKINSON, B., P. TOTTERDELL, R.B. BRINER & S. REYNOLDS. 1996. Changing Moods: The Psychology of Mood and Mood Regulation. Longman, London.

3. PLUTCHIK, R. 1997. The circumplex as a general model of the structure of emotions and personality. *In* Circumplex Models of Personality and Emotions. R. Plutchik & H.R. Conte, Eds.: 17–45. APA Press, Washington, DC.
4. FRIJDA, N.H. 1994. Emotions are functional most of the time. *In* The Nature of Emotion: Fundamental Questions. P. Ekman & R.J. Davidson, Eds.: 112–122. Oxford University Press, New York.
5. AMERICAN PSYCHIATRIC ASSOCIATION. 1994. Diagnostic and Statistical Manual of Mental Disorders (4th edit., DSM-IV). Author. Washington, DC.
6. BAREFOOT, J.C. & M. SCHROLL. 1996. Symptoms of depression, acute myocardial infarction, and total mortality in a community sample. Circulation **93:** 1976–1980.
7. KAWACHI, I., D. SPARROW, P.S. VOKONAS, *et al.* 1994. Symptoms of anxiety and risk of coronary heart disease: the normative aging study. Circulation **90:** 2225–2229.
8. PLUTCHIK, R. 1980. Emotion: A Psychoevolutionary Synthesis. Harper & Row, New York.
9. RUSSELL, J.A. 1997. How shall an emotion be called? *In* Circumplex Models of Personality and Emotion. R. Plutchik & H. Conte, Eds.: 205–220. APA Press, Washington, DC.
10. WATSON, D. & A. TELLEGEN. 1985. Toward a consensual structure of mood. Psychol. Bull. **98:** 219–235.
11. BARLOW, D.H. 1988. Anxiety and Its Disorders: The Nature and Treatment of Anxiety and Panic. Guilford Press, New York.
12. CLARK, L.A. & D. WATSON. 1991. Theoretical and empirical issues in differentiating depression from anxiety. *In* Psychosocial Aspects of Depression. J. Becker & A. Kleinman, Eds.: 39–65. Lawrence Erlbaum Associates, Hillsdale.
13. FELDMAN, L.A. 1995. Variations in the circumplex structure of mood. Pers. Soc. Psychol. Bull. **21:** 806–817.
14. WATSON, D. & L.A. CLARK. 1984. Negative affectivity: the disposition to experience aversive emotional states. Psychol. Bull. **96:** 465–490.
15. DOHRENWEND, B.S. 1973. Social status and stressful life events. J. Pers. Soc. Pscyhol. **28:** 225–235.
16. MCLEOD, J.D. & R.C. KESSLER. 1990. Socioeconomic status differences in vulnerability to undesirable life events. J. Health Soc. Behav. **31:** 162–172.
17. BROWN, G.W., M.N. BHROL-CHAIN & T. HARRIS. 1975. Social class and psychiatric disturbance among women in an urban population. Sociology **9:** 225–254.
18. KESSLER, R.C. 1979. Stress, social status, and psychological distress. J. Health Soc. Behav. **20:** 259–272.
19. TAYLOR, S.E. & T.E. SEEMAN. 1999. Psychosocial resources and the SES–Health relationship. Ann. N.Y. Acad. Sci. **896:** this volume.
20. ALDARONDO, E. & D.B. SUGARMAN. 1996. Risk marker analysis of the cessation and persistence of wife assault. J. Consult. Clin. Psychol. **64:** 1010–1019.
21. CHRISTMAS, A.L., J.S. WODARSKI & P.R. SMOKOWSKI. 1996. Risk factors for physical child abuse: a practice theoretical paradigm. Fam. Ther. **23:** 233–248.
22. HELZER, J.E., A. BURNAM & L.T. MCEVOY. 1991. Alcohol Abuse and Dependence. *In* Psychiatric Disorders in America. L.N. Robins & D.A. Regier, Eds.: 81–116. The Free Press, New York.
23. KESSLER, R.C., K.A. MCGONAGLE, Z. SHANYANG, *et al.* 1994. Lifetime and 12-month prevalence of DSM-III-R psychiatric disorders in the United States. Arch. Gen. Psychiatry **51:** 8–19.
24. BELLE, D.E. 1982. The impact of poverty on social networks and supports. Marriage Fam. Rev. **5:** 89–103.
25. HOUSE, J.S. 1987. Social support and social structure. Sociol. Forum **2:** 135–146.
26. RUBERMAN, W., E.J.D. WEINBLATT, D.E. GOLDBERG, *et al.* 1984. Psychosocial influences on mortality after myocardial infarction. N. Engl. J. Med. **311:** 552–559.
27. MIROWSKY, J. & C.E. ROSS. 1986. Social patterns of distress. Ann. Rev. Sociol. **12:** 23–45.
28. KESSLER, R.C. & P.D. CLEARY. 1980. Social class and psychological distress. Am. Sociol. Rev. **45:** 463–478.

29. CARNEY, R.M., K.E. FREEDLAND, M.W. RICH, *et al.* 1995. Depression as a risk factor for cardiac events in established coronary heart disease: a review of possible mechanisms. Ann. Behav. Med. **17:** 142–149.
30. BOOTH-KEWLEY, S. & R.R.VICKERS. 1994. Associations between major domains of personality and health behavior. J. Pers. **62:** 281–298.
31. HOEHN-SARIC, R. & D.R. MCCLEOD. 1988. The peripheral sympathetic nervous system: its role in normal and pathologic anxiety. Psychiatr. Clin. N. Am. **11:** 375–386.
32. WATKINS, L.L., P. GROSSMAN, R. KRISHNAN & A. SHERWOOD. 1998. Anxiety and vagal control of heart rate. Psychosom. Med. **60:** 498–502.
33. HERBERT, B. & S. COHEN. 1993. Depression and immunity: a meta-analytic review. Psychsom. Med. **55:** 364–379.
34. MCEWEN, B. S. & T. SEEMAN. 1999. Protective and damaging effects of mediators of stress: elaborating and testing the concepts of allostasis and allostatic load. Ann. N.Y. Acad. Sci. **896:** this volume.
35. ASELTINE, R.G. & R.C. KESSLER. 1993. Marital disruption and depression in a community sample. J. Health Soc. Behav. **34:** 237–251.
36. WEISSMAN, M.M. 1987. Advances in psychiatric epidemiology: rates and risks for major depression. Am. J. Public Health **77:** 445–451.
37. MILLER, T.Q., R.S. MARKSIDES, D.A.CHIRIBOGA & L.A. RAY. 1995. A test of the psychosocial vulnerability and health behavior models of hostility: results from an 11-year follow-up study of Mexican Americans. Psychosom. Med. **57:** 572–581.
38. NEWTON, T.L. & J.R. KIECOLT-GLASER. 1995. Hostility and erosion of marital quality during early marriage. J. Behav. Med. **18:** 601–619.
39. ASARNOW, J.R., G.A. CARLSON & D. GUTHRIE. 1987. Coping strategies, self-perceptions, hopelessness, and perceived family environments in depressed and suicidal children. J. Consul. Clin. Psychol. **55:** 361–366.
40. BECK, A.T., R.A. STEER, N. EPSTEIN, *et al.* 1990. Beck self-concept test. Psychol. Assess. **2:** 191–197.
41. GREENBERG, M.S. & A.T. BECK. 1989. Depression versus anxiety: a test of the content-specificity hypothesis. J. Abnorm. Psychol. **98:** 9–13.
42. BECK, A.T. 1971. Cognition, affect, and psychopathology. Arch. Gen. Psychiatry. **24:** 495–500.
43. HAAGA, D.A.F., M.J. DYCK & D. ERNST. 1991. Empirical status of cognitive theory of depression. Psychol. Bull. **110:** 215–236.
44. LICHTENSTEIN, P. 1992. Socioeconomic status and physical health, how are the related? An empirical study based on twins reared apart and twins reared together. Soc. Sci. Med. **36:** 441–450.
45. KESSLER, R.C. 1982. A disaggregation of the relationship between socioeconomic status and psychological distress. Am. Psychol. Rev. **47:** 752–764.
46. FAWCETT, J. & H.M. KRAVITZ. 1983. Anxiety syndromes and their relationship to depressive illness. J. Clin. Psychiatry **44:** 8–11.
47. GLASSMAN, A.H. & P.A. SHAPIRO. 1998. Depression and the course of coronary artery disease. Am. J. Psychiatry. **155:** 4–11.
48. MUSSELMAN, D.L., D.L. EVANS & C.B. NEMEROFF. 1998. The relationship of depression to cardiovascular disease. Arch. Gen. Psychiatry **55:** 580–592.
49. EVERSON, S.A., R.E. ROBERTS, D.E. GOLDBERG, *et al.* 1998. Depressive symptoms and increased risk of stroke mortality over a 29-year period. Arch. Intern. Med. **158:** 1133–1138.
50. SIMONSICK, E.M., R.B. WALLACE, D.G. BLAZER, *et al.* 1995. Depressive symptomatology and hypertension-associated morbidity and mortality in older adults. Psychosom. Med. **57:** 427–435.
51. CARNEY, R.M., M.W. RICH, K.E. FREEDLAND, *et al.* 1988. Major depressive disorder predicts cardiac events in patients with coronary artery disease. Psychosom. Med. **50:** 627–633.
52. FRASURE-SMITH, N., F. LESPÉRANCE & J. TALJIC. 1993. Depression following myocardial infarction: impact on 6-mo survival. JAMA **270:** 1819–1825.
53. FRASURE-SMITH, N., F. LESPÉRANCE & J. TALJIC. 1995. Depression and 18-month prognosis after myocardial infarction. Circulation **91:** 999–1005.

54. AHERN, D.K., L. GORKIN, J.L. ANDERSON, et al. 1990. Biobehavioral variables and mortality or cardiac arrest in the cardiac arrhythmia pilot study (CAPS). Am. J. Cardiol. **66:** 59–62.
55. BAREFOOT, J.C., M.S. HELMS, D.B MARK, et al. 1996. Depression and long term mortality risk in patients with coronary artery disease. Am. J. Cardiol. **78:** 613–617.
56. AROMAA, A., R. RAITASALO, A. REUNANEN, et al. 1994. Depression and cardiovascular diseases. Acta. Psychiatr. Scand. Suppl. **377:** 77–82.
57. PRATT, L.A. D.E. FORD, R.M. CRUM, et al. 1996. Coronary heart disease/myocardial infarction: depression, psychotropic medication, and risk of myocardial infarction: prospective data from the Baltimore ECA follow-up. Circulation **94:** 3123–3129.
58. SESSO, H.D., I. KAWACHI, P.S. VOKONAS, et al. 1998. Depression and the risk of coronary heart diseases in the normative aging study. Am. J. Cardiol. **82:** 851–856.
59. GOLDBERG, E.L., G.W. COMSTOCK & R.K. HORNSTRA. 1979. Depressed mood and subsequent physical illness. Am. J. Psychiatry **136:** 530–534.
60. VOGT, T., C. POPE, J. MULLOOLY, et al. 1994. Mental health status as a predictor of morbidity and mortality: a 15-year follow-up of members of a health maintenance organization. Am. J. Public Health **84:** 227–231.
61. BURACK, J.H., D.C. BARRETT, R.D. STALL, et al. 1993. Depressive symptoms and CD4 lymphocyte decline among HIV-infected men. JAMA **270:** 2568–2573.
62. VEDHARA, K., K.H. NOTT, C.S. BRADBEER, et al. 1997. Greater emotional distress is associated with accelerated CD4+ cell decline in HIV infection. J. Psychosom. Res. **42:** 379–390.
63. LYKETSOS, C.G., D.R. HOOVER, M. GUCCIONE, et al. 1993. Depressive symptoms of medical outcomes in HIV infection. JAMA **270:** 2563–2567.
64. PERRY, S., B. FISHMAN, L. JACOBSBERG, et al. 1992. Relationships over 1 year between lymphocyte subsets and psychosocial variables among adults with infection by human immunodeficiency virus. Arch. Psychiatry **49**(5): 396–401.
65. SHEKELLE, R.B., W.J. RAYNOR, A.M. OSTFELD, et al. 1981. Psychological depression and 17-year risk of death from cancer. Psychosom. Med. **43:** 117–125.
66. KAPLAN, G.A. & P. REYNOLDS. 1986. Depression and cancer mortality and morbidity: prospective evidence from the Alameda County Study. J. Behav. Med. **11:** 1–13.
67. BRUCE, M.L., P.J. LEAF, G.P. ROZAL, et al. 1994. Psychiatric status and 9-year mortality data in the New Haven epidemiologic catchment area study. Am. J. Psychiatry **151:** 716–721.
68. MURPHY, J.M. R.R. MONSON, D.C. OLIVIER, et al. 1987. Affective disorders and mortality: A general population study. Arch. Gen. Psychiatry **44:** 473–480.
69. WULSIN, L.R., G.E. VAILLANT & V.E. WELLS. 1999. A systematic review of the mortality of depression. Psychosom. Med. **61:** 6–17.
70. BROWN, G.W. & T. HARRIS. 1978. Social Origins of Depression. Tavistock, London.
71. EVERSON, S.A., D.E. GOLDBERG, G.A. KAPLAN, et al. 1996. Hopelessness and risk of mortality and incidence of myocardial infarction and cancer. Psychosom. Med. **58:** 113–121.
72. ANDA, R., D. WILLIAMSON, D. JONES, et al. 1993. Depressed affect, hopelessness, and the risk of ischemic heart disease in a cohort of U.S. adults. Epidemiology **4:** 285–294.
73. EVERSON, S.A., G.A. KAPLAN, D.E. GOLDBERG, et al. 1997. Hopelessness and 4-year progression of carotid atherosclerosis. The Kuopio ischemic heart disease risk factor study. Arterioscler. Thromb. Vasc. Biol. **17:** 1490–1495.
74. CLARK, L.A. & D. WATSON. 1994. Distinguishing functional from dysfunctional affective responses. In The Nature of Emotion: Fundamental Questions. P. Ekman, R.J. Davidson & D. Watson, Eds.: 131–137. Oxford University Press, New York.
75. JONAS, B.S., P. FRANKS & D.D. INGRAM. 1997. Are symptoms of anxiety and depression risk factors for hypertension? Longitudinal evidence from the national health and nutrition examination survey I epidemiologic follow-up study. Arch. Fam. Med. **6:** 43–49.
76. MARKOVITZ, J.H., K.A. MATTHEWS, W.B. KANNEL, et al. 1993. Psychological predictors of hypertension in the Framingham study. Is there tension in hypertension? JAMA **270**(20): 2439–2443.

77. RUSSEK, L.G., S.H. KING, S.J. RUSSEK, et al. 1990. The Harvard mastery of stress study 35-year follow-up: prognostic significance of patterns of psychophysiological arousal and adaptation. Psychsom. Med. **52:** 271–285.
78. JENKINS, C.D., P.D. SOMERVELL & C.G. HAMES. 1983. Does blood pressure usually rise with age? Or with stress? J. Hum. Stress. **9:** 4–12.
79. MOSER, D.K. & K. DRACUP. 1996. Is anxiety early after myocardial infarction associated with subsequent ischemic and arrhythmic events? Psychsom. Med. **58:** 395–401.
80. HAINES, A. P., J.D. IMESON & T.W. MEADE. 1987. Phobic anxiety and ischaemic heart disease. Br. Med. J. **295:** 297–299.
81. KAWACHI, I., G.A. COLDITZ, A. ASCHERIO, et al. 1994. Prospective study of phobic anxiety and risk of coronary heart disease in men. Circulation **89:** 1992–1997.
82. KUBZANSKY, L.D., I. KAWACHI, A. SPIRO, et al. 1997. Is worrying bad for your heart? A prospective study of worry and coronary heart disease in the normative aging study. Circulation **95:** 818–824.
83. EAKER, E.D., J. PINSKY & W.P. CASTELLI. 1992. Myocardial infarction and coronary death among women: psychosocial predictors from a 20-year follow-up of women in the Framingham study. Am. J. Epidemiol. **135:** 854–864.
84. CORYELL,W., R. NOYES & J. CLANCY. 1982. Excess mortality in panic disorder. Arch. Gen. Psychiatry **39:** 701–703.
85. CORYELL, W., R. NOYES & J.D. HOUSE. 1986. Mortality among outpatients with anxiety disorders. Am. J. Psychiatry **143:** 508–510.
86. ALLGULANDER, C. & P.W. LAVORI. 1991. Excess mortality among 3302 patients with "Pure" anxiety neurosis. Arch. Gen. Psychiatry **48:** 599–602.
87. MARTIN, R.L., R. CLONINGER, S.B. GUZE, et al. 1985. Mortality in a follow-up of 500 psychiatric outpatients. Arch. Gen. Psychiatry **42:** 58–66.
88. KUBZANSKY, L.D., I. KAWACHI, S.T. WEISS, et al. 1998. Anxiety and coronary heart disease: a synthesis of epidemiological psychological, and experimental evidence. Ann. Behav. Med. **20:** 47–58.
89. MILLER, T.Q., T.W. SMITH, C.W. TURNER, et al. 1996. A meta-analytic review of research on hostility and physical health. Psychol. Bull. **119:** 322–348.
90. SMITH, T.W. 1994. Concepts and methods in the study of anger, hostility, and health. In Anger, Hostility and the Heart. A.W. Siegman & T.W. Smith, Eds.: 23–42. Lawrence Erlbaum, Hillsdale.
91. BAREFOOT, J.C. & I.M. LIPKUS. 1994. The assessment of anger and hostility. In Anger, Hostility, and the Heart. A.W. Siegman & T.W. Smith, Eds.: 43–66. Lawrence Erlbaum, Hillsdale.
92. SMITH, T.W. 1992. Hostility and health: current status of a psychosomatic hypothesis. Health Psychol. **11:** 139–150.
93. DEMBROSKI, T.M., J.M. MACDOUGALL, R.B. WILLIAMS, et al. 1985. Components of type A, hostility, and anger in relationship to angiographic findings. Psychosom. Med. **47:** 219–233.
94. DEMBROSKI, T.M., J.M. MACDOUGALL, P.T. COSTA, et al. 1989. Components of hostility as predictors of sudden death and myocardial infarction in the multiple risk factor intervention trial. Psychosom. Med. **51:** 514–522.
95. HECKER, M.H.L., M.A. CHESNEY, G.W. BLACK, et al. 1988. Coronary-prone behaviors in the western collaborative group study. Psychosom. Med. **50:** 153–164.
96. MATTHEWS, K.A., D.C. GLASS, R.H. ROSENMAN, et al. 1977. Competitive drive, pattern A, and coronary heart disease: a further analysis of some data from the western collaborative group study. J. Chron. Dis. **30:** 489–498.
97. BAREFOOT, J.C., W.G. DAHLSTROM & R.B. WILLIAMS. 1983. Hostility, CHD incidence, and total mortality: a 25-year follow-up study of 255 physicians. Psychosom. Med. **45:** 59–63.
98. KOSKENVUO, M., J. KAPRIO, R.J. ROSE, A. KESANIEMI, et al. 1988. Hostility as a risk factor for mortality and ischemic heart disease in men. Psychosom. Med. **50:** 330–340.
99. SHEKELLE, R.B., M. GALE, A.M. OSTFELD, et al. 1983. Hostility, risk of coronary heart disease, and mortality. Psychosom. Med. **45:** 109–114.

100. HEARN, M.D., D.M. MURRAY & R.V. LUEPKER. 1989. Hostility, coronary heart disease, and total mortality: a 33-year follow-up study of university students. J. Behav. Med. **12:** 105–121.
101. LEON, G.R., S.E. FINN, D. MURRAY, *et al.* 1988. Inability to predict cardiovascular disease from hostility scores or MMPI items related to type A behavior. J. Consult. Clin. Psychol. **56:** 597–600.
102. MCRANIE, E.W., L.O. WATKINS, J.M. BRANDSMA, *et al.* 1986. Hostility, coronary heart disease (CHD) incidence, and total mortality: lack of association in a 25-year follow-up study of 478 physicians. J. Behav. Med. **9:** 119–125.
103. KAWACHI, I., D. SPARROW, A. SPIRO, *et al.* 1996. A prospective study of anger and coronary heart disease: the normative aging study. Circulation **94:** 2090–2095.
104. JULKENEN, J., R. SALONEN, G.A. KAPLAN, *et al.* 1994. Hostility and the progression of carotid atherosclerosis. Psychosom. Med. **56:** 519–525.
105. MATTHEWS, K.A, J.F. OWENS, L. KULLER, *et al.* 1998. Are hostility and anxiety associated with carotid atherosclerosis in healthy postmenopausal women? Psychosom. Med. **60:** 633–638.
106. BLUMENTHAL, J.A., R.S. WILLIAMS, A.G. WALLACE, *et al.* 1982. Physiological and psychological variables predict compliance to prescribed exercise therapy in patients recovering from myocardial infarction. Psychosom. Med. **44:** 519–527.
107. GUIRY, E., R.M. CONROY, N. HICKEY, *et al.* 1987. Psychological response to an acute coronary event and its effect on subsequent rehabilitation and lifestyle change. Clin. Cardiol. **10:** 256–260.
108. ANDA, R.F., D.F. WILLIAMSON, L.G. ESCOBEDO, *et al.* 1990. Depression and the dynamics of smoking. A national perspective. JAMA **264:** 1541–1545.
109. HUGHES, J.R., D.K. HATSUKAMI, J.E. MITCHELL, *et al.* 1986. Prevalence of smoking among psychiatric outpatients. Am. J. Psychiatry **143:** 993–997.
110. FARMER, M.E., B.Z. LOCKE, E.K. MOSCICKI, *et al.* 1988. Physical activity and depressive symptoms: the NHANES I epidemiologic follow-up study. Am. J. Epidemiol. **128:** 1340–1351.
111. BRESLAU, N., M. KILBEY & P. ANDRESKI. 1991. Nicotine dependence, major depression, and anxiety in young adults. Arch. Gen. Psychatriy **48:** 1069–1074.
112. POHL, R., V.K. YERAGANI, R. BALON, *et al.* 1992. Smoking in patients with panic disorder. Psychiatry Res. **43:** 253–262.
113. SIEGLER, I.C. 1994. Hostility and risk: Demographic and lifestyle variables. *In* Anger, Hostility, and the Heart. A.W. Siegman & T.W. Smith, Eds.: 199–214. Lawrence Erlbaum, Hillsdale.
114. MARKOVITZ, J.H., K.A. MATTHEWS, R.R. WING, *et al.* 1991. Psychological, biological and health behavior predictors of blood pressure changes in middle-aged women. J. Hypertens. **9:** 399–406.
115. WELLS, K.B., J.M. GOLDING & M.A. BURNAM. 1989. Chronic medical conditions in a sample of the general population with anxiety, affective, and substance use disorders. Am. J. Psychiatry. **146:** 1440–1446.
116. EATON, W.W., H. ARMENIAN, J. GALLO, *et al.* 1996. Depression and risk for onset of type II diabetes: a prospective population-based study. Diabetes Care **19:** 1097–1102.
117. HAYWARD, C. 1995. Psychiatric illness and cardiovascular disease risk. Epidemiol. Rev. **17:** 129–138.
118. EHLERT, U. & R. STRAUB. 1998. Physiological and emotional response to psychological stressors in psychiatric and psychosomatic disorders. Ann. N.Y. Acad. Sci. **851:** 477–486.
119. SMITH, T.W. & L.C. GALLO. 1999. Personality and Health. *In* The Handbook of Health Psychology. A. Baum, T. Revenson & J. Singer, Eds. Lawrence Erlbaum, Hillsdale. In press.
120. MARKOVITZ, J.H. & K.A. MATTHEWS. 1991. Platelets and coronary heart disease: potential psychophysiologic mechanisms. Psychosom. Med. **53:** 643–668.
121. CHRISTENSEN, A.J., D.L. EDWARDS, J.S. WIEBE, *et al.* 1996. Effect of verbal self-disclosure on NK cell activity: moderating influence of cynical hostility. Psychosom. Med. **58:** 150–155.

122. CRAIG, T.J. & P.A. VAN NATTA. 1979. Influence of demographic characteristics on two measures of depressive symptoms. Arch. Gen. Psychiatry **36:** 149–154.
123. FISCELLA, K. & P. FRANKS. 1997. Does psychological distress contribute to racial and socioeconomic disparities in mortality? Soc. Sci. Med. **45:** 1805–1809.
124. ICKOVICKS, J.R., C.M. VISCOLI & R.I. HORWITZ. 1997. Functional recovery after myocardial infarction in men: the independent effects of social class. Ann. Intern. Med. **127:** 518–525.
125. KAPLAN, G.A., R.E. ROBERTS, T.C. CAMACHO, *et al.* 1987. Psychosocial predictors of depression. Am. J. Epidemiol. **125:** 206–220.
126. LYNCH, J.W., G.A. KAPLAN, R.D. COHEN, *et al.* 1996. Do cardiovascular risk factors explain the relation between socioeconomic status, risk of all-cause mortality, cardiovascular mortality, and acute myocardial infarction? Am. J. Epidemiol. **144:** 934–942.
127. LYNCH, J.W., G.A. KAPLAN & J.T. SALONEN. 1997. Why do poor people behave poorly? Variation in adult health behaviours and psychosocial characteristics by stages of the socioeconomic lifecourse. Soc. Sci. Med. **44:** 809–819.
128. MURPHY, J.M., D.C. OLIVIER, R.R. MONSON, et al. 1991. Depression and anxiety in relation to social status. Arch. Gen. Psychiatry. **48:** 223–229.
129. SALOKANGAS, R.K.R. & O. PUTANEN. 1998. Risk factors for depression in primary care findings of the TADEP project. J. Affect. Disord. **48:** 171–180.
130. STEELE, R.E. 1978. Relationship of race, sex, social class, and social mobility to depression in normal adults. J. Soc. Psychol. **104:** 37–47.
131. WARHEIT, G.J., C.E. HOLZER & S.A. AREY. 1975. Race and mental illness: an epidemiologic update. J. Health Soc. Behav. **16:** 243–256.
132. WEST, C.G., D. REED & G. GILDENGORIN. 1998. Can money buy happiness? Depressive symptoms in an affluent older population. Am. Geriatr. Soc. **46:** 49–57.
133. WEISSMAN, M.M., M.L. BRUCE, P.J. LEAF, *et al.* 1991. Affective disorders. *In* Psychiatric Disorders in America. L.N. Robins & D.A. Regier, Eds.: 53–80. The Free Press, New York.
134. BRUCE, M.L., D.T. TAKEUCHI & P.J. LEAF. 1991. Poverty and psychiatric status. Arch. Gen. Psychiatry **48:** 470–474.
135. COMSTOCK, G.W. & K.J. HELSING. 1975. Symptoms of depression in two communities. Psychol. Med. **6:** 551–563.
136. WEISSMAN, M.M. & J.K. MYERS. 1978. Rates and risks of depressive symptoms in a United States urban community. Acta Psychiat. Scand. **57:** 219–231.
137. HIMMELFARB, S. & MURRELL, S.A. 1984. The prevalence and correlates of anxiety symptoms in older adults. J. Psychol. **116:** 159–167.
138. WARHEIT, G.J., R.A. BELL, J.J. SCHWAB & J.M. BUHL 1986. An epidemiologic assessment of mental health problems in the southeastern United States. *In* Community Surveys of Psychiatric Disorders. M.M. Weissman, J.K. Meyers & C.E. Ross, Eds.: 191–208. Rutgers University Press, New Brunswick.
139. MYERS, J.K., J.J. LINDENTHAL & M.P. PEPPER. 1974. Social class, life events and psychiatric symptoms: a longitudinal study. *In* Stressful Life Events. B.P. Dohrenwend & B.S. Dohrenwend, Eds.: 191–206. Wiley, New York.
140. EATON, W.W., A. DRYMAN & M.M. WEISSMAN. 1991. Panic and phobia. *In* Psychiatric Disorders in America. L.N. Robins & D.A. Regier, Eds.: 155–179. The Free Press, New York.
141. BLAZER, D.G., D. HUGHES, L.K. GEORGE, *et al.* 1991. Generalized anxiety disorder. *In* Psychiatric Disorders in America. L.N. Robins & D.A. Regier, Eds.: 180–203. The Free Press, New York.
142. MAGEE, W.J., W.W. EATON, H.U. WITTCHEN, *et al.* 1996. Agoraphobia, simple phobia, and social phobia in the national comorbidity survey. Arch. Gen. Psychiatry **53:** 159–168.
143. WITTCHEN, H.U., S. ZHAO, R.C. KESSLER, *et al.* 1994. DSM-III-R generalized anxiety disorder in the national comorbidity survey. Arch. Gen. Psychiatry **51:** 355–364.
144. BAREFOOT, J.C., B.L. PETERSON, W.G. DAHLSTROM, *et al.* 1991. Hostility patterns and health implications: correlates of Cook-Medley hostility scale scores in a national survey. Health Psychol. **10:** 18–24.

145. CARMILLI, D., R.H. ROSENMAN & G.E. SWAN. 1988. The Cook and Medley hostility scale: a heritability analysis in adult male twins. Psychosom. Med. **50:** 165–170.
146. SCHERWITZ, L., L. PERKINS, M. CHESNEY, *et al.* 1991. Cook-Medley hostility scale and subsets: relationship to demographic and psychosocial characteristics in young adults in the CARDIA study. Psychosom. Med. **53:** 36–49.
147. MATTHEWS, K.A., S.F. KESLEY, E.N. MEILAHN, *et al.* 1989. Educational attainment and behavioral and biologic risk factors for coronary heart disease in middle-aged women. Am. J. Epidemiol. **129:** 1132–1144.
148. GUMP, B.B., K.A. MATTHEWS & K. RÄIKKÖNEN. 1999. Modeling relationships among socioeconomic status, hostility, cardiovascular reactivity, and left ventricular mass in African American and white children. Health Psychol. **18:** 140–150.
149. MITTELMAN, M.M., M. MACLURE, M. NACHNANI, *et al.* 1997. Educational attainment, anger, and the risk of triggering myocardial infarction onset. Arch. Intern. Med. **157:** 769–775.
150. DOHRENWEND, B.P., I. LEVAV, P.E. SHROUT, *et al.* 1992. Socioeconomic status and psychiatric disorders: the causation–selection issue. Science **255:** 946–952.
151. LINK, B.G., B.P. DOHRENWEND & A.E. SKODOL. 1986. Socio-economic status and schizophrenia: noisome occupational characteristics as a risk factor. Am. Sociol. Rev. **51:** 242–258.
152. MANUCK, S.B. 1994. Cardiovascular reactivity in cardiovascular disease: "Once more unto the breach." Int. J. Behav. Med. **1:** 4–31.
153. KAPLAN, G.A. 1995. Where do shared pathways lead? Some reflections on a research agenda. Psychosom. Med. **57:** 208–212.

Social Status and Susceptibility to Respiratory Infections

SHELDON COHEN[a]

Department of Psychology, Carnegie Mellon University,
Pittsburgh, Pennsylvania 15213-3890, USA

ABSTRACT: Adults and children of lower socioeconomic status (SES) are at higher risk for a wide range of communicable infectious diseases, especially respiratory infections. Greater risk for infectious illness among people with lower SES is thought to be attributable to increased exposure to infectious agents and decreased host resistance to infection. We summarize three studies that examine the prospective association of several markers of social status (unemployment, perceived and observed social status) with host resistance to upper respiratory infections. Unemployment was associated with increased susceptibility to infection in adult humans. Lower social status in male monkeys was also associated with increased susceptibility, as was lower perceived social status in humans. The association of social status and susceptibility was accounted for primarily by increased risk in the lowest social status groups. However, further increases in social status were associated with further decreases in susceptibility in both monkeys and humans.

INTRODUCTION

Adults and children of lower socioeconomic status (SES) are at higher risk for a wide range of communicable infectious diseases, especially respiratory infections. For example, in China low income and poor living conditions were associated with greater incidence of acute upper respiratory tract infections.[1] In Guatemala, children of parents with lower levels of education had higher rates of respiratory illnesses than those with less educated parents.[2] Similarly, in India acute respiratory episodes among children were greater for those from families with lower per capita income and lower literacy rates.[3] British children from lower social classes were found to be absent from school more often as a result of upper respiratory and ear infections.[4] U.S. studies have found similar relations. Lower levels of formal education and unemployment have been associated with greater incidence of acute lower respiratory tract infections[5] and otitis media.[6–8] Similarly, U.S. children from poor families missed more days of school and spent more days in bed as a result of acute respiratory illnesses.[6] Children (up to 17 years old) from families who received federal assistance were also more likely to die of pneumonia or influenza compared to those from families not receiving federal assistance.[9]

The evidence discussed so far is primarily from studies comparing those below the poverty level to others in the population. However, there is substantial evidence

[a]Address for correspondence: 412-268-2336 (voice); 412-268-3294 (fax).
e-mail: scohen@cmu.edu

for a graded relation between SES and health with each increase in SES associated with increased health and lessened mortality.[10] A study of tuberculosis in an adult U.S. sample provides some evidence for a graded relation between SES and incidence of an infectious respiratory illness. Although the link between tuberculosis and poverty has been established for many years,[11] in this study, risk of contracting tuberculosis was found to increase uniformly with decreases in income and education and increases in poverty and public assistance.[12]

Why are people with lower SES at greater risk for infectious illness? There are two categories of explanation (see TABLE 1). One attributes greater incidence to increased *exposure* to infectious agents with decreased SES. Lower SES families often have more children and live in more crowded quarters, both environmental conditions conducive to transmission of infectious agents.[5,13] Poor environmental sanitation and poor hygienic practices might also increase exposure among poorer and less educated groups. Alternatively, SES may increase risk of infection and infectious illness because it alters the *body's ability to fight off infection*. For example, those with lower SES may lack information about vaccination, lack access to medical care, or be unable to afford vaccinations.[14] Vaccinations boost the immune system's ability to respond to specific infectious agents and hence reduce incidence and severity of illness. Inadequate nutrition among lower SES groups may also contribute to poorer host resistance. Malnutrition is known to suppress the immune system's ability to fight off infections and has been identified as a pathway linking poor children to disease risk.[3] Health practices that worsen with decreasing education are also thought to act as pathways linking SES to infectious susceptibility. For example, greater rates of smoking contribute to greater susceptibility to respiratory infectious illness among teenagers and adults,[1,15,16] whereas passive smoke exposure increases susceptibility among children.[16] Other health practices associated with increased risk of respiratory infection such as inadequate physical exercise and poor sleep quality are also more prevalent among those lower on the SES gradient.[15,17] Occupational exposure to immune-altering substances can also alter host resistance. For example, workers in occupations associated with low socioeconomic status have higher risk for tuberculosis, presumably because of higher occupational exposure to agents that increase the risk of progressing from latent infection to active TB.[18] Finally, lower levels of SES are associated with reporting more stressful life events,

TABLE 1. Pathways linking lower socioeconomic status to increased risk for infectious illness

Increased Exposure to Infectious Agents

    greater crowding and family size

    poorer sanitation

    poorer hygienic practices

Decreased Host Resistance to Infection

    less access to immunizing vaccinations

    poorer nutrition

    more smoking (passive and active)

    more psychological stress

perceptions of stress, and negative affective states including depression and anger.[17] Greater stress and negative affect are risk factors for upper respiratory infections in community studies,[19,20] as well as in viral-challenge studies where exposure to the pathogenic agent is controlled.[21–23]

SES EFFECTS IN THE VIRAL-CHALLENGE MODEL

As discussed earlier, greater incidence of infectious illness among those with lower SES may be attributable to either greater exposure to infectious agents or to lower host resistance. In this article, we discuss three viral-challenge studies that investigated the role of SES in host resistance. In all three studies we use an upper respiratory disease model that allows us to experimentally control exposure to a virus and to monitor the development of both infection and clinical illness. In short, *after* characterizing subjects on markers of social status (as well as behavioral, endocrine, and immune factors), we inoculate them with an upper respiratory virus. After exposure they are closely monitored (in quarantine) for the development of infection and illness. There is considerable variability in response to these viruses in terms of both whether subjects become infected, and whether they express symptoms. This paradigm eliminates the possibilities that associations we find between social status and susceptibility are attributable to any of the following: *previous exposure* to the virus (we measure prechallenge antibody to the experimental virus); *differential exposure* to the virus (we expose subjects to controlled doses of the virus); or *illness-causing changes* in social status (we accept only healthy subjects into the trials and assess social status before viral exposure).

We will briefly discuss two studies with human subjects and one with nonhuman primates. The distributions of income, education, and occupational status in our human studies tend to be constrained and somewhat unrepresentative. Many of our volunteers have relatively low incomes, and about 30% are college students. Because the traditional markers of SES are not well represented in our samples, we have pursued other markers of SES as predictors of infectious illness. In the first (human) study, we examine under- and unemployment, and in the second (monkey) and third (human) studies we examine observed (monkeys) and perceived (humans) social status.

UNEMPLOYMENT AND SUSCEPTIBILITY TO CLINICAL COLDS

The data on unemployment derive from a study of 276 volunteers.[22] The major focus of the study was identifying the types of stressful life events that increased risk for infectious illness. We assessed life events before exposing volunteers to one of two rhinoviruses and then followed them for five days after exposure to monitor infection (viral shedding) and signs/symptoms (e.g., mucus weights, congestion) of the common cold. The major outcome in the study was clinical illness, which was defined as both infection by the challenge virus and expression of symptoms (see Ref. 22).

We used an interview, the Life Events and Difficulties Schedule[24] (LEDS), to assess the existence of enduring (one month or longer) and consensually threatening (agreement by judges) stressful events. Twenty-eight (9%) of the volunteers were identified as being unemployed or underemployed according to these criteria. (To simplify presentation, we will refer to this group as unemployed.) This is a different approach than just asking about employment status. For example, instead of treating all unemployed persons the same, the LEDS differentiates leaving an unsatisfying job because of lack of financial need (not coded as an unemployment stressor) from being fired following 20 years of dedicated and fulfilling service (coded as unemployment stressor).

The data were analyzed to determine whether unemployment predicted who developed clinical colds. The analyses included eight control variables that might provide alternative explanations for the relation between unemployment and colds. These included antibody to the experimental virus before inoculation, age, body mass index (weight in kilograms divided by height in meters^2), season (fall or spring), race (Caucasian or not), gender, education (high school graduate or less, some college, and bachelor's degree or greater), and virus type (RV39 or Hanks). The result indicated that even after accounting for all of these variables, those who were unemployed were 3.4 times ($p < 0.03$) more likely to develop colds than the remainder of the volunteers.

We also attempted to identify possible behavioral and biological pathways that might link unemployment to susceptibility. The analyses indicated that at least part of the association could be attributed to unemployed people smoking, having poorer sleep quality, and elevated levels of norepinephrine (a stress hormone).

SOCIAL STATUS AND SUSCEPTIBILITY TO INFECTION: THE MONKEY STUDY

Several years ago, we conducted a study in which the objective was to assess the roles of social stress and social status in susceptibility to upper respiratory infection.[23] Sixty male cynomolgus monkeys were randomly assigned to stable or unstable social conditions for fifteen months. Two markers of social status, social rank (based on who wins encounters with other animals) and percent of behaviors that were submissive, were assessed at independent observation periods. Social rank was assessed monthly, and submissive behaviors were measured during intensive monitoring of the animals' behavior during the 11th and 14th months of the study. Endocrine and immune responses were each assessed at three-month intervals. At the beginning of the 15th month, all animals were exposed to a virus (adenovirus) that causes a common cold-like illness. The primary outcome was whether or not an animal developed a biologically verifiable infection (shed adenovirus) following viral exposure.

Although the social stability manipulation was associated with increased agonistic behavior (as indicated by minor injuries) and elevated norepinephrine responses to social reorganizations, the manipulation did not influence the probability of being infected by the virus. However, low social status (as assessed by either rank or percent of behaviors that were submissive) was associated with a substantially greater

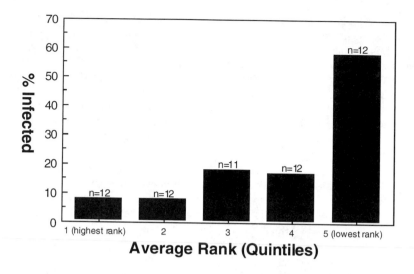

FIGURE 1. Percentage of animals infected by the virus presented by average social rank (quintiles); *1* refers to the highest rank and *5* to the lowest. Adapted from the original figure (see Ref. 23), with permission from the American Psychological Association.

probability of being infected. As apparent from FIGURE 1, although the association of social status and susceptibility was accounted for primarily by increased risk in the lowest social status groups, there was evidence for a graded relation with further increases in social status associated with further decreases in susceptibility. Lower social status was also associated with less body weight, greater elevated cortisol responses to social reorganizations, and less aggressive behavior. However, none of these characteristics could account for the relation between social status and infection.

SOCIAL STATUS AND SUSCEPTIBILITY TO INFECTION: THE HUMAN STUDY

The relationship between social status in the animals and susceptibility led us to consider the possibility that a similar relationship might occur in humans. However, it was not entirely clear how social status in monkeys (based on winning confrontations with other animals in their social group) might apply to humans. One possibility was that the traditional measures of SES—income, education, and occupational status—are the appropriate analogues in humans. However, these are all measures of status in relation to the larger society as opposed to the individuals' own social groups.[25] Instead, we used a measure of perceived social status in one's own community developed by the MacArthur Foundation's Network on Socioeconomic Status and Health. This measure is very simple to complete. The subject is presented with the picture of a ladder with nine rungs and is asked to indicate (with an X) where they stand in their own community.

This study design was similar to the human study described earlier. One hundred and six subjects were administered the ladder as well as other psychological, behavioral, and biological measures. They were then exposed to a rhinovirus (RV23) and followed in quarantine for five days and monitored for the development of infection (viral shedding or fourfold increase in RV23 antibody titer). We have just begun to analyze these data. Our initial analyses focused on the association between perceived social status and infection. Control variables were the same as described in the previous study. The preliminary results were surprisingly similar to those of the monkey study. Lower perceived social status was associated with greater susceptibility to infection. This association was accounted for primarily by increased risk in the lowest social status groups. However, there was also evidence for a graded relation with further increases in social status associated with further decreases in susceptibility. Interestingly, perceived social status was not associated with smoking status, sleep efficiency, alcohol consumption, or exercise. Nor was it associated with circulating levels of catecholamines. Consequently, we currently do not have any evidence for a behavioral or biological pathway linking perceived status to susceptibility to infection.

CONCLUSIONS

We have provided evidence from three prospective studies for the relation between markers of SES and susceptibility to upper respiratory infectious illness. This includes a substantial association between unemployment and greater susceptibility. Unemployment has been associated with a broad range of disease risk in past studies,[26] and documenting its relation to host resistance to infection further justifies the centrality of work in our lives and the magnitude of stress generated when we lose our livelihood. We have also found provocative evidence in regard to the relation of social status and host resistance to infectious disease. This includes greater susceptibility among monkeys who tend to lose encounters with other animals and people who rate themselves as having relatively lower status in their own communities. Although it is those of the lowest social status who are at greatest risk, for both monkeys and man there is some evidence for a graded relation with increased status associated with less risk. This work raises many interesting questions that have not yet been addressed. For example, to what degree is perceived social status a function of traditional measures of SES such as income, education, and occupational status? To what degree does it reflect components of status among one's own social network that are not highly correlated with traditional measures? To what degree is it a biased report reflecting dispositional characteristics such as neuroticism or depression? What are the pathways that link social status (real or perceived) to susceptibility to infectious agents? Does it operate through stress and stress hormones or through other biological or behavioral concomitants of social status?

ACKNOWLEDGMENTS

The studies reported in this article were supported by Grants MH47234; MH50429 and a Senior Scientist Award (MH00721) to Dr. Cohen from the National Institute of Mental Health. Supplemental support was provided by the John D. and Catherine T. MacArthur Foundation Network of Social Economic Status and Health.

REFERENCES

1. WANG, J., Q. WANG & Z. BI. 1990. Epidemiology of acute respiratory tract infections among Guatemalan ambulatory preschool children. Rev. Infect. Dis. **12**(Suppl. 8): S1029–1034.
2. CRUZ, J.R., G. PAREJA, A. DE FERNANDEZ, F. PERALTA, P. CACERES & F. CANO. 1990. The epidemiology of acute respiratory infections in children and adults: a global perspective. Epidemiol. Rev. **12**: 149–178.
3. DEB, S.K. 1998. Acute respiratory disease survey in Tripura in case of children below five years of age. J. Indian Med. Assoc. **96**(4): 111–116.
4. POWER, C. 1992. A review of child health in the 1958 birth cohort: National Child Development Study. Ped. Perinat. Epidemiol. **6**: 81–110.
5. SIMS, S., M.A. DOWNHAM, J. MCQUILLIN & P.S. GARDNER. 1976. Respiratory syncytial virus infection in North-East England. Br. Med. J. **2**(6044): 1095–1098.
6. EGBUONU, L. & B. STARFIELD. 1982. Child health and social status. Pediatrics **69**: 550–557.
7. PARADISE, J.L., H.E. ROCKETTE, D.K. COLBORN, et al. 1997. Otitis media in 2253 Pittsburgh-area infants: prevalence and risk factors during the first two years of life. Pediatrics **99**(3): 318–333.
8. STAHLBERG, M.R., O. RUUSKANEN & E. VIROLAINEN. 1986. Risk factors for recurrent otitis media. Pediatr. Infect. Dis. **5**(1): 30–32.
9. NELSON, M.D., JR. 1992. Socioeconomic status and childhood mortality in North Carolina. Am. J. Public Health **82**: 1131–1133.
10. ADLER, N.E., T. BOYCE, M. A. CHESNEY, S. COHEN, S. FOLKMAN, R.L. KAHN & S.L. SYME. 1994. Socioeconomic status and health: the challenge of the gradient. Am. Psychol. **49**: 15–24.
11. SPENCE, D.P., J. HOTCHKISS, C.S. WILLIAMS & P.D. DAVIES. 1993. Tuberculosis and poverty. Br. Med. J. **307**: 759–761.
12. CANTWELL, M.F., M.T. MCKENNA, E. MCCRAY & I.M. ONORATO. 1998. Tuberculosis and race/ethnicity in the United States: impact of socioeconomic status. Am. J. Respir. Crit. Care Med. **157**(4PT1): 1016–1020.
13. TABER, L.H., A. PAREDES, W.P. GLEZEN & R.B. COUCH. 1981. Infection with influenza A/Victoria virus in Houston families, 1976. J. Hyg. (London) (IEF) **86**(3): 303–313.
14. SOLBERG L.I., M.L. BREKKE & T.E. KOTTKE. 1997. Are physicians less likely to recommend preventive services to low-SES patients? Prev. Med. (PM4) **26**(3): 350–357.
15. COHEN, S., W.J. DOYLE, D.P. SKONER, B.S. RABIN & J.M. GWALTNEY, JR. 1997. Social ties and susceptibility to the common cold. JAMA **277**: 1940–1944.
16. GRAHAM, N.M. 1990. The epidemiology of acute respiratory infections in children and adults: A global perspective. Epidemiol. Rev. **12**: 149–178.
17. COHEN, S., G.A. KAPLAN & J.T. SALONEN. 1999. The role of psychological characteristics in the relation between socioeconomic status and perceived health. J. Appl. Soc. Psychol. **29**: 551–574.
18. MMWR. 1995. Proportionate mortality from pulmonary tuberculosis associated with occupation—28 states, 1979–1990. Morb. Mortal. Wkly. Rep. (NE8) **44**(1): 14–19.
19. GRAHAM, N.M.H., R.B. DOUGLAS & P. RYAN. 1986. Stress and acute respiratory infection. Am. J. Epidemiol. **124**: 389–401.

20. MEYER, R.J. & R.J. HAGGERTY. 1962. Streptococcal infections in families. Pediatrics **29:** 539–549.
21. COHEN, S., D.A.J. TYRRELL & A.P. SMITH. 1991. Psychological stress in humans and susceptibility to the common cold. N. Engl. J. Med. **325:** 606–612.
22. COHEN, S., E. FRANK, W.J. DOYLE, D.P. SKONER, B.S. RABIN & J.M. GWALTNEY, JR. 1998. Types of stressors that increase susceptibility to the common cold in adults. Health Psychol. **17:** 214–223.
23. COHEN, S., S. LINE, S.B. MANUCK, B.S. RABIN, E. HEISE & J.R. KAPLAN. 1997. Chronic social stress, social status and susceptibility to upper respiratory infections in nonhuman primates. Psychosom. Med. **59:** 213–221.
24. BROWN, G.W. & T.O. HARRIS, Eds. 1989. Life Events and Illness. Guilford Press, New York.
25. KAPLAN, J. & S. MANUCK. 1999. Status, stress, and atherosclerosis: the role of environment and individual behavior. Ann. N.Y. Acad. Sci. **896:** this volume.
26. KASL, S.V. 1978. Epidemiological contributions to the study of work stress. *In* Stress at work. C.I. Cooper & R. Payne, Eds.: 3–48. Wiley, New York.

Sleep as a Mediator of the Relationship between Socioeconomic Status and Health: A Hypothesis

EVE VAN CAUTER[a] AND KARINE SPIEGEL

Department of Medicine, University of Chicago,
5841 South Maryland Avenue, Chicago, Illinois, USA

Laboratory of Experimental Medicine, Université Libre de Bruxelles, Belgium

ABSTRACT: This article discusses the hypothesis that the adverse impact of low socioeconomic status (SES) on health may be partly mediated by decrements in sleep duration and quality. Low SES is frequently associated with a diminished opportunity to obtain sufficient sleep or with environmental conditions that compromise sleep quality. In a recent study, we examined carbohydrate metabolism, endocrine function, and sympatho-vagal balance in young, healthy adults studied after restricting sleep to four hours per night for six nights as compared to a fully rested condition obtained by extending the bedtime period to 12 hours per night for six nights. The state of sleep debt was associated with decreased glucose tolerance, elevated evening cortisol levels, and increased sympathetic activity. The alterations in glucose tolerance and hypothalamo–pituitary–adrenal function were qualitatively and quantitatively similar to those observed in normal aging. These results indicate that sleep loss can increase the "allostatic load" and facilitate the development of chronic conditions, such as obesity, diabetes, and hypertension, which have an increased prevalence in low SES groups.

THE SES–HEALTH GRADIENT AND SLEEP LOSS: A HYPOTHESIS

The pathways underlying the relationship between socioeconomic status (SES) and health are likely to involve multiple physiological systems. In this volume, pathways involving cardiovascular mechanisms, immune mechanisms, and neuroendocrine and metabolic effects of stress are discussed. As indicated in other chapters, the burden of negative emotions in low-SES groups and the erosion of psychosocial resources that often accompany low-SES status are also thought to be involved in the linear gradient between SES and health. In recent years, evidence has rapidly accumulated to indicate that sleep loss may have adverse effects on cardiovascular function, on immune function, on endocrine function (particularly on the stress-responsive hypothalamo–pituitary–adrenal [HPA] system) and on carbohydrate metabolism. The negative impact of sleep loss on mood and affect has been long recognized. Increased irritability has also been noted in a majority of studies involving

[a]Address for correspondence: Eve Van Cauter, Ph.D., Department of Medicine, MC 1027, University of Chicago, 5841 South Maryland Ave., Chicago, IL 60637, USA. 773-702-0169 (voice); 773-702-9194 (fax).
e-mail: evcauter@medicine.bsd.uchicago.edu

prolonged sleep deprivation. In short, sleep loss has a negative impact on most, if not all, mechanisms that have been proposed as implicated in the association between low SES and poor health.

Sleep curtailment is a hallmark of modern society. "Normal" sleep duration has decreased from approximately 9 hours in 1910 to an average of 7.5 hours today.[1] Many persons voluntarily choose to curtail their sleep to the shortest amount tolerable to maximize the time available for work and leisure activities.[2] Social pressures, and particularly the pressures of the working environment, impose curtailed bedtimes to an increasingly large number of persons in Western societies. These constraints on time available to sleep seem to be more prevalent in low-SES occupations. Millions of shift workers sleep on average less than 6 hours per work day to meet the demands of around-the-clock operations.[3] Sleep times of 5.25 to 5.5 hours per day have been reported in rotating night workers.[4] Electrophysiologically verified sleep times of 3.83 to 5.38 hours have been recorded in truck drivers.[5] Even in the absence of work pressure, members of low-SES groups are also likely to have fewer opportunities to obtain sufficient amounts of restorative sleep because of adverse environmental conditions, including crowded and/or unsafe living quarters, noise, and temperatures either too hot or too cold. Last, but not least, anxiety and stress are notorious for their negative impact on sleep. In support of the notion that sleep in low-SES groups may be more affected by adverse economic circumstances is a study that has indicated that, during severe economic depression, sleep quality is not drastically deteriorated, except among unemployed blue-collar workers.[6]

The evidence summarized in the two previous paragraphs has led us to formulate the hypothesis that the adverse impact of low socioeconomic status (SES) on health may be partly mediated by decrements in sleep duration and quality. This hypothesis is amenable to rigorous scientific testing, which we hope will be undertaken in the near future. A number of instruments to monitor sleep duration and quality outside of the laboratory have become available during the past few years. These include well-standardized questionnaires and scales such as the Pittsburgh Sleep Quality Questionnaire[7] and the Karolinska Sleepiness Scale,[8] the use of wrist activity monitoring (using devices the size and weight of a wristwatch) to accurately estimate sleep onset and offset,[9] and ambulatory sleep-monitoring devices such as the "Nightcap," a simple, portable system combining measurements of head movements and eyelid movements to differentiate between wake, REM sleep, and non-REM sleep.[10] These techniques have already been used in field studies of social isolation,[11] social support of cancer patients,[12] and carbohydrate metabolism in short and long sleepers (unpublished data of our group) and could thus be used to monitor sleep across SES groups and test the hypothesis that some of the adverse health impacts of low SES are partly caused by chronic sleep loss. Importantly, if sleep loss was indeed identified as a contributing factor to the SES–health gradient, corrective strategies could be designed and tested.

ENDOCRINE AND METABOLIC CONSEQUENCES OF A "SLEEP DEBT"

Despite the fact that sleep is known to modulate metabolic and endocrine regulation, immune function, and cardiovascular parameters, the consensus that prevailed until recently is that sleep is for the brain, not for the rest of the body,[13,14] and that sleep loss results in increased sleepiness and decreased cognitive performance but has little or no effect on peripheral function.[13–15] The vast majority of studies of sleep deprivation have examined acute total sleep deprivation for one or more days, but the much more common condition of chronic partial sleep loss has only been addressed in a handful of studies.[16–18] We recently measured metabolic and hormonal parameters in subjects studied during one week of sleep restriction and after one week of sleep recovery. Following a period of baseline conditions with a standard bedtime duration of 8 hours, as typically used in studies of normal human sleep, a group of young, healthy men were studied after six nights of sleep restriction to four hours per night and after six nights of sleep extension to 12 hours per night. The protocol is schematically represented in FIGURE 1.

Sleep was monitored during each of the 16 nights of the study. Naps were not allowed. Compliance was verified by analysis of recordings of wrist activity, which were obtained continuously throughout the study. On the fifth day of sleep restriction and sleep extension, the subjects underwent an intravenous glucose tolerance test (IVGTT) at 09:00, and saliva samples for the measurement of free cortisol levels were collected at 30-min intervals from 15:00 until bedtime. On the sixth day of

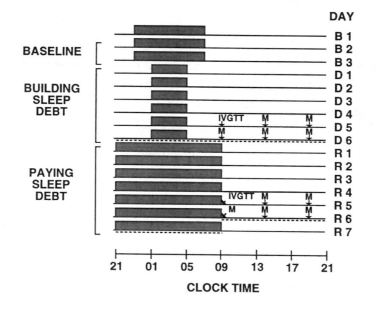

FIGURE 1. Schematic representation of the protocol. The *shaded bars* represent the sleep periods. M: carbohydrate-rich meals given at 5-hour intervals. IVGTT: intravenous glucose tolerance test. The study period included three nights with bedtime from 23:00 to 07:00 (B1-B3), six nights with bedtimes from 01:00 to 05:00 (D1-D6; sleep restriction), and seven nights with bedtime from 21:00 to 09:00 (R1-R7; sleep recovery). In the morning of D5 and R5, an IVGTT was administered at 09:00. The dashed lines show the 24-hour sampling periods at 10–30-minute intervals at the end of sleep restriction and sleep recovery.

sleep restriction and sleep extension, blood sampling was initiated, and samples were collected at frequent intervals for 24 hours to measure hormonal levels. Identical carbohydrate-rich (62%) meals were consumed at 09:00, 14:00, and 19:00 on the fifth and sixth days of both sleep restriction and sleep recovery. Beat-to-beat heart-rate interval was recorded continuously via a polar chest belt.

The upper panels of FIGURE 2 show the mean glucose and insulin profiles following ingestion of a carbohydrate-rich breakfast on the sixth day of both conditions.

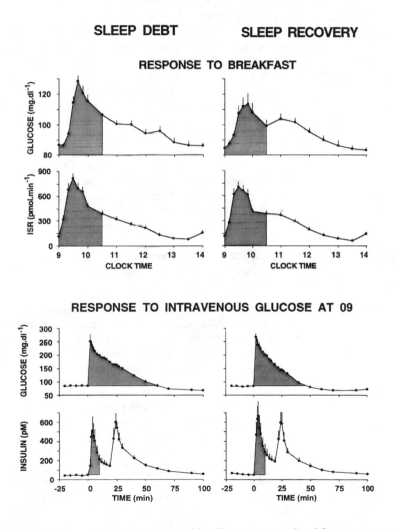

FIGURE 2. Mean (+ SEM) glucose and insulin responses to breakfast (*upper panels*) and mean (+ SEM) profiles of blood glucose and serum insulin during the IVGTT (*lower panels*) at the end of one week of sleep restriction (*left panels*) and one week of sleep extension (*right panels*).

The glucose response to breakfast was higher when sleep was curtailed than when sleep was extended ($p = 0.05$), although insulin secretory responses were similar under both conditions. The difference in peak glucose levels in response to breakfast between the sleep restriction and sleep recovery conditions (i.e., ± 15 mg·dl^{-1}) translates into an approximate 20 mg·dl^{-1} difference in glucose levels 120 min after the beginning of a standard glucose tolerance test.[19] This comparison suggests that, under the sleep debt condition, the young, lean subjects who participated in this study would have responded to a standard oral glucose tolerance test in a manner consistent with current diagnostic criteria for impaired glucose tolerance. The lower panels of FIGURE 2 show the glucose and insulin responses to the intravenous glucose injection. The parameters of glucose tolerance measured at the end of the recovery period were in the normal range for young, healthy men, but the parameters measured in the state of sleep debt were consistent with a clinically significant impairment of carbohydrate tolerance. Thus, the rate of disappearance of glucose postinjection (K_G) was nearly 40% slower in the sleep debt condition than after recovery (1.45 ± 0.31 versus $2.40 \pm 0.41\%\cdot\text{min}^{-1}$; $p < 0.02$). K_G values around $1.60\%\cdot\text{min}^{-1}$ are typical of older adults with impaired glucose tolerance[20] whereas values of 2.2–$2.9\%\cdot\text{min}^{-1}$ are typical of fit young subjects.[21] The acute insulin response to glucose (AIR_G), shown on the lowest panel of FIGURE 2 as a shaded area, was reduced by 30% in the sleep debt condition as compared to postrecovery (AIR_G; 304 ± 95 versus 432 ± 110 pM·min; $p < 0.04$). A decrease in acute insulin response to glucose is an early marker of diabetes.[22] Differences in AIR_G of similar magnitude have been previously described in aging.[23] Finally, another parameter of glucose tolerance, glucose effectiveness, a measure of noninsulin-dependent glucose utilization, was also markedly decreased in the state of sleep debt. A likely explanation for this decrease in glucose effectiveness is that brain glucose uptake was decreased in the very sleepy subjects at the end of the period of sleep curtailment (upper panels of FIGURE 3; $p < 0.0.0005$).

A measure of the relative importance of sympathetic (inhibitory) and parasympathetic (stimulatory) activity was derived from analyses of the recordings of heart rate variability. Sympatho-vagal balance was significantly higher in the sleep restriction than in the sleep recovery condition (mean rRR during the period 09:00–14:00 was 0.77 ± 0.02 versus 0.66 ± 0.04, $p < 0.02$; mid-upper panels of FIGURE 3).

When compared to the fully rested condition, the state of sleep debt was also associated with alterations of cortisol secretion, whether estimated by total cortisol levels in plasma or free cortisol levels in saliva. The primary alteration was an elevation of cortisol concentrations in the afternoon and early evening (shaded area in lower panels of FIG. 3; $p = 0.0001$). This later disturbance, which we have previously observed in conditions of acute total and partial sleep loss,[24] may reflect decreased efficacy of the negative-feedback regulation of the HPA axis. Based on the analysis of the levels of free cortisol in saliva, the rate of decrease of free cortisol concentrations between 16:00 and 21:00 was approximately six-fold slower during the sleep debt condition than after full sleep recovery (0.024 ± 0.048 versus 0.156 ± 0.047 ng·ml^{-1} per hour; $p < 0.01$). An elevation of plasma cortisol levels in the afternoon and early evening similar to that observed in our subjects under the sleep debt condition has been previously reported in several studies of normal aging.[25,26]

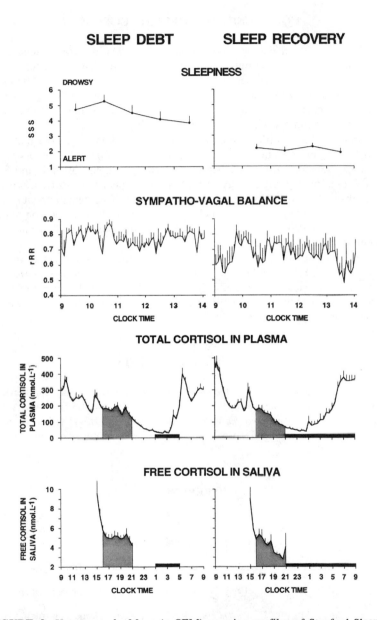

FIGURE 3. *Upper panels*: Mean (+ SEM) morning profiles of Stanford Sleepiness Scores (SSS; 1: "feeling active and vital; alert; wide awake"; 6: "sleepiness; prefer to be lying down; fighting sleep; woozy") and sympatho-vagal balance (rRR). *Lower panels*: Mean (+ SEM) profiles of total cortisol levels in plasma and free cortisol levels in saliva. The afternoon and early evenings levels of cortisol (*shaded areas*), whether estimated from total plasma concentrations or from free saliva levels, were higher in the sleep debt condition than after recovery.

CONCLUSIONS AND PERSPECTIVES

Our findings indicate that one week of partial sleep loss has consequences for peripheral function that, if maintained chronically, could have long-term adverse health effects. Indeed, decreased carbohydrate tolerance and increased sympathetic tone are well-recognized risk factors for the development of insulin resistance, obesity, and hypertension.[27] An elevation of evening cortisol is thought to be involved in age-related insulin resistance and memory impairments.[28,29]

Ongoing studies in our laboratory are examining vigilance, glucose metabolism, and glucocorticoid levels in subjects who report usual bedtimes of 6 hours or less as compared to subjects with usual bedtimes between 7 hours 30 min and 8 hours 30 min. Preliminary findings suggest that short sleepers tend to be more insulin resistant than persons with more standard sleep habits. The development of insulin resistance in a state of chronic sleep debt is consistent with an adaptation of pancreatic function to the alteration in glucose tolerance demonstrated after one week of sleep curtailment.

In conclusion, chronic sleep curtailment and a reduced opportunity to recover from sleep loss are likely to be highly prevalent conditions in low-SES groups. Recent research indicates that the resulting state of chronic sleep debt is associated with metabolic alterations that could partly underlie the association between low SES and increased morbidity.

ACKNOWLEDGMENTS

This work was partially supported by grants from the Mind–Body Network of the MacArthur Foundation (Chicago, IL), Grant F49620-94-1-0203 from the Air Force Office of Scientific Research to E. Van Cauter, and Grant DK-41814 from the NIH. The University of Chicago General Clinical Research Center is supported by NIH Grant RR-00055.

REFERENCES

1. WEBB, W.B. & H.W. AGNEW. 1975. Are we chronically sleep deprived? Bull. Psychon. Soc. **6:** 47–48.
2. BROMAN, J.E., L.G. LUNDH & J. HETTA. 1996. Insufficient sleep in the general population. Neurophysiol. Clin. **26:** 30–39.
3. BLIWISE, D.L. 1996. Historical change in the report of daytime fatigue. Sleep **19:** 462–464.
4. BONNET, M. & D. ARAND. 1995. We are chronically sleep deprived. Sleep **18:** 908–911.
5. MITLER, M., J. MILLER, J. LIPSITZ, *et al.* 1997. The sleep of long-haul truck drivers. N. Engl. J. Med. **337:** 755–761.
6. HYYPPA, M.T., E. KRONHOLM & E. ALANEN. 1997. Quality of sleep during economic recession in Finland: a longitudinal cohort study. Soc. Sci. Med. **45:** 731–738.
7. BUYSSE, D.J., C.F.D. REYNOLDS, T.H. MONK, *et al.* 1989. The Pittsburgh Sleep Quality Index: a new instrument for psychiatric practice and research. Psychiatry Res. **28:** 193–213.
8. GILLBERG, M., G. KECKLUND & T. AKERSTEDT. 1994. Relations between performance and subjective ratings of sleepiness during a night awake. Sleep **17:** 236–241.

9. BORBELY, A.A. 1986. New techniques for the analysis of the human sleep–wake cycle. Brain Dev. **8:** 482–488.
10. AJILORE, O., R. STICKGOLD, C.D. RITTENHOUSE, *et al.* 1995. Nightcap: laboratory and home-based evaluation of a portable sleep monitor. Psychophysiology **32:** 92–98.
11. CACIOPPO, J.T., J.M. ERNST, M.H. BURLESON, *et al.* 1999. Lonely traits and concomitant physiological processes: The MacArthur social neurosciences studies. Submitted.
12. SPIEGEL, D. 1999. In press.
13. HORNE, J. 1988. Why We Sleep. Oxford University Press, Oxford.
14. BENINGTON, J.H. & H.C. HELLER. 1995. Restoration of brain energy metabolism as the function of sleep. Progr. Neurobiol. **45:** 347–360.
15. BONNET, M.H. 1994. Sleep deprivation. *In* M.H. Kryger, T. Roth & W.C. Dement, Eds.: 50–67. Principles and Practice of Sleep Medicine. W.B. Saunders, Philadelphia.
16. BRUNNER, D.P., D.J. DIJK & A.A. BORBELY. 1993. Repeated partial sleep deprivation progressively changes the EEG during sleep and wakefulness. Sleep **16:** 100–113.
17. DINGES, D., F. PACK, K. WILLIAMS, *et al.* 1997. Cumulative sleepiness, mood disturbance, and psychomotor vigilance performance decrements during a week of sleep restricted to 4–5 hours per night. Sleep **20:** 267–277.
18. SPIEGEL, K., R. LEPROULT & E. VAN CAUTER. 1999. Impact of a sleep debt on metabolic and endocrine function. Lancet **354:** 1435–1439.
19. GUMBINER, B., K.S. POLONSKY, W.F. BELTZ, *et al.* 1989. Effects of aging on insulin secretion. Diabetes **38:** 1549–1556.
20. GARCIA, G.V., R.V. FREEMAN, M.A SUPIANO, *et al.* 1997. Glucose metabolism in older adults: a study including subjects more than 80 years of age. J. Am. Geriatr. Soc. **45:** 813–817.
21. PRIGEON, R.L., S.E. KAHN & D. PORTE, JR. 1995. Changes in insulin sensitivity, glucose effectiveness, and B-cell function in regularly exercising subjects. Metabolism **44:** 1259–1263.
22. KAHN, C.R. 1995. Etiology and pathogenesis of type II diabetes mellitus and related disorders. *In* K. Becker, Ed.: 1210–1216. Principles and Practice of Endocrinology and Metabolism. 2nd edit. J.B. Lippincott, Philadelphia.
23. KAHN, S.E., R.L. PRIGEON, D.K. MCCULLOCH, *et al.* 1993. Quantification of the relationship between insulin sensitivity and B-cell function in human subjects: evidence for a hyperbolic function. Diabetes **42:** 1663–1672.
24. LEPROULT, R., G. COPINSCHI, O. BUXTON, *et al.* 1997. Sleep loss results in an elevation of cortisol levels the next evening. Sleep **20**(10): 865–870.
25. VAN CAUTER, E., R. LEPROULT & D.J. KUPFER. 1996. Effects of gender and age on the levels and circadian rhythmicity of plasma cortisol. J. Clin. Endocrinol. Metab. **81:** 2468–2473.
26. KERN, W., C. DODT, J. BORN, *et al.* 1996. Changes in cortisol and growth hormone secretion during nocturnal sleep in the course of aging. J. Gerontol. **51A:** M3–M9.
27. REAVEN, G.M., H. LITHELL & L. LANDSBERG. 1996. Hypertension and associated metabolic abnormalities: the role of insulin resistance and the sympathoadrenal system. N. Engl. J. Med. **334:** 374–381.
28. DALLMAN, M.F., A.L. STRACK, S.F. AKANA, *et al.* 1993. Feast and famine: critical role of glucocorticoids with insulin in daily energy flow. Front. Neuroendocrinol. **14:** 303–347.
29. MCEWEN, B.S. 1998. Protective and damaging effects of stress mediators. N. Engl. J. Med. **338:** 171–179.

Cardiovascular Pathways: Socioeconomic Status and Stress Effects on Hypertension and Cardiovascular Function

THOMAS PICKERING[a]

Hypertension Center, New York Presbyterian Hospital,
520 East 70th Street, New York, NY 10021, USA

ABSTRACT: In westernized societies there is a consistent and continuous gradient between the prevalence of cardiovascular disease (including both coronary heart disease and stroke) with SES, such that people from lower SES have more disease. Several studies have examined the roles of the major cardiovascular risk factors for explaining this gradient. There is a strong SES gradient for smoking, which parallels the gradient in disease, but the gradients for hypertension and cholesterol are weak or absent. Central obesity and physical inactivity may also be contributory factors. In the United States there is a strong association between SES and race, and it is suggested that the higher prevalence of hypertension and cardiovascular disease in blacks may be attributed to psychosocial factors, including those related to SES. The possible pathways by which SES affects cardiovascular disease include effects of chronic stress mediated by the brain, differences in lifestyles and behavior patterns, and access to health care. At the present time, the second of these is the strongest candidate; the effects of stress have been little studied.

INTRODUCTION

Studies conducted in several countries have shown a continuous gradient between SES, as measured by income, education, or professional grade, and cardiovascular morbidity and mortality. This has been shown for total cardiovascular morbidity, coronary heart disease, and stroke. In some cases, such as the Whitehall Civil Servants Study conducted in England, the ratio of death rates from the lowest to the highest professional grade may be as much as 3 to 1[1] (see FIG. 1). It was not always thus: in the United Kingdom coronary heart disease was commoner in the affluent classes in 1931 and 1951, but since 1961 it has been commoner in the lower classes, and the difference appears to be increasing.[2] It is relatively rare in traditional and non-westernized societies, but studies of migrants from African villages to cities and of Japanese moving from Japan to the United States[3] have shown a consistent trend for cardiovascular disease (CVD) to increase as a western lifestyle is adopted.

[a]Address for correspondence: 212-746-2149 (voice) 212-746-2685 (fax).
e-mail: tpicker@mail.med.cornell.edu

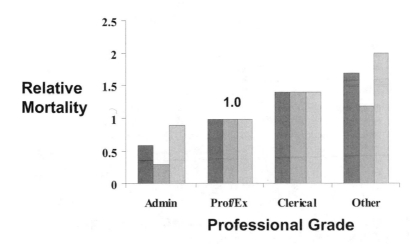

FIGURE 1. Data from the Whitehall Study showing the gradient in cardiovascular (CV) disease according to professional grade in British civil servants. *Admin,* administrators (the highest grade); *Prof/Ex,* professional and executive; *Other,* the lowest grade. Key: ■, coronary heart disease (CHD); ■, stroke; ■, other CV. Rates are normalized to Prof/Ex grade. Data from Marmot *et al.*[1]

THE ROLE OF THE MAJOR RISK FACTORS.

Studies such as the Framingham Heart Study have shown that about 50% of coronary heart disease can be explained by the three major cardiovascular risk factors—blood cholesterol, blood pressure, and smoking. The first Whitehall Study[1] found that about one quarter of the SES–CVD gradient could be explained by these major CVD risk factors, which are reviewed below.

Smoking

Almost all studies have found that there is a gradient in the prevalence of smoking that parallels the gradient of cardiovascular disease. An analysis of three cohorts in Chicago (the Chicago Heart Association Detection Project in Industry, the Peoples Gas Company Study, and the Western Electric Study) found a significant and graded inverse relation between education and cigarette use in all three.[4] In the Whitehall Study the prevalence of smokers was approximately twice as high in the lowest grade as compared to the highest[1] (FIG. 2).

Cholesterol and Lipid Factors

There is often little or no SES gradient in total blood cholesterol. Thus, none of the three Chicago cohorts showed any association between cholesterol and education.[4] In the first Whitehall Study, in which there was a nearly threefold gradient of coronary heart disease deaths, blood total cholesterol was slightly *higher* in the highest grade of civil servants[1] (FIG. 2). In the second study, conducted several years lat-

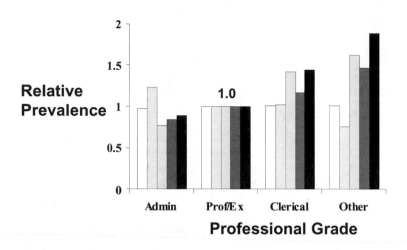

FIGURE 2. Data from the Whitehall study showing relative prevalence (normalized to Prof/Ex grade) of the major risk factors for cardiovascular disease according to professional grade (see FIG. 1). □, hypertension; □, hypercol; □, smokers; ■, obese; ■, sedentary. Data from Marmot *et al.*[1]

er, there was no gradient of LDL cholesterol, but a much stronger gradient with HDL cholesterol (in which low SES was associated with low HDL).[5] The Whitehall Study has also examined some of the other lipid factors that are known to relate to atherosclerosis: thus apolipoprotein A1, the major apoprotein of HDL cholesterol, shows the same gradient with SES as HDL, and the ratio of apo B to apo A1, which is also regarded as an index of atherogenicity, shows an inverse gradient. Both of these observations are consistent with the higher prevalence of disease in lower SES groups.[6] In contrast, the Tromso Heart Study in Norway found a negative relation between educational level and blood total cholesterol in both men and women,[7] and a study of middle-aged women in Pittsburgh found the same: less educated women had higher levels of LDL cholesterol, apolipoprotein B, and triglycerides than more highly educated women.[8] These differences may be the result of cultural differences in diets.

Blood Pressure

The literature on the relationship between blood pressure and SES is also mixed. The three Chicago cohorts mentioned above exhibited an inverse association between blood pressure and education that was independent of body weight.[4] In the Intersalt Study, which was a multinational study of the relationship between salt intake and blood pressure, negative relations between years of education and blood pressure were found for men in 28 out of 47 populations, and for women in 38.[9] However, in many of the studies in which the SES–CVD gradient was observed, there was no corresponding gradient of blood pressure.[10] Colhoun *et al.* reviewed studies of the relationship between SES and blood pressure and found 57 studies from developed countries and 13 from less developed countries.[11] Almost all studies from the United States and Canada found a relation between SES and blood pressure, and in

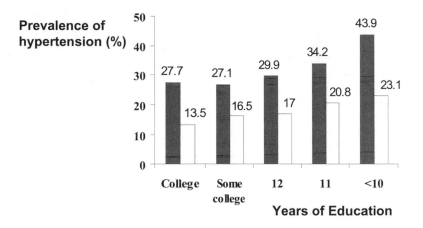

FIGURE 3. Prevalence of hypertension according to educational level in the Hypertension Detection and Follow-up Program (HDFP). ■, black; □, white. Data replotted from Ref. 12.

one biracial study, the Hypertension Detection and Follow-up Program (HDFP), the relationship was stronger for blacks than for whites.[12] In Europe and the United Kingdom this relationship is less marked or absent.[11] These differences could not be attributed to different treatment rates of hypertension. In the Whitehall Study, which found a nearly threefold gradient in coronary heart disease and stroke, the gradient in systolic pressure was 4 mmHg.[1] In less developed countries such as India and Kenya, the association goes the other way: this may reflect the well-known effects of acculturation, whereby moving from a traditional village life to a westernized urban center is associated with a rise of blood pressure.[13–15] Thus, blood pressure differences cannot explain much, if any, of the SES–CVD gradient.

Relatively little is known about the determinants of the SES–blood pressure gradient. As described above, the gradient cannot be accounted for by differences in treatment rates or access to health care, although in the HDFP the SES gradient was seen in the patients who were randomized to Usual Care, but was absent in the active treatment (Special Intervention) group[12] (FIG. 3). In the Intersalt study the predictors of the SES–blood pressure gradient included a high salt intake (measured by 24-hour urine collections), a low potassium intake, a greater BMI, and alcohol intake.[9] A few prospective studies have looked at the association between SES and blood pressure. The CARDIA Study of 5000 young black and white men and women identified a number of predictors of blood pressure increase over a 10-year follow-up.[16] These included education, BMI, waist circumference, alcohol intake, pulse rate, smoking, and several measures of the insulin resistance syndrome, particularly fasting insulin, low HDL, and triglycerides.

Body Mass Index

In the Whitehall Study there was a marked negative relationship between SES and BMI.[1] In the Chicago cohorts the gradient was marginal and statistically insignificant.[4] The Pittsburgh study of middle-aged women found that although there was an inverse relationship between education and BMI, and between BMI and several of the major cardiovascular risk factors, controlling for BMI did not eliminate these relations.[8] In the Whitehall Study there was also a strong negative relationship between SES and the metabolic syndrome, characterized by central obesity (a high waist–hip ratio), relative glucose intolerance, high blood pressure, high triglycerides, and low HDL cholesterol.[5]

Physical Inactivity

Most studies have shown an inverse relationship between SES and physical activity during leisure time. An example is the Whitehall Study, where 26% of the highest SES grade (administrators) reported that they did not take regular exercise, in contrast to 56% of the lowest grade.[1] Physical inactivity is clearly linked to obesity, and the combination may thus contribute to the SES–disease gradient.

THE ROLE OF HEALTH CARE FACTORS.

Access to health care is one of the possible factors that might explain the SES–CVD gradient, particularly in the United States. However, the gradient is also seen in countries such as Sweden where there is universal health insurance. Thus an analysis of the Gothenberg Primary Prevention Study found that the odds ratio for coronary heart disease morbidity was 2.2 between the lowest and highest of five professional grades.[10] After adjusting for known risk factors (including blood pressure, smoking, cholesterol, BMI, exercise habits, and alcohol intake) this only decreased to 1.9. Interestingly, the stroke rate showed no SES gradient. In one subgroup of the Beta Blocker Heart Attack Trial (BHAT) study, having less than 10 as opposed to 12 or more years of education resulted in a twofold difference in mortality during the three years following a heart attack, despite the fact that all the patients were members of the Health Insurance Plan of New York and were presumably receiving the same quality of health care.[17]

Several studies have examined the possibility that the SES differences in blood pressure could be due to differences in treatment rates.[11] Although in some cases the relationship was modified by controlling for treatment rates, in no case could it be explained.

THE ROLE OF BEHAVIORAL FACTORS

The inability of the traditional CVD risk factors to explain more than 25% of the SES–CVD gradient in the British Whitehall Civil Servants Study led Marmot *et al.* to suggest that other factors related to the working conditions might contribute.[18] In the second Whitehall Study, some of these factors were investigated: the job strain model of Karasek was incorporated, on the grounds that it had been shown to predict CHD morbidity in several studies and also appeared to be related to SES.[18] Measures of social support in the workplace were also included. For men, adjusting for support made very little difference to the SES–CVD gradient (reducing the odds ratio between the lowest and highest professional grades from 1.5 to 1.43), whereas adjusting for control at work reduced it from 1.5 to 1.18. When all the adjustment factors were combined (including risk factors and height) the gradient was eliminated (to 0.95). Similar results were found for women. Thus perceived control at the workplace may be a factor that deserves further study for explaining the SES–disease gradient.

One of the most comprehensive analyses of the determinants of the SES–cardiovascular disease gradient was undertaken by Lynch *et al.* using data from the Kuopio Study[19] performed with 2,272 Finnish men, in which SES was classified by income. The rate of cardiovascular mortality was 2.66 times higher in the lowest income group in comparison to the highest; this ratio was reduced to 1.24 by adjusting for "biologic" risk factors (including cholesterol, blood pressure, fibrinogen, and BMI among others), to 1.83 by adjusting for "behavioral" factors (smoking, alcohol consumption, and physical activity), and to 1.71 for psychosocial factors (depression, hopelessness, and social support). When all the 23 evaluated risk factors were included, the SES gradient for cardiovascular mortality was eliminated. The gradient for myocardial infarction, however, was reduced only from 4.34 to 2.83 by adjusting for these same 23 factors. Control was not included in the Kuopio Study.

The importance of behavioral or "nontraditional" risk factors relating to SES is well illustrated by the BHAT in which patients were randomized to receive either a beta blocker (propranolol) or placebo following a heart attack.[17] Over a three-year follow-up period, the mortality was about 30% lower in the propranolol-treated group, but this effect pales into insignificance in comparison to the effect of education: those with less than 10 years of education had a mortality of 12%, whereas in those with 12 years or more it was about 5%, a difference of more than twofold.

TO WHAT EXTENT IS THE SES–CVD GRADIENT IN THE U.S. EXPLAINED BY RACE AND ETHNICITY?

In the United States there is such a strong association between ethnicity and SES that it is virtually impossible to study the effects of ethnicity separately from SES. In an analysis of the Multiple Risk Factor Intervention Trial (MRFIT) data, Davey Smith *et al.* compared the mortality differences in black and white men after adjustment for SES and the major cardiovascular risk factors.[20] For stroke, the relative risk in blacks compared with whites was 2.23 (adjusted for age); after adjustment for age and income it fell to 1.78, and after adjustment for age, income, and risk factors (blood pressure, smoking, cholesterol, known CHD, and diabetes) to 1.57. For CHD mortality, the corresponding figures were 1.12, 0.91, and 0.88 (see FIG. 4). These figures emphasize the importance of SES factors in comparison with the traditional cardiovascular risk factors. A somewhat similar analysis was performed by Goralnick *et al.*, who looked at the life expectancies of blacks and whites as a function of age, education, and gender.[21] At age 65, when years of education were controlled for, the range of differences in life expectancy according to race was between 0.3 and 1.7 years in the four groups (black and white men and women). But when race was controlled for, the differences according to education were much bigger (2.5 to 4.6 years). Thus education appeared to be more important than race. In the United

States, African-Americans bear a greater burden of cardiovascular disease than whites, and the prevalence of hypertension among blacks is approximately double.[22] This difference is, however, much greater in the United States than in other countries.[23] Several studies have documented that hypertension is relatively rare in Africa, with the exception of the big cities.[24] It is also clearly established in longitudinal studies conducted mostly in Africa that moving from village to city life is associated with an increase of blood pressure,[14] which suggests that environmental factors are predominantly responsible. A major unresolved issue is whether the higher prevalence of hypertension seen in blacks in the United States compared to whites is genetic or environmental. So far, attempts to identify genes or physiological processes that distinguish "black hypertension" from "white hypertension" have proved disappointing.[23] Several studies have found that blacks with darker skin color have higher pressures than those with light skin,[25,26] which could be explained by either genetic or cultural factors. Although there have been reports of racial differences in physiological regulatory processes such as sodium sensitivity, the renin–angiotensin system, and kallikrein,[27] there is no evidence that these differences, which are usually subtle, are causally related to the differing prevalence of hypertension.

At the present time, the higher prevalence of hypertension in U.S. blacks can best be explained by environmental factors. A proportion of the differential can be explained by obesity (particularly in black women) and mineral intake, but potentially stronger and also less well-defined factors are psychosocial stress and racism. The low prevalence of hypertension in rural Africa has already been referred to, and there are populations where a black–white blood pressure difference is absent or very small. One example is Cuba[28] and another is a study of factory workers in En-

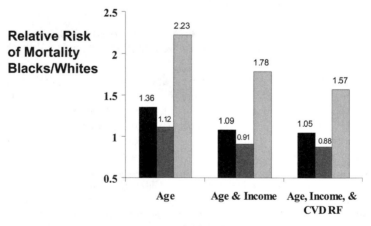

Adjustments for Risk Estimates

FIGURE 4. Data from MRFIT study, showing relative mortality in blacks versus whites for: ■, all cardiovascular disease (CVD); ■, coronary heart disease (CHD); and ▨, stroke. Adjustment for income virtually eliminates the SES gradient for all CVD and CHD; the major CVD risk factors (RF) account for little further reduction in the gradient. Data from Davey *et al.*[20]

gland,[29] in both of which it was concluded that the similarities of social class between the ethnic groups might account for the similarity of blood pressures. Studies
of blacks conducted in American cities have shown a subtle SES gradient of blood
pressure (and other risk factors). Thus there is substantial evidence for a "neighborhood" effect on blood pressure,[30] which is related to psychosocial factors independently of the traditional environmental influences,[31,32] such that people living in
poor neighborhoods tend to have higher blood pressures than those living in more
affluent areas.

Further evidence for the role of environmental and SES factors comes from an
analysis of cardiovascular mortality in New York City,[33] which compared the rates
in blacks and whites, but which also classified the blacks according to their place of
birth—the Southern United States, the Northeast, or the Caribbean. For men aged 45
to 64, the death rates from CVD were 836 per 100,000 of population for blacks born
in the South, 654 for blacks born in the Northeast, and 345 for blacks born in the Caribbean. The rate for whites was 493. Thus the range of mortality among the different
groups of blacks was much greater than the black–white difference. These results
point to the importance of early influences on cardiovascular health, since it is likely
that the environments in which the different groups were living in New York were
similar. Differences in the cardiovascular risk factors between the groups have not
been examined.

The role of racial discrimination has been largely ignored in studies of hypertension in blacks, and yet it seems likely that it could be very important. The CARDIA
study has found that racial discrimination can account for some of the black–white
differences in blood pressure,[34] but in ways that are not easy to interpret: thus black
women who reported no discrimination, and who responded to unfair treatment by
accepting it and keeping it to themselves, had higher pressures than women who did
report that they had experienced discrimination. This is an area that clearly needs
more research.

WHAT ARE THE BIOLOGICAL PATHWAYS
OF THE SES–CVD RELATIONSHIP?

The ability to monitor surrogate markers of CVD and also to visualize atherosclerotic plaque directly should greatly improve our ability to evaluate the biological
pathways by which SES may exert its effects. A good example of this comes from
the Kuopio Ischemic Heart Disease Risk Factor Study,[35] where it has been possible
to monitor the progression of atherosclerosis in the carotid artery over a four-year
period. It has been found that psychosocial factors such as job demands predict this
progression,[36] and an analysis of blood pressure reactivity (measured as the anticipatory increase of pressure before an exercise test) showed that the greatest progression of atherosclerosis occurred in men who showed increased reactivity and were
from low SES.[35]

The pathways by which SES affects cardiovascular disease are almost certainly
multiple, and likely to be somewhat different in different populations. Leaving aside
differences in access to or utilization of health care, the two major pathways may
be presumed to be a direct effect of chronic stress on the disease process, presumably

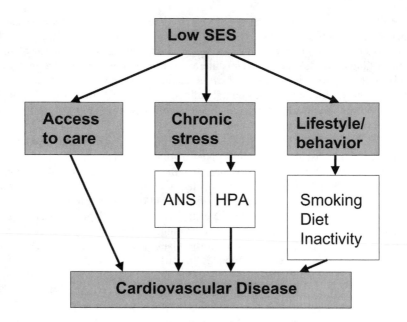

FIGURE 5. Schematic of pathways by which SES might influence cardiovascular disease. *ANS*, autonomic nervous system; *HPA*, hypothalamic–pituitary–adrenal cortex axis.

acting through the brain, and indirect effects acting through changes in health-related behaviors (FIG. 5).

It is presumed that any effects of psychosocial stress must be mediated through the central nervous system, so it is relevant to consider those pathways by which the brain affects bodily processes, principal among which are the symptomatic nervous system, the hypothalamic–pituitary–adrenal axis, and the renin–angiotensin–aldosterone system.

The Sympathetic Nervous System

The autonomic nervous system regulates a number of bodily functions, including all aspects of the cardiovascular system. The autonomic nervous system was conceptualized many years ago as the organ of "fight or flight responses" by Cannon,[37] and it is certainly the dominant mechanism for mediating acute cardiovascular and metabolic responses. Whether it also contributes to chronic changes is less certain, but the possibility exists. Thus there is extensive evidence that increased sympathetic activity is a feature of many cases of hypertension in young adults. This is supported by direct evidence: muscle sympathetic nerve activity is increased; norepinephrine spillover rates are increased; and there is an augmented response to alpha- and beta-adrenergic blockade.[38] Sympathetic activity could affect the development of atherosclerosis in a number of ways: by increasing insulin resistance (see below), by its hemodynamic effects on the arterial wall (see below), or by direct metabolic effects, such as increasing plasma triglycerides through its effect on lipoprotein lipase and altering the metabolism of low-density lipoproteins.[39] Other effects of increased sympathetic activity that could increase the risk of cardiovascular disease are the effects of epinephrine on platelet aggregation and the development of left ventricular hypertrophy, another risk factor for cardiovascular morbidity. There is a correlation between increased sympathetic activity and insulin resistance, which is itself a risk factor for heart disease. Julius has suggested two ways by which chronically increased sympathetic activity could lead to insulin resistance: the first is by conversion from fast-twitch to slow-twitch fibers in skeletal muscle (the latter are predominant in hypertensives and more insulin resistant); and the second is by causing capillary rarefaction, which is also associated with insulin resistance.[39]

The Parasympathetic Nervous System

The vagus nerve slows the heart, but has little effect on contractility. Although activation of the sympathetic nervous system is usually accompanied by inhibition of the parasympathetic, this is not always the case. At rest, both heart rate and heart rate variability are predominantly under parasympathetic control, but during challenge sympathetic influences predominate. Blood pressure variability, which some hypothesize may contribute to endothelial damage and atherosclerosis, is also influenced by parasympathetic activity, but in this case parasympathetic activity increases blood pressure variability at rest, but buffers or decreases it during challenge.[40] It has been proposed that vagal tone, or the lack of it, may be a physiologic index of stress.[41]

Heart Rate Variability as a Marker of Autonomic Tone

It has been proposed that spectral analysis of heart rate variability may provide a means for the quantification of sympathetic and parasympathetic tone, on the grounds that there are cyclical variations of heart rate with different periodicities determined by the sympathetic and parasympathetic nerves. The analysis is performed by recording an ECG during a period of stable heart rate and then performing either Fourier analysis or autoregression to detect peaks with different frequencies. Two peaks of interest are the high-frequency peak (0.15–0.4 Hz) with the same periodicity as respiration and caused mainly by parasympathetic activity, and a low- or mid-frequency peak (0.1 Hz), which is proposed to represent sympathetic activity but which certainly includes parasympathetic and other components. The ratio of the low- to high-frequency peaks has been proposed as a marker of sympathetic to parasympathetic balance. This remains controversial, however, because there are many situations in which there is a discrepancy between other measures of sympathetic and vagal activity and the heart rate variability.[42] Although the relative roles of the two limbs of the autonomic nervous system remain controversial, there is agreement that decreased heart rate variability per se is associated with the presence of coronary heart disease and is also a risk factor for cardiovascular morbidity. What is not clear is whether this association is causal. It could be, for example, that reduced heart rate variability is a consequence of atherosclerotic damage to the carotid sinuses and hence the baroreceptor reflexes. Heart rate variability would be relatively easy to study in relation to SES, but so far there is little information on this.

The Hypothalamic–Pituitary–Adrenal (HPA) Axis

The pituitary is the principal gland by which the brain controls the endocrine system, and one of the pathways involved in the stress response is the release of ACTH, which in turn leads to release of cortisol by the adrenal cortex. Activation of the HPA axis is usually evaluated using cortisol measurements; these can be made from the plasma, saliva, or urine. There is no doubt that the experience or anticipation of acute stress activates the HPA axis and leads to increased cortisol secretion,[43] but with repeated exposure there is great interindividual variation in the extent to which the cortisol response habituates.[44] Studies of chronic stress have given inconsistent findings, some showing activation, and others suppression.[46] The HPA axis is a potential candidate for mediating some of the effects of SES on CVD, but has so far not been studied extensively in this regard. One study[46] found a positive association between salivary cortisol levels and SES, with the highest values being found among administrative civil servants, and the lowest among unskilled workers and unemployed subjects. Another study[47] compared salivary cortisols in employed and unemployed subjects and found no differences in the overall levels, although the unemployed showed higher early morning and lower evening levels than the employed subjects.

Beta-Endorphin

Beta-endorphin is co-secreted with ACTH in response to stress. There is evidence that opioids buffer stress-induced blood pressure responses by combating the activity of the sympathetic nervous system. It has also been suggested that deficient opioids might lead to hostile behavior.[48]

The Renin–Angiotensin–Aldosterone System

The release of renin from the kidney stimulates the production of angiotensin and aldosterone, which have multiple influences on cardiovascular function. Renin release is stimulated by the sympathetic nerves innervating the kidney, as well as by changes in renal perfusion pressure and sodium balance.[49]

WHAT ARE THE BIOLOGICAL MARKERS OF THE SES–CVD RELATIONSHIP?

Another way of investigating the links between SES and cardiovascular disease is by looking for biological markers of the relationship, without necessarily knowing which pathway is activating them. These could be at several different levels, as shown in FIGURE 6, and range from hemodynamic factors such as blood pressure and heart rate to markers of endothelial damage such as von Willebrand factor (one of the clotting factors in blood). Although genetic factors are certainly going to be important, it seems unlikely at the present time that they will play a major role in determining the SES–disease gradient.

Fibrinogen

In the Whitehall Study it was found that fibrinogen, which is a recognized risk factor for coronary heart disease, showed an inverse gradient with SES that was more pronounced in women than in men.[50] The levels were higher in smokers, and lower in drinkers of alcohol. More interestingly, high fibrinogen levels were also related to psychosocial factors: men whose jobs combined low control, monotony, and under-utilization of skills had higher values. There was also evidence for an effect of early life experiences on fibrinogen, such as father's social class and years of education. The mechanisms by which fibrinogen levels are influenced by these factors are unknown.

The Insulin Resistance Syndrome

As described above, central obesity, or the insulin resistance syndrome, is strong-ly associated both with SES and cardiovascular disease,[5] and is another biological marker of the association. There is some evidence that it may be associated with chronic life stress (measured by type A behavior, anger, and hostility),[51] and Bjorn-torp has suggested that it may provide a "missing link" between psychosocial factors and cardiovascular disease through activation of the HPA axis.[52]

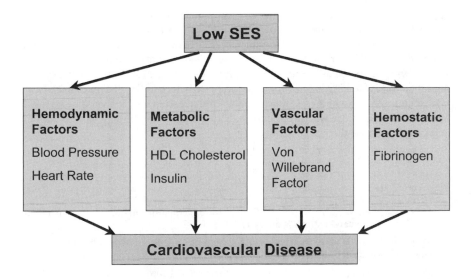

FIGURE 6. Some of the biological markers that have been implicated in the relation between SES and cardiovascular disease.

CONCLUSIONS

The SES–cardiovascular disease gradient has been found wherever it is sought and appears to apply to both coronary heart disease and stroke. As with many other diseases, the relationship appears to be continuous across all grades of SES. Because cardiovascular disease is the end result of a wide variety of pathological processes, it is fair to assume that any explanation of the ways by which SES affects it will also be multifactorial. The causal chain between SES and disease can be looked at in a number of ways. The principal mechanisms could be the direct effects of stress on the disease processes, which might include activation of the sympathetic nervous system to raise blood pressure, for example. At the present time, direct evidence of the links between SES as a stressor acting via the central nervous system to cause disease are lacking, although in many cases the individual components have been identified. A second mechanism, which is much better established, is through the influence of SES on lifestyles and behavior patterns. In this case, SES can be regarded more as a cultural influence acting, for example, through health beliefs and habits, rather than as a source of chronic stress. Third, the possibility must also be considered that access to, or utilization of, health care is a factor.

A second way of examining the problem is to divide the known and suspected risk factors for cardiovascular disease into categories such as "biological," "behavioral," and "psychological," as was done in the Kuopio Study, for example. Although much useful information can and has been obtained with this method, it does not directly address the causal links. Thus the finding that high blood pressure (a "biological" factor) is a potential mediator of the relationship could be explained in a variety of ways, including behavioral factors (e.g., diet and alcohol intake) and psychological factors (e.g., racial discrimination or job strain). Ultimately, the pathways by which SES affects cardiovascular disease must have a behavioral or social explanation. Although genetic factors undoubtedly will be found to contribute in some ways, the bulk of evidence (such as the migrant studies, for example) strongly favor environmental factors. Smoking is one of the major contributors to the SES gradient of cardiovascular disease, which raises the unanswered question why it should be so much more prevalent in those who are socially disadvantaged. Finding the answer should help us to minimize the gradient.

REFERENCES

1. MARMOT, M.G., M.J. SHIPLEY & G. ROSE. 1984. Inequalities in death—specific explanations of a general pattern? Lancet 1: 1003–1006.

2. MARMOT, M.G., A.M. ADELSTEIN, N. ROBINSON & G.A. ROSE. 1978. Changing social-class distribution of heart disease. Br. Med. J. 2: 1109–1112.

3. MARMOT, M.G. & S.L. SYME. 1976. Acculturation and coronary heart disease in Japanese-Americans. Am. J. Epidemiol. 104: 225–247.

4. LIU, K., L.B. CEDRES, J. STAMLER, A. DYER, R. STAMLER, S. NANAS, et al. 1982. Relationship of education to major risk factors and death from coronary heart disease, cardiovascular diseases and all causes. Findings of three Chicago epidemiologic studies. Circulation 66: 1308–1314.

5. BRUNNER, E.J., M.G. MARMOT, K. NANCHAHAL, M.J. SHIPLEY, S.A. STANSFELD, M. JUNEJA, et al. 1997. Social inequality in coronary risk: central obesity and the metabolic syndrome. Evidence from the Whitehall II study. Diabetologia 40: 1341–1349.

6. BRUNNER, E.J., M.G. MARMOT, I.R. WHITE, J.R. O'BRIEN, M.D. ETHERINGTON, B.M. SLAVIN, et al. 1993. Gender and employment grade differences in blood cholesterol, apolipoproteins and haemostatic factors in the Whitehall II study. Atherosclerosis 102: 195–207.

7. JACOBSEN, B.K. & D.S. THELLE. 1988. Risk factors for coronary heart disease and level of education. The Tromso Heart Study. Am. J. Epidemiol. 127: 923–932.

8. MATTHEWS, K.A., S.F. KELSEY, E.N. MEILAHN, L.H. KULLER & R.R. WING. 1989. Educational attainment and behavioral and biologic risk factors for coronary heart disease in middle-aged women. Am. J. Epidemiol. 129: 1132–1144.

9. STAMLER, R., M. SHIPLEY, P. ELLIOTT, A. DYER, S. SANS & J. STAMLER. 1992. Higher blood pressure in adults with less education. Some explanations from INTERSALT. Hypertension 19: 237–241.

10. ROSENGREN, A., H. WEDEL & L. WILHELMSEN. 1988. Coronary heart disease and mortality in middle aged men from different occupational classes in Sweden. Br. Med. J. 297: 1497–1500.

11. COLHOUN, H.M., H. HEMINGWAY & N.R. POULTER. 1998. Socio-economic status and blood pressure: an overview analysis. J. Hum. Hypertens. 12: 91–110.

12. HYPERTENSION DETECTION AND FOLLOW-UP PROGRAM COOPERATIVE GROUP. 1987. Educational level and 5-year all-cause mortality in the hypertension detection and follow-up program. Hypertension 9: 641–646.

13. GILBERTS, E.C., M.J. ARNOLD & D.E. GROBBEE. 1994. Hypertension and determinants of blood pressure with special reference to socioeconomic status in a rural south Indian community. J. Epidemiol. Commun. Health 48: 258–261.

14. POULTER, N.R., K.T. KHAW, B.E. HOPWOOD, M. MUGAMBI, W.S. PEART, G. ROSE, et al. 1990. The Kenyan Luo migration study: observations on the initiation of a rise in blood pressure. Br. Med. J. 300: 967–972.

15. POULTER, N.R., K.T. KHAW & P.S. SEVER. 1988. Higher blood pressures of urban migrants from an African low-blood pressure population are not due to selective migration. Am. J. Hypertens. 1: 143S–145S.

16. DYER, A.R., K. LIU, M. WALSH, C. KIEFE, D.R. JACOBS & D.E. BILD. 1999. Ten-year incidence of elevated blood pressure and its predictors: The CARDIA Study. J. Hum. Hypertens. 13: 13–21.

17. RUBERMAN, W., E. WEINBLATT, J.D. GOLDBERG & B.S. CHAUDHARY. 1984. Psychosocial influences on mortality after myocardial infarction. N. Engl. J. Med. 311: 552–559.

18. MARMOT, M.G., H. BOSMA, H. HEMINGWAY, E. BRUNNER & S. STANSFELD. 1997. Contribution of job control and other risk factors to social variations in coronary heart disease incidence [see comments]. Lancet 350: 235–239.

19. LYNCH, J.W., G.A. KAPLAN, R.D. COHEN, J. TUOMILEHTO & J.T. SALONEN. 1996. Do cardiovascular risk factors explain the relation between socioeconomic status, risk of all-cause mortality, cardiovascular mortality, and acute myocardial infarction? Am. J. Epidemiol. 144: 934–942.

20. DAVEY, S.G., J.D. NEATON, D. WENTWORTH, R. STAMLER & J. STAMLER. 1988. Mortality differences between black and white men in the USA: contribution of income and other risk factors among men screened for the MRFIT. [MRFIT Research Group. Multiple Risk Factor Intervention Trial.] Lancet 351: 934–939.

21. GURALNIK, J.M., K.C. LAND, D. BLAZER, G.G. FILLENBAUM & L.G. BRANCH. 1993. Educational status and active life expectancy among older blacks and whites. N. Engl. J. Med. 329: 110–116.

22. ANONYMOUS. 1997. The sixth report of the Joint National Committee on prevention, detection, evaluation, and treatment of high blood pressure. Arch Intern. Med. 157: 2413–2446.

23. COOPER, R. & C. ROTIMI. 1997. Hypertension in blacks. Am. J. Hypertens. 10: 804–812.

24. COOPER, R. & C. ROTIMI. 1994. Hypertension in populations of West African origin: is there a genetic predisposition? [Editorial]. J. Hypertens. **12:** 215–227.
25. HARBURG, E., L. GLEIBERMANN, P. ROEPER, M.A. SCHORK & W.J. SCHULL. 1978. Skin color, ethnicity, and blood pressure I: Detroit blacks. Am. J. Public Health **68:** 1177–1183.
26. KLAG, M.J., P.K. WHELTON, J. CORESH, C.E. GRIM & L.H. KULLER. 1991. The association of skin color with blood pressure in US blacks with low socioeconomic status [see comments]. JAMA **265:** 599–602.
27. FALKNER, B. 1990. Differences in blacks and whites with essential hypertension: biochemistry and endocrine. State of the art lecture. Hypertension **15:** 681–686.
28. ORDUNEZ-GARCIA, P.O., A.D. ESPINOSA-BRITO, R.S. COOPER, J.S. KAUFMAN & F.J. NIETO. 1998. Hypertension in Cuba: evidence of a narrow black–white difference. J. Hum. Hypertens. **12:** 111–116.
29. CRUICKSHANK, J.K., S.H. JACKSON, D.G. BEEVERS, L.T. BANNAN, M. BEEVERS & V.L. STEWART. 1985. Similarity of blood pressure in blacks, whites and Asians in England: the Birmingham Factory Study. J. Hypertens. **3:** 365–371.
30. DIEZ-ROUX, A.V., F.J. NIETO, C. MUNTANER, H.A. TYROLER, G.W. COMSTOCK, E. SHAHAR, *et al.* 1997. Neighborhood environments and coronary heart disease: a multilevel analysis. Am. J. Epidemiol. **146:** 48–63.
31. HARBURG, E., L. GLEIBERMAN, M. RUSSELL & M.L. COOPER. 1991. Anger-coping styles and blood pressure in black and white males: Buffalo, New York. Psychosom.Med **53:** 153–164.
32. HARBURG, E., E.H.J. BLAKELOCK & P.R. ROEPER. 1979. Resentful and reflective coping with arbitrary authority and blood pressure: Detroit. Psychosom. Med. **41:** 189–202.
33. FANG, J., S. MADHAVAN & M.H. ALDERMAN. 1996. The association between birthplace and mortality from cardiovascular causes among black and white residents of New York City [see comments]. N. Engl. J. Med. **335:** 1545–1551.
34. KRIEGER, N. & S. SIDNEY. 1996. Racial discrimination and blood pressure: the CARDIA Study of young black and white adults. Am. J. Public Health **86:** 1370–1378.
35. LYNCH, J.W., S.A. EVERSON, G.A. KAPLAN, R. SALONEN & J.T. SALONEN. 1998. Does low socioeconomic status potentiate the effects of heightened cardiovascular responses to stress on the progression of carotid atherosclerosis? Am. J. Public Health **88:** 389–394.
36. EVERSON, S.A., J.W. LYNCH, M.A. CHESNEY, G.A. KAPLAN, D.E. GOLDBERG, S.B. SHADE, *et al.* 1997. Interaction of workplace demands and cardiovascular reactivity in progression of carotid atherosclerosis: population based study. Br. Med. J. **314:** 553–558.
37. CANNON, W.C. 1929. Bodily Changes in Pain, Hunger, Fear, and Rage. Charles T Brandford, Boston.
38. JULIUS, S. & S. NESBITT. 1996. Sympathetic overactivity in hypertension. A moving target. Am. J. Hypertens. **9:** 113S–120S.
39. JULIUS, S. 1993. Insulin, insulin resistance, and blood pressure elevation. Arch. Intern. Med. **153**(3): 290–291.
40. SLOAN, R.P., P.A. SHAPIRO, E. BAGIELLA, M.M. MYERS & J.M. GORMAN. 1999. Cardiac autonomic control buffers blood pressure variability responses to challenge: a psychophysiologic model of coronary artery disease. Psychosom. Med. **61**(1): 58–68.
41. PORGES, S.W. 1995. Cardiac vagal tone: a physiological index of stress. Neurosci. Biobehav. Rev. **19**(2): 225–233.
42. BERNTSON, G.G., J.T. BIGGER, JR., D.L. ECKBERG, et al. 1997. Heart rate variability: origins, methods, and interpretive caveats. Psychophysiology **34**(6): 623–648.
43. SMYTH, J., M.C. OCKENFELS, L. PORTER, *et al.* 1998. Stressors and mood measured on a momentary basis are associated with salivary cortisol secretion. Psychoneuroendocrinology **23**(4): 353–370.
44. KIRSCHBAUM, C., J.C. PRUSSNER, A.A. STONE, *et al.* 1995. Persistent high cortisol responses to repeated psychological stress in a subpopulation of healthy men. Psychosom. Med. **57**(5): 468–474.

45. BRANDTSTADTER, J., B. BALTES-GOTZ, C. KIRSCHBAUM & D. HELLHAMMER. 1991. Developmental and personality correlates of adrenocortical activity as indexed by salivary cortisol: observations in the age range of 35 to 65 years. J. Psychosom. Res. **35:** 173–185.
46. OCKENFELS, M.C., L. PORTER, J. SMYTH, C. KIRSCHBAUM, D.H. HELLHAMMER & A.A. STONE. 1995. Effect of chronic stress associated with unemployment on salivary cortisol: overall cortisol levels, diurnal rhythm, and acute stress reactivity. Psychosom. Med. **57:** 460–467.
47. BRUEHL, S., C.R. CARLSON, J.F. WILSON, J.A. NORTON, G. COLCLOUGH, M.J. BRADY, J.J. SHERMAN & J.A. MCCUBBIN. 1996. Psychological coping with acute pain: an examination of the role of endogenous opioid mechanisms. J. Behav. Med. **19**(2): 129–142.
48. DI BONA, G.F. & U.C. KOPP. 1997. Neural control of renal function. Physiol. Rev. **77:** 75–197.
49. BRUNNER, E., S.G. DAVEY, M. MARMOT, R. CANNER, M. BEKSINSKA & J. O'BRIEN. 1996. Childhood social circumstances and psychosocial and behavioural factors as determinants of plasma fibrinogen. Lancet **347:** 1008–1013.
50. RAIKKONEN, K., L. KELTIKANGAS-JARVINEN, H. ADLERCREUTZ & A. HAUTANEN. 1996. Psychosocial stress and the insulin resistance syndrome. Metabolism **45:** 1533–1538.
51. BJORNTORP, P. 1991. Visceral fat accumulation: the missing link between psychosocial factors and cardiovascular disease? J. Intern. Med. **230:** 195–201.

Part V Summary: What Is to Be Done?

KATHERINE NEWMAN

Kennedy School of Government, Harvard University,
79 John F. Kennedy Street, Cambridge, Massachusetts 02138, USA

There is much left to be done to understand the mechanisms whereby social and economic inequality "get under the skin." Yet as the papers in this volume underscore, the existence of a gradient connecting stratification to health outcomes is hardly in question any more. Hence, the chapters that follow assume the relationship between inequality and health and go on to pose the next question: What should our society do to counteract these forces? How should government, the private sector, public health officials, the nonprofit world, our educational leadership, and social service agencies intervene in the transmission that leads from inequality to deleterious health outcomes that disadvantage those who lie in the middle and the bottom of the continuum?

At least three options are worthy of debate: (1) address inequality "head on," through the redistribution of wealth, income, education, housing, and exposure to environmental hazards; (2) develop ameliorative interventions that leave the basic distribution of resources untouched, but redress some of the consequences of inequality; or (3) leave the status quo undisturbed and accept that inequalities in basic resources will cause the outcomes we see in our society at present.

In practice, as the papers in this section suggest, the United States has invoked all three of these strategies. As Philip Lee points out, the Social Security Act was a fundamental intervention that redistributed income in a way that virtually broke the connection between old age and poverty, beginning in the 1930s. Unemployment insurance, Aid to Families with Dependent Children, and even the introduction of the progressive income tax system were and remain today redistributive programs that—at least in theory—reduced socioeconomic inequality. More contemporary examples might include college scholarship programs or affirmative action, both of which seek to open access to higher education or employment that will, in turn, reduce inequality through redistribution. In theory, absent these interventions, we would see even starker degrees of inequality in the United States and attendant increases in morbidity and mortality toward the lower end of the class spectrum.

Significant investment in anti-smoking or sex education programs, civic recreation programs that encourage exercise, the creation of the Medicare and Medicaid system, and public health measures designed to inform the public about health-promoting behaviors are well-known examples of interventions that do nothing to alter socioeconomic inequality itself, but may go some distance toward arresting the impact of stratification on health. The United States has pursued these ameliorative measures for decades as a means of opening access to resources that the less fortunate might otherwise have to forego entirely.

Finally, there have been many periods in our history when inequality was accepted as a natural condition of our economic system, and intervention either resisted or dismantled in an effort to return the social order to a purer version of a laissez-faire economy or a privatized social order. Some would argue that just such a set of assumptions is making a comeback now. After 60 years of experience with the redistributive reforms of the 1930s, the United States has embarked on an experiment in welfare reform, for example, which effectively ends the federal commitment to the support of the indigent poor. The theory behind this reform is that the discipline of the market will work more effectively to channel personal behavior toward positive ends. If inequalities persist, on this account, they are the price we pay for living in a free market social system.

Unlike the other parts of this volume, which are based primarily on scientific evidence, this section reminds us that the problem of inequality and health is at least partly an issue of political will. At various points in our history, public commitments to the reduction of inequality, or to blunting its impact, have made meaningful contributions to improving the life chances and health profiles of millions of Americans. The results are visible in the form of economic well-being, particularly among the elderly (who have benefited considerably from social policies designed to lift retirees out of poverty and to guarantee their access to health care). We have done less for the nation's children, among whom poverty has increased by a considerable margin in the past 20 years. Minority families have also been on the receiving end of several decades of widening inequality, with black and latino youth particularly hard hit in a changing economy that leaves the less skilled with fewer opportunities for occupational mobility. Middle class families have weathered the storms of downsizing, the increasing pressures on dual-career households to balance the demands of work and family, and the concomitant reduction in leisure time among professionals. All along the SES continuum, social pressures are building that may be related in systematic ways to the health outcomes this volume is designed to address.

Alvin Tarlov's paper examines the conditions under which the political will can be harnessed toward both redistribution and amelioration and takes as a case study a recent attempt to garner support for both forms of policy intervention in England— the Atcheson Report. Tarlov argues for the importance of a parallel effort in the United States in order to redress the fundamental maldistribution of resources that seems to underlie inequalities in health outcomes.

The section ends with a call for interdisciplinary research that will help to guide the social policies necessary to come to grips with inequality and health. Appropriate policies will have to address not only *patterns* of health inequality, but also the *pathways* that lead from the distribution of wealth, education, and opportunity to the health gradient that is so clear in the data. The National Institutes of Health stand ready to further this field so that, in the end, national initiatives will be based on sound scientific findings. As Norman Anderson explains in his contribution, the NIH is poised to embark on a number of major initiatives, supported by the federal government, whose purpose is to explore systematically the relationship between racial, economic, ethnic, regional, and class-based forms of inequality that appear to have an impact on health outcomes. Anderson argues that the kind of interdisciplinary approach represented in this volume is vital to developing a clear understanding of the causes, effects, and pathways that we must map in order to ground social, economic, and medical interventions in firm scientific research.

Policy responses to the research represented in this book are still "under construction." However, the seriousness with which the task is being undertaken is reflected clearly in these three papers, which link the scholarship building up in laboratories, national surveys, animal studies, and cross-national comparisons to what may be the hardest question of all: What is to be done?

Public Policy Frameworks for Improving Population Health

ALVIN R. TARLOV[a,b]

The Health Institute, New England Medical Center, Harvard School of Public Health, Tufts University School of Medicine, USA

ABSTRACT: Four conceptual frameworks provide bases for constructing comprehensive public policy strategies for improving population health within wealthy (OECD) nations. (1) *Determinants* of population health. There are five broad categories: genes and biology, medical care, health behaviors, the ecology of all living things, and social/societal characteristics. (2) *Complex systems*: Linear effects models and multiple independent effects models fail to yield results that explain satisfactorily the dynamics of population health production. A different method (complex systems modeling) is needed to select the most effective interventions to improve population health. (3) *An intervention framework* for population health improvement. A two-by-five grid seems useful. Most intervention strategies are either ameliorative or fundamentally corrective. The other dimension of the grid captures five general categories of interventions: child development, community development, adult self-actualization, socioeconomic well-being, and modulated hierarchical structuring. (4) *Public policy development process*: the process has two phases. The initial phase, in which public consensus builds and an authorizing environment evolves, progresses from values and culture to identification of the problem, knowledge development from research and experience, the unfolding of public awareness, and the setting of a national agenda. The later phase, taking policy action, begins with political engagement and progresses to interest group activation, public policy deliberation and adoption, and ultimately regulation and revision. These frameworks will be applied to help understand the 39 recommendations of the *Independent Inquiry into Inequalities in Health,* the Sir Donald Acheson Report from the United Kingdom, which is the most ambitious attempt to date to develop a comprehensive plan to improve population health.

INTRODUCTION

Copious data, confirmed in practically every study and society examined, has identified with sufficient confidence many of the key social and societal factors that if improved would elevate population health. Further research undoubtedly will broaden, add important insights, and refine the texture of our understanding. Nonetheless, the knowledge base that exists in 1999 is sufficiently comprehensive and

[a]Current address for correspondence: Alvin R. Tarlov, M.D., James A. Baker III Institute for Public Policy, Rice University, 6100 Main St., Houston, TX 77005-1892. 713-527-4063 (voice).

[b]This manuscript is a slightly modified version of Chapter 17 by Tarlov and St. Peter in *Society and Population Health; A Reader. Volume II: A State Perspective.* Alvin R. Tarlov & Robert F. St. Peter, Eds. 1999. The New Press, New York.

robust to support the beginning of selected aspects of a population health improvement program.

The improvement of certain societal features would at a minimum improve the general quality of living overall, but would likely improve population health as well. These features include improved opportunities for the following: successful child development, strengthened community cohesion, enhanced self-fulfillment, increased socioeconomic well-being, and modulated hierarchical structuring.

Multipronged actions initiated by multiple sectors are likely to be most effective. The sectors include nonprofit community and national organizations; faith organizations; philanthropies; schools; the recreational, entertainment, and media groups; business; political parties; public policy interests; and local, regional, and national governments. This paper is limited to public policies to improve population health, but the public policies are unlikely to be effective, or even adopted, unless there is in parallel an activation of multiple sectors and synergism is achieved. Social currents, directions, and norms become embedded in expectations, behaviors, and operations. Accepted paradigms ultimately become encoded in laws and regulations. Even relatively modest shifts in social norms, say five degrees out of a whole circumference, will be difficult to achieve. Movement toward more healthful societal circumstances will require multiple approaches and the mobilization of understanding, concern, and commitment of multiple sectors. Public policy development usually does not lead, but rather follows broad public concern.

Four conceptual frameworks, when integrated, can provide guidance for constructing public policy ideas and developing strategies for improving population health within developed nations: (1) determinants of population health, (2) complex system modeling, (3) intervention framework, and (4) public policy development process. The four conceptual frameworks will be described, and then applied to an assessment of the 39 recommendations made in *Independent Inquiry into Inequalities in Health*,[1] the 1998 Sir Donald Acheson report from the United Kingdom, the most ambitious research-based attempt to date to formulate a comprehensive plan to improve population health. Although many chapters in this book advance policy recommendations, the comprehensiveness and coherency of the *Independent Inquiry* provide an opportunity to illustrate the conceptual frameworks for policy developed for this chapter.

DETERMINANTS OF POPULATION HEALTH

There are five major categories of influence on health: genes and associated biology; health behaviors such as dietary habits, tobacco, alcohol and drug use, and physical fitness; medical care and public health services; the ecology of all living things; and social and societal characteristics (FIG. 1). To summarize, the relative proportional influence of each of the five categories is unknown in precise quantitative terms. FIGURE 1 should be interpreted as a crude approximation at this stage of the science. The dashed radii are intended to convey rough estimates, as well as the interdependence/interactivity of the various influences. The absence of a radial line separating total ecology from social/societal characteristics reflects the lack of quantitative knowledge on these two categories of determinants at this time. Genes,

DETERMINANTS OF POPULATION HEALTH

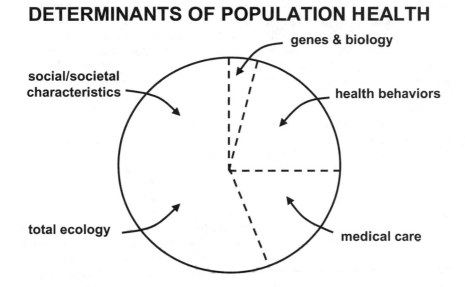

FIGURE 1. Relative influence of the five major determinant categories of population health: rough approximations.

health behaviors, medical care, total ecology, and social/societal characteristics comprise a big, complex, and dynamic network of interactive variables that is understood in a general sense but not understood in a precise, quantitative way. A large body of evidence indicates that social/societal factors exert a major influence on population health. Efforts to improve population health through policies to modify the other four categories of influence while leaving social/societal characteristics unchanged are unlikely to be successful.

COMPLEX SYSTEM MODELING

Mention is made above of the interactivity of most of the factors that influence population health. Changes in one induce responses in the others. Positive and negative feedbacks and cancellation and synergistic effects are predominant features of hugely complex systems exemplified by the influence of surrounding factors on population health. When added to the surrounding factors the physiological systems within the human being that mediate the social effects with uncountable numbers and kinds of adaptations and adjustments, the health production system reveals itself as almost incomprehensibly complex. Linear effects models, multiple independent effects models, and multivariate analytic methods that have driven the social determinants of health field up to this time fail to yield results that satisfactorily explain the dynamics of population health production. Population health production is unlikely to be understood from analyses of individual components. Sociobiologic system complexity cannot be explained mechanistically or predictably as can the internal combustion engine or chemical equations. The social determinants of health field, and most particularly the ability to predict with greater certainty the multitudinous consequences of interventions, require that the concepts and measures of complex systems be applied. It is noteworthy that 30 pages of a recent issue of *Science*[2] have been devoted to exploring complex systems related not only to chemistry and the nervous system but also to social systems such as the grouping behavior of animals and the economy.

Yet, despite quantitative shortcomings in our ability to assign precise numerical causal roles to each class of population health determinant and our inability to isolate with precision the impact on population health of each variable in the complex social-health system, there are several broad categories of interventions that could beneficially be applied now. Improvements in child development, community cohesion, self-fulfillment, total ecology, and socioeconomic mobility would result generally in improved quality of life, and at the same time these improvements would likely be salutary to population health. Reasonable evidence, not certainty of knowledge, permitted tobacco control to move forward 40 years ago. Existing data is adequate for formulating policies and other actions that could affect population health importantly. Awaiting new analytic methods and quantitatively more precise information will delay by decades or longer attempts to improve population health.

AN INTERVENTION FRAMEWORK FOR POPULATION HEALTH IMPROVEMENT

The intervention framework (TABLE 1) identifies five broad intervention objectives that are likely to be salutary for population health. The five are improved child development, strengthened community cohesion, enhanced self-fulfillment, increased socioeconomic well-being, and modulated hierarchical structuring; that is, interventions aimed at children, the community, adults, the economy, and arrangements for social positioning. Each intervention can be classified as either ameliorative or fundamentally corrective. For example, ameliorative interventions to improve child development might include approval of a city ordinance that allows surplus space in public school buildings to be used for day care while parents are working, or to reinvigorate the YMCAs and the YWCAs so that supervised after-school recreational activities for children and youths become generally available. Fundamentally

TABLE 1. Intervention framework to improve population health

Intervention Objectives	Ameliorative	Fundamentally Corrective
Improve *child* development		
Strengthen *community cohesion*		
Enhance opportunities for *self-fulfillment*		
Increase *socioeconomic* well-being		
Modulate *hierarchical* structuring		

corrective programs to improve child development might include programs to train fathers and mothers in parenting skills and in establishing home environments conducive to positive cognitive, emotional, and behavioral development, and developing day care programs having high standards, well-trained and culturally diverse professionals who earn professional wages, transportation that makes the program within practical reach of families, and financial foundations to make the programs affordable to all. The intervention framework could help a community or organization develop short- and long-range planning and identify a combination of ameliorative and fundamentally corrective strategies to provide some near-term accomplishments as well as long-term restructuring that addresses the population health program at its roots.

Other examples can be chosen for strengthening community cohesion, enhancing opportunities for self-fulfillment, increasing socioeconomic mobility, or for modulating the effects of hierarchical structuring. The examples are likely to include combinations of public policies, private sector actions, and community programs, and the active involvement of multiple sectors as presented earlier in this chapter. We will return to this intervention framework in reference to the *Independent Inquiry into Inequalities in Health.*

PUBLIC POLICY DEVELOPMENT PROCESS

This framework separates policy development into two phases (FIGURE 2), an initial phase leading to the development of a public consensus and a later political phase when specific policy actions are taken. Before political action, a broad public understanding needs to be acquired that population health problems have origins in real issues that can be addressed remedially to everyone's advantage. Once that understanding has been assimilated, an evident desire must develop at a high enough priority among a sufficient proportion of the population to create a national agenda, or an authorizing environment and momentum for action. When sufficient momentum has developed, the political process will be authorized to pursue policies to address the problem. This framework helps decide where to apply energy in implementing strategies for population health improvement.

In the example of improved child development used above, all aspects of the initial phase have already been accomplished. That is, a public consensus has formed, a national agenda has been developed, and an authorizing environment has developed that will make it natural and acceptable to engage the political process in thinking through alternative proposals to improve opportunities for successful child development. However, although early childhood experiences are commonly known to be related to cognitive, emotional, and behavioral development, it is not well known that the quality of early childhood development is closely tied to adult health. Americans also place a high value on adult health. Therefore, while the issue of child development is ready for political engagement, the policy action phase might be advanced with greater force if the adult health issue is joined.

On the other hand, a plan to elevate socioeconomic well-being that includes a component of income redistribution should acknowledge that the startling rise in income inequality in the United States has been well documented in books and reports

FRAMEWORK

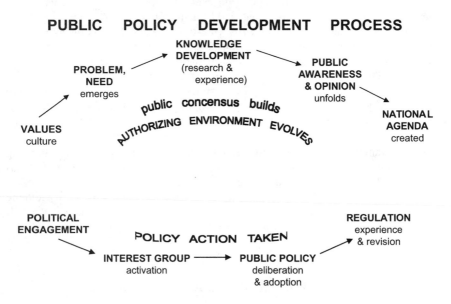

PUBLIC POLICY DEVELOPMENT PROCESS

KNOWLEDGE
DEVELOPMENT
(research &
experience)

PROBLEM,
NEED
emerges

PUBLIC
AWARENESS
& OPINION
unfolds

public concensus builds

AUTHORIZING ENVIRONMENT EVOLVES

VALUES
culture

NATIONAL
AGENDA
created

POLITICAL
ENGAGEMENT

POLICY ACTION TAKEN

REGULATION
experience
& revision

INTEREST GROUP ⟶ PUBLIC POLICY
activation   deliberation
& adoption

FIGURE 2. Conceptual framework for the two phases of the public policy development process: public consensus/national agenda building, and political/public policy actions taken.

from universities, research organizations, some nonprofit organizations, and journalists. Yet, the relationship of income inequality to gross inequalities in health has not yet stimulated a broad and sustained dialogue in the U.S. media and on the political campaign trails. Nor has the problem risen to occupy a position on the national agenda as has been achieved for issues in education, social security, Medicare, patient bill of health care rights, and international finance and trade. In contrast to the child development issue that is ripe for political action, the income distribution issue should start in the public awareness and public consensus arena. Political productivity is the end game of social transformation.

All four conceptual frameworks should be integrated into a coherent strategy for improving population health. Although the emphasis in this chapter is on public policies, surely corporate policies, community programs, medical care, and health behaviors have important roles to play in child development and adult health. We would lose important potential allies if we ignored the corporate, community, health care, and behavior change public health sectors. Likewise, an understanding of complex systems, even at a low level of sophistication, will be important in anticipating the likelihood of multiple effects of interventions and in maintaining an early alertness and watchful eye for unintended and undesired consequences of interventions. Further, desired outcomes in complex systems can be accomplished through several routes, allowing the selection of an alternate public policy initiative that has a greater public and political chance of being adopted and sustained. The intervention framework provides the key choices in relatively neutral terms for specific objective setting and intervention concentration, while the public policy development framework can help design the strategy and select the venue in which to initiate the strategy.

INDEPENDENT INQUIRY INTO INEQUALITIES IN HEALTH

The New Labor Party government of Prime Minister Tony Blair, United Kingdom, in July, 1997, requested Sir Donald Acheson, former Chief Medical Officer of the National Health Service, to review and summarize inequalities in health in England, and to identify priority areas for future policy development likely to offer opportunities for government to develop beneficial cost-effective and affordable interventions to reduce health inequalities.

The charge of the inquiry instructed that the policy proposals were to be based on "scientific and expert evidence" and "within the broad framework of Government's financial strategy"(Ref. 1, pp.155–157). The report was to be completed in about a year, and indeed was submitted to the government in September, 1998.

Several limitations were imposed at the outset. The report was to be focused on government opportunities, as opposed to private sector initiatives. The recommendations were to be framed in the context of the new governments' financial plans for the country. Only one year was allowed for a project that many of us would have regarded as a three or more year undertaking.

A salient feature of the inquiry is its consistent insistence that the summarization of knowledge be based on science and that the recommendations be supportable by the scientific evidence and by peer review by scientists expert in this field. The process and the report were overseen by a five-member Scientific Advisory Group.

The inquiry was guided by a socioeconomic model of health initially proposed by Dahlgren and Whitehead in 1991 (Ref. 1, pp.5–6). The model emphasizes the context in which we live and by which health or disease is generated. The context is depicted by concentric rings with people at its center enveloped successively by the influences of lifestyle, social and community characteristics, and finally an array of macro-socioeconomic, cultural, and environmental conditions. The influence of this contextual conceptualization, sometimes referred to as socioecologic, is evident in the report.

The report is in two parts. Part 1 contains a summary of research data on inequalities in health. Part 2 consists of reviews of the evidence, amplified from the data cited in Part 1, upon which the policy formulations are discussed. A list of 39 policy recommendations is given at the end of Part 2.

Readers might tend to turn directly to the list of recommendations, but it is a mistake if one's analysis of the report ends there. Out of context, the recommendations can be interpreted as a war on poverty or as a welfare program for disadvantaged mothers and children. A reading of the entire Part 2, however, adds background, content, depth, and texture to the recommendations. They become a comprehensive, integrated, and plausible set of recommendations for government policies designed to reduce inequalities in population health. The recommendations address population health inequalities induced by health behaviors, by deficiencies in medical care planning and delivery, or by the pervasive influence of social and societal character-istics. Although the principal emphasis is on social and societal factors, the argument is well made that inequalities in medical services often sustain or amplify inequali-ties in health.

The Recommendations

Most of the 39 recommendations have multiple sub-recommendations, and many recommendations are cross-listed under several of the 13 recommendation catego-ries devised for the report (TABLE 2). For simplicity in this chapter, the recommen-dation categories can usefully be collected into four "groupings" (TABLE 3). The groupings will only be scanned briefly here.

Group A, Scope and Emphasis

Recommendations 1 and 2 set a comprehensive tone by indicating that all gov-ernment policies should be examined for their possible impact on health inequalities, and indicates that the report gives special emphasis to the less well-off with highest (but not exclusive) priority to women of child-bearing age, expectant mothers, and children.

Group B, Sociostructural Improvements

Recommendations 3 through 20 will perhaps be of greatest interest to this book's readers; they are summarized in TABLE 4. Assessment of *all* public policies for their

TABLE 2. Thirteen categories used for the 39 recommendations in the *Independent Inquiry into Inequalities in Health*, United Kingdom, 1998

1. General	8. Mothers, children, families
2. Poverty, income, benefits	9. Young people and workers
3. Education	10. Older people
4. Employment	11. Ethnic minorities
5. Housing	12. Gender
6. Mobility, transport, pollution	13. National health services
7. Nutrition and agriculture policy	

TABLE 3. Four groupings (by the author of this chapter) for the 39 recommendations in the *Independent Inquiry into Inequalities in Health*, United Kingdom, 1998

Group	Number of Recommendations
A. Scope and emphasis	(2)
B. Sociostructural improvements	(18)
C. Disadvantaged emphasis	(16)
D. Health services	(3)

impact on health inequalities appears in TABLE 4 with specific attention to employment and nutrition (agricultural) policies. Income transfers are invoked to lift the bottom out of poverty, to ameliorate the effects of unemployment, and to assure the affordability of wholesome foods for all. Benefits strategies are advanced by the report with respect to expanding preschool opportunities, improving job training, increasing the availability and quality of public housing, and increasing public transport. Again, a full understanding of the sweep of the report should be achieved by reading the texts of both Parts 1 and 2.

Group C, Disadvantaged Emphasis

Recommendations 21 through 36, specify the report's emphasis on mothers, children, and families; young people and workers; older people; ethnic minorities; and young men and young women separately. To cite just a few examples, for families the report recommends elimination of poverty by income transfers, the elimination of food poverty through distribution of surpluses and assuring affordability, greater opportunities for day care and preschool education, and social and emotional support services for parents through increasing the role of "health visitors." The issue of material inequality is addressed for older people through income transfers and benefits, and for ethnic minorities the report recommends that socioeconomic inequalities be reduced. The span of the recommendations for the disadvantaged can be appreciated by reading the full report. A large fraction of the specific recommendations under Groups A, B, and D would also be beneficial to the disadvantaged.

TABLE 4. Recommendations for sociostructural improvements, Group B, 18 recommendations, in the *Independent Inquiry into Inequalities in Health*, United Kingdom, 1998

Needing Improvement	Recommendations
Poverty and income inequality	Income transfers Benefits
Education	Increase funds for preschools and less well-off schools, and expand health promotive schools
Employment	Improve training and job quality Study impact of all employment policies Ameliorate affects unemployment
Housing	Increase availability and quality of public housing
Mobility, transportation, pollution	Increase public transportion Decrease motor vehicle use Lower speed limits Increase cycling and walking
Nutrition	Study impact of agricultural policies Improve distribution surplus Wholesome foods in grocery stores Ensure affordability of foods

Group D, Health Services

Recommendations 37 through 39 seek to promote equity of access and quality of services. The report recommends that resource allocation for health services be differentially determined by needs weighting for each specific population. Monitoring of improved equity should be facilitated by adequate data systems and triennial audits.

A brief summary of the report does not do justice to its expanse. Its objective is to reduce inequalities in health through a reassessment of all government policies that might have a direct or indirect effect on health inequality. It uses all avenues including medical care, preventative public health measures, encouragement of more salutary health behaviors, and a large measure of sociostructural remodeling. The latter includes direct actions for diminishing income inequality (income transfers) and recommends a wide range of expanded benefits intended to reduce inequalities in health. The comprehensiveness of the report's attention to a wide panoply of structurally embedded societal features commands attention by everyone concerned about the recalcitrant problem of health inequalities within societies.

A U.S. PERSPECTIVE (INTERVENTION FRAMEWORK) APPLIED TO THE INDEPENDENT INQUIRY'S RECOMMENDATIONS

The cultural, social, and political contexts of the United Kingdom and the United States are sufficiently dissimilar to justify skepticism that conceptual frameworks for action are cross-applicable. Nonetheless, as scientists and others working in the field of society and population health turn attention to the practical work of fostering development of actual programs and social policies to improve population health, concepts and theories will be needed to guide the formulations and to ground imaginations in reality. Two conceptual frameworks (interventions, public policy development) offered in this chapter are works in progress. There is no empiric evidence of their validity or their practical usefulness. These works in progress might be sharpened and made more useful by applying them to the independent inquiry's recommendations in a test more or less of the validity of the concepts within the frameworks. TABLE 5 is an attempt to do that.

In this depiction we have placed each of the report's recommendations on sociostructural remodeling into the grid of intervention objectives and assigned them as most likely to be in the ameliorative or fundamentally corrective category. Using child development as an example, expanding preschool opportunities for children aged 0–5 and using financial support allocation formulas that are weighted according to the needs of the particular students of each school are both fundamentally corrective. For increasing socioeconomic well-being, income transfers and benefits programs are fundamentally corrective. For enhancing opportunities for self-fulfillment using employment policies, assessing and responding supportively to the effects of unemployment can be ameliorative of a problem that already is in existence, whereas elevating skill levels of workers by institutionalizing training and undertaking a comprehensive assessment of all employment policies regarding their direct and indirect effects on health inequalities could be fundamentally corrective actions.

TABLE 5. Recommendations for sociostructural improvements made by the *Independent Inquiry into Inequalities in Health* (U.K.) placed into the conceptual framework for interventions advanced in this paper (U.S.)

Intervention	Ameliorative	Fundamentally Corrective
Improve *child* development		EDU: preschools weighted funding
Strengthen *community cohesion*		MOB: ↑ public transport ↓ motor vehicles ↑ cycling, walking
Enhance opportunities for *self-fulfillment*	EMP: unemployment effects HOU: public housing NUT: distribute surplus grocery stores	EMP: training/skills policies review
Increase *socioeconomic* well-being		PII: income transfers benefits
Modulate *hierarchical* structuring		

ABBREVIATIONS: EDU, education; EMP, employment; HOU, housing; MOB, mobility; NUT, nutrition, PII, poverty, income inequality.

What does the intervention framework reveal about the recommendations of the report? Our interpretations should be regarded as tentative, and perhaps even foolhardy, because of our ignorance of the British value structure, politics, present and long-range currents in social transformation, and the present state of laws and regulations. With reservations, and in the spirit of a desire to understand whether the framework has any utility, two interpretations are offered. First, the report advances relatively few recommendations that are ameliorative, at least with respect to sociostructural modifications. Ameliorative actions respond to the present population's needs and sufferings and in many ways are reflections of a society's empathy and humanitarianism toward its fellow citizens. The empty spaces in the ameliorative column can possibly be explained by the fact that the charge to the inquiry specifically circumscribed the attention to "…government…interventions to reduce health inequalities." Private sector organizations and communities are more likely to take ameliorative actions. Perhaps the report's relatively greater emphasis on fundamentally corrective policies should be lauded, especially in light of the report's recommendation No. 1 that *all* policies be reviewed for their possible impact on health inequalities.

Second, the report offers no recommendations to modulate hierarchical structuring. This might be the most difficult target area to restructure. Most of the research and published attention on social inequality has concentrated on the most easily measured social variable, that is, per capita or household income. But other elements of hierarchical social structures might be fundamentally and more profoundly causative of health inequalities. Some of these include hierarchically graded distributions within a social structure of status, opportunity, privilege, power, and authority. These variables have not been addressed in the research and have been absent from the public discourse, little as it has been, on social characteristics and population health inequalities.

How do the independent inquiry's recommendations on sociostructural improvements fit into the framework for the public policy development process (FIG. 3)? To reiterate, the conceptualization of the process for the United States is not likely to be transferable to the United Kingdom. However, perhaps something can be learned from doing so.

To begin, all of the recommendations of the report are framed as recommendations for government action because the inquiry was conceived of and framed by the government elected to office at that time. As a result all recommendations enter the process at a late phase of the public policy development process—at the public policy deliberation stage.

I would think that, in the hypothetical exercise of applying the inquiry's report to America, a preferred strategy would be to enter the process at an earlier phase, as

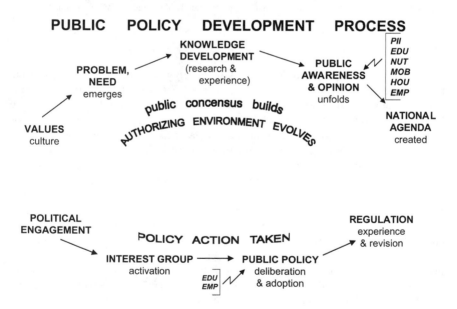

FRAMEWORK

PUBLIC   POLICY   DEVELOPMENT   PROCESS

FIGURE 3. Recommendations for sociostructural improvements made by the *Independent Inquiry into Inequalities in Health* (UK) inserted into in the public policy development process in places (*italics*) that the author of this chapter believes would be appropriate for the circumstances of the United States.

depicted in FIGURE 3. Political, media, and public awareness of the causative connection of social position to inequalities in health does not exist in the U.S. The national popular agenda does not include health related to hierarchical structuring except as an issue of poverty. A public consensus on this subject does not exist. An authorizing environment has not been created. Social–health inequalities cannot be engaged as a political issue.

In the United States, political engagement has begun for small parts of the inquiry's recommendations. For example, expanding preschool availability receives consistent attention in policy discussions related both to working mothers and to children being raised in poverty. Several large and influential nonprofit advocacy organizations promote and sustain these issues. Consistent media attention is directed. The environment has evolved, a national agenda has developed, political engagement and interest groups have been activated, and public policy deliberations are taking place.

But the larger agenda, acquisition by the U.S. society of an understanding of the dynamics of health production through sociostructural influences, has not even begun. Therefore, a strategy more likely to succeed in the United States according to this framework and depicted in FIGURE 3 would start with continued research connected to a national program of elevating public awareness to the level of concern that lifts the issue to the national agenda. The strategy for the United States would begin with research to understand just what the American public, by subpopulations, already knows about the relationship of social features to population health. It is probably very little, except as related to poverty. Knowledge would also have to be gained about specific values and beliefs already held by the public that might be sparked into reverberation with the social-health gradient subject. This would provide a focus for a national public information program using multiple channels of communication and education.

The British report, *Independent Inquiry into Inequalities in Health,* given its purpose, is a highly valuable and progressive source of information and recommendations. It sets out a comprehensive policy agenda to improve population health, at least for developed nations. With individual nations building their own conceptual frameworks to select social restructuring targets for intervention, and with knowledge of the public attitude development process in their country and with approaches that activate the public sector, the private sector, and community action, the independent inquiry provides a treasure of summarized knowledge and comprehensive approaches that other nations will find valuable.

The conceptual frameworks developed in this chapter with some modifications might be salient for health improvement planning at the national, state, or smaller geopolitical unit level. The independent inquiry from the United Kingdom sets a useful example by its comprehensiveness and its attention to the need for sociostructural revision if meaningful population health improvement is to be attained.

REFERENCES

1. INDEPENDENT INQUIRY. 1998. Inequalities in Health: Report. Her Majesty's Stationery Office, London. With the permission of the Department of Health.
2. 1994. Complex systems. Science **284**(5411): 79–109.

Socioeconomic Status and Health

Policy Implications in Research, Public Health, and Medical Care

PHILIP R. LEE

Institute for Health Policy Studies, University of California, San Francisco,
3333 California Street, Suite 265, San Francisco, California 94143-0936, USA

ABSTRACT: The role of public policy in research, public health, and medical care is discussed as well as the extent to which public policy has been informed by increased knowledge about the relationship between SES and health and to what extent policy has affected SES-related health disparities. Observations on current healthcare policy and recommendations for the future are offered.

INTRODUCTION

The subject of this paper is the role of public policy related to research, public health, and medical care—how these have been based on the growing body of knowledge related to socioeconomic status (SES) and health or have affected the health status disparities related to SES. The relationships are not clear-cut, and the solutions are not obvious.

Public policies in the United States during this century have dealt with the full range of factors discussed by George Kaplan[1] including the following:

- Economic and social policies (e.g., income tax, social security, federal grants-in-aid to the states);

- Neighborhoods (community action program of the Office of Economic Opportunity);

- Work (occupational health and safety, mine safety, minimum wage, worker's compensation);

- Education (elementary and secondary education act, head start);

- Family, friends, and social groups (many grant-in-aid programs and projects supporting mediating organizations in the nonprofit sector);

- Health behaviors (e.g., smoking, diet, and exercise have been stressed in the Healthy People initiative since this process was initiated by the Assistant Secretary/Surgeon General Dr. Julius Richmond and his deputy, Dr. Mike McGinnis); and

- Biological mediators (NIH, Medicare).

While this review will not follow the conceptual framework provided by Alvin Tarlov,[2] he does provide another framework for analysis, as he has so brilliantly demonstrated in his chapter. Policies can also be viewed from Norman Anderson's "level of analysis" framework[3]: social/environmental; behavioral/psychological; and organ system, cellular, and molecular. Although this framework is not used in my review, I would note the shift downward toward the molecular in biomedical research; the growing emphasis on organ systems in medical care (e.g., specialization); and the focus of social policies (e.g., Social Security) on the social/environmental level.

When one examines the dramatic change in the health status of the population since 1900 in the context of the major convulsions in this country since the turn of the century—

- Two world wars;

- The Korean, Vietnam, and Gulf Wars;

- The Cold War;

- The deep economic depression of the 1930s, and the recurrent recessions and economic recoveries since;

- The dramatic change in the role of the federal government that began in the 1930s;

- The periods of progressive politics under Teddy Roosevelt, Woodrow Wilson, Franklin Roosevelt, John Kennedy, and Lyndon Johnson and the conservative periods under Harding, Coolidge, and Hoover, as well as Nixon, Carter, Reagan, Bush, and Clinton;

- The end of child labor;

- The rise of the trade unions;

- The industrialization of the nation to become the preeminent economic superpower;

- Urbanization;

- Immigration;

- The Civil Rights Act of 1964 and the Voting Rights Act of 1965;

- The end of segregation in health care;

- The civil rights movement;

- The tumult of the 1960s;

- The tax cuts of the 1980s;

- The shift from the industrial age to the information age;

- The economic expansion of the 1990s with globalization of the economy and other changes too numerous to mention

—it is difficult to sort out what policies, especially at the federal level, had an impact on the health of the population, particularly in narrowing the disparities of health status related to SES.[4–6]

One thing is clear, however. Despite the dramatic shift in burden of illness and causes of death since the turn of the century, inequalities in health status related to SES remain and may have even grown larger in the past 100 years.

RESEARCH POLICIES

Research and the technologies spawned by research have been major factors contributing to the advances in public health and medical care for the past 120 years. It was in 1878 that Pasteur presented his germ theory of infection to the French Academy of Medicine. Later that year in a paper with Jules Joubert and Charles Cumberland, he spelled out his views in more detail, particularly the role of microorganisms as a cause of specific diseases, as well as fermentation and putrefaction.[7]

The most significant development of this period was the development of bacteriology as a scientific field. Of the contributions of Pasteur and Koch to this development, Porter wrote: "Pasteur was a wizard, both within the lab and beyond, but bacteriology's consolidation into a scientific discipline was due mainly to Robert Koch (1843–1910) and his team and pupils, whose painstaking microscopic work definitively established the germ concept of disease and systematically developed its potential."(See Ref. 7, p. 436.) It is hard to overstate the impact of germ theory and bacteriology on research, medical education, medical care, and public health in the 20th century.

Medicine had its scientific roots in anatomy, physiology, and pathology before the scientific revolution spawned by bacteriology in the late 19th century. Public health had its scientific base in statistics and epidemiology before its transformation by bacteriology. While public health measures spawned by the sanitary revolution that began in the United States about 1850 had a significant impact on reducing mortality, medicine had little impact until the mid 1930s with the introduction of the sulfanimides.

While bacteriology was being developed in Europe, the roots of biomedical research policy were established in the United States with the creation of the Hygiene Laboratory, a small bacteriology laboratory at the Marine Hospital on Staten Island, New York. The evolution of biomedical research policy in the early years after its founding were evident in the mandates established by Congress over the years. In 1891, the laboratory was moved to Washington, D.C., and in 1901 it was recognized in law when Congress authorized $35,000 to build a new building to house the laboratory, which could "investigate infectious and contagious diseases and matters pertaining to the public health."[8] The Hygiene Laboratory was expanded in 1902 to add divisions of chemistry, pharmacology, and zoology. The mandate was expanded in 1912 when the Public Health–Marine Hospital Service was renamed the U.S. Public Health Service, and the laboratory was authorized to conduct research into noninfectious diseases. This broader mandate permitted a young public health service officer, Dr. Joseph Goldberger, to investigate and identify the cause of pellagra in the South. When he found it was due to a dietary deficiency, rather than an infectious agent, steps were taken to improve the diets of the poor blacks and soon after to dramatically reduce the ravages of pellagra (see Ref. 8, p. 410).

In 1931, when the name of the Hygiene Laboratory was changed to the National Institutes of Health (NIH), its mandate was expanded to include fellowships for research into basic biological and medical problems. The legislation marked a major transition in research policy from dependence on private philanthropy to a willingness of private institutions to seek public funds. The process evolved further with the enactment of the National Cancer Act in 1937, which provided for the creation of the National Cancer Institute (NCI) and the funding of extramural research and training grants (see Ref. 8, p. 411).

The basic policy framework for the support of biomedical research for the remainder of the 20th century was provided by the Public Health Service Act of 1944. The extramural granting authority of the NCI was expanded to the NIH, and subsequent acts provided this authority for a number of categorical institutes provided over the next 45 years. By 1960, there were 10 components of the NIH; there were 15 by 1970; and 24 institutes, centers, and divisions by 1995. The budget had grown from $8 million in 1947, with one-half of the expenditures for intramural research, to more than $100 million by 1957 and more than $1 billion by 1967, with only about 15% intramural (see Ref. 8, p. 412).

Many areas of research and their application to clinical medicine and public health (e.g., rubella vaccine, smoking and lung cancer) have been directly related to NIH funding. More than 80 Nobel prizes have been awarded to investigators supported by the NIH, including one by the current NIH Director, Dr. Harold Varmus, when he was one of the faculty at the University of California San Francisco.

Has the investment in research had an impact on medicine and public health in the 120 years since the establishment of the Hygiene Laboratory? The answer is yes. Will research be a major factor influencing medicine and public health in the future? Again, the answer is yes. The emphasis, however, has shifted from bacteriology to molecular biology and genetics, and the future is likely to produce major advances cross a broad front, including the neurosciences.

Will the biomedical paradigm dominate the future direction of biomedical research policy? I don't think so. It is likely to be increasingly influenced by the social and behavioral sciences, including the kind of studies reported over the past two days. Future progress will depend not only on advancing knowledge, but also on applying what we know. The NIH needs to move from such a heavy emphasis on the biological processes to what George Kaplan called "proximate pathways" and health behaviors to the upstream determinants of health such as social support, factors affecting early childhood development, education, neighborhood, social capital, and community or population-based interventions, not just clinical interventions.[1]

PUBLIC HEALTH

Let me turn to public health, where the relationship between policies and improvements in health are more clear-cut. Public health must increasingly be viewed in the context of the broad definition by the Institute of Medicine in its 1988 Report on the Future of Public Health, not narrowly from the role of government agencies alone.[9] The Centers for Disease Control and Prevention (CDC), U.S. Public Health

Service, has recently announced that it will issue a series of reports on the great public health accomplishments of this century.[10] These will include:

1. Vaccination;
2. Improvements in motor vehicle safety;
3. Work-related health problems;
4. Safer workplaces;
5. Control of infectious diseases;
6. Decline in deaths from coronary heart disease and stroke;
7. Safer and healthier food;
8. Healthier mothers and babies;
9. Fluoridation of drinking water; and
10. Recognition of tobacco use as a health hazard.

Policies at the state, local, and federal levels have contributed to these accomplishments as well as research related to infectious diseases, occupational illness, auto and occupational safety, coronary artery disease, hypertension, fluoridation, and nutrition. In many cases (e.g., decline in deaths from coronary heart disease and stroke, control of infectious diseases, healthier mothers and children) both medicine and public health contributed to the achievement of these advances. While most reduced mortality and increased life expectancy, others (e.g., fluoridation) contributed to reduced morbidity and a better quality of life.

Despite the progress and substantial accomplishments, many problems remain related to the infectious diseases, including:

1. HIV/AIDS;
2. Emerging and re-emerging infections;
3. Influenza;
4. Nosocomial infection; and
5. Antibiotic resistance.

Other problems include:

1. Old diseases with new causes (e.g., peptic ulcer, cervical cancer);
2. Chronic illness; and
3. Problems with a strong social complement (e.g., teen pregnancy, family violence, and substance abuse).

These problems are being addressed both by the traditional categorical public health programs as well as through the Healthy People process launched 20 years ago by Dr. Julius Richmond when he was serving as the Assistant Secretary/ Surgeon General. The process set health goals and objectives for the nation for 1990, 2000, and now for 2010. The process is beginning to give more emphasis to SES and health disparities, but it must give these more emphasis. Recently, Nancy Moss recommended: "Healthy People should move from framing health goals for the poor and non-poor populations to targeting health disparities across the socioeconomic spectrum, while recognizing the disproportionate disadvantage borne by vulnerable populations, including the poor."[11] The President's Initiative to close the gap of health disparities, stimulated by the current Assistant Secretary/ Surgeon General, Dr. David Satcher, is a move in the right direction.[12]

Regulations since the passage of the Biologies Control Act in 1902 at the local, state, and national levels have played a critical role in reducing the morbidity and mortality for infectious diseases; promoting worker health and safety; reducing auto fatalities; providing for chlorination and fluoridation of water supplies; requiring pasteurization of milk; assuring the vaccination of children; promoting food, drug, and devices safety; requiring nutrition labeling; reducing cigarette smoking in hospitals and public buildings and the workplace; and establishing a system of health statistics and infectious disease reporting.

Although it is impossible to accurately estimate the impact of public health policies in this century, there is no doubt that they have played a major role in reducing morbidity and mortality and in improving the quality of life for the people of the United States.

MEDICAL CARE

Although it is impossible to estimate the overall effectiveness in narrowing health disparities related to socioeconomic status during the past 60 years, special programs, such as TBC control, can be assessed.

In his review of trends in mortality in the 20th century, Rothstein noted that while American physicians tend to view the improvements as due to medical interventions, British physicians believe that "more general social changes, in broad public health measures, in standard of living, in life style are responsible."[13]

Policy makers, like physicians, seem to have greater faith in medical care than in other interventions that are susceptible to policies at the federal, state, and local levels. Historically the hospital—first just the inpatient service, then the outpatient clinics and emergency room—were viewed as a means to provide the poor with some level of medical care in the face of illness.

Federal policies related to medical care were among the first enacted by Congress. An act of July 16, 1798, passed by the Fifth Congress of the United States, taxed employers of merchant seamen to fund arrangements for their medical care through the Marine Hospital Service. The Act included authorization for the President "to provide the temporary relief and maintenance of sick or disabled seamen in hospitals or other proper institutions now established in several ports."[14] The Marine Hospital Service became the U.S. Public Health Service, and PHS hospitals continued to provide for merchant seamen until the administration of President Reagan in the early 1980s.

Medical care has been provided for members of the armed forces since the Revolutionary War. Care for veterans in a separate VA Hospital system was authorized after World War I. The Synder Act of 1920 authorized health care for American Indians to be provided by the Bureau of Indian Affairs. The Maternity and Infant Care Act of 1921 provided grants to states allowing them to develop health services for mothers and children. The act lapsed in 1929 because of opposition from the AMA, but it became Title V of the Social Security Act in 1935. During WWII health insurance was provided for the wives and children of enlisted service men. Despite its success this was promptly terminated after WWII because of AMA opposition.

Although President Eisenhower was not considered an advocate of progressive legislation, the Dependents Medical Care Act authorizing the CHAMPUS Program was enacted in 1956, the Federal Employees Health Benefits Program in 1959, and the Kerr Mills Act in 1960. The most important federal medical care financing legislation occurred in 1965 with the enactment of Medicare and Medicaid.

Health care expenditures have risen for the past 70 years, but the rate of increase accelerated after the enactment of Medicare and Medicaid and the recent advances in medical technology including drugs, devices, and procedures. Medicare and Medicaid expenditures in 1996 were $351 billion, more than one-third of the nation's health care bill. Public expenditures for medical care now exceed 45% of total expenditures for medical care. Clearly, medical care is where the money is, but the impact on mortality rates and on closing disparities in health status have been less dramatic and less important than the contributions of public health.

Medical care, while benefiting some individuals greatly in terms of their survival as well as their quality of life, has contributed relatively little to the overall improvement in the health status of the population. Improvements in the health of the population are likely to increase in importance in the future, particularly if there is a closer collaboration between medicine and public health and if both work together closely with the community.[15]

CONCLUDING OBSERVATIONS

A few concluding observations:

- Research policies are likely to continue to drive the advances in medical care and public health;

- Public health investments—both regulatory policies and infrastructure support to deal broadly with determinants of health are not popular in the present climate, but will continue to be of critical importance. Categorical public health programs continue to give more emphasis to care than to primary prevention and population-based interventions;

- Medical care expenditures will continue to increase and will limit the availability of funds for investment in all areas, such as early childhood development, that might deliver far more benefit in terms of the health of populations than the increasing expenditures for medical care;

- SES-related health disparities have, to date, had little influence on policy, but they are likely to be the focus of increased attention and action;

- Improvements in the health status of the population can be significantly advanced with increased collaboration between medicine and public health.

REFERENCES

1. KAPLAN, G. 1999. Part III summary: what is the role of the social environment in understanding the inequalities in health? Ann. N.Y. Acad. Sci. **896:** this volume.
2. TARLOV, A.R. 1999. Public policy frameworks for improving population health. Ann. N.Y. Acad. Sci. **896:** this volume.
3. ANDERSON, N.R. 1999. Solving the puzzle of SES and health: the need for interdisciplinary, multilevel research. Ann. N.Y. Acad. Sci. **896:** this volume.

4. EVANS, H. 1998. The American Century. 710. Alfred A. Knopf, New York.
5. JENNINGS, P. & T. BREWSTER. 1998. 605. The Century, Doubleday, New York.
6. JOHNSON, P. 1997. A History of the American People. 1088. Harper Collins, New York.
7. PORTER, R. 1997. The Greatest Benefit to Mankind: A Medical History of Humanity. 433. W.W. Norton, New York.
8. HARDEN, V.A. 1998. National Institutes of Health. *In* A Historical Guide to the U.S. Government. G.T. Kurian, Ed.: 409. Oxford University Press, New York.
9. INSTITUTE OF MEDICINE. 1988. The Future of Public Health. 255. National Academy Press, Washington, DC.
10. CENTERS FOR DISEASE CONTROL AND PREVENTION. 1999. Ten great public health achievements—United States 1900–1999. JAMA **281:** 1481.
11. MOSS, N. 1999. Socioeconomic disparities in health in the United States: an agenda for action. Soc. Sci. Med. Provisionally accepted for publication.
12. HAMBURG, M. 1998. Eliminating Racial and Ethnic Disparities in Health: Response to the Presidential Initiative on Race. July 17. U.S. Department of Health and Human Services, Washington, DC.
13. ROTHSTEIN, W.G. 1995. Readings in American Health Care. 85. University of Wisconsin Press, Madison, WI.
14. LONGEST, B.B., JR. 1998. Health Policymaking in the United States. 2nd edit. 267. Health Administration Press, Chicago.
15. LASKER, R.D. 1997. Medicine and Public Health—The Power of Collaboration. 178. Health Administration Press, Chicago.

Solving the Puzzle of Socioeconomic Status and Health: The Need for Integrated, Multilevel, Interdisciplinary Research

NORMAN B. ANDERSON[a]

Office of Behavioral and Social Sciences Research,
National Institutes of Health, Bethesda, Maryland 20892, USA

The Office of Behavioral and Social Sciences Research (OBSSR) was pleased to be a cosponsor of this important meeting on socioeconomic status and health. One of the principal goals of the OBSSR is to integrate sociobehavioral and biomedical research across the National Institutes of Health (NIH) through the stimulation of cross-disciplinary research. It is clear from the papers in this volume that to fully understand the links between SES and health, research that cuts across disciplinary boundaries is of the utmost importance. Although research from single disciplines has produced a body of knowledge on many of the components and processes associated with the SES–health relationship (e.g., health behaviors, social support, neighborhood environment, endocrine activity, psychological stress), it is also clear that these components and processes are inextricably linked. In other words, the social, behavioral, and biological processes that might mediate the SES–health relationship are interdependent. Failure to conduct research across disciplinary lines precludes the discovery of these interdependent processes.

A substantial body of research exists that demonstrates the manifold connections across what might be termed "levels of analysis" of health science. Research that integrates the various levels of analysis represents one of the next great frontiers in the health sciences, with the potential to accelerate advances in both basic and clinical research and in public health. The hallmark of such integrated, multilevel research is interdisciplinary collaborations, which use the expertise of several disciplines to address complex health issues. The next two sections provide an outline of the notion of multilevel research and some of the principles on which it is based. This discussion draws heavily from Anderson[1] and Anderson and Scott.[2] The final section describes current activities at N.I.H. related to advancing interdisciplinary research.

THE CONCEPT OF LEVELS OF ANALYSIS

The notion of levels of analysis is not new to the health sciences. For example, it has been applied quite productively to cognitive and behavioral neuroscience, where both theoretical models and empirical findings have emerged.[3–5] Cacioppo

[a]Address for correspondence: Norman B. Anderson, Ph.D., Office of Behavioral and Social Sciences Research, National Institutes of Health, Building 1, Room 326, One Centre Drive, Bethesda, MD 20892. 301-402-1146 (voice); 301-402-1150 (fax).
e-mail: Norman_Anderson@nih.gov

and Berntson[6] have provided one of the most detailed overviews of the concept of multilevel analyses in their discussion of the interdependence of social psychological and neuroscience research. The success of this approach in neuroscience research suggests that it might be a useful heuristic in other areas of the health science enterprise, especially in understanding SES and health. In fact, an integrated, multilevel approach to research may represent a unifying framework for all of the health sciences.

FIGURE 1 illustrates one potentially useful way of categorizing the various levels of analysis in health research: the social/environmental, behavioral/psychological, organ systems, cellular, and molecular. Each of these levels contains a large number of indices that have been used to study specific health outcomes or pathogenic sociobehavioral or biological processes. Some of these indices are shown in TABLE 1. The social/environmental level includes such variables as stressful life events, social support, economic resources, neighborhood characteristics, and environmental hazards. The behavioral/psychological level may include emotion, cognition, memory, dietary practices, stress coping styles, and tobacco use. The organ systems level of analysis includes the cardiovascular, endocrine, immune, and central nervous systems and their outputs. On the cellular level, variables include receptor number and sensitivity, dendritic branches, synapse number, and electrical conductance. Finally, the molecular or genetic level includes such variables as DNA structure, proteins, mRNA, and transcription factors.

The determination of which indices fall within which levels of analysis is admittedly somewhat arbitrary (e.g., do stressful life events fall in the social/environmental or behavioral/psychological levels?). The point, however, is that the majority of

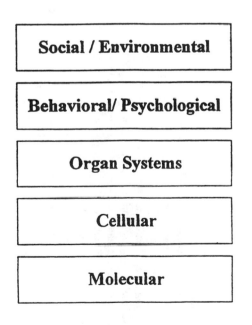

FIGURE 1. Levels of analysis in health research.

TABLE 1. Some indices of various levels of analysis[a]

Social/environmental	Behavioral/psychological	Organ systems	Cellular	Molecular
Stressful life events	Emotion	Cardiovascular	Receptor number	DNA structure
Social support	Memory	Blood pressure	Receptor sensitivity	Proteins
Sociocultural groupings	Learning	Heart rate	Cell number	mRNA
Occupational status	Cognition	Ejection fraction	Dendritic branches	tRNA
Economic resources	Diet	Occlusion	Synapse number	rRNA
Family environment	Exercise	Endocrine	Cortical reorganization	Proto-oncogenes
Neighborhood characteristics	Smoking	Catecholamines	Electrical conductance	Translation factors
Environmental stimulation and enrichment	Alcohol intake	Cortisol	(e.g., cell firing)	Second messengers
Reinforcement contingencies	Drug abuse	ACTH		
National income distribution	Perception	GH		
Environmental hazards	Attention	Insulin		
Natural and human disasters	Stress appraisal and coping	Immune		
Social hierarchies	Language	Lymphocytes		
	Expectations	Phagocytes		
	Motivation	Cytokines		
	Personality	CNS		
	Aggression	Evoked potentials		
	Mental illnesses	Cortical weight		
		Blood flow		
		Metabolic rate		
		ANS		
		SNS		
		PNS		

[a]Adapted from Anderson.[1]

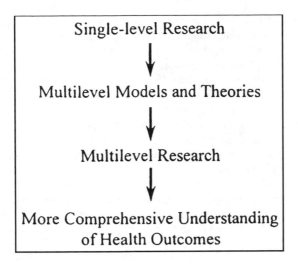

FIGURE 2. Processes involved in an integrated, multilevel approach to health sciences research.

research in the health sciences occurs within a single level of analysis, closely tied to specific disciplines. Even when interdisciplinary research occurs in an area in which scientists from different disciplines are working together on the same problem, it is not always *multilevel* research. This type of interdisciplinary research focuses on a single level of analysis, with no exploration of influences from higher or lower levels on the problem of interest. As mentioned, the single-level approach clearly has been successful, with important contributions made from each level. At the same time, knowledge produced at one level has not always been used to inform research at other levels. Moreover, the science in some areas has progressed to a point where a more integrated, multilevel approach to research design and analysis could pay dividends. As shown in FIGURE 2, it is possible that single-level research could lead to the development of multilevel models and theories, which in turn would stimulate multilevel research activities. The ultimate goal of such an approach would be more comprehensive understanding of health outcomes.

PROCESSES AND PRINCIPLES OF
INTEGRATED, MULTILEVEL RESEARCH

In their discussion of an integrated, multilevel approach to social psychological and neuroscience research, Cacioppo and Berntson[6] state that "analysis of a phenomenon at one level of organization can inform, refine, or constrain inferences based on observations at another level of analysis and, therefore, can foster comprehensive accounts and general theories of complex psychological phenomena." That is, the *interpretation* of findings from single-level research might benefit from the consideration of relevant factors from other levels. Applied to health sciences research more generally, an integrated, multilevel approach involves two types of processes. The first, following from Cacioppo and Berntson, involves the use of findings from one level of analysis to inform, refine, and constrain inferences from observations at another level of analysis. This process might be thought of as "multilevel model or hypothesis development." Here, the objective is a more complete conceptualization of the phenomenon of interest by developing multilevel models or hypotheses, which necessitates the incorporation of findings from other levels. The researcher is asking the question, "What are the variables at higher or lower levels of analysis that might influence or be influenced by the phenomenon that I am studying?" The second process logically follows the first and involves the simultaneous study of a phenomenon across levels of analysis to foster a more comprehensive understanding of the determinants of health outcomes or pathogenic processes. This second process is epitomized by integrated, multilevel, cross-disciplinary research designed to test well-articulated multilevel models or hypotheses.

Several principles and a corollary of multilevel research have been proposed that may be adapted for the broader domain of health research. These include the principle of parallel causation, the principle of convergent causation, the principle of

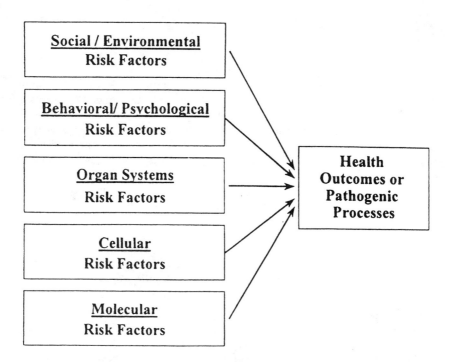

FIGURE 3. Principle of parallel causation. Each factor may be sufficient but not necessary for the prediction of health outcomes or pathogenic processes.

reciprocal causation, and the corollary of proximity. Each of these concepts is defined in the following.

The Principle of Parallel Causation

The principle of parallel causation holds that each level of analysis may contain risk factors for a single health outcome or pathogenic process (FIG. 3). Each of these risk factors may be sufficient, but not necessary, for the prediction of outcomes or processes. For example, in the prediction of coronary heart disease (CHD), social-level risk factors include socioeconomic status and social support; behavioral-level risk factors include physical inactivity and smoking; and organ systems-level risk factors include low-density lipoproteins and hypertension. Each level of analysis contains variables that alone are sufficient to account for a significant proportion of the variance in CHD, though no particular level is necessary for the prediction of CHD.

The Principles of Convergent and Reciprocal Causation

With convergent causation, a convergence or interaction of variables from at least two levels of analysis lead to a health outcome or pathogenic process (FIG. 4). Thus, variables within a single level may be necessary, but not sufficient, to produce an out-

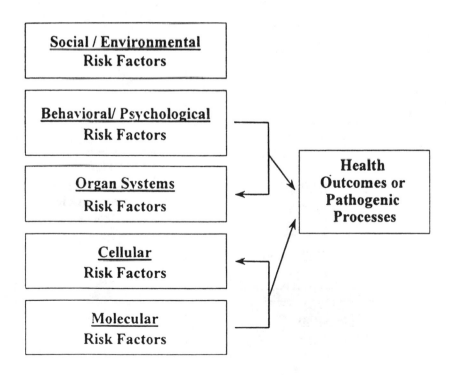

FIGURE 4. Principle of convergent causation. Each factor may be necessary but not sufficient for the prediction of health outcomes or pathogenic processes.

come. Here, factors from one level of analysis affect factors at another level, and this cross-level causation ultimately influences outcomes. The principle of reciprocal causation is similar to convergent causation, but posits bidirectional influences across levels, involving negative- and positive-feedback loops (FIG. 5). For example, the initiation of cigarette smoking (behavioral level) in adolescents may be strongly tied to such social and environmental factors as peer influences and advertising (convergent causation); smoking behavior in turn could later affect biological processes leading to a biological addiction (convergent causation); and this biological addiction contributes to the maintenance of smoking behavior (reciprocal causation). Thus, the behavior of smoking leads to biological changes that further serve to maintain this behavior. The principles of convergent and reciprocal causation are the foundations of integrated, multilevel research in that they highlight the critical importance of interactions across levels of analysis in fostering more complete accounts of health phenomena.

The Corollary of Proximity

This corollary holds that the mapping of elements or variables across levels of organization increases in complexity as the number of intervening levels increases.[5] That is, research aimed at exploring interactions between variables at adjacent levels

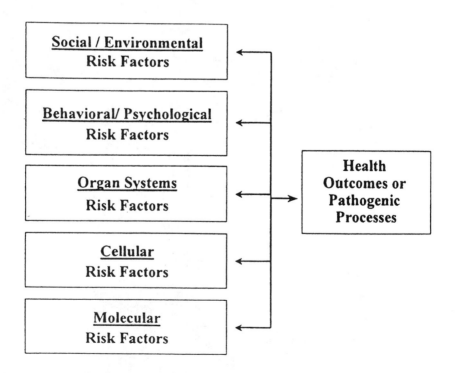

FIGURE 5. Principle of reciprocal causation. Factors have bidirectional influences on each other across levels of analysis.

of analysis will typically be less complex than that examining variables at nonadjacent levels. This is because events at any level of analysis (e.g., the cellular level) can be influenced by events within the same or at adjacent levels (e.g., organ systems level), which in turn may be affected by events at the next level of organization (e.g., behavioral level). This added complexity does not preclude research across multiple levels, but suggests that an incremental approach may be the most useful one.[6] Churchland and Scjnowski[3] voiced a similar perspective, stating that: "The ultimate goal of a unified account does not require that it be a single model that spans all levels of organization. Instead, the integration will probably consist of a chain of models linking adjacent levels. When one level is explained in terms of a lower level, this does not mean that the higher level theory is useless or that high-level phenomena no longer exist. On the contrary, explanations will coexist at all levels...."

MEETING THE NEED FOR MULTILEVEL, INTERDISCIPLINARY RESEARCH ON SES AND HEALTH: THE ROLE OF THE NIH

From the papers in this volume, it is clear that integrated, multilevel, interdisciplinary research on SES and health represents an extraordinary scientific opportunity—one that may pay dividends in improving the public's health. The NIH obviously has an important role to play in assisting researchers in capitalizing on this opportunity. Outlined below are just a few of the activities at NIH relevant to SES and health.

- The Fogarty International Center will soon host a planning workshop on international health and economic development. The purpose of this workshop is to determine the feasibility and scope of a proposed program to investigate the economic implications of disease burden and demographic status in developing nations.

- The National Institute of Dental and Craniofacial Research (NIDCR) is planning a Request for Applications (RFA) for Centers for Research on Health Disparities. The Centers will focus on health disparities based on race/ethnicity, SES, and potentially others, and address research, training, and interventions.

- The National Institute on Environmental Health Sciences (NIEHS) is developing a research agenda and RFA on environmental aspects of SES and health. Many other Institutes and Centers at NIH will also participate in the RFA.

- The National Institute on Aging (NIA), in collaboration with Dr. Keith Whitfield of Pennsylvania State University, is planning a new emphasis on SES, ethnicity, and health as part of its Baltimore Longitudinal Study of Aging (part of the NIA Intramural Program).

- NIH Director Harold Varmus has designated research on health disparities—which include SES and race/ethnic, among other types of disparities—as one of his Areas of Emphasis beginning in fiscal year 2000.

- As part of this Areas of Emphasis designation, Dr. Varmus has appointed a panel of Directors of NIH Institutes, Centers, and Offices to develop a trans-NIH plan for addressing health disparities.

In addition to the above activities, it should be noted that a number of Institutes and Centers of the NIH have had a long standing interest and commitment to research on SES and health. These include:

- The National Cancer Institute;
- The National Heart, Lung, and Blood Institute;
- The National Institute on Child Health and Human Development;
- The National Institute on Aging;
- The National Institute on Mental Health;
- The National Institute on Drug Abuse;
- The National Institute on Alcoholism and Alcohol Abuse; and
- The National Institute of Nursing Research.

Relevant Activities of the OBSSR

The OBSSR also has a number of ongoing activities designed to increase interdisciplinary research more generally. Some of these activities are listed below.

Funding Educational Workshops in Interdisciplinary Research

The OBSSR organized two trans-NIH RFAs to facilitate the advancement of interdisciplinary research. Specifically, proposals were sought for workshops that would provide training for junior investigators interested in the integration of different fields of social and behavioral sciences research and/or the integration of these areas with more biological levels of analysis. The short-term goal of this initiative was to encourage social, behavioral, and biomedical scientists at an early stage of their careers to learn each other's methods, procedures, and/or theoretical perspectives. The long-term goal of this RFA is to enable researchers to develop cross-disciplinary collaborations and to submit high-quality biobehavioral grant applications. Ten workshops were funded under this RFA following the initial solicitation, and it is anticipated that a similar number will be funded on the second round.

Identifying and Documenting Successful Models for Interdisciplinary Research

In collaboration with the Social Science Research Council (SSRC), the OBSSR has organized a working group to document and understand the factors and circumstances that foster successful collaborations between biomedical researchers and those from the social and behavioral sciences. The working group will examine barriers to such collaboration (e.g., scientific language differences and disincentives for collaboration) and ways in which these difficulties can be overcome. This process will be informed by in-depth case studies of successful interdisciplinary collaborations. Key research domains that will form these case studies are:

- Aging and the life course,
- Affective and cognitive neuroscience,
- Behavioral cardiology,
- Positive health, and
- Prevention and management of HIV/AIDS.

Identifying Interdisciplinary Training Needs in the Neurosciences

The OBSSR is collaborating with the National Institute of Mental Health, the National Institute on Aging, and the National Institute of Nursing Research to fund an Institute of Medicine (IOM) study on the training of biobehavioral investigators in the neurosciences. The goal of the study is to develop recommendations on the types of training and funding necessary to create scientists who are broadly trained to conduct research at the nexus of the behavioral and brain sciences. The study would also make recommendations on how to overcome barriers to the development and support of interdisciplinary educational programs.

Developing Methods for the Behavioral Testing of Transgenic Mice

In recent years, there has been increased interest among molecular biologists in examining behavioral phenotypes in knockout and transgenic animal models. In response to this interest, the OBSSR formed a working group of behavioral scientists, chaired by Jackie Crawley of NIMH. The Working Group will develop a comprehensive, standardized battery of behavioral testing procedures for transgenic mice that will be accessible over the Internet. This battery will consist of diagnostic screening procedures to assess for general sensory deficits and physical limitations and a set of specialized tests to assess specific behavioral features. For example, tests may be outlined for animal models of depression, anxiety, cognitive functioning, and regulatory behavior. It is hoped that the development of such a standardized test battery will help foster interdisciplinary, multilevel research in the field of behavior genetics.

Setting Priorities for Behavioral and Social Sciences Research at the NIH

At the request of NIH Director, Harold Varmus, the OBSSR has commissioned the National Research Council (NRC) of the National Academy of Sciences (NAS) to identify priorities for research in the behavioral and social sciences at NIH. This request occurs in a context of increased recognition at NIH of the importance of behavioral and social factors to health and the potential for large increases in the NIH budget. The identification of research priorities in the behavioral and social sciences will help the NIH apply current and future research resources strategically, so as to balance the goals of reducing the burden of disease and capitalizing on scientific opportunities. More specifically, these priorities will be used to guide OBSSR in the development of trans-NIH funding initiatives, workshops, and conferences. The priorities may also be included in the NIH Director's Areas of Research Emphasis activities and may be used by the NIH Institutes in developing special funding activities. Although the specific priorities have not been announced, it is likely that they will include research topics relevant to multilevel research. The NRC Committee on Future Directions in the Behavioral and Social Sciences, chaired by Burt Singer of Princeton University, will issue a report early in 2000.

REFERENCES

1. ANDERSON, N.B. 1998. Levels of analysis in health science: a framework for integrating sociobehavioral and biomedical research. Ann. N.Y. Acad. Sci. **840:** 563–576.

2. ANDERSON, N.B. & P. SCOTT. 1999. Making the case for psychophysiology during the era of molecular biology. Psychophysiology **36:** 1–13.
3. CHURCHLAND, P.S. & T.J. SEJNOWSKI. 1988. Perspectives on cognitive neuroscience. Science **242:** 741–745.
4. KOOB, G.F. & F.E. BLOOM. 1988. Cellular and molecular mechanisms of drug dependence. Science **242:** 715–723.
5. FODOR, J.A. 1968. Psychological explanation. Random House, New York.
6. CACIOPPO, J.T. & G.G. BERNTSON. 1992. Social psychological contributions to the decade of the brain: the doctrine of multilevel analysis. Am. Psychol. **47**(8): 1019–1028.

Social Class Differences in Morbidity Using the New U.K. National Statistics Socio-Economic Classification

Do Class Differences in Employment Relations Explain Class Differences in Health?

TARANI CHANDOLA[a,b] AND CRISPIN JENKINSON[c]

[b]Nuffield College, New Road, Oxford OXI INF, United Kingdom

[c]Health Services Research Unit, University of Oxford, Institute of Health Sciences, Headington, Oxford OX3 7LF, United Kingdom

Although there have been a number of studies on social class differences in health and mortality in the U.K., the mechanisms underlying these class differences remain debatable. Social class differences in material and lifestyle factors have been identified as part of the main mechanisms underlying inequalities in health.[1] Some studies have hypothesized that class differences in work characteristics and employment conditions may also explain part of the observed class differences in health.[2] Differences between classes in job control in particular, have been singled out as a mechanism that could explain some of the association between class and health outcomes.[3]

The new U.K. National Statistics Socio-Economic Classification (NS-SEC) is explicitly based on differences between employment conditions and relations.[4] Part of the reason for replacing the existing Registrar General's social classification (RGSC) with the NS-SEC is the nonspecific basis for classifying occupations into the Registrar General's classes. Bartley *et al.*[5] suggest that the examination of the relationship of the NS-SEC to health outcomes tests the hypothesis that occupations having employment relations and conditions characterized by a wage rather than salary, little or no prospects for promotion, and lower levels of autonomy would experience lower life expectancy. If differences between social classes in employment relations have an important role in explaining social class differences in mortality and morbidity, one may expect significant social class differences to remain in the NS-SEC even after adjusting for more established explanatory mechanisms such as lifestyle and material factors.

This study investigates the associations of the NS-SEC with morbidity in the Oxford Healthy Lifestyles Survey III (OBLSIII, $n = 6454$), a cross-sectional survey of adult men and women aged 18–64 years randomly selected from the counties of Berkshire, Buckinghamshire, Northamptonshire, and Oxfordshire. The associations of the Short Form health survey (SF-36) physical and mental summary scores with the NS-SEC are analyzed in a series of multiple regression models adjusting for age,

[a]Address for correspondence: +44 1865 278615 (voice); +44 1865 278621 (fax).
e-mail: tarani.chandola@nuf.ox.ac.uk

TABLE 1. Multiple regression of SF-36 physical and mental scores in the OHLS III data for men and women separately: estimates (standard errors) and F-test of social class in different models

NS-SEC	Model I	Model II	N
SF-36 physical score—men			
Higher manager	54.59 (0.55)	46.11 (2.26)	1009
Lower manager	−0.39 (0.45)	−0.04 (0.44)	407
Intermediate employee	−0.14 (0.57)	0.25 (0.57)	225
Small employer	−1.87 (0.49)	−1.18 (0.49)	330
Lower supervisor	−1.30 (0.48)	−0.54 (0.48)	344
Semi-routine employee	−1.97 (0.43)	−1.06 (0.43)	507
Routine employee	−1.74 (0.80)	−0.65 (0.79)	106
Rsq	0.31	0.34	
F-test for NS-SEC	5.63[a]	2.03	
SF-36 physical score—women			
Higher manager	53.26 (0.57)	37.54 (2.13)	747
Lower manager	−0.13 (0.50)	0.02 (0.48)	493
Intermediate employee	−0.50 (0.42)	0.00 (0.40)	1058
Small employer	−1.38 (0.70)	−0.78 (0.68)	192
Lower supervisor	−1.43 (0.92)	−0.10 (0.89)	98
Semi-routine employee	−1.30 (0.48)	−0.08 (0.48)	638
Routine employee	−2.08 (0.60)	−0.27 (0.60)	300
Rsq	0.28	0.33	
F-test for NS-SEC	3.15[a]	0.94	
SF-36 Mental score—men			
Higher manager	50.50 (0.65)	31.00 (2.64)	1009
Lower manager	−0.05 (0.53)	0.18 (0.52)	407
Intermediate employee	−0.03 (0.68)	0.49 (0.66)	225
Small employer	0.07 (0.58)	0.67 (0.57)	330
Lower supervisor	0.09 (0.57)	0.92 (0.56)	344
Semi-routine employee	−0.59 (0.50)	0.38 (0.51)	507
Routine employee	1.28 (0.94)	2.44 (0.93)	106
Rsq	0.06	0.11	
F-test for NS-SEC	0.72	1.48	
SF-36 mental score—women			
Higher manager	47.37 (0.67)	25.92 (2.47)	747
Lower manager	0.66 (0.58)	0.93 (0.56)	493
Intermediate employee	−0.93 (0.48)	−0.57 (0.47)	1058
Small employer	0.23 (0.81)	0.69 (0.78)	192
Lower supervisor	−0.52 (1.07)	0.80 (1.03)	98
Semi-routine employee	−0.99 (0.56)	0.40 (0.55)	638
Routine employee	−1.88 (0.70)	0.06 (0.69)	300
Rsq			
F-test for NS-SEC	2.89[b]	1.80	

NOTE: Model I includes age and employment status; Model II includes age, employment status, lifestyles, and housing/environment conditions
[a]$p < 0.01$.
[b]$p < 0.05$.

employment status, lifestyle factors (smoking, exercise, obesity, diet, and alcohol consumption), housing problems (with cold and damp), and neighborhood conditions (an index of problems with traffic, public transport, burglaries, litter and rubbish, noise and vandalism, lack of open spaces, assaults, etc.). Model I includes age, employment status, and the NS-SEC, while Model II includes age, employment status, lifestyle factors, housing/neighborhood conditions, and the NS-SEC.

In TABLE 1, there are significant social class differences in the SF-36 physical and mental scores for women and in the SF36 physical score for men (Model I). In general, the higher and lower managerial social classes have the highest estimated scores (or the best health) whereas the semi-routine and routine employee class have the lowest estimated scores (or the worst health). In Model II (which adjusts for age, employment status, health behaviors, and housing/neighborhood factors), there are no significant social class differences in the SF-36 physical and mental scores.

The new National Statistics Social Classification (NSSC) demonstrates social class differences in the SF-36 physical and mental health scores. The results also suggest that these social class differences can, to a large extent, be "explained" away by a combination of material and lifestyle factors. The reduction of the social class differences in physical and mental health to nonsignificance when adjusted for health behaviors and housing/neighborhood factors suggests that differences in employment relations and conditions may not have a large explanatory role in relation to inequalities in health.

REFERENCES

1. DEPARTMENT OF HEALTH AND SOCIAL SECURITY (DHSS). 1980. Inequalities in Health, Report of a Research Working Group, DHSS, London.
2. FITZPATRICK, R., M. BARTLEY, B. DODGEON, D. FIRTH & K. LYNCH. 1997. Social variations in health: relationship of mortality to the interim revised social classification. *In* Constructing Classes. D. Rose & K. O'Reily, Eds. ESRC/ONS, Swindon.
3. MARMOT, M.G., H. BOSMA, H. HEMINGWAY, E. BRUNNER & S. STANSFELD. 1997. Contribution of job control and other risk factors to social variations in coronary heart disease incidence [see comment]. Lancet 350: 235–239.
4. ROSE, D. & K. O'REILY. 1997. Constructing Classes. ESRC/ONS, Swindon.
5. BARTLEY, M., K. LYNCH, A. SACKER & B. DODGEON. 1998. Social variations in health: relationship of mortality to the OS socio-economic class (SEC) schema. Presented at SEC Validation Workshop, University of Essex, Essex, U.K.

Orthostatic Blood Pressure Responses as a Function of Ethnicity and Socioeconomic Status: The ARIC Study

RODNEY CLARK,[a,b] HERMAN A. TYROLER,[c] AND GERARDO HEISS[c]

[b]Department of Psychology, Wayne State University,
71 West Warren, Detroit, Michigan 48202, USA

[c]Department of Epidemiology, University of North Carolina at Chapel Hill,
School of Public Health, Chapel Hill, North Carolina 27514, USA

According to a recent definition devised by the Joint National Committee on High Blood Pressure, approximately 51 million Americans, 17 years of age and older, meet diagnostic criteria for hypertension.[1] One controversial line of research aimed at delineating the putative causes of hypertension has examined the relationship between cardiovascular responses to standardized stressors (e.g., orthostasis) and cardiovascular outcomes.[2–5] Research also suggests that cardiovascular responses to these stressors vary as a function of ethnicity[6] and socioeconomic status.[7]

This study examined the effects of ethnicity and education on orthostatic blood pressure responses in a normotensive sample of participants free of clinical cardiovascular disease and diabetes ($n = 6{,}412$). Average supine–standing blood pressure measurements were calculated and were used for stratified and logistic analyses. Prevalence odds ratios (POR) and 95% confidence intervals (CI) were calculated as the measures of effect in the multivariate logistic analyses. Sitting systolic and diastolic blood pressure levels were associated with the magnitude of orthostatic blood pressure responses. African-Americans were more likely to exhibit exaggerated systolic (POR = 1.22, CI = 1.08, 1.38) and diastolic (POR = 1.32, CI = 1.15, 1.50) blood pressure responses to orthostasis. Relative to participants with 12 years of education, participants with less than 12 years of education were more likely to have exaggerated increases or exaggerated decreases in systolic blood pressure on standing (12% and 20%, respectively). A significant interaction between ethnicity and education was not observed in these data. There was no evidence of modification of ethnicity and education effects by any of the covariates.

The observed orthostatic blood pressure differences may be attributable to differential exposures to chronic psychosocial stressors in African-Americans and those of low educational achievement.[8,9] Future studies might extend the finding here by (1) obtaining individual information on environmental factors like perceived racism, chronic stress, and job strain to quantify psychosocial stress exposure; (2) examining the possible mediating effects of psychosocial factors like John Henryism, life style

[a]Address for correspondence: Rodney Clark, Department of Psychology, Wayne State University, 71 West Warren, Detroit, MI 48202, USA. 313-577-7640 (voice); 313-577-7636 (fax). e-mail: rclark@sun.science.wayne.edu

incongruity, and anger-coping styles, and (3) investigating the efficacy of psychosocial stress exposure as a predictor of subsequent hypertension development.

REFERENCES

1. SCHWARTZ, L.M. & S. WOLOSHIN. 1999. Changing disease definitions: implications for disease prevalence. Analysis of the Third National Health and Nutrition Examination Survey, 1988–1994. Eff. Clin. Prac. **2:** 76–85.
2. MATTHEWS, K.A., K.L. WOODALL & M.T. ALLEN. 1993. Cardiovascular reactivity to stress predicts future blood pressure status. Hypertension. **22:** 479–485.
3. MANUCK, S.B., A.L. KASPROWICZ & M.F. MULDOON. 1990. Behaviorally evoked cardiovascular reactivity and hypertension: conceptual issues and potential associations. Ann. Behav. Med. **12:** 17–29.
4. SPARROW, D., B. ROSNER, V. VOKOMAS & S.T. WEISS. 1986. Relationship of blood pressure measurement in several positions. Am. J. Cardiol. **57:** 218–221.
5. SPARROW, D., C.P. TIFFT, B. ROSENER & S.T. WEISS. 1984. Postural changes in diastolic blood pressure and the risk of myocardial infarction: the normative aging study. Circulation **70:** 533–537.
6. GOLDSTEIN, I.B. & D. SHAPIRO. 1995. The cardiovascular response to postural change as a function of race. Bio. Psycho. **19:** 173–186.
7. ARMSTEAD, C.A., N.B. Anderson & K.A. Lawler. 1994. The interaction of socioeconomic status, ethnicity, and cardiovascular reactivity among women. *In* Program and Abstracts of the Annual Meeting of the Psychosomatic Society, Boston, MA.
8. CLARK, R., N.B. ANDERSON, V.R. CLARK & D.R. WILLIAMS. 1999. Racism as a stressor for African Americans: a biopsychosocial model. Am. Psychol. **54:** 805–816.
9. ANDERSON, N.B. & C.A. ARMSTEAD. 1995. Toward understanding the association of socioeconomic status and health: a new challenge for the biopsychosocial approach. Psychosom. Med. **57:** 213–225.

Social Class as a Moderator of Income Effects on Stress and Health Outcomes across Nine Years

DAVID S. DeGARMO[a] AND DEBORAH M. CAPALDI

Oregon Social Learning Center, 160 E. 4th, Eugene, Oregon 97401, USA

Socioeconomic status (SES) is consistently associated with better health outcomes. This relationship is identified as the SES–health gradient.[1] *Social causation* models argue that social structure (e.g., class, income, networks) explains the SES–health gradient. *Social selection* or *social drift* models argue that persons with biological predispositions for poor health become downwardly mobile, and this effect explains the SES–health gradient. With the exception of schizophrenia, however, social causation models are consistently supported both for mortality and major health outcomes.[2,3]

From a social causation perspective, the question still remains whether the SES–health gradient is linear or nonlinear. A *linear gradient* model suggests that an association of SES and health occurs at every level of SES. Not only do those in poverty have poorer health than those with higher SES, but also those at the highest level enjoy better health than do those just below.[1] A *differential vulnerability* model argues that the association between SES and health is nonlinear because of qualitative differences in social class experiences. Those in lower SES or below an income threshold are exposed to more stress and negative life events. In turn, these persons are more vulnerable to the effects of stress than are their upperclass counterparts.[4] This analysis tests a vulnerability hypothesis by examining SES differences in stress exposure and change in income as predictors of health over time.

Participants were 206 parents from the Oregon Youth Study (OYS), a longitudinal study of antisocial behavior in boys. The sample was selected from a catchment area with the highest per capita police arrests in a Northwest metropolitan area. Parents were assessed annually when the focal boy was in grades 4 through 12. Parents' reports of stress and health were obtained from interviews and questionnaires. Scores were the mean of the mother and father variables. *Depression* was measured with the CES-D,[5] the *Negative Life Events* component was measured with the Life Experience Survey,[6] *Family Stress* was measured with the Family Events Checklist,[7] and *Substance Use* was scored from a questionnaire.[8] *Income* was indicated by categories 1–9, ranging from "below $5,000" (1) to "above $50,001" (9). The sample was classified into high ($n = 117$) and low ($n = 88$) SES with the Hollingshead 4-Factor Index of Social Status[9] combining the lower two and the upper three social strata. Models were tested with directional hypotheses.

[a]Address for correspondence: 541-485-2711 (voice); 541-485-7087 (fax).
e-mail: davidd@oslc.org

For time-averaged levels, the low-SES group had more negative life events ($M = 2.49$ and 2.25), higher depression ($M = 18.6$ and 16.6) and higher substance use ($M = 2.6$ and 2.4). No significant differences were found for family stress. For change, no mean differences were found except for income growth for high SES compared to low SES ($M = 20.1$ and 16.3 for change, $M = 4.8$ and 3.8 for average). Effects of income change are shown in FIGURE 1. Standardized path models indicated that an increase in income was associated with a decrease in negative life events ($\beta = -0.25$), decrease in depression ($\beta = -0.23$), and decrease in family stress ($\beta = -0.36$) for high-SES but not for low-SES groups. Additionally, an increase in life events and family stress predicted an increase in depression for low-SES ($\beta = 0.29$ and 0.36) but not for high-SES groups.

Plots (not shown) of change in income with change in health indicated a nonlinear relation for each outcome. Both an income threshold and social class differences explain a nonlinear relation. That is, accelerated income growth and income growth in higher social strata are associated with reductions in poor health, but not for lower SES families. Therefore, a final model regressing health slopes on (a) income change squared and (b) income change multiplied by social class is shown in TABLE 1.

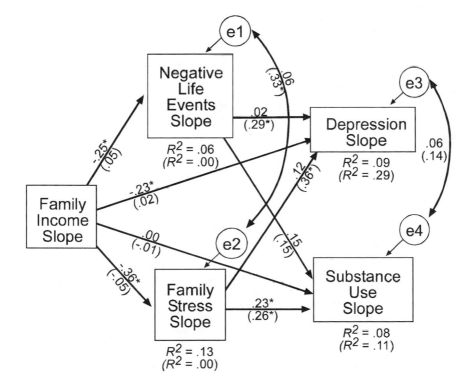

FIGURE 1. Nine-year change in income as a predictor of stress and mental health by social class. Social class: high SES, (low SES). $*p < 0.05$.

TABLE 1. Nine year linear slopes regressed on income and SES predictors[a]

	Life Events Slope	Family Stress Slope	Depression Slope	Substance Use Slope
Income slope	0.21	0.16	0.07	0.37^c
SES	0.05	0.14	0.07	0.03
Threshold hypothesis				
Income slope^2	-0.36^c	-0.44^b	-0.22	-0.49^b
Social class hypothesis				
Income slope × SES	-0.13^c	-0.16^c	-0.13^c	-0.00

[a]Paths are standardized.
[b]$p < 0.01$.
[c]$p < 0.05$ one-tailed.

Independent effects of both an income threshold and social class differences were found for prediction of change in negative life events and change in family stress, whereas social class was related to change in depression and a threshold model was supported for change in substance use.

These data supported an income threshold model and differential vulnerability for SES. There were more negative life events, depression, and substance use in the lower social strata suggesting greater stress exposure. Although both groups increased in income over nine years, beneficial effects of income growth were found in path models for the high-SES group only, indicating that the process or effects of stress differ by SES. The regression models supported a nonlinear association for the SES–Health gradient showing independent effects for an income growth threshold hypothesis and a social class vulnerability explanation. These data underscore the importance of understanding differential processes for social class in future research to identify mechanisms linking SES and health.

REFERENCES

1. ADLER, N.E., T. BOYCE, M.A. CHESNEY, S. COHEN, S. FOLKMAN, R.L. KAHN & S.L. SYME. 1994. Socioeconomic status and health: the challenge of the gradient. Am. Psychol. **49:** 15–24.
2. DOHRENWEND, B.P., I. LEVAV, P.E. SHROUT, S. SCHWARTZ, G. NAVEH, B.G. LINK, A.E. SKODOL & A. STUEVE. 1998. Ethnicity, socioeconomic status, and psychiatric disorders: a test of the social causation–social selection issue. *In* Adversity, Stress, and Psychopathology. B.P. Dohrenwend, Ed.: 285–318. Oxford, New York.
3. MIROWSKY, J. & C.E. ROSS. 1989. Social Causes of Psychological Distress. Aldine de Gruyter, New York.
4. MCLEOD, J.D. & R.C. KESSLER. 1990. Socioeconomic status differences in vulnerability to undesirable life events. J. Health Soc. Beh. **31:** 162–172.
5. RADLOFF, L.S. 1977. The CES-D scale: a self-report depression scale for research in the general population. Appl. Psychol. Meas. **1:** 385–401.
6. SARASON, I.G., J.H. JOHNSON & J.M. SIEGEL. 1978. Assessing the impact of life changes: development of the life experiences survey. J. Consult. Clin. Psychol. **46:** 932–946.

7. PATTERSON, G.R. 1982. Coercive family process. Castilia, Eugene, OR.
8. CAPALDI, D.M. & G.R. PATTERSON. 1991. Relation of parental transitions to boys' adjustment problems: I. A linear hypothesis. II. Mothers at risk for transitions and unskilled parenting. Dev. Psychol. **27:** 489–504.
9. HOLLINGSHEAD, A.B. 1975. Four factor index of social status. Yale University. Unpublished manuscript.

Socioeconomic Disparities in Adult Oral Health in the United States

T.F. DRURY,[a] I. GARCIA, AND M. ADESANYA

National Institute of Dental and Craniofacial Research, National Institutes of Health, Building 45, Room 3AN-44, Bethesda, Maryland 20892, USA

INTRODUCTION

Socioeconomic status (SES) inequalities in health and health care utilization are receiving increasing attention in current U.S. policy initiatives. To stimulate discussion of inequalities in oral health and oral health care in this policy context, the present study describes and evaluates SES disparities in oral health among adults in the United States.

METHODS

Information on clinical parameters of oral health for 14,000+ persons 18 years and over obtained through the 1988–1994 National Health and Nutrition Examination Survey (NHANES III) was analyzed. SES was measured by a composite index based on individual educational attainment and family economic status (based on the ratio of annual family income to the poverty threshold). This index was grouped into four approximately equal categories describing persons with *lower, lower middle, upper middle,* and *higher* SES index scores. SES disparities in the prevalence of each oral health characteristic studied were quantified by the ratio between the odds for persons in each of the three lower SES categories and the odds for persons in the *higher* SES category. Particular attention was given to the ratios between the odds for the lowest and highest SES categories. Both stratified and multiple logistic regression analyses were carried out using SUDAAN software (Release 7.0). *t*-Tests were used in evaluating pairwise comparisons; the Satterthwaite adjusted *F* statistic was used in the context of the logistic analyses to evaluate potential two-way interactions between SES and age, gender, race/ethnicity, and (when appropriate) a recent dental visit. A 0.01 level of significance was used in evaluating statistical results.

RESULTS

SES gradients in aspects of adult oral health occurred across a broad spectrum of indicators reflective of unmet needs (TABLE 1). Logistic analyses that controlled for age, gender, and race/ethnicity revealed that, compared to persons in the *higher* SES category, those in the *lower* SES category were 6.1 times more likely to have untreat-

[a]Address for correspondence: 301-594-4916 (voice); 301-480-8254 (fax).

TABLE 1. Percent of persons 18 years and over with selected oral diseases and conditions, and standard error (S.E.) of percent, by socioeconomic status: United States, 1988–1994[a]

Oral disease or condition[b]		Socioeconomic status			
	All	Lower	Lower middle	Upper middle	Higher
All persons 35+ years					
Completely edentulous	15.1 (0.8)	32.8 (1.6)	20.2 (1.1)	9.8 (1.0)	4.5 (0.5)
Dentate persons 18+ years					
Untreated coronal decay	27.9 (1.1)	49.9 (1.3)	35.7 (1.8)	23.0 (1.3)	13.1 (1.0)
Untreated root decay	11.0 (0.5)	24.0 (1.3)	14.5 (1.0)	9.7 (0.9)	4.7 (0.5)
Any gingivits	52.9 (2.1)	63.4 (2.0)	57.1 (3.0)	50.3 (2.1)	45.7 (2.6)
LOA 4+ mm	24.9 (0.8)	33.3 (1.2)	26.6 (1.3)	22.7 (1.2)	20.6 (1.3)
1+ RTCs[c] involving pulpal pathology or a retained root[d]	7.4 (0.5)	17.7 (1.2)	8.7 (0.7)	5.1 (0.8)	2.4 (0.5)
A dental visit in the past 12 months	54.7 (1.0)	34.6 (1.7)	46.0 (1.5)	58.5 (1.5)	69.8 (1.9)

[a]Source: NHANES III. Data given as percent of persons (SE of percent).

[b]Definitions for oral health indicators: *edentulous status,* person has no natural teeth; *untreated coronal decay,* person has one or more coronal tooth surfaces with untreated decay; *untreated root decay,* person has one or more root tooth surfaces with untreated decay; *gingivitis,* person has one or more gingival bleeding sites; *loss of attachment of 4+ mm,* person has one or more sites with LOA of 4+ mm; *any tooth condition involving pulpal pathology or a retained root,* person has one or more RTCs involving pulpal pathology or a retained root; *recent dental visit,* person reported visiting a dentist or dental hygienist in past 12 months.

[c]*RTCs* stands for restorations and tooth conditions that might benefit from treatment.

[d]Data shown are for dentate persons 18–74 years of age.

ed coronal decay, were 7.2 times more likely to have untreated root decay, and were 7.5 times more likely to have a restoration or tooth condition involving pulpal pathology or a retained root that might benefit from treatment (*p* values less than 0.0001). On only two indicators (gingivitis and loss of attachment of 4+ mm) was a lower threshold reached among persons with *upper middle* SES scores. For gingivitis, persons in the *lower* and *lower middle* SES categories also were similar. There was an SES gradient in the recent use of dental services (TABLE 1), but these latter differentials did not account for any of the SES disparities in adult oral health. In one instance (edentulism among persons 35 years and over), the effects of SES were conditional on racial/ethnic background: there was a strong SES gradient in edentulism among white non-Hispanics, but not among Mexican-Americans nor black non-Hispanics (TABLE 2). Racial/ethnic background also was an important effect modifier of the relative frequency of edentulism among the *lower* and *lower middle* SES categories, and partly as well among the *upper middle* SES category (TABLE 2).

TABLE 2. Likelihood of being edentulous by SES categories conditional on racial/ethnic background among persons 35 years and over: United States, 1988–1994[a]

Interaction between SES and race/ethnicity	Likelihood of being edentulous, compared to higher SES white non-Hispanic females of average age by SES index score			
	Lower	Lower middle	Upper middle	Higher
I. Ignored[b]	9.2[c]	5.1[c]	2.3[c]	1.0
II. Taken into account[b]				
Mexican-American	1.5	1.6	0.77[d]	0.132[e]
Black non-Hispanic	4.9[c]	3.2[c]	3.0[c]	1.5
White non-Hispanic	10.3[c]	5.3[c]	2.3[c]	1.0
Pairwise comparisons[f]				
M-A vs. Bn-H	0.0000	0.011	0.0003	0.02
M-A vs. Wn-H	0.0000	0.0000	0.002	0.04
Bn-H vs. Wn-H	0.0001	0.003	0.16	0.17

[a]Source: NHANES III.
[b]Figures given are adjusted odds ratios.
[c]$p \leq 0.0001$.
[d]Mexican-Americans in the upper-middle SES category were observed to be 1.3 times less likely to be edentulous than the reference population (p value, 0.46).
[e]Mexican-Americans in the higher SES category were observed to be 7.6 times less likely to be edentulous than the reference population (p value, 0.04).
[f]Figures given are p values.

CONCLUSIONS

SES disparities in adult oral health occur across a broad spectrum of unmet oral health needs. These disparities mostly take the form of a gradient that is not mediated by recent use of dental services. SES interacts with race/ethnicity in regard to edentulism. Race/ethnicity also modifies the effect of SES on the prevalence of edentulism. Future research needs to clarify the social, psychological, and biological pathways articulating SES and unmet oral health needs. Parallel analyses need to be carried out for key unmet oral health needs of children and adolescents.

Income Inequality, Social Trust, and Self-Reported Health Status in High-Income Countries

GEORGE T.H. ELLISON[a]

Equity and Health Research Programme, Department of Biological Anthropology, University of Cambridge, CB2 3DZ, United Kingdom

INTRODUCTION

A growing number of studies have found a statistical association between income inequality and average health status, both among[1] and within[2] high-income countries. An increasingly popular explanation for this association is that income inequality undermines social cohesion and has a detrimental psychosocial impact on health.[3,4] A recent analysis of income inequality, social distrust, and mortality rates among 39 U.S. states seems to support this explanation.[2] Given the constraints of their cross-sectional analysis, Kawachi *et al.*[2] used a path analysis to investigate the role of social distrust in the relationship between income inequality and age-adjusted mortality rates. If, as their analysis suggests,[2] income inequality leads to worse health status through "disinvestment in social capital" (as measured by the weighted prevalence of social distrust), we would expect to find a similar effect among different high-income countries. We would also expect to find clearer evidence of such an effect on self-reported health status, as this should be more sensitive to psychosocially unhealthy situations.[1,5]

METHODS

Information on social trust and self-reported health status was taken from the 1980 World Values Survey, for which face to face interviews were conducted with representative national samples in 23 countries; a weighting variable was included to compensate for any deviation from population parameters in the households surveyed.[6] The prevalence of social trust and self-reported good/very good health were measured using weighted responses to two items, namely: "Generally speaking, would you say that most people can be trusted or that you can't be too careful in dealing with people?" and "All in all, how would you describe your state of health these days?" Information on average income and income distribution were taken from the 1982, 1983, and 1997 World Development Report, which contained data on GNP per capita (in international dollars) and six measures of income distribution from surveys conducted between 1979 and 1981 for 12 of the high-income (GNP$_{1995}$

[a]Address for correspondence: +44(0)1223 335454(voice); +44(0)1223 335460(fax).
e-mail: gthe2@cam.ac.uk

greater than \$9,700) countries covered by the 1980 World Values Survey.[7] (These countries were Belgium, Canada, Denmark, France, Finland, Japan, the Netherlands, Norway, Spain, Sweden, the United Kingdom, and the United States.) The measures of income distribution comprised the percentage share of equivalized household income received by the lowest 20%, 40%, 60%, and 80% and highest 20% and 10% of each country's households. To provide comparable estimates of average income for countries surveyed in different years, GNP per capita was expressed as a percentage of U.S. GNP in each respective year (GNP_{US100}). Bivariate Spearman's correlation analyses were used to select which measure of income distribution was most strongly correlated with self-reported health status. Forward sequential analyses of covariance (ANCOVAs) were then used to assess the statistical strength of any association between self-reported health status, income distribution, and social trust, independent of differences in average income (GNP_{US100}), after transforming any of those variables with significantly skewed distributions.

RESULTS

Only two of the six measures of income distribution (the proportion of income received by the poorest 60% and 80% of households) displayed statistically significant correlations with the weighted prevalence of good/very good health ($r_s > 0.601$; $p < 0.039$). Both measures were positively correlated with better self-reported health, suggesting that income inequality was associated with an increased prevalence of poor health. Before evaluating the effect of average income and social trust on the strongest of these associations, both GNP_{US100} and the weighted prevalence of good/very good health were squared to adjust their negatively skewed distributions ($g_1 < -1.310$; $p < 0.05$). After controlling for $(GNP_{US100})^2$, there remained a significant positive association between (the weighted prevalence of good/very good health)^2 and the proportion of income received by the poorest 80% of households [B(SEM) = 1232.2 (441.6); $p = 0.021$; see TABLE 1]. There was also a statistically

TABLE 1. Forward sequential analyses of covariance (ANCOVAs) to evaluate the relationship[a] between the proportion of income received by the lowest 80% of households, the weighted prevalence of social trust, and (the weighted prevalence of good/very good health)^2 in 12 high-income countries, after controlling for $(GNP_{US100})^2$

Independent variables	Step 1 B(SEM)	Step 2 B(SEM)	Step 3 B(SEM)
$(GNP_{US100})^2$	−0.04 (0.10)	0.049 (0.11)	−0.04 (0.11)
Income received by lowest 80%	1232.16 (441.57)[b]	—	1201.40 (694.64)[c]
Prevalence of social trust	—	70.49 (39.26)[c]	3.16 (52.71)
Unadjusted r^2	49.2%	30.2%	49.2%
Adjusted r^2	37.9%	14.7%	30.1%

NOTE: Dependent variable: (the weighted prevalence of good/very good health)^2.
[a]Coefficient estimates, B(SEM), and total model unadjusted and adjusted variance, r^2.
[b]$p < 0.05$.
[c]$p < 0.2$.

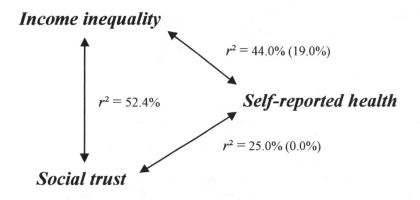

FIGURE 1. The unadjusted variance (r^2) in (self-reported health status)^2 explained by the prevalence of social trust and income inequality, after controlling for $(GNP_{US100})^2$, and one another ($\cdot$).

significant positive association between the weighted prevalence of social trust and the proportion of income received by the poorest 80% of households, even after controlling for $(GNP_{US100})^2$ [B(SEM) = 9.7 (3.0), $p = 0.009$]. However, there was no evidence of a statistical association between social trust and (the weighted prevalence of good/very good health)^2 after controlling for $(GNP_{US100})^2$ [B(SEM) = 70.5 (39.3); $p = 0.106$; see TABLE 1]. Indeed, after controlling for $(GNP_{US100})^2$ and income inequality, the percentage of unadjusted variance (r^2) in (the weighted prevalence of good/very good health)^2 explained by the prevalence of social trust fell to 0.0%, whereas income inequality explained 19.0% of the unadjusted variance in (the weighted prevalence of good/very good health)^2, even after controlling for $(GNP_{US100})^2$ and the prevalence of social trust (see FIG. 1).

DISCUSSION

These results support the idea that income inequality undermines the prevalence of social trust in high-income countries,[2,3] although differences in social trust do not appear to be responsible for international differences in self-reported health status. This suggests that social trust may not mediate the effect of income inequality on average health status *between* high-income countries. However, because perceptions of trust and self-reported health status depend on the sociocultural context of the settings in which they are measured,[5] sociocultural factors might modify the impact of social trust on self-reported health in different countries.

Given the strong association between self-reported health status and objective measures of morbidity and mortality at the *individual* level,[7] it is tempting to infer that aggregate measures of self-reported health at the *population* level accurately reflect disparities in *average* health status. Yet this would represent an "ecological fallacy" if different populations perceive morbidity and mortality differently, even though individuals within each population accurately perceive their own morbidity or mortality risk in comparison to other individuals within their own population.

Indeed, using the weighted prevalence of self-reported health status from 18 high-income countries examined by the 1990/91 World Values Survey, along with matching data on age- and sex-standardized mortality rates (SMR, deaths per 100,000) between 1995 and 2000 from the 1997 World Health Report and estimates of life expectancy at birth in 1990 from the 1992 World Development Report, there is little evidence of any statistical association between self-reported health status and either SMR ($r_s = 0.030$; $p = 0.906$) or life expectancy ($r_s = 0.070$; $p = 0.783$).[8] Even limiting these analyses to European and Scandinavian countries by excluding Canada, Japan, and the United States provides no clearer indication of an association between self-reported health status and either SMR ($r_s = -0.075$; $p = 0.791$) or life expectancy ($r_s = 0.209$; $p = 0.455$). These results suggest that applying comparisons of self-reported health status, morbidity and mortality at the individual level to international comparisons of self-reported health status at the population level may be an "ecological fallacy."

REFERENCES

1. JUDGE, K. et al. 1998. Income inequality and population health. Soc. Sci. Med. **46:** 567–569.
2. KAWACHI, I. et al. 1997. Social capital, income inequality, and mortality. Am. J. Public Health **87:** 1491–1498.
3. WILKINSON, R.G. 1996. Unhealthy Societies. Routledge, London.
4. MARMOT, M.G. 1998. Improvement of social environment to improve health. Lancet **351:** 57–60.
5. MARTIKAINEN, P. et al. 1999. Reliability of perceived health by sex and age. Soc. Sci. Med. **48:** 1117–1122.
6. INGLEHART, R. 1990. Cultural Shift. Princeton University Press, Princeton.
7. IDLER, E.L. & Y. BENYAMINI. 1997. Self-rated health and mortality: a review of twenty-seven community studies. J. Health Soc. Behav. **38:** 21–37.
8. ELLISON, G.T.H. 2000. Mortality, life expectancy and self-reported health status in high-income countries: an ecological fallacy exposed. Ann. Human. Biol. **27:** in press.

The Human Development Index and Per Capita Gross National Product as Predictors of Dental Caries Prevalence in Industrialized and Industrializing Countries

M.H. HOBDELL,[a,b] R. LALLOO,[c] AND N.G. MYBURGH[c]

[b]University of Texas-Houston, Dental Branch,
6516 John Freeman Avenue, Houston, Texas 77030, USA

[c]University of the Western Cape, Faculty of Dentistry, Oral Health Centre,
Private Bag X08, 7785, Mitchells Plain, South Africa

High prevalence of dental caries in children in industrialized communities has been associated with high levels of available sugar. More recently, however the relationship between dental caries and sugar availability in industrialized countries has come into question, because of the effectiveness of different methods of dental caries prevention, despite continuing high levels of available sugar. As there has been a decline in overall dental caries prevalence in industrialized countries, so material deprivation has emerged as a contributing or associated factor of high dental caries prevalence. Factors indicative of material deprivation in preschool children that have been investigated are low birth weight, low uptake of polio vaccination, and being a part of a single parent family. This study was undertaken to explore two issues: first, whether the relationship between sugar availability and dental caries prevalence demonstrated by Screebny in 1982[1] still holds, given the reductions in dental caries levels that have occurred in industrialized countries since then. Second, whether the relationship between dental caries and deprivation could be demonstrated internationally, between countries, at different levels of socioeconomic development. Data were obtained from three separate sources: dental caries data from the World Health Organization Global Oral Epidemiology Data Bank,[2] sugar data from the United Nations Food and Agricultural Organization (UNFAO),[3] calculated as the mean sugar availability for the five years preceding the date of the dental epidemiological survey given in the 1994 WHO report; and socioeconomic data from the United Nations Development Programme (UNDP).[4] Additional dental caries and sugar availability data were obtained from the 1982 paper of Screebny, which contained comparable data for 47 countries. Complete 1982 and 1994 sets of data were available for 26 of Screebny's original 47 countries. These were grouped according to their 1978 GNP classification. The composition of the HDI was not finalized in 1982, so it was not used in this comparison. The Human Development Index (HDI score) and annual per capita share of the Gross National Product (GNP in US$) were used as proxy measures of economic and material disadvantage. The 1994 WHO

[a]Address for correspondence: 713-500-4022 (voice); 713-500-4100 (fax).
e-mail: mhobdell@mail.db.uth.tmc.edu

TABLE 1. Comparison of the mean 12-year-old DMFT and available sugar in grams/ day in 26 countries in 1982 and 1994, by socioeconomic group (high, medium, low)

Year	High		Medium		Low	
	Sugar	DMFT	Sugar	DMFT	Sugar	DMFT
GNP (1994)	114.1	2.0	84.1	2.2	25.7	1.1
GNP (1982)	113.5	4.9	76.8	2.9	27.6	1.6

mean 12-year-old DMFT score with the UNDP, HDI score, together with the 1991 World Bank per capita GNP, were obtained for 101 countries. These were then grouped according to the UNDP and World Bank 1994 classifications of their HDI and GNP values (high-H, medium-M, and low-L). In addition to the DMFT, HDI, and GNP data, the mean annual urban population growth rate (1960–1992), mean years of schooling (1992), mean percentage of low-weight births (1985–1990), daily caloric availability as a percentage of requirements (1988–1990), infant mortality rate (1992), under-five mortality rate (1992), and mean annual growth in per capita GNP (1980–1991) were abstracted from the 1994 UNDP Report. Despite the inherent weaknesses of the WHO epidemiological data, there is good evidence in these findings that the relationship between sugar availability and dental caries, demonstrated by Screebny in 1982, no longer exists, at least in the high and low socioeconomic groups (TABLE 1). It is suggested that this could be for two very different yet not unrelated reasons. Prevention of dental caries has increased significantly in industrialized countries in this time period, since the introduction of fluoridated toothpastes and other regimes. These are less available in low-income countries. In the low-income countries, the social disruptions of war and civil unrest and externally driven macroeconomic changes have significantly increased the numbers of people living below the poverty line during this same time period. Historically under these circumstances, dental caries prevalence has decreased. The data presented here suggest that the increasing urbanization and national wealth (found mainly in those countries experiencing economic transformation) may be important factors in determining changes in caries prevalence (TABLE 2). Many communities in the United States, particularly those along the Rio Grande Valley and in certain areas elsewhere

TABLE 2. Regression analyses: dependent variable—DMFT score for 12 year olds

Independent variables	r	p
HDI	0.33	0.001
GNP	−0.6	0.1
HDI + GNP (multiple regression)	0.001	
Growth in urban population	−0.26	0.025
Mean years of schooling	0.22	0.05
Infant mortality rate	−0.23	0.05
Under-five mortality rate	−0.28	0.01

in large cities, are passing through similar changes. It is suggested that it is these communities that are more at risk of increased levels of dental caries than are those who have been resident for longer and have traditionally stayed longer in school. Decreasing infant and under-five mortality rates in a population would also seem to signal a possible rise in dental caries, prevalence, unless population-wide preventive measures are in place.

REFERENCES

1. SCREEBNY, L.M. 1982. Sugar availability, sugar consumption and dental caries. Commun. Dent. Oral Epidemiol. **10:** 1–7.
2. BARMES, D.E. & J. SARDO-INFIRRI. 1977. WHO activities in oral epidemiology. Commun. Dent. Oral Epidemiol. **5:** 22–29.
3. UNFAO. 1999. Food Balance Sheets Reports. <http:www.fao.org/waicent/waicent .htm> 1984/96.
4. UNDP. 1994. Human Development Report. Oxford University Press, New York.

Pathways between Area-Level Income Inequality and Increased Mortality in U.S. Men

H.S. KAHN,[a,b] A.V. PATEL,[b] E.J. JACOBS,[b] E.E. CALLE,[b]
B.P. KENNEDY,[c] AND I. KAWACHI[c]

[b]American Cancer Society, Atlanta, Georgia 30329, USA

[c]Department of Health and Social Behavior, Harvard School of Public Health, 677 Huntington Avenue, Boston, Massachusetts 02115, USA

CONTEXT

In multilevel epidemiologic analysis, independent variables may be defined at the geographic area level or at the individual level. Area-level income inequality is associated with increased all-cause mortality rates. In the American Cancer Society's prospective Cancer Prevention Study-II (CPS-II), we found such an association only among men at attained ages 30–74 years old whose education was not above high school graduation (TABLE 1), but not among women or men with higher education. To explore the biologic or social mechanisms underlying this observed association, we wished to learn if adjustment for any individual-level behavior or characteristic would reduce the effect on mortality of area-level income inequality. If it did, this would suggest that the individual-level factor might play a role in the increased mortality risk associated with living in areas of high income inequality.

DESIGN

CPS-II is a 14-year mortality follow-up study including participants from all 318 U.S. standard metropolitan statistical areas (SMSAs; described in the 1980 U.S. Census). For each SMSA we calculated the area-level income inequality as the decile ratio of household incomes, that is, the top 10% versus the bottom 10% within the SMSA. Using Cox proportional-hazards analyses, we assessed the change in the SMSA-level mortality risk resulting from adjustment for various individual-level characteristics.

PARTICIPANTS

Our analytic cohort included 76,628 men in CPS-II with attained ages 30–74 years and education not beyond high school graduate who provided personal, indi-

[a]Address for correspondence: Henry S. Kahn, M.D., Centers for Disease Control, Division of Diabetes Translation, MS K-68, 4770 Buford Highway, Atlanta, Georgia 30341-3724, USA. 770-488-1052 (voice); 770-488-1148 (fax).

e-mail: hsk1@cdc.gov

TABLE 1. All-cause mortality experience in CPS-II of male, modestly educated (not above high school graduate), SMSA residents (n = 76,628) during 14-year follow-up

Area-level income inequality	30–64 years[a]		65–74 years[a]		30–74 years[a]	
	Mortality rate	RR (95% CI)	Mortality rate	RR (95% CI)	Mortality rate	RR (95% CI)
Low	809.2	1.00	2442.7	1.00	1356.5	1.00
Moderate	906.7	1.12 (1.05–1.20)	2598.3	1.06 (1.01–1.12)	1473.5	1.09 (1.04–1.13)
High	879.5	1.09 (1.00–1.18)	2693.6	1.10 (1.04–1.17)	1487.4	1.10 (1.04–1.15)

NOTE: Mortality rates are presented as age-adjusted (5-year intervals) annual deaths per 100,000, by area-level income inequality (low, moderate, high) and by attained age (30–64 years, 65–74 years, 30–74 years).

[a] Attained age.

TABLE 2. Age-adjusted rate ratios and 95% CI for all-cause mortality by area-level income inequality after adjustments for individual-level variables with adjustment for alternative individual-level variables

Area-level income inequality	—	Smoking	Exercise	Alcohol intake	Body mass index	Civic participation	Friends and relatives	Marital status	Vegetable intake	Prevalent disease
Low	1.00 —	1.00 —	1.00 —	1.00 —	1.00 —	1.00 —	1.00 —	1.00 —	1.00 —	1.00 —
Moderate	1.08 1.03–1.12	1.05 1.01–1.09	1.06 1.02–1.10	1.07 1.03–1.12	1.07 1.03–1.12	1.06 1.02–1.11	1.08 1.03–1.12	1.07 1.03–1.12	1.08 1.04–1.12	1.06 1.02–1.10
High	1.09 1.04–1.15	1.05 1.00–1.10	1.06 1.01–1.11	1.09 1.04–1.14	1.09 1.03–1.14	1.07 1.02–1.13	1.09 1.04–1.14	1.09 1.04–1.14	1.09 1.04–1.14	1.08 1.03–1.13

NOTE: Participants were 72,628 modestly educated men in CPS-II, attained ages 30–74.

vidual-level information at baseline in 1982. This predominantly white cohort excluded men who did not reside in a SMSA, those who had changed residential neighborhoods between 1980 and 1982, and those who reported a history of cancer at baseline.

RESULTS

In our proportional-hazards model adjusted only for age (1-year intervals), men from the 63 SMSAs of greatest income inequality (decile ratio, 23.0 to 39.4) had higher age-adjusted, all-cause mortality rates (rate ratio [RR] = 1.09, 95% CI 1.04–1.15) than men from the 111 SMSAs of least income inequality (decile ratio, 12.8 to 17.9). This high/low inequality RR was reduced by further adjustment for individual-level smoking (RR = 1.05, 95% CI 1.00–1.10) or for exercise (RR = 1.06, 95% CI 1.01–1.11) (TABLE 2). Smaller reductions were found with adjustments for individual-level civic participation (attendance at church, clubs, and groups) or for prevalent chronic disease (self-reported heart disease, stroke or diabetes).

INTERPRETATIONS

Among modestly educated men, smoking or limitation of exercise may play a role in the excess mortality associated with living in areas of high income inequality. Other individual characteristics, perhaps reflecting psychosocial stress or diminished life opportunities, may also participate in multiple pathways from area-level inequality to mortality, but their impacts on the area-level effects appear to be weak. Interruption of any single pathway is unlikely to eliminate the risk associated with living in areas of income inequality.

Education, Income, Wealth, and Health among Whites and African Americans

JOAN M. OSTROVE[a,b] AND PAMELA FELDMAN[c]

[b]Health Psychology Program, University of California, San Francisco, San Francisco, California 94143, USA

[c]Carnegie Mellon University, Pittsburgh, Pennsylvania 15213, USA

This investigation explored the relationship of socioeconomic status (SES) to physical and mental health in two nationally representative samples of whites and African Americans. In general, as SES levels increase, rates of morbidity and mortality decrease.[1] SES also shows a linear association with mental health.[2] Although this association has been demonstrated in many countries and across time, the nature of the association may not be the same in different populations even within the United States. It has been suggested that African Americans may not benefit equally in terms of attaining better physical health as their SES levels rise.[3]

We used data from the American's Changing Lives (ACL) and the Health and Retirement (HRS) surveys, which included large subsamples of African Americans and whites to examine the meaning of several SES indicators (income, education, employment) and their relation to health in each racial group. We also assessed the contribution of a less traditional indicator of SES—wealth—in the SES–health relationship. Assessment of wealth, or net worth, has been suggested as an additional and potentially more comprehensive measure of SES than education and income.[4]

In both studies, African Americans had lower levels of education, household income, and wealth than whites. Unexpectedly, however, the strength of the interrelationships among the three SES indicators did not differ for African Americans and whites. In addition, we found that SES operated to affect physical and mental health in a very similar fashion for African Americans and whites. (See TABLES 1 and 2.) We found that wealth, in addition to more traditional indicators of SES, made a unique and significant contribution to explaining both physical and mental health for African Americans and whites. Thus, different indicators of SES including wealth appear to have a similar impact on the health of both racial groups. Examining the relations of different SES indicators to health across groups is critical to eliminating persistent social inequalities in health.

REFERENCES

1. ADLER, N.E., T. BOYCE, M.A. CHESNEY, S. COHEN, S. FOLKMAN, R.L. KAHN & S.L. SYME. 1994. Socioeconomic status and health: the challenge of the gradient. Am. Psychol. **49:** 15–24.

[a]Current address for correspondence: Joan M. Ostrove, Ph.D., Department of Psychology, Macalester College, St. Paul, Minnesota 55105, USA.

2. Brown, H.D. & N.E. Adler. 1998. Socioeconomic status. *In* Encyclopedia of Mental Health. 555–561. Academic Press, San Diego.
3. Anderson, N.B. & C.A. Armstead. 1995. Toward understanding the association of socioeconomic status and health: a new challenge for the biopsychosocial approach. Psychosom. Med. **57:** 213–225.
4. Oliver, M.L. & T.M. Shapiro. 1995. Black Wealth, White Wealth. Routledge, New York.

TABLE 1. Individual and simultaneous regression models predicting self-reported health

	Americans Changing Lives		Health and Retirement Survey	
	Individual model Bs	Simultaneous model Bs	Individual model Bs	Simultaneous model Bs
Step 1				
Age	-0.29^c	-0.29^c	-0.09^c	-0.09^c
Gender[a]	-0.05^c	-0.05^c	-0.08^c	-0.08^c
Step 2				
Race[b]	-0.07^c	-0.07^c	-0.16^c	-0.16^c
Step 3				
Education	0.18^c	0.12^c	0.34^c	0.19^c
Employment status	0.23^c	0.19^c	0.23^c	0.20^c
Household income	0.19^c	0.06	0.39^c	0.13^c
Wealth	0.12^c	0.04	0.38^c	0.25^c
Step 4				
Race * Education	0.00	-0.03	0.01	0.01
Race * Employment status	0.06	0.03	0.07^c	0.04
Race * Household income	0.04	0.05	0.01	0.00
Race * Wealth	0.02	-0.01	-0.01	-0.03
Overall R[b]	0.09^c to 0.12^c	0.14^c	0.10^c to 0.14^c	0.22^c

NOTE: All continuous independent variables are standardized. Unstandardized betas are reported for these variables; standardized betas are reported for categorical variables.
[a]Gender is dummy coded, 0 = male, 1 = female.
[b]Race is dummy coded, 0 = white, 1 = African American.
[c]$p < 0.01$.

TABLE 2. Individual and simultaneous regression models predicting depression

	Americans Changing Lives		Health and Retirement Survey	
	Individual model Bs	Simultaneous model Bs	Individual model Bs	Simultaneous model Bs
Step 1				
Age	0.03	0.03	-0.01	-0.01
Gender[a]	0.08^c	0.08^c	0.14^c	0.14^c
Step 2				
Race[b]	0.13^c	0.13^c	0.09^c	0.09^c
Step 3				
Education	-0.16^c	-0.07^c	-0.08^c	-0.03^c
Employment status	-0.17^c	-0.14^c	-0.19^c	-0.15^c
Household income	-0.25^c	-0.10^c	-0.12^c	-0.05^c
Wealth	-0.18^c	-0.08^c	-0.12^c	-0.08^c
Step 4				
Race * Education	-0.01	0.01	-0.03	-0.02
Race * Employment status	-0.03	0.01	-0.08^c	-0.03
Race * Household income	-0.02	-0.03	-0.03	-0.01
Race * Wealth	-0.03	-0.02	-0.01	0.02
Overall R^b	0.04^c to 0.08^c	0.09^c	0.06^c to 0.10^c	0.15^c

NOTE: All continuous independent variables are standardized. Unstandardized betas are reported for these variables; standardized betas are reported for categorical variables.
[a]Gender is dummy coded, 0 = male, 1 = female.
[b]Race is dummy coded, 0 = white, 1 = African American.
[c]$p < 0.01$.

Income Inequality and Mortality in Canada and the United States

An Analysis of Provinces/States

NANCY A. ROSS[a] AND MICHAEL C. WOLFSON

Statistics Canada, Ottawa, Ontario, Canada K1A 0T6

The "big idea" published in the April 20th, 1996 edition of the *British Medical Journal* is that what matters for mortality and health in an industrial society is not the absolute wealth of that society but rather how equitably wealth is distributed. Studies in support of this idea have examined data from different countries,[1] U.S. states,[2,3] and U.S. metropolitan areas.[4]

To extend this work, measures of inequality and age-group specific mortality for the 10 Canadian provinces and 53 Canadian metropolitan areas were calculated. Inequality was measured as the amount of income belonging to households earning less than the median income of the state/province or metropolitan area (the "median share").[b] The analyses consisted of age-group specific multiple regression models (weighted by population size) for the U.S. states and the Canadian provinces. For details of the metropolitan area analysis see Ross *et al.*[5] The multiple regression modeling proceeded incrementally with models fit first for the 50 U.S states only, then with the Canadian provinces and finally with a dummy variable to take account of mortality differences between Canada and the United States after accounting for median share and mean state/provincial income.

For U.S. states, after controlling for mean state income, the median share was a significant explanatory variable in models of infant (less than 1 year), children/youth (1 to 24 years), working-age male and female (25–64 years) and all-age mortality (TABLE 1). The effect was largest for working-age males where a 1% increase in the proportion of income going to the bottom half of households was associated with a mortality decline, independent of mean state income, of approximately 49 deaths per 100,000.

The overall explanatory significance of the models improved with the addition of the 10 Canadian provinces. This was not surprising given that the provinces tended to have lower mortality and greater equality than the U.S. states. In the models

---

[a]Address for correspondence: Nancy A. Ross, RH Coats Bldg., 24th Floor, Statistics Canada, Ottawa, ON Canada K1A 0T6. 1-613-951-3735 (voice); 1-951-5643 (fax).

e-mail: rossnan@statcan.ca

[b]The inequality measures for the U.S. states and metropolitan areas are from Kaplan *et al.*[2] and Lynch *et al.*,[4] respectively. U.S. state-level mortality rates are three-year averages (1989–1991) and were calculated based on counts downloaded from the Centers for Disease Control's Wonder web site. The U.S. metropolitan area mortality rates are from Lynch *et al.*[4] Corresponding Canadian income inequality measures were derived from 1991 census microdata; and three-year average Canadian mortality rates (1990–1992) were calculated from Statistics Canada's National Mortality Database. All mortality rates were standardized to the age distribution of the Canadian population in 1991.

TABLE 1. Regression results for U.S.-only models ($n = 50$), combined Canada and U.S. models ($n = 60$), and models ($n = 60$) incorporating a dummy country indicator, by age grouping

Age group	Model	Intercept	Median share (%)	Mean income (in thousands of dollars)	Country flag	Adjusted R^2
Infants	U.S. only	**1773**	**−31.94**	−4.50	—	0.13
	U.S. and Canada	**2189**	**−50.72**	**−5.60**	—	0.36
	U.S. and Canada w/ dummy	**1660**	**−31.22**	−4.20	**85.00**	0.42
Children and youth	U.S. only	**161**	**−3.76**	**−0.60**	—	0.53
	U.S. and Canada	**163**	**−3.85**	**−0.60**	—	0.66
	U.S. and Canada w/ dummy	**160**	**−4.85**	**−0.60**	0.48	0.65
Working-age men	U.S. only	**1526**	**−49.07**	−0.10	—	0.61
	U.S. and Canada	**1567**	**−50.70**	−0.30	—	0.67
	U.S. and Canada w/ dummy	**1511**	**−48.63**	−0.20	8.99	0.73
Working-age women	U.S. only	**630**	**−16.98**	−0.20	—	0.46
	U.S. and Canada	**690**	**−19.60**	−0.40	—	0.64
	U.S. and Canada w/ dummy	**612**	**−16.75**	−0.20	**12.44**	0.59
Elderly men	U.S. only	**8186**	−76.45	**−21.00**	—	0.15
	U.S. and Canada	**8113**	−72.70	**−21.00**	—	0.21
	U.S. and Canada w/ dummy	**8140**	−73.68	**−21.10**	−4.28	0.20
Elderly women	U.S. only	**5360**	−56.41	0.90	—	0.03
	U.S. and Canada	**6032**	**−85.83**	−1.30	—	0.18
	U.S. and Canada w/ dummy	**5139**	−52.87	1.00	**143.67**	0.23
All ages	U.S. Only	**1407**	**−26.86**	−1.30	—	0.32
	U.S. and Canada	**1481**	**−30.07**	−1.60	—	0.49
	U.S. and Canada w/ dummy	**1379**	**−26.30**	−1.30	16.45	0.49

NOTE: Bold numbers indicate statistical significance at $p < 0.05$.

containing the country dummy variable, there were significantly higher infant and female mortality rates in the U.S. than in Canada, after accounting for both the distribution of state/provincial income and the mean state/provincial income.

Like the state/provincial level comparison shown here, Canadian metropolitan areas generally had more equal distributions of income and lower mortality rates than U.S. metropolitan areas. The unemployment rate was strongly positively associated with mortality in Canada (data not shown) at both the provincial and metropolitan area levels. Although unemployment was also related to mortality in the same way in the United States, states with high unemployment also tended to have relatively unequal income distributions.[2] In Canada, unemployment was unrelated to provincial inequality.

Overall, the general location of Canadian provinces and metropolitan areas with respect to U.S. states and metropolitan areas supported the association of higher (lower) inequality with higher (lower) mortality. Within Canada, however, there was no relationship between inequality and mortality. One important difference between the two countries is that unemployment and inequality go hand-in-hand at the state level in the United States but they do not, at the provincial level, in Canada. Even after accounting for income distribution and mean income, infant and female mortality was lower in Canada than in the United States. Infants and women are the heaviest users of health care services so it is plausible that differences in mortality attributable to universal access would be most apparent in these groups.

REFERENCES

1. WILKINSON, R.G. 1992. Income distribution and life expectancy. Br. Med. J. **304:** 165–168.
2. KAPLAN, G.A., E.R. PAMUK, J.W. LYNCH, *et al.* 1996. Inequality in income and mortality in the United States: analysis of mortality and potential pathways. Br. Med. J. **312:** 999–1003.
3. KENNEDY, B.P., I. KAWACHI & D. PROTHROW-STITH. 1996. Income distribution and mortality: cross-sectional ecological study of the Robin Hood Index in the United States. Br. Med. J. **312:** 1004–1007.
4. LYNCH, J.W., G.A. KAPLAN, E.R. PAMUK, *et al.* 1998. Income inequality and mortality in metropolitan areas of the United States. Am. J. Public Health **88:** 1074–1080.
5. ROSS, N.A., M.C. WOLFSON, J.R. DUNN, J.-M. BERTHELOT, G.A. KAPLAN & J.W. LYNCH. Income inequality in Canada and the United States. Br. J. Med. Submitted.

For Richer, for Poorer, in Sickness and in Health: Socioeconomic Status and Health among Married Couples

DIANE S. SHINBERG[a]

Center for Demography and Ecology and Department of Sociology,
University of Wisconsin—Madison,
1180 Observatory Drive, Madison, Wisconsin 53706, USA

Do socioeconomic status (SES) gradients differ between husbands and wives? Marital status has been linked to health through material support, through psychosocial support, through social control, and through health selection into (and out of) marriage. Marriage is one social institution in which many interpersonal, social, and environmental characteristics of the participants are shared. Distinguishing between the characteristics shared by married spouses and the unshared or personal characteristics within the couple may aid in understanding social influences on health. The measurement of SES sometimes blurs this distinction between shared and unshared characteristics within couples. Often so-called "individual" level SES (education, occupation, and income) is measured at the family or couple level, rather than at the personal level. For example, when measuring SES for married women who lack current or continuous employment, researchers often source the SES of the husband as though it was the same as the SES of the wife.

For this paper, I differentiate the personal SES of wives from the personal SES of husbands in order to examine SES and health among married couple pairs using a sample of midlife adults followed for over thirty-five years in the Wisconsin Longitudinal Study (WLS). In the WLS, data were collected on family background, education, occupation, income, and other social characteristics from a cohort of high school graduates since 1957. The most recent rounds of the study surveyed some 8500 high school graduates at ages 53 and 54 in 1992–1993. Through the 1975 and 1992 interviews, extensive data on the socioeconomic characteristics of respondents and their spouses were collected. The analytic sample used in this research is limited to study participants who responded in both the 1975 and the 1992 waves and who were currently married to the same spouse at both waves, yielding a sample of 4698 couples who were in stable marriages for at least 17 years (the inter-wave period). Because the original respondents of the WLS are Wisconsin high school seniors in the class of 1957, they are almost exclusively non-Hispanic white.

For this paper, I include measures of the SES characteristics for *each* spouse. Both husbands and wives in this study are coded according to their own educational attainment as of 1975, their own individual 1974 earnings, and their own employ-

[a]Current address for correspondence: D. Shinberg, Division of Health Interview Statistics, Centers for Disease Control and Prevention, 6525 Belcrest Rd., Room 875, Hyattsville, MD 20782, USA. 301-458-4669 (voice); 301-458-4035 (fax).
e-mail: zik1@cdc.gov

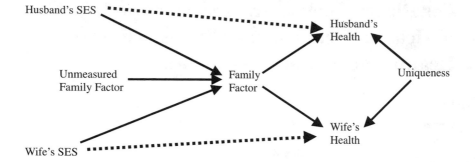

FIGURE 1. MIMIC model of couples' health at midlife: The Wisconsin Longitudinal Study.

ment status (whether or not they worked) and their own occupational status (based on the 1970 Duncan Socioeconomic Index) for their current or last job as of 1975. Health is measured for *each* spouse with self-reported health status for primary respondents in the WLS, and with respondents' proxy reports of health for their husbands or wives. Health status is measured categorically as very poor, poor, fair, good, or excellent.

TABLE 1. Parameter estimates for preferred model of couples' socioeconomic status and couple's health: The Wisconsin Longitudinal Study

Exogenous 1974–1975 SES variables	Husband's health in 1992	Wife's health in 1992
Husband's educational attainment[a]	**0.150** (0.017)	**0.054** (0.008)
Wife's educational attainment[a]	**0.032** (0.006)	**0.054** (0.008)
Husband's earnings[b]	**0.032** (0.007)	**0.055** (0.009)
Wife's earnings[b]	**0.032** (0.007)	**0.055** (0.009)
Husband's employment status[c]	−0.008 (0.015)[e]	**0.124** (0.009)
Wife's employment status[c]	**0.073** (0.008)	**0.026** (0.014)
Husband's occupational status[d]	**0.057** (0.009)	**0.096** (0.013)
Wife's occupational status[d]	**0.027** (0.007)	**0.046** (0.011)

NOTE: Estimated total effects and their (standard errors) are reported. **Bolded** coefficients are more than twice their standard errors.

[a]Educational attainment by 1975 is reported in years.

[b]Earnings for 1974 reported in $100's.

[c]Employment status for 1975 coded 1 for no job and 0 for employed.

[d]Occupational status for 1975 is Duncan SEI score for current/last job.

[e]The only parameter sensitive to respondent-proxy status is the direct influence of husband's employment status on husband's health. The total effect of husband's employment status on husband's health is **−0.0935** (0.0148) when husbands' characteristics are reported by wives. The direct effect given in the table is for when husbands report their own characteristics.

Using this sample of primary respondents and their spouses as couple pairs, first I examined the correlation of general health status between couples. Next, I estimated a modified MIMIC (multiple indicator, multiple cause) model to predict the general health outcomes for couples (using LISREL 8).[1] That is, in a structural equation framework, I specified a common latent couple factor that affects the 1992 health of the husband and wife in each couple (FIG. 1). Measures of socioeconomic status (e.g., educational attainment, earnings, and employment and occupational status) derived from the 1975 interview are modeled to affect the common latent factor. I consider whether and how the SES characteristics of *each* spouse jointly influence the health of *each* spouse within married couples. Each individual socioeconomic status measure is tested for whether or not it directly affects the individual spouse's health status, net of the shared couple factor.

All the measures of husbands' and wives' SES from early midlife tested in these models were significantly and positively related to *both* spouses' health at later midlife (TABLE 1). The educational attainment, employment status, and earnings of husbands contribute equally to the common family factor as do the educational attainment, employment status, and earnings of wives. Although both husbands' and wives' occupational status contribute to the common family factor, husbands' occupational status contributes more than wives'. Both husbands' and wives' employment status is related directly to their own health status. Husbands' educational attainment directly influences husbands' health over and above its indirect effects through the common family factor. However, wives' educational attainment does not contribute directly to wives' health. There were almost no differences in the relationships among health and SES by respondent-proxy status. Gender differences (between husbands and wives) were much more important in these models for these data than respondent-proxy status. The preferred model explained 62–64% of the variance in wives' health, but only 26% of the variance in husbands' health.

The socioeconomic status of individuals and their significant family members, viz., spouses, shape their health in later life. Investigations of SES differentials in adult health should include the socioeconomic characteristics of individuals and their spouses. Where possible, such investigations should use couple models to take advantage of the shared aspects of the family socioeconomic environment.

REFERENCE

1. JÖRESKOG K.G. & D. SÖRBOM. 1996. LISREL 8: User's Reference Guide. Scientific Software International, Inc. Chicago.

Determinants of Health:
Testing of a Conceptual Model

BARBARA STARFIELD[a] AND LEIYU SHI

Department of Health Policy and Management,
Johns Hopkins University School of Hygiene and Public Health,
624 North Broadway, Baltimore, Maryland 21205-1996, USA

Systematic exploration of the relative strength of the many determinants of health requires a framework or model for organizing research endeavors. Despite the 150-year-old literature on social determinants of health, there have been few efforts at developing such a model. The Lalonde Report (1974),[1] which popularized a prior conceptualization of health as being determined by biological, environmental, life style, and health care organization, is still cited and even repeated in various incarnations as a prototype, despite the fact that much greater specificity is required if policy decisions are to result from scholarly inquiry.

In this presentation we provide an example of the evolution of causal diagrams from the early 1970s to the late 1990s.[2–5] This example shows how discrete lines of scholarly endeavors can shape the way these diagrams are formed. For example, in the 1970s and 1980s Aaron Antonovsky's work[6] on social coherence influenced the specification of pathways; in the 1990s, social cohesion has replace social coherence, even though it is a variable more related to social context than to individual psychological representation of 'feelings.' Very few empirical studies address more than two steps in a postulated pathway.[6,7]

More recent models (FIG. 1) explicitly represent the ecological context that influences individuals primarily indirectly through more proximate social and environmental phenomena, and even more proximate individual manifestations of these contextual phenomena. Virtually absent from most of the recent literature is consideration of the contextual variables related to health services organization and delivery and their translation into individual experiences of quality of services received.

When these more comprehensive models are used, it becomes evident that no single pathway is responsible for manifestation of a population's health. Rather, the interaction between a variety of types of domains, including the biological, social, behavioral, environmental, and medical become clear. As noted by Greenland *et al.,*[9] conventional multivariate techniques for assessing the strength of relationships become problematic as the interactions among variables overwhelms the ability of these techniques to accurately characterize the interactions.

A simple example of these interactions is provided by the work of Shi *et al.,*[10] who used a path analytic strategy informed by FIGURE 1 to examine the relative impact of the contextual variables of income inequality and the supply of primary care versus specialty physicians in the 50 U.S. states. They found that both income inequality and the supply of primary care physicians directly influenced most of the

[a]Address for correspondence: 410-614-3737 (voice); 410-614-9046 (fax).
e-mail: bstarfie@jhsph.edu [*or*] Ishi@jhs.edu

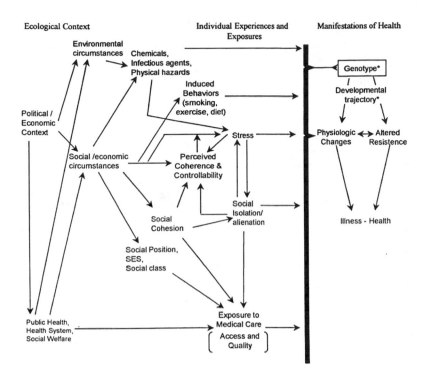

FIGURE 1. Prevention of death, disease, and disability. (Adapted from B. Starfield.[8])

population health indicators and that income equality acted, in part, through primary care physician, to population ratios. Some health care resources (primary care physicians) but not others (specialty physicians) partly compensated for the adverse effect of income inequality.

REMAINING CHALLENGES

The following are important remaining challenges in the development and application of causal diagrams.

1. Specification and standardization of measures of the important variables in the pathway, as well as possible modifiers and interaction effects with other and possibly unknown factors;
2. Standardization of measures of health as appropriate "outcomes";
3. Cohort effects and latencies, and critical periods, that is, within cohorts, historical influences on different cohorts, cumulative effects over time within cohorts, and presence of critical periods;
4. More appropriate statistical techniques for path analyses;
5. Specification of causal pathways for "positive health" as a complement to those for determinants of mortality, morbidity, and disability.

REFERENCES

1. EVANS, R., M. BARER & T. MARMOR. 1994. Why Are Some People Healthy and Others Not? The Determinants of Health of Populations. Aldine de Gruyter, New York.
2. STARFIELD, B. 1973. Health services research: a working model. N. Engl. J. Med. **289:** 132–136.
3. BLUM, H.L. 1981. Planning for Health. Human Sciences Press, New York.
4. ACHESON, SIR DONALD. 1998. Independent Inquiry into Inequalities in Health. The Stationery Office, London.
5. BOSMA, H., H. DIKE VAN DE MHEEN & J.P. MACKENBACH. 1999. Social class in childhood and general health in adulthood: questionnaire study of contribution of psychological attributes. Br. Med. J. **318:** 18–22.
6. ANTONOVSKY, A. 1979. Health, Stress, and Coping. Jossey-Bass, San Francisco.
7. KAWACHI, I., B.P. KENNEDY, S.M. LOCHNER & D. PROTHROW-STITH. 1997. Social capital, income inequality, and mortality. Am. J. Public Health **87:** 1491–1495.
8. STARFIELD, B. 1998. Primary Care: Balancing Health Needs, Services and Technology. Oxford University Press, New York.
9. GREENLAND, S., J. PEARL & J. ROBINS. 1999. Causal diagrams for epidemiologic research. Epidemiology **10:** 37–48.
10. SHI, L. B. STARFIELD, B. KENNEDY & I. KAWACHI. 1999. Income, inequality, primary care, and health indicators. J. Fam. Pract. **4:** 275–284.

The Direct and Indirect Effects of Metropolitan Area Inequality on Mortality

A Hierarchical Analysis

NORMAN J. WAITZMAN,[a,b] KEN R. SMITH,[c] AND ANTOINETTE STROUP[c]

[b]Department of Economics, University of Utah, Salt Lake City, Utah 84112, USA

[c]Department of Family and Consumer Studies, University of Utah, Salt Lake City, Utah 84112USA

BACKGROUND

In previous research, we delineated several of the conceptual issues regarding the pathways by which socioeconomic characteristics of areas might affect individual health[1] and constructed first-time empirical analyses of the effects of poverty-area residence[2,3] and of residential economic segregation in metropolitan areas[1] on individual mortality using national samples. These analyses showed that area characteristics independently influenced mortality rather than serving as mere proxies for socioeconomic characteristics of individual residents. They also suggested that both the *level* and spatial *distribution* of resources in relatively large metropolitan areas significantly affected the life chances of residents. In this analysis, we extended our earlier research by considering (1) the extent to which the health effects associated with *spatial economic segregation* might be attributable to the *statistical distribution* of area income, and also by providing (2) a preliminary assessment as to hierarchical structure, that is, the extent to which area effects indirectly affect mortality by modifying the effects on mortality of individual socioeconomic status.

METHODS

The data for our analysis, described in detail elsewhere,[1] comprised nine successive annual National Health Interview Surveys (NHIS) from 1986 to 1994 matched to death certificates through 1995. Metropolitan statistical area (MSA) identifiers were appended to the data for respondents residing in thirty-four of the largest metropolitan statistical areas (MSAs) in the United States. The sample was restricted to 136,956 respondents aged 35 to 65 years residing in one of those MSAs, of which 3,715 had died by 1996.

Economic segregation, or *spatial inequality*, in each area was gauged by the so-called "*p* index" of poverty, roughly the average across tracts of the probability of within-tract encounters between residents above and below the poverty line in each MSA in 1990. *Statistical inequality* was measured by the 1990 Gini coefficient on family income in each MSA. Incorporation of both measures provided a test of the

[a]Address for correspondence: Norman J. Waitzman, Ph.D., Department of Economics, University of Utah, 1645 E. Central Campus Dr. Front, Salt Lake City, UT 84112, USA. 801-581-7600 (voice); 801-585-5649 (fax).

e-mail: waitzman@econ.sbs.utah.edu

extent to which each characteristic provides distinct effects on mortality. In addition, a measure of MSA-level median income was incorporated in a full model to assess the extent to which the effects of area *inequality* were distinct from the effects of the *level* of area economic development.

A two-stage, hierarchical model was constructed and statistically estimated using hierarchical linear modeling (HLM). The HLM procedure consisted of running a first-stage logistic regression analysis of mortality on individual covariates and then running a second-stage equation analyzing the extent to which area features shift and modify the estimated coefficients from the first level. The individual characteristics incorporated in level one of our model included age, race, education, and household income.

RESULTS

The direct effects on mortality of these area characteristics are shown in fitted regression lines in FIGURE 1 (income inequality) and FIGURE 2 (residential economic segregation). The upper line in both figures reflects the separate area effects when no stage-one individual characteristics were included in the model. The middle curve shows those area effects when all stage-one individual covariates are incorporated, whereas the bottom line shows the results for the same model, but with both area measures of inequality as well as a measure of area median income incorporated in the stage-two analysis.

Both *spatial* and *statistical inequality* in the MSA significantly increased the risk of mortality of residents. The higher income inequality in New York City, for example, relative to Norfolk, Virginia, was associated with more than a 50% increase in the annual probability of mortality (FIG. 1, top line). The magnitude of this relationship was actually strengthened after control for individual-level characteristics (FIG. 1, middle line). Similar results are shown in FIGURE 2 for measures of *spatial inequality*. The significant upward slope in the bottom line of the figures demon-

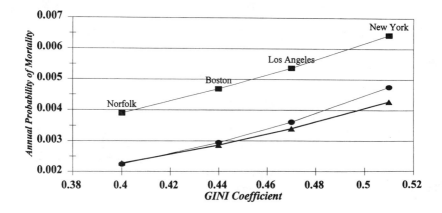

FIGURE 1. Area level influences on risk of mortality (ages 30–64): income inequality. Symbols: —■—, no individual-level controls; —●—, individual-level controls; —▲—, all-area/individual-level controls.

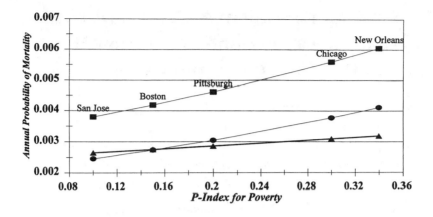

FIGURE 2. Area level influences on risk of mortality (ages 30–64): economic segregation. Symbols: —■—, no individual-level controls; —●—, individual-level controls; —▲—, all-area/individual-level controls.

strates that resource *distribution* affects mortality independent of the *level* of economic development in the area (as measured by median income) and that the two measures of *distribution* capture distinct effects related to perhaps different underlying pathways.

The area measures that were incorporated in this analysis also indirectly affected mortality through modifying the effects of individual socioeconomic status on mortality, generally in the expected direction (not shown).

CONCLUSION

Metropolitan area statistical and spatial economic inequalities significantly increased mortality for residents, both directly and indirectly. To reduce these effects, economic policies aimed at revitalizing urban areas ought to be directed at the distributional patterns of income and space that are invariably altered by economic growth.

ACKNOWLEDGMENT

This research was supported in part by a grant from the Economic Policy Institute, Washington, DC.

REFERENCES

1. WAITZMAN, N.J. & K.R. SMITH. 1998. Separate but lethal: the effects of economic segregation on mortality in metropolitan America. Milbank Q. **76**(3): 341–373.
2. SMITH, K.R. & N.J. WAITZMAN. 1997. Effects of marital status on the risk of mortality in poor and non-poor neighborhoods. Ann. Epidemiol. **7**: 343–349.
3. WAITZMAN, N.J. & K.R. SMITH. 1998. Phantom of the area: poverty-area residence and mortality in the United States. Am. J. Public Health **88**(6): 973–976.

Unbundling Education: A Critical Discussion of What Education Confers and How It Lowers Risk for Disease and Death

IRENE H. YEN[a,b] AND NANCY MOSS[c]

[b]Behavioral Risk Factors Program, School of Public Health,
University of California, Berkeley, California 94720, USA

[c]Pacific Institute for Women's Health, Los Angeles, California 90064, USA

Understanding what education confers is important for understanding the influence of socioeconomic status on health. Along with income and occupation, education is one of the three most common measures of socioeconomic status in the epidemiology research literature. For adults, the literature suggests that education is inversely related to risk for mortality,[1-3] cardiovascular disease,[4] certain cancers,[4,5] smoking,[6] physical inactivity,[6] and body mass index.[7] Analyses of national survey data from less industrialized countries have also demonstrated that maternal education is a consistent predictor of lower fertility and infant and child mortality, even after adjusting for other socioeconomic factors.[8,9] In the context of less developed countries, analyses have shown that maternal education is not a marker for household income or use of health services.[10] Researchers have proposed mechanisms through which maternal education affects child health: ideational change,[11] socialization,[12] and a combination of increased access to external services and information.[13] Yet for the United States setting, the mechanisms through which education influences lower risk for disease and death are not understood.

This paper "unbundles" the meaning of measures of education in the United States and discusses the possible skills and social benefits of education that would confer lower risk on individuals. Skills may include (1) ability to process certain kinds of information or critical thinking[14] and (2) ability to interact with bureaucracies, institutions, and health practitioners. Social benefits may include (1) credentials and the economic access they provide; (2) social networks and extension of cultural capital[15,16]; (3) socialization to adopt health-promoting behaviors; and (4) enhanced expectations for the future leading to hopefulness, planning, self-efficacy, and a sense of control. The interpretation of education effects may be period- and cohort-specific. It is important that public health researchers develop a systematic research program to test which of these meanings of education are key to different health outcomes.

Understanding the mechanisms through which education affects health may further elucidate the socioeconomic status and health gradient and the interaction between social and physiological factors.

[a]Current address for correspondence: Irene H. Yen, Ph.D., M.P.H., Institute for Health and Aging, 3333 California St., Suite 270, San Francisco, California 94143, USA. 415-502-4587 (voice); 415-476-9030 (fax).
e-mail: ihyen@itsa.ucsf.edu

REFERENCES

1. KITAGAWA, E.M. & P.M. HAUSER. 1973. Differential mortality in the United States: a study in socioeconomic epidemiology. Harvard University Press, Cambridge, MA.
2. MANTON, K.G., E. STALLARD & L. CORDER. 1987. Education-specific estimates of life expectancy and age-specific disability in the U.S. elderly population: 1982 to 1991. J. Aging Health **9:** 419–450.
3. MUSTARD, C.A., S. DERKSEN, J.M. BERTHELOT, M. WOFLSON & L.L. ROOS. 1997. Age-specific education and income gradients in morbidity and mortality in a Canadian province. Soc. Sci. Med. **45:** 383–397.
4. BUCHER, H.C. & D.R. RAGLAND. 1995. Socioeconomic indicators and mortality from coronary heart disease and cancer: a 22-year follow-up of middle-aged men. Am. J. Public Health **85:** 1231–1236.
5. LA VECCHIA, C., E. NEGRI & S. FRANCESCHI. 1992. Education and cancer risk. Cancer **70:** 2935–2941.
6. WINKLEBY, M.A., H.C. KRAEMER, D.K. AHN & A.N. VARADU. 1998. Ethnic and socioeconomic differences in cardiovascular disease risk factors: findings for women from the Third National Health and Nutrition Examination Survey, 1988–1994. JAMA **280:** 356–362.
7. IRIBARREN, C., R.V. LUEPKER, P.G. MCGOVERN, D.K. ARNETT & H. BLACKBURN. 1997. Twelve-year trends in cardiovascular disease risk factors in the Minnesota Heart Survey. Are socioeconomic differences widening? Arch. Intern. Med. **157:** 873–881.
8. HOBCRAFT, J., J. MCDONALD & S.O. RUTSTEIN. 1984. Socio-economic differentials in infant and child mortality: a cross-national comparison. Popul. Stud. **38:** 193–223.
9. BICEGO, G.T. & J.T. BOERMA. 1993. Maternal education and child survival: a comparative study of survey data from 17 countries. Soc. Sci. Med. **36:** 1207–1227.
10. CLELAND, J.G. & J.K. VAN GINNEKEN. 1988. Maternal education and child survival in developing countries: the search for pathways of influence. Soc. Sci. Med. **27:** 1357–1368.
11. CALDWELL, J.C. 1979. Education as a factor in mortality decline: an examination of Nigerian data. Popul. Stud. **33:** 395–413.
12. LINDENBAUM, S. 1990. Maternal education and health care processes in Bangladesh: the health and hygiene of the middle classes. *In* What We Know about Health Transition: The Cultural, Social and Behavioural Determinants of Health. J. Caldwell, S. Findley, P. Caldwell, G. Santow, W. Cosford, J. Braid & D. Broers-Freeman, Eds.: 425–440. Health Transition Centre, The Australian National University, Canberra, Australia.
13. LEVINE, R.A., S.E. LEVINE, A. RICHMAN, F.M.T. URIBE, C. SUNDERLAND CORREA & P.M. MILLER. 1991. Women's schooling and child care in the demographic transition: a Mexican case study. Popul. Develop. Rev. **17:** 459–496.
14. WINSHIP, C. & S. KORENMAN. 1997. Does staying in school make you smarter? The effect of education on IQ in *The Bell Curve*. *In* Intelligence, Genes, and Success: Scientists Respond to *The Bell Curve*. B. Devlin, S.E. Fienberg, D.P. Resnick & K. Roeder, Eds.: Springer-Verlag, New York.
15. BOURDIEU, P. 1977. Cultural reproduction and social reproduction. *In* Power and Ideology in Education. J. Karabel & A.H. Halsey, Eds.: Oxford University Press, New York.
16. MACLEOD, J. 1995. Ain't No Makin' It: Aspirations and Attainment in a Low-Income Neighborhood. Westview Press, Boulder.

Socioeconomic Disparities in Adolescent Health: Contributing Factors

KATHLEEN THIEDE CALL[a] AND JAMES NONNEMAKER

School of Public Health, University of Minnesota, Box 729 Mayo,
420 Delaware Street S.E., Minneapolis, Minnesota 55455, USA

Using the first wave of the Add Health (the National Longitudinal Study of Adolescent Health)[1] public use data, we examined the relationship between socioeconomic status (SES) and adolescent self-rated health and mental health status. This research is guided by a theoretical framework first discussed by House[2] and later expanded by Williams.[3] According to this perspective, individual behaviors and values are shaped by social structures, such that SES has a direct impact on health outcomes, in addition to indirect and interactive effects through both psychosocial factors and medical care.

Most investigations of the relationship between SES and health focus on the very young or adult samples. Certainly, some of the behavior patterns established during adolescence—health-threatening behavior and inappropriate use of health care—may not manifest themselves as poor physical health outcomes until much later in life. However, we expect that behavior patterns and experiences during childhood and adolescence will have immediate impacts on mental health. It is precisely because the health-related behaviors, personal experiences, and access to health care during this period have both short- and long-term implications for health status that they should command more attention from the research community.

Using regression analyses, we first examine the direct impact of parental socioeconomic status and its components (education and income) on adolescent health (controlling age, gender, birth weight, family size, and parental marital status). We then study the indirect and moderating effects of psychosocial factors (e.g., self-esteem, social stressors, health-related behaviors such as smoking and drinking, and social ties with parents, peers, and in school) on the relationship between SES and health outcomes. Finally, we examine the indirect and moderating influence of access to medical care (e.g., parent's and adolescent's reports of access to medical care) on adolescent health.

As presented in TABLE 1, adolescents from advantaged families report less depressive affect. The association between SES and adolescent depressed mood remains significant even when the impact of psychosocial factors (e.g., self-esteem, social stressors, health-related behaviors such as smoking and drinking, and social ties with parents, peers, and in school) and access to medical care are taken into account. Adolescents with high self-esteem are less likely to report depressive affect. Those who have had a friend or family member attempt or commit suicide, or who have themselves witnessed or experienced violence in the previous year indicate

[a]Address for correspondence: 612-624-3922 (voice); 612-624-2196 (fax).
e-mail: callx001@tc.umn.edu

TABLE 1. Effects of socioeconomic status, psychosocial factors, and access to medical care on adolescent depressive affect

	Unstandardized regression coefficients							
	1	2	3	4	5	6	7	8
Socioeconomic status + controls (low to high)	-0.55***	-0.56***	-0.47***	-0.41***	-0.43***	-0.43***	-0.45***	-0.40***
Personal resources:								
Self esteem (low to high)		-0.26***	-0.23***	-0.22***	-0.21***	-0.13***		-0.13***
Stressors:								
Friend suicidality (none, attempt, commit)			0.36***	0.35***	0.27**	0.22**		0.21*
Family member suicidality (none, attempt, commit)			0.56***	0.55***	0.52***	0.51***		0.48**
Feel safe in neighborhood (low to high safety)			-0.15***	-0.15***	-0.14***	-0.09***		-0.08***
Witness/experience violence in past year (none to several events)			0.24***	0.24***	0.18***	0.13***		0.11**
Parent: reports financial problems (0 = no, 1 = yes)			NS	NS	NS	0.24*		0.25*
Parent: self rated health (poor to excellent)				NS	-0.09*	-0.09*		NS
Parent: generally happy (0 = no, 1 = yes)				-0.51*	-0.47*	NS		NS
Health behaviors:								
Cigarette use (none to more frequent)					0.14***	0.11***		0.11***
Alcohol use (none to more frequent)					NS	NS		NS
Marijuana use (none or more frequent)					0.11***	0.08**		0.07*
Social ties:								
School connectedness (low to high)						-0.08***		-0.08***
Family connectedness (low to high)						-0.20***		-0.19***
Friend connectedness (low to high)						NS		NS
Access to medical care:								
Parent: family access (hard to easy)							-0.12*	NS
Needed, did not get medical care (0 = yes, 1 = no)							-1.44***	-0.88***
Adjusted R-square (sample size, 3573)	0.05***	0.11***	0.15***	0.15***	0.17***	0.20***	0.09***	0.21***

NOTE: * $p < 0.05$, ** $p < 0.01$, *** $p < 0.001$, NS = not significant. All equations control for adolescent age, race, sex, birth weight, family size, and parental marital status.

TABLE 2. Effects of parental education, psychosocial factors, and access to medical care on adolescent self-rated health status

	Unstandardized regression coefficients							
	1	2	3	4	5	6	7	8
Parental education + controls (low to high)	0.14***	0.14***	0.12***	0.10***	0.09***	0.09***	0.13***	0.09***
Personal resources:								
Self esteem (low to high)	0.09***	0.08***	0.08***	0.08***	0.07***		0.07***	0.09***
Stressors:								
Friend suicidality (none, attempt, commit)			−0.07*	−0.07*	NS	NS		NS
Family member suicidality (none, attempt, commit)			NS	NS	NS	NS		NS
Feel safe in neighborhood (low to high safety)			0.03***	0.03***	0.03***	0.02*		0.02*
Witness/experience violence in past year (none to several events)			−0.04***	−0.04***	NS	NS		NS
Parent: reports financial problems (0 = no, 1 = yes)				NS	NS	NS		NS
Parent: self rated health (poor to excellent)				0.07***	0.07***	0.06***		0.06***
Parent: generally happy (0 = no, 1 = yes)				NS	NS	NS		NS
Health behaviors:								
Cigarette use (none to more frequent)					−0.07***	−0.06***		−0.06***
Alcohol use (none to more frequent)					NS	NS		NS
Marijuana use (none or more frequent)					NS	NS		NS
Social ties:								
School connectedness (low to high)						0.02***		0.02***
Family connectedness (low to high)						NS		NS
Friend connectedness (low to high)						NS		NS
Access to medical care:								
Parent: family access (hard to easy)							NS	NS
Needed, did not get medical care (0 = yes, 1 = no)							0.27***	0.14***
Adjusted R-square (sample size, 3573)	0.03***	0.10***	0.11***	0.12***	0.13***	0.14***	0.04***	0.14***

NOTE: *$p < 0.05$, **$p < 0.01$, ***$p < 0.001$, NS = not significant. All equations control for adolescent age, race, sex, birth weight, family size and parental marital status.

higher levels of depressed mood. More frequent smoking and use of marijuana are associated with depressive affect. Feelings of depression are lower among adolescents who feel connected at school and report warm and supportive relationships with family members. Adolescents who report they needed, but did not get medical care are more depressed than those who perceive having access to services. The relationships between SES, psychosocial factors, medical access, and depressed mood presented in TABLE 1 are slightly less potent for both parental income and education.

Education is a more salient predictor of adolescent self-rated health status than income or the composite indicator of SES. (In fact, SES and income become insignificant when self-esteem and stressors are added to the model.) Specifically, adolescents whose parents are more highly educated rate their health better than adolescents whose parents have attained less formal education (see TABLE 2). Adolescents who have a positive self-image, whose parents report being healthy, and who live in a safe neighborhood report being in better health. In contrast, adolescents who smoke rate their health lower. Feeling connected at school and perceiving that medical care is available when needed is associated with higher self-reported health status among adolescents.

Using conditional analyses, we explored whether the influence of psychosocial factors or access to medical care on adolescent depressed mood and self-rated health varies within SES, income, or educational strata. The data do not indicate moderating effects.

In summary, we find that parental SES and its components have strong and persistent effects on adolescent's depressive affect, even after taking self-esteem, stressors, social supports, health behaviors, and access to care into account. High parental SES and income are related to high self-rated health among adolescents, but their effect fades once psychosocial factors and access to medical care are taken into account. In contrast, parental education has direct as well as indirect (through psychosocial factors and access to care) implications for adolescent health status.

REFERENCES

1. <http://talltoad.cpc.unc.edu/projects/addhealth/>
2. HOUSE, J.S. 1981. Social structure and personality. *In* Social Psychology: Sociological Perspectives. M. Rosenberg & R.H. Turner, Eds.: 525–561. Basic Books, New York.
3. WILLIAMS, D.R. 1990. Socioeconomic differentials in health: a review and redirection. Soc. Psychol. Q. **53:** 81–99.

Effects of Socioeconomic Status and Psychosocial Stress on the Development of the Fetus

JANET A. DiPIETRO,[a,b] KATHLEEN A. COSTIGAN,[c]
STERLING C. HILTON,[d] AND EVA K. PRESSMAN[c]

[b]Department of Population and Family Health Sciences, Johns Hopkins University,
Baltimore, Maryland 21205, USA

[c]Division of Maternal–Fetal Medicine, Johns Hopkins University,
Baltimore, Maryland 21205, USA

[d]Department of Statistics, Brigham Young University, Provo, Utah 84601, USA

Recent studies have revealed a relationship between higher levels of maternal psychosocial stress during pregnancy and reduced birth weight and length of gestation. Previously, we have documented poorer fetal neurobehavioral development from mid-gestation in fetuses of healthy women with normal pregnancies who were of low socioeconomic status (SES).[1] Fetuses of low-SES women were found to move less often and with less vigor, display reduced neural integration between cardiac and motor function, and have lower variability in heart rate. Neurobehavioral measures provide information about the nature of the developing nervous system. These data suggest that fetuses of poor but otherwise healthy women with good prenatal care may display indications of developmental immaturity at birth. Although there are many potential mediators of this relationship (e.g., exposure to environmental agents, nutrition), the current analysis was undertaken to determine the role of maternal psychosocial stressors and affect in mediating fetal development.

This study included a sample of 103 women with normal pregnancies who were assessed at three gestational ages (24, 30, and 36 weeks), stratified by SES ($n = 52$ middle/high SES; $n = 51$ low SES). The upper SES group consisted of employed, older, well-educated ($M = 16.3$ years education) and primarily nonminority (77%) women; subjects in the lower SES group were predominantly unemployed, less educated ($M = 11.8$ years), and African American. At each visit, 50 minutes of fetal heart rate and movement data were digitized from an actocardiograph fetal monitor into a computerized analysis system; these data were used to construct measures of neurobehavioral function. Maternal report scales of emotional intensity, daily stressors, and pregnancy-specific hassles and uplifts were administered at each visit. Generalized estimating equation techniques (GEE) were used to model the longitudinal relations between stress and fetal development separately for each SES group. Each equation includes adjustment for maternal education, age, and parity. The de-

[a]Address for correspondence: Janet DiPietro, Johns Hopkins University, Department of Population and Family Health Sciences, Hampton House, Rm. 397, 624 N. Broadway, Baltimore, MD 21205. 410-955-8536 (voice); 410-955-2303 (fax).
e-mail: jdipietr@jhsph.edu.

TABLE 1. Results of GEE analysis modeling (Z scores) for fetal measures at 24, 30, and 36 weeks with maternal psychosocial measures

Psychosocial measure	Fetal activity level		Heart rate accelerations	
	High SES (n = 52)	Low SES (n = 51)	High SES (n = 52)	Low SES (n = 51)
Daily stress inventory[a]	1.98*	2.78**	1.78~	1.87~
Pregnancy hassles/uplifts[b]	4.60***	2.19*	1.85~	−0.42
Affective intensity[c]	1.95~	−3.13**	1.79~	−2.23*

NOTE: ~$p < 0.10$. **$p < 0.05$. ***$p < 0.01$. ***$p < 0.001$. (two-sided)
[a]From Brantley, P.J. *et al.*[3]
[b]From DiPietro, J.A. *et al.*[4]
[c]From Larsen, R.J. *et al.*[5]

pendent measures represent two aspects of fetal well-being: fetal motor activity and accelerations in fetal heart rate.

Results indicate that aspects of maternal stress systematically affect fetal development. Some relations are similar across SES: fetuses of women who are more hassled or negative about their pregnancy (higher intensity of hassles relative to uplifts) and report more daily stressors move more often (TABLE 1). Similar, although less robust, associations exist for heart rate accelerations and are consistent with an interpretation that maternal stress increases sympathetic activation of the fetus. However, maternal emotional intensity is associated with increased fetal activity in the upper SES group, but reduced activity in the lower SES group. A composite measure based on each of the three measures of affect and stress near the end of pregnancy (36 weeks) extends and confirms these results (FIG. 1). In the higher SES

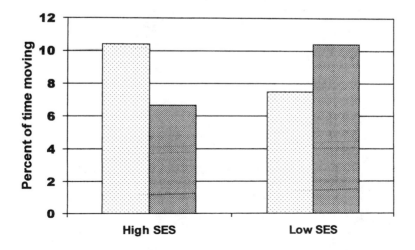

FIGURE 1. Fetal movement by SES and stress composite score at 36 weeks gestation. Symbols: ▨, high stress; ▨, low stress.

group, stress is associated with greater fetal activity, movement duration, vigor, and periods of continuous, high-amplitude movement (r ranges from 0.27 to 0.34). These associations are consistently inverse in the low-SES group (r ranges from -0.26 to -0.34).

Contrary to expectations, women in the low-SES group reported lower daily stressors than the upper SES group and were more uplifted about their pregnancy (see Hawkins, DiPietro and Costigan[2]). Within the high-SES group, GEE results indicate that pregnancy-related uplifts are negatively associated with fetal movement ($Z = -2.67$), a finding that parallels the SES difference and suggests emotional valence is an important consideration. These data indicate significant complexity in how the social environment interacts with maternal psychosocial functioning to influence fetal development.

ACKNOWLEDGMENT

This research was support by 2R01 HD27592, NICHD, awarded to Janet A. DiPietro.

REFERENCES

1. DiPIETRO, J.A., et al. 1998. Fetal neurobehavioral development: associations with socioeconomic class and fetal sex. Dev. Psychobiol. **33:** 79–91.
2. HAWKINS, M., J.A. DiPIETRO & K.A. COSTIGAN. 1999. Social class differences in maternal stress appraisal during pregnancy. Ann. N.Y. Acad. Sci. **896:** this volume.
3. BRANTLEY, P.J., et al. 1987. A daily stress inventory: development, reliability, and validity. J. Behav. Med. **10:** 61–73.
4. DiPIETRO, J.A., et al. 1999. Psychosocial stress in pregnancy: development and validation of the Pregnancy Experience Scale. Submitted.
5. LARSEN, R.J., et al. 1986. Affect intensity and reactions to daily life events. J. Pers. Soc. Psychol. **51:** 803–814.

Social Position, Age, and Memory Performance in the Whitehall II Study

R. FUHRER,[a,b] J. HEAD,[b] AND M.G. MARMOT[c]

[b]Department of Epidemiology and Public Health,
Royal Free and University College Medical School, University College London,
1-19 Torrington Place, London WC1E 6BT, United Kingdom

[c]Centre for Health and Society, Department of Epidemiology and Public Health,
University College London, WC1E 6BT, United Kingdom

INTRODUCTION

Cognitive performance varies across the life span in normal development and aging. Memory loss is the first recognizable symptom of dementia, but memory decline is also a feature of normal aging. Although factors such as poor physical and mental health have an impact on memory, age is the best predictor of memory decline. There is evidence that educational attainment affects performance on cognitive tests,[1] as well as the rate of memory decline[2] and the occurrence of dementia.[3] Education is often used as a measure of social stratification, but it is only a partial indicator of social position. This paper examines whether social position as measured by British Civil Service employment grade: (1) affects the relationship of age and memory performance and (2) has an effect that is independent of the effect of education.

METHODS

The British Civil Service provides a valuable population for studying the social determinants of health and aging. Within one set of institutions, where broad similarities in the environment might be expected to minimize differences in morbidity and mortality, quite the reverse is found to be true. The grade classification identifies a clear hierarchy in the social and material circumstances of the men and women in the Civil Service. Grade of employment reflects income, education, and status; and for the analyses reported here, jobs were grouped into three levels—administrative, professional/executive, and clerical/support.

At Phase 1 (1985–1987), 10,308 men and women 35 to 55 years of age participated in a medical screening examination and completed a psychosocial, health behavior and health questionnaire.[4] About halfway through Phase 3 screening (1991–1993), a battery of cognitive tests was introduced, and 3398 persons complet-

[a]Address for correspondence: +44 207 391 1685 (voice); +44 207 813 0242 (fax).
e-mail: r.fuhrer@public-health.ucl.ac.uk

ed the full test battery. Educational attainment was defined by the age when full-time education was terminated based on English school leaving policies. These were classified as finishing beyond age 18 (i.e., higher education), finishing between the ages of 17 and 18 (i.e., starting and/or completing the General Certificate of Education—Advanced Levels), and finishing at or before age 16 (i.e., before or at the school leavers examination, the General Certificate of Education—Ordinary Levels examinations).

The cognitive battery included a measure of verbal and numerical reasoning (fluid intelligence), a vocabulary or word recognition test, which is considered to measure crystallized intelligence; a 20-word list learning test, which is a measure of short-term verbal memory or immediate recall; and two measures of verbal fluency.

RESULTS

FIGURE 1 shows that increasing age is associated with poorer memory performance and that social position does not modify the age–memory performance relationship. The effect of education on memory is removed when current social position (employment grade) is included in the model (TABLE 1). These findings are observed in both men and women.

TABLE 1. Linear regression of memory performance on age, grade, and education

	Beta coefficients			
	Age	Age + Education	Age + Grade	Age + Education + Grade
Men ($n = 2247$)				
Age	-0.30^a	-0.27^a	-0.32^a	-0.30^a
Education		-0.22^a		-0.10
Employment grade			-0.58^a	-0.47^a
Women ($n = 853$)				
Age	-0.33^a	-0.26^b	-0.23^b	-0.23^a
Education		-0.29^c		-0.10
Employment grade			-0.54^a	-0.47^b

NOTE: Employment grade and education are coded from highest (reference group) to lowest.
[a]$p < 0.0001$.
[b]$p < 0.001$.
[c]$p < 0.01$.

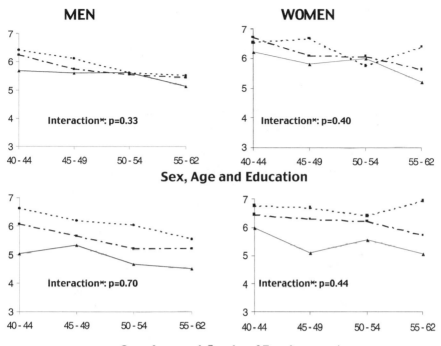

FIGURE 1. *Upper panels*, mean memory score by sex, age, and education: ●, beyond age 18; ■, age 17–18; ▲, at or before age 16. *Lower panels*, mean memory score by sex, age, and grade of employment: ●, administrative; ■, professional/executive; ▲, clerical/support. * Tests whether the linear age decline differs by education or grade of employment.

DISCUSSION

These findings confirm that memory declines with age in a linear fashion even among middle-aged adults. Furthermore, as has been shown in studies of middle-aged and older samples, education is inversely related to memory performance.[5] However, in contrast to other studies, social position as measured by employment grade is a dominant predictor of age-related memory function. Although, education is correlated with employment grade, the two measures are not synonymous. Education may reflect early influences on both brain and social development, whereas present social position may reflect current behaviors, exposures, and/or experiences that may influence rate of decline.[6] An alternative explanation might be that employment grade is a better measure than education of overall cognitive aptitude, which has been shown to be correlated with memory performance.[7] Access to more education is in part determined by ability, but also by other social factors; whereas in this sample, grade of employment may mirror cognitive activity throughout the life course. Our longitudinal data will be used to confirm these results.

ACKNOWLEDGMENTS

The Whitehall II study was supported by grants from the Medical Research Council; British Heart Foundation, Health and Safety Executive; National Heart Lung and Blood Institute (HL36310); National Institute on Aging (AG13196); Agency for Health Care Policy Research (HS06516); The New England Medical Center; Division of Health Improvement, Institute for Work and Health, Toronto; and the John D. and Catherine T. MacArthur Foundation Research Networks on Successful Midlife Development and Socio-economic Status and Health. MGM is supported by an MRC Research Professorship.

We also thank all participating civil service departments and their welfare, personnel, and establishment officers; the Occupational Health and Safety Agency; the Council of Civil Service Unions; all participating civil servants in the Whitehall II study; and all members of the Whitehall II study team.

REFERENCES

1. LEZAK, M.D. 1995. Neuropsychological Assessment. Oxford University Press, Oxford.
2. SCHMAND, B., J. SMIT, J. LINDEBOOM, C. SMITS, C. JONKER & B. DEELMAN. 1997. Low education is a genuine risk factor for accelerated memory decline and dementia. J. Clin. Epidemiol. 50: 1025–1033.
3. EVANS, D.A., L.E. HEBERT, L.A. BECKETT, P.A. SCHERR, M.S. ALBERT, M.J. CHOWN, D.M. PILGRIM & J.O. TAYLOR. 1997. Education and other measures of socioeconomic status and risk of incident Alzheimer disease in a defined population of older persons. Arch. Neurol. 54: 1399–1405.
4. MARMOT, M.G., G. DAVEY SMITH, S.A. STANSFELD, C. PATEL, F. NORTH, J. HEAD, I. WHITE, E.J. BRUNNER & A. FEENEY. 1991. Health inequalities among British civil servants: the Whitehall II study. Lancet 337: 1387–1393.
5. NILSSON, L.G., L. BAECKMAN, K. ERNGRUND, L. NYBERG, R. ADOLFSSON, G. BUCHT, S. KARLSSON, M. WIDING & B. WINBLAD. 1997. The Betula prospective cohort study: memory, health and aging. Aging Neuropsychol. Cognit. 4: 1–32.
6. WHITE, L., R. KATZMAN, K. LOSONCZY, M. SALIVE, R. WALLACE, L. BERKMAN, J. TAYLOR, G. FILLENBAUM & R. HAVLIK. 1994. Association of education with incidence of cognitive impairment in three established populations for epidemiologic studies of the elderly. J. Clin. Epidemiol. 47: 363–374.
7. SCHMAND, B., J.H. SMIT, M.I. GEERLINGS & J. LINDEBOOM. 1997. The effects of intelligence and education on the development of dementia. A test of the brain reserve hypothesis. Psychol. Med. 27: 1337–1344.

Social Dominance and Cardiovascular Reactivity in Preschoolers

Associations with SES and Health

LAUREN HEIM GOLDSTEIN,[a,b] ANIKA TRANCIK,[c] JENNIFER BENSADOUN,[d]
W. THOMAS BOYCE,[d] AND NANCY E. ADLER[e]

[b]Harold E. Jones Child Study Center, Institute for Human Development,
University of California, Berkeley, California 94720, USA

[c]Department of Psychology, University of Washington, Seattle, Washington 98105, USA

[d]School of Public Health, University of California, Berkeley, California 94720, USA

[e]Health Psychology Program, Center for Health and Community,
University of California, San Francisco, California 94143, USA

The link between socioeconomic status (SES) and health has been clearly established: individuals with low SES have poorer health than those individuals with high SES.[1,2] There is also evidence of a graded association at all levels of SES.[3] In the child development literature, very little is known about what factors in children's lives may contribute to the SES–health association. One domain that may be important is a child's peer relationships. Is a child's position in the peer group hierarchy analogous to an adult's position in the socioeconomic status hierarchy? If so, would hierarchy position in preschool be related to health? In addition, perhaps individual differences in children's cardiovascular reactions to stress mediate the association between SES and health. These two factors, social dominance and cardiovascular reactivity, can be measured in very young children with valid research methods. The objective of this cross-sectional study was to examine relations among SES, social dominance, cardiovascular reactivity, and physical and mental health outcomes in preschool children.

Seventy 3–5-year-olds (62% boys; 47% Caucasian, 10% African American, 15% Asian, and 28% multiethnic) and their parents participated. Families came primarily from the middle and upper class with 9% reporting a family income of less than $20,000, 6% between $20,000 and $40,000, 23% between $40,000 and $60,000, 26% between $60,000 and $80,000, 13% between $80,000 and $100,000, and 23% over $100,000. Children completed a 30-minute physiologic protocol composed of developmentally challenging tasks during which their heart rate and blood pressure were monitored.[4,5] To assess social dominance, children were observed in naturally occurring peer interactions at the preschools.[6,7] Parents completed questionnaires assessing family demographics and their children's physical and mental health and behavior. For this paper, family income was used as the SES indicator. A six-item

[a]Address for correspondence: Lauren Heim Goldstein, Ph.D., Harold E. Jones Child Study Center, Institute for Human Development, University of California, Berkeley, 2425 Atherton Street, Berkeley, CA 94720-6070. 510-643-2523 (voice); 510-643-7350 (fax).
e-mail: LHG@uclink4.berkeley.edu

global physical health scale was created (higher scores indicate worse physical health). Two cardiovascular reactivity variables were computed: a heart rate intensity score (mean heart rate during tasks) and a heart rate recovery difference score (mean heart rate during number recall task minus mean heart rate during rest).

Findings revealed that children from lower income families had poorer physical health ($r = -0.24$, $p < 0.05$) and more internalizing behavior problems ($r = -0.29$, $p < 0.05$) than children from higher income families. Regression analyses were conducted testing for significant main and interactive effects. Results for the three models tested are presented in TABLE 1. Results suggest that in different family contexts, different profiles of dominance and cardiovascular reactivity may be adaptive. For children from high-income families, *more* cardiovascular reactivity was associated with more externalizing symptoms, whereas for children from low-income families, *less* reactivity was associated with more externalizing symptoms (beta for SES–

TABLE 1. Results for three models tested

Model 1: Income and reactivity as predictors

Predictors	Global physical health		Externalizing symptoms	
	Beta	R^2Ch	Beta	R^2Ch
Gender	—	—	-0.36^b	0.12^a
Family income	-0.22	0.06	-0.17	0.02
Reactivity	-0.42^a	0.12^a	0.02	0.01
Income × Reactivity	-0.14	0.02	-0.39^b	0.14^b
R^2 total		0.19^a		0.28^b

Model 2: Income and social dominance as predictors[c]

Predictors	Global physical health		Externalizing symptoms	
Gender	—	—	-0.37^b	0.13^b
Family income	-0.17	0.06	0.02	0.00
Dominance	0.15	0.02	0.15	0.02
Income × Dominance	-0.27^a	0.07^a	-0.19	0.03
R^2 total		0.15^a		0.18^a

Model 3: Dominance and reactivity as predictors

Predictors	Global physical health		Externalizing symptoms	
Gender	—	—	-0.36^b	0.11^a
Family income	-0.27	0.04	-0.10	0.01
Dominance	-0.05	0.01	0.01	0.00
Reactivity	-0.47^b	0.10^a	0.01	0.00
Reactivity × dominance	0.38^a	0.10^a	-0.20	0.04
R^2 total		0.25^a		0.28^b

NOTE: Standardized regression coefficients shown.
[a] $p < 0.05$.
[b] $p < 0.01$.
[c] See FIGURE 1.

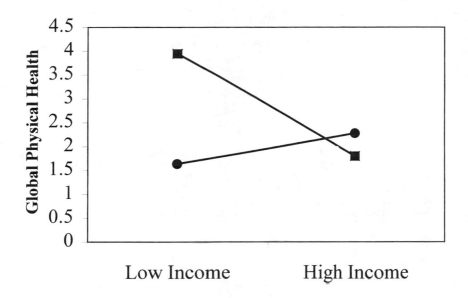

FIGURE 1. Family income by social dominance predicting global physical health. ●, low dominance; ■, high dominance.

reactivity interaction, 0.39, $p < 0.01$). For children from low-income families, high social dominance was associated with poor global physical health. For children from high-income families, dominance status was not associated with global physical health (beta for SES–dominance interaction, $-0.27, p < 0.05$; see FIGURE 1). Perhaps the incongruity in status position between home and school poses a risk for some children. Children who were both low on the dominance hierarchy and highly reactive had the poorest global physical health (beta for dominance–reactivity interaction, 0.38, $p < 0.05$). These findings highlight the importance of exploring biology-environment interactive associations in predicting health in children. Cardiovascular reactivity and social dominance may be *mediating* the SES–health association in preschool children. Gaining a more complete understanding of how social dominance and cardiovascular reactivity may mediate the SES–health association can help us to identify children at risk for physical health problems and psychopathology at an early age.

ACKNOWLEDGMENTS

Support for this research was funded by the MacArthur Foundation Research Network on Psychopathology and Development, and the MacArthur Foundation Research Network on SES and Health.

REFERENCES

1. MARMOT, M.G. *et al.* 1984. Inequalities in death: specific explanations of a general pattern. Lancet **1:** 1003–1006.
2. MARMOT, M.G. *et al.* 1991. Health inequalities among British civil servants: the Whitehall II study. Lancet **337:** 1387–1393.
3. ADLER, N.E. *et al.* 1994. Socioeconomic status and health: the challenge of the gradient. Am. Psychol. **49:** 15–24.
4. BOYCE, W.T. *et al.* 1995. Dimensions of psychobiologic reactivity: cardiovascular responses to laboratory stressors in preschool children. Ann. Behav. Med. **17:** 315–323.
5. BOYCE, W.T. *et al.* 1995. Psychobiologic reactivity to stress and childhood respiratory illnesses: results of two prospective studies. Psychosom. Med. **57:** 411–422.
6. STRAYER, F.F. & J. STRAYER. 1976. An ethological analysis of social agonism and dominance relations among preschool children. Child Dev. **47:** 980–989.
7. STRAYER, F.F. & M. TRUDEL. 1984. Developmental changes in the nature and function of social dominance among young children. Ethol. Sociobiol. **5:** 279–295.

Markers of Transition to Adulthood, Socioeconomic Status of Origin, and Trajectories of Health

CAROLYN HARLEY[a,b] AND JEYLAN T. MORTIMER[c]

[b]*Division of Health Service Research and Policy, School of Public Health, University of Minnesota, Minneapolis, Minnesota 55455, USA*

[c]*Life Course Center, Department of Sociology, University of Minnesota, Minneapolis, Minnesota 55455, USA*

This study examines the processes by which the transition to adulthood may impact mental health and result in the social gradient in health. The transition to adulthood is a formative time in the life course when young people relinquish the roles and obligations of adolescence and youth and take on the responsibilities of adulthood. Studies consistently show that the transition to adulthood can have both deleterious and beneficial effects on health.[1–4] We hypothesize that the socioeconomic health gradient emerges in early adulthood as a result of the differential timing, spacing, and sequencing of major transitional events.

Our data source is the Youth Development Study (YDS). An initial panel of 1,000 adolescents, chosen randomly from students registered in the St. Paul, Minnesota public school district, has been surveyed since the ninth grade of high school (1988–1998). The transitional events of interest here are: (1) independence from the parental home; (2) marriage or cohabitation; and (3) parenthood. *Timing* is indicated by the period in which a particular transition occurred. *Sequencing* references the degree of departure from the normative sequence, of leaving the parental home, then marrying (or cohabiting), and becoming a parent. *Pile-up* is defined by the number of transitions occurring in a single year. Following House *et al.*,[5] socioeconomic status of origin was measured by a composite of parental income and education during the first year of data collection. The mental health outcome is depressive affect measured in 1995, four years after high school. Race, gender, and depressive affect in the 9th grade (prior health status) are controlled.

In the YDS, a social gradient in depressive affect emerged in early adulthood, when panel members were mostly four years beyond high school. Despite the presumed individualization of the life course across social classes, we still find significant differences in the experience of transition to adulthood by social class, including precocious family transitions for those of lower socioeconomic status, and more problematic transition to adulthood, as indicated by the experience of pile-up and non-normative sequencing.

[a]Address for correspondence: Carolyn Harley, Division of Health Service Research and Policy, Box 729, Mayo Building, Minneapolis, MN 55455, USA. 612-624-9507 (voice); 612-624-7020 (fax).
e-mail: harl0027@tc.umn.edu

TABLE 1. Timing of transition and depressive affect (standardized coefficients, OLS regression)

	Depressive affect four years after high school		
	Timing of leaving home model	Timing of marriage model	Timing of parenthood model
Socioeconomic status	-0.160^a	-0.142^c	-0.087^c
Race	-0.095^b	-0.088^b	-0.117^b
Gender	-0.028	-0.016	0.035
9th grade depressive affect	0.162^a	0.170^a	0.162^c
Early transition	0.071	0.053	0.173^c
Intermediate transition	0.003	0.021	-0.011
	$n = 577$	$n = 557$	$n = 425$
	$R^2 = 0.078^a$	$R^2 = 0.072^a$	$R^2 = 0.097^a$

$^a p < 0.001.$
$^b p < 0.05.$
$^c p < 0.01.$

TABLE 2. Timing of transition, pile-up, sequencing, and depressive affect (standardized coefficients, OLS regression)

	Depressive affect four years after high school		
	Leaving home interaction model	Marriage interaction model	Parenthood interaction model
Socioeconomic status	-0.079	-0.081	-0.079
Race	-0.127^a	-0.131^b	-0.130^b
Gender	0.036	0.025	0.032
9th grade depressive affect	0.162^b	0.165^b	0.154^b
Early transition	-0.227	-0.495^a	0.017
Intermediate transition	0.035	-0.074	-0.052
Pile-up	-0.012	0.064	0.040
Sequencing	0.086	0.099	0.033
Pile-up × Early	0.352^b	0.589^a	0.189^a
	$n = 412$	$n = 412$	$n = 412$
	$R^2 = 0.098^c$	$R^2 = 0.102^c$	$R^2 = 0.108^c$

$^a p < 0.01.$
$^b p < 0.05.$
$^c p < 0.001.$

Our analysis strategy involved the sequential inclusion of variables representing features of the transition to adulthood in OLS models to assess potential mediators of the social class–health relationship. We find that the social gradient in health remains evident when the timing of the three family-related transitions are taken into account (TABLE 1). However, inclusion of interaction terms in the models, expressing the combination of early timing and pile-up, renders the effect of social status statistically insignificant (TABLE 2). This analysis illuminates the underlying processes that may explain the emerging socioeconomic gradient in mental health. That is, this phenomenon appears to be tied to the stressors that arise when early transitions are coupled with a pile-up of transitions. Young people from lower socioeconomic backgrounds, whose transitions are early and "piled-up," are likely to face many responsibilities and stressors without sufficient time to adapt to them.

ACKNOWLEDGMENTS

This research was supported by the National Institute of Mental Health, MI-142843, "Work Experience and Mental Health: A Panel Study of Youth." This paper was completed while the second author was a Fellow at the Center for Advanced Study in the Behavioral Sciences. She is grateful for the support provided by the Center, as well as by the Hewlett Foundation and the W.T. Grant Foundation (Grant 95167795) for the fellowship. The authors would like to thank Michael Finch, Michael Shanahan, Chris Uggen, Barbara McMorris, and Sabrina Oesterle for helpful advice in the development of this paper.

REFERENCES

1. BROWN, C.H., R.G. ADAMS & S.G. KELLAM. 1981. A longitudinal study of teenage motherhood and symptoms of distress: the Woodlawn Community Epidemiological Project. Res. Commun. Mental Health **2:** 183–213.
2. SCHULENBERG, J., K.N. WADSWORTH, P.M. O'MALLEY, J.G. BACHMAN & L.D. JOHNSTON. 1996. Adolescent risk factors for binge drinking during the transition to young adulthood: variable and pattern-centered approaches to change. Dev. Psychol. **32:** 659–674.
3. MILLER-TUTZAUER, C., K.E. LEONARD & M. WINDLE. 1991. Marriage and alcohol use: a longitudinal study of maturing out. J. Studies Alcohol **52:** 434–440.
4. NURMI, J.E. 1997. Self-definition and mental health during adolescence and young adulthood. *In* Health Risks and Developmental Transitions During Adolescence. J. Schulenberg, J.L. Maggs & K. Hurrelmann, Eds.: 395–419. Cambridge University Press, Cambridge.
5. HOUSE, J.S., *et al.* 1990. Age, socioeconomic status, and health. Milbank Q. **68:** 383–411.

Racial Differences in Education, Obesity, and Health in Later Life

CHRISTINE L. HIMES[a]

Center for Policy Research, Syracuse University,
426 Eggers Hall, Syracuse, New York 13244, USA

A better understanding of the mechanisms through which SES may influence health status can be gained by examining specific risk factors associated both with disease and with SES. One such risk factor is obesity. Obesity is currently defined as a body mass index (BMI) of 30.0 Kg/m^2 or greater.[1] Body size in this range has been associated with a variety of chronic diseases, including diabetes[2,3] and arthritis.[2,4] Obesity also is linked to education and race. An inverse relationship between education and obesity has been found repeatedly in developed countries, particularly among women.[5] The prevalence of obesity in the U.S. population also differs by race. African Americans exhibit higher rates of obesity, a difference that may be the result of a combination of cultural, dietary, and economic factors.[5] Although the relationships among health, obesity, and education have been established for most adults, very few studies have examined these relationships late in life. Research on mortality has shown that at ages over 70, high BMIs are not strongly related to increased risks of death.[6] However, the relationship to chronic diseases at older ages has not been examined.

This research uses data from the Assets and Health Dynamics of the Oldest Old (AHEAD) Survey to examine the relationships between obesity, race, and education at very old ages. The survey interviewed 7,274 community-dwelling respondents age 70 and older in 1994. In addition to sociodemographic information, respondents were asked to report their current height and weight, presence of medical conditions, and disabilities. Logistic regression models are estimated to determine the effects of race and education on obesity, and then to examine the effects of race, education, and obesity on the prevalence of arthritis and diabetes.

Increasing age among those 70 and older and male gender are both associated with lower odds of obesity for both whites and African Americans (TABLE 1). However, only among whites is education a significant predictor of obesity. The effects of obesity and education on the reported prevalence of arthritis and diabetes also vary by race (TABLE 2). Among the white elderly, higher levels of education reduce the odds of reporting both arthritis and diabetes; however for African Americans, higher levels of education affect only arthritis. Similarly, obesity is linked to both diabetes and arthritis among white elderly, but only to arthritis for African Americans.

Obesity is related to later life health, especially among white elderly. These results also indicate that education is not clearly related to obesity and at least some health conditions among elderly African Americans. Because educational levels are

---

[a]Address for correspondence: 315-443-9064 (voice); 315-443-1081 (fax).
e-mail: clhimes@maxwell.syr.edu

TABLE 1. Effects of education on the odds of being obese (BMI $\geq$ 30.0 kg/m^2) for the AHEAD population by race

	African American	White
Age	0.942[a]	0.923[a]
Female	2.333[a]	1.387[a]
Married	0.894	0.941
Years of education	0.983	0.922[a]
Parents' education	0.793	0.852
Current smoker	0.626	0.497[a]
Former smoker	0.832	1.001
Number of cases	871	5,839

[a]Significant at 0.01 level.

generally low for African Americans in this age cohort, approximately 40% have less than eight years of school, education may not be a good discriminator of socioeconomic status for this group. The selective survival of African Americans into later life may also contribute to the lack of effect of education on late life health.

TABLE 2. Effects of education and obesity on the odds of reporting arthritis and diabetes in the AHEAD population by race

	Arthritis		Diabetes	
	African American	White	African American	White
Age	1.022	1.012[a]	0.953[b]	0.965[b]
Female	1.308	1.520[b]	1.136	0.731[b]
Married	0.629[b]	0.930	1.069	0.833[a]
Years of education	0.954[b]	0.956[b]	0.992	0.941[b]
Parents' education	1.006	0.912	1.374	0.876
Current smoker	1.232	0.773[a]	0.773	0.564[b]
Former smoker	1.139	0.952	0.752	0.973
Obese	2.222[b]	1.735[b]	1.323	2.138[b]

[a]Significant at 0.05 level.
[b]Significant at 0.01 level.

REFERENCES

1. NATIONAL HEART LUNG AND BLOOD INSTITUTE. 1998. Clinical Guidelines on the Identification, Evaluation, and Treatment of Overweight and Obesity in Adults. Public Health Service, Washington, DC.
2. PI-SUNYER, F.X. 1991. Health implications of obesity. Am. J. Clin. Nutr. **53:** 1595S–1603S.
3. COLDITZ, G.A. *et al.* 1990. Weight as a risk factor for clinical diabetes in women. Am. J. Epidemiol. **132:** 501–513.
4. DAVIS, M.A. *et al.* 1990. Body fat distribution and osteoarthritis. Am. J. Epidemiol. **132:** 701–707.
5. WORLD HEALTH ORGANIZATION. 1998. Obesity: Preventing and Managing the Global Epidemic. WHO, Geneva.
6. ALLISON, D.B. *et al.* 1997. Body mass index and all-cause mortality among people age 70 and over; the Longitudinal Study of Aging. Int. J. Obes. **21:** 424–431.

Limitations to the Use of Education as an SES Indicator in Studies of the Elderly

Confounding by Cognition

DIANE S. LAUDERDALE[a] AND KATHLEEN A. CAGNEY

Department of Health Studies, The University of Chicago, Chicago, Illinois, USA

OBJECTIVES

Educational attainment has consistently been shown to predict performance on cognitive function tests among the elderly.[1–5] Separating the extent to which education indicates socioeconomic status (SES) and the extent to which it is an independent predictive factor is difficult given the paucity of data sources that include both measures of cognition and wealth. We have examined the relative contributions of education and economic factors to cognitive function in later life and the degree to which they vary by race and Latino ethnicity.

METHODS

Using the Asset and Health Dynamics of the Oldest Old (AHEAD) study, a national study of those aged 70+ that oversampled African Americans and Latinos, we examined the effects of education and wealth on cognitive impairment for African Americans, whites, and Latinos using OLS regression. AHEAD's comprehensive set of wealth and cognition measures provide a unique opportunity to elucidate the sociodemographic determinants of cognitive well-being in later life.

RESULTS

For African Americans and whites, there is a strong monotonic relationship between education and cognition (TABLE 1). For Latinos there is a threshold, with no gain in cognitive function associated with education above high school. Adjusting for wealth, the difference in cognitive function score between the highest and lowest educational levels is greater for African Americans (11.5/35 points) than whites (9/35 points) or Latinos (6/35 points). Adjusting for education, the difference in cognitive function scores between the highest and lowest wealth categories is only 1 to 3 points (TABLE 2). A subgroup analysis of Latino ethnicity by nativity indicates no evidence of an education effect for Latinos born within the United States, but for those born outside the United States the effects of both educational attainment and higher wealth on cognitive ability are significant.

[a]Address for correspondence: 773-834-0913 (voice); 773-702-1979 (fax).
e-mail: lauderdale@health.bsd.uchicago.edu

TABLE 1. Bivariate results

	Black (n = 876)	White (n = 5360)	Latino (n = 341)
Age	-0.37^a	-0.39^a	-0.39^a
Female	0.08	0.05	-0.37
Education			
Below 4th grade	-12.43^a	-11.26^a	-7.59^a
4th to 8th grade	-8.88^a	-7.63^a	-4.36^b
Some high school	-6.52^a	-4.46^a	-1.55
High school graduate	-2.95^b	-1.55^a	-0.62
Some college	-1.38	-0.65^c	-2.73
College	—	—	—
Income			
Below 5,000	-4.64^a	-5.44^a	-2.74
5,000 to 14,999	-3.23^b	-3.43^a	-1.49
15,000 to 24,999	-2.13^c	-2.08^a	1.42
25,000 to 49,999	-0.81	-0.95^a	1.86
At least 50,000	—	—	—
Net worth			
Not above 0	-5.84^a	-5.99^a	-5.59^a
0 to 24,999	-3.73^a	-4.08^a	-4.34^b
25,000 to 74,999	-2.46^b	-2.89^a	-3.95^b
75,000 to 200,000	-1.36	-1.43^a	-1.27
At least 200,000	—	—	—

[a] $p < 0.001$.
[b] $p < 0.01$.
[c] $p < 0.05$.

DISCUSSION

We conclude that education is serving only minimally as a proxy for SES in studies of cognitive function. Further, education does not translate equally across race/ethnicity and, for Latino ethnicity, varies by nativity. These data suggest that education may be a poor indicator of SES in studies of the elderly in which the outcome of interest has a cognitive component, such as Instrumental Activity of Daily Living deficits.

TABLE 2. Multivariate results: education and wealth

	Black	White	Latino
Age	-0.28^a	-0.32^a	-0.32^a
Female	0.20	0.54	-0.57
Education			
Below 4th grade	-11.52^a	-8.99^a	-6.30^a
4th to 8th grade	-7.93^a	-6.25^a	-3.63^c
Some high school	-6.16^a	-3.59^a	-1.06
High school graduate	-3.03^a	-1.56^a	-0.96
Some college	-1.69^d	-0.68^b	-1.85
College	—	—	—
Net worth			
Not above 0	-0.93	-3.02^a	-1.27
0 to 24,999	0.54	-1.85^a	-1.44
25,000 to 74,999	0.77	-0.87^a	-1.33
75,000 to 200,000	1.04	-0.48^b	0.10
At least 200,000	—	—	—

[a] $p < 0.001$.
[b] $p < 0.01$.
[c] $p < 0.05$.
[d] $p < 0.10$

REFERENCES

1. DARTIGUES, J., M. GAGNON, L. LETENNEUR, P. BARBERGER-GATEAU, D. COMMENGES, M. EVALDRE & R. SALAMON. 1992. Principal lifetime occupation and cognitive impairment in a French elderly cohort (Paquid). Am. J. Epidemiol. **135:** 981–988.
2. EVANS, D.A., L.A. BECKETT, M.S. ALBERT, L.E. HEBERT, P.A. SCHERR, H.H. FUNKENSTEIN & J.O. TAYLOR. 1993. Level of education and change in cognitive function in a community population of older persons. Ann. Epidemiol. **3:** 71–77.
3. HERZOG, A.R. & R.B. WALLACE. 1997. Measures of cognitive functioning in the AHEAD study. J. Gerontol. Soc. Sci. **52B:** 37–48.
4. SCHERR, P.A., M.S. ALBERT, H.H. FUNKENSTEIN, N.R. COOK, C.H. HENNEKENS, L.G. BRANCH, L.R. WHITE, J.O. TAYLOR & D.A. EVANS. 1988. Correlates of cognitive function in an elderly community population. Am. J. Epidemiol. **128:** 1084–1101.
5. WHITE, L., R. KATZMAN, K. LOSONCZY, M. SALIVE, R.B. WALLACE, L. BERKMAN, J. TAYLOR, G.G. FILLENBAUM & R.J. HAVLIK. 1994. Association of education with incidence of cognitive impairment in three established populations for epidemiologic studies of the elderly. J. Clin. Epidemiol. **47:** 363–374.

Parenting Behavior and Emotional Health as Mediators of Family Poverty Effects upon Young Low-Birthweight Children's Cognitive Ability

MIRIAM R. LINVER,[a,b] JEANNE BROOKS-GUNN,[b] AND DAFNA KOHEN[c]

[b]Center for Children and Families, Teachers College, Columbia University, 525 W. 120th St., Box 39, New York, New York 10027-6696, USA

[c]University of British Columbia, Vancouver, British Columbia, Canada V6T 1Z3

The negative consequences for families living in poverty have been demonstrated for both parents and children. Researchers have found that living in poverty has negative effects on child outcomes such as cognitive and emotional development.[1] Researchers have documented connections between living in poverty and maternal depression and emotional health,[2] as well as between poverty and parenting practices.[3] Few researchers, however, have linked all these constructs in a single model to test the possible direct and indirect effects of living in poverty on young children's cognitive and emotional outcomes, as mediated by maternal emotional health and parenting practices. Groups lead by Conger, Elder, and McLoyd provide exemplary models for how this research may be performed.[4–6] They have developed models that examine the effects of poverty on outcomes in the context of family influences. We wish to extend these models, which link family poverty, maternal emotional health, parenting, and older children's and adolescents' cognitive ability, to younger children's cognitive ability. It is our premise that a large portion of the association between low income and child cognitive ability found for young children is mediated through familial pathways, specifically through maternal mood and parenting. We developed models that represented the effects of poverty on child cognitive ability at ages three and five.

To test our models, we used data from the Infant Health and Development Program (IHDP).[7] Our sample included 817 white and African American infants weighing between 1000 and 2500 grams at birth, and their mothers. Predictor measures included a composite measure of income and an income-to-needs ratio, maternal emotional health, and observational measures of maternal parenting; outcome measures included child cognitive ability and behavior problems at ages three and five years; control variables included maternal education, verbal ability, marital status, race, and age at child's birth, as well as child's gender, birthweight, site, and intervention status.

Structural equation models with nested model comparisons were used to select the model that best fit the data. FIGURES 1 and 2 present the standardized parameter

[a]Address for correspondence: 212-678-3479 (voice); 212-687-3676 (fax).
e-mail: MRL23@columbia.edu

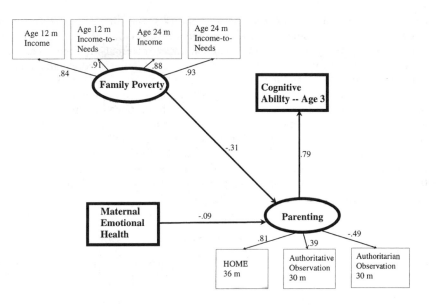

FIGURE 1. Standardized parameter estimates for child cognitive ability at age three years as outcome. *Note*: Controls include IHDP sit, treatment group, maternal age, race, marital status, education, PPVT score, as well as child birth weight and gender.

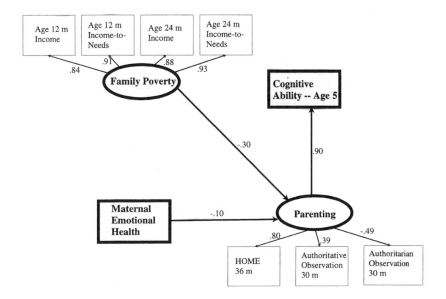

FIGURE 2. Standardized parameter estimates for child cognitive ability at age five years as outcome. *Note*: Controls include IHDP sit, treatment group, maternal age, race, marital status, education, PPVT score, as well as child birth weight and gender.

estimates for our final models for cognitive ability at ages three years (FIG. 1) and five years (FIG. 2). Parenting was found to mediate the relation between poverty and child cognitive ability, as well as the relation between maternal emotional health and child cognitive ability. Maternal emotional health did not mediate the relation between family poverty and low-birthweight children's cognitive ability.

Our findings are compelling for a number of reasons. First, our sample is larger than previous studies; with 817 children we had more power to find associations among our constructs, and we could include many control variables. A second strength of our study is that our models were empirically and theoretically based. Finally, our sample was quite diverse. We included both single- and two-parent families as well as African American and white families across the income spectrum. In this sense, our sample is more diverse than Conger's Iowa rural farm sample or McLoyd's Michigan urban African American sample.

REFERENCES

1. KORENMAN, S., J.E. MILLER & J.E. SJAASTAD. 1995. Long-term poverty and child development in the United States: results from the NLSY. Child. Youth Serv. Rev. **17:** 127–155.
2. ADLER, N.E., T. BOYCE, M.A. CHESNEY, S. COHEN, S. FOLKMAN, R.L. KAHN & S.L. SYME. 1994. Socioeconomic status and health: the challenge of the gradient. Am. Psychol. **49:** 15–24.
3. KELLEY, M.L., T.G. POWER & D.D. WIMBUSH. 1992. Determinants of disciplinary practices in low-income black mothers. Child Dev. **63:** 573–582.
4. CONGER, R.D., X. GE, G.H. ELDER, F.O. LORENZ & R.L. SIMONS. 1994. Economic stress, coercive family process, and development problems of adolescents. Child Dev. **65:** 541–561.
5. ELDER, G.H. 1974. Children of the great depression: social change in life experience. University of Chicago Press, Chicago.
6. MCLOYD, V.C. 1990. The impact of economic hardship on black families and children: psychological distress, parenting, and socioemotional development. Child Dev. **61:** 311–346.
7. INFANT HEALTH AND DEVELOPMENT PROGRAM. 1990. Enhancing the outcomes of low-birth-weight, premature infants: a multisite, randomized trial. J. Am. Med. Assoc. **263:** 3035–3042.

Socioeconomic Factors and Emergency Pediatric ICU Admissions

ANNE L. NACLERIO,[a,b] JOHN W. GARDNER,[c] AND MURRAY M. POLLACK[d]

[b]Department of Pediatrics, George Washington University and
Critical Care Medicine, Children's National Medical Center,
Lackland AFB, Texas 78236, USA

[c]Department of Epidemiology and Biostatistics,
Uniformed Services University of the Health Sciences, Bethesda, Maryland, USA

[d]Department of Pediatrics, George Washington University School of Medicine, and
Department of Critical Care, Children's National Medical Center, Washington, DC, USA

INTRODUCTION

Socioeconomic status (SES) has long been known as a strong predictor of morbidity and premature mortality.[1] Today 22% of children in the United States are below the federal poverty level (FPL),[2] and 10 million are uninsured. Adults with lower SES suffer disproportionately from many diseases with mortality rates above those in the higher socioeconomic strata.[3] Although fewer studies have been done in children, children of low SES have higher morbidity from diseases such as asthma[4] and sickle cell disease,[5] poorer immunization status,[6] poorer nutrition, and lower rates of immunization. Patterns of health care utilization also differ between the classes. For instance, poor children with asthma have 40% fewer visits to the doctor but have 40% more hospitalizations. Utilization, however, cannot be equated with health care "needs." Studies have shown large variations in resource consumption even after controlling for illness severity.[7] The literature is scarce on the use of ICU resources among the social classes and are nonexistent for the pediatric population. A cohort study of 847 adult ICU patients found that patients from the lower socioeconomic groups had both higher severity of illness on ICU admission and higher ICU mortality.[8] We hypothesized that the lower socioeconomic groups would disproportionately utilize emergent pediatric intensive care unit (PICU) care and their severity of illness would be higher.

METHODS

All five PICUs serving the Washington, DC metropolitan statistical area (DC-MSA) collaborated on this project. Emergency patients were included from January 1, 1997 through May 31, 1997. Elective admissions and children over 14 years or from outside the DC-MSA were excluded. This area includes Washington DC, 11

[a]Address for correspondence: Anne L. Naclerio, M.D., M.P.H., Pediatric Critical Care Medicine, Wilford Hall Medical Center, 2200 Bergquist Dr., Suite 1, Lackland AFB, TX 78236, USA. 210-292-7279 (voice); 210-292-3836 (fax).
e-mail: Anaclerio@aol.com

surrounding counties, and five independent cities in Maryland and Virginia. Patients were identified upon admission, and data were collected by chart review. Patients were assigned to a census tract based on their address. Data for patient and population SES variables were obtained from the 1990 Census Bureau Data. Five SES variables were defined for each tract; median household income, percent below the FPL, percent of work force in working class occupations, percent unemployed, and percent with less than a high school education. Means for the SES variables were compared between the population and the cases with t-tests. Incidence of emergent PICU admission was defined for the region. Admission rates by tract were correlated with each continuous SES variable using Pearson's correlation coefficient. PICU admission rates were compared for all dichotomized SES variables using a chi-square analysis on both a crude level and an age adjusted level. All analyses were done on three severity levels.

RESULTS

One thousand four hundred twenty two cases were identified, 545 met inclusion criteria, and 526 were included in this analysis. The rate of emergency PICU admission in the DC-MSA for children less than 14 years of age was 6.9 per 10,000 children for the five-month study period. This equates to an annual incidence of emergency PICU admission in our population of 16.6/10,000 children. Comparison of the cases and the population on the SES variables is shown in TABLE 1 on two severity levels. Severe admissions are defined as those cases that have a PRISM-III score of greater than or equal to five at 12 or 24 hours. All cases considered, the cases were significantly different from the population on median household income and percent below poverty level. The children admitted to the PICU were from tracts with a significantly lower median household income ($p < 0.001$) and a greater proportion of persons living below the federal poverty level ($p < 0.04$). When only the severe admissions are considered, differences from the population on median household income and percent below poverty level become more pronounced and cases become significantly different from the population on measures of education and unemployment as well ($p < 0.05$). Median household income was significantly correlated with admission rates on all levels of severity ($p < 0.01$). For every $10,000 increase in median household income, PICU admission rates dropped by 9% ($p < 0.002$) for all admissions and by 12.4% for severe admissions over the study period. Percent below poverty was also positively correlated with admission rate. For every 10% increase in the number of families below the FPL, severe PICU admissions rose by 21% ($p < 0.05$). When the SES variables were dichotomized and compared, we found that children from tracts where the median household income was less than $50,000 were 1.3 times as likely to be admitted than children from tracts where the average income was above that level ($p < 0.0016$). If only severe admissions were included, the relative risk of admission rose to 1.5 ($p < 0.004$). Similarly, children from tracts where 10% or more of the families were living below the FPL were 1.5 times as likely to be admitted to the PICU than those who were not ($p < 0.00006$). If only severe admissions were included, the relative risk of admission rose to over 2 ($p < 0.000001$). The relationship between categorized SES variables and severe PICU admission rates are shown in TABLE 2.

TABLE 1. Cases compared to population on SES variables

	Below poverty level	Working class	Unemployed	Below high school education	Median household income
Cases					
All	7.2%	54.8%	3.9%	16.2	$47,234
Severe	7.9%	55.8%	4.3%	17.1%	$46,081
Population	6.5%	54.6%	3.8%	15.6%	$49,903
Ratio					
All	1.11	1.0	1.03	1.04	0.95
Severe	1.22	1.1	1.13	1.10	0.92
p-Value					
All	0.04	NS	NS	NS	< 0.001
Severe	0.01	0.19	0.03	0.03	0.001

TABLE 2. Relative risk of admission

	Cases[a]	Rate[b]	Rate Ratio	*p*-Value
Poverty level				
More than 10% below FPL	62	4.78	2.04**	0.000001
Less than 10% below FPL	148	2.34		
Education level				
At least 15% below high school	96	3.05	1.20	0.19
Less than 15% below high school	114	2.54		
Working class				
50% of more	133	2.85	1.10	0.52
Less than 50%	77	2.59		
Income class				
Low, less than $50,000	136	3.26	1.52**	0.004
High, at least $50,000	74	2.14		

[a]Severe cases (PRISM ≥ 5), $n = 210$.
[b]Admits/10,000 children.

DISCUSSION

Socioeconomically deprived children are disproportionately represented in the PICU. Children admitted to the PICU were poorer than the local population, income correlated with admission rates and as severity of illness increased, so did the magnitude of this relationship. Occupation and education were less important. Admission to a PICU represents either the failure of primary prevention efforts, treatment failures, or complications of treatment and reflects on the effectiveness of the societal health care system. ICU admission is at the end of the spectrum of illness severity and cost. In an era of health care reform and redesign, knowledge of the relationships between resource utilization and social class are relevant. Improved understanding of these relationships will guide our prevention programs, training programs and future health policy initiatives.

REFERENCES

1. SYME, S.L. *et al.* 1976. Social class, susceptibility and sickness. Am. J. Epidemiol. **104:** 1–8.
2. STATISTICAL ABSTRACTS OF THE UNITED STATES. 1993. Census Bureau Library Reference Desk. Government Printing Office, Washington, DC.
3. ANTONOVSKY, A. 1967. Social class, life expectancy and overall mortality. Milbank Mem. Fund Q. **45:** 31–73.
4. LESON, S. *et al.* 1995. Risk factors for asthmatic patients requiring intubation: observations in children. J. Asthma **32:** 285–294.
5. OKANY, C.C. *et al.* 1993. The influence of socio-economic status on the severity of sickle cell disease. Afr. J. Med. Sci. **22:** 57–60.
6. WILLIAMS, I.T. *et al.* 1995. Interaction of socioeconomic status and provider practices as predictors of immunization coverage in Virginia children. Pediatrics **96:** 439–446.
7. GOLDBERG, K.C. *et al.* 1992. Racial and community factors influencing coronary artery bypass graft surgery rates for all 1986 Medicare patients. JAMA **18:** 1473–1477.
8. LATOUR, J. *et al.* 1991. Inequalities in health in ICU patients. Am. J. Epidemiol. **44:** 889–894.

Socioeconomic Status and Health among Elderly People in Sweden

M.G. PARKER,[a,b] K. AHACIC,[b] M. THORSLUND,[b] AND O. LUNDBERG[c]

[b]Department of Social Work, Stockholm University, 10691 Stockholm, Sweden

[c]Swedish Institute for Social Research, Stockholm University, Stockholm, Sweden

INTRODUCTION

The older the age group studied, the more mechanisms have had a chance to influence health at various time during the life span, and therefore the more complex the pathways to inequalities in health. As the average age of the population increases, it becomes more important to understand how these inequalities express themselves—both in efforts to provide appropriate services to those who need them, and also in the search to understand the pathways to inequalities. These studies are based on the Swedish Panel Study of Living Conditions of the Oldest Old (SWEOLD), an interview survey of a representative sample ($n = 537$) aged 77 to 99. Two studies include data from the Level of Living Survey (LLS), a sample of over 6000 residents interviewed in 1968, 1974, 1981, and 1991. SES is based on occupation.

STUDIES

Lundberg and Thorslund[1] found SES to be significantly correlated with joint pain, circulatory problems, and low peak flow. The strongest correlation was with peak flow. SES was not significantly correlated with self-rated health (SRH) (TABLE 1.)

Parker et al.[2] found that SES is strongly correlated with several function measures (ADL, mobility, and performance tests) and that the relationship is more distinct among men than women (TABLE 2.)

Ahacic, Parker, and Thorslund[3] examined mobility limitations in the population between 1968 and 1992. During this time there was general improvement in mobility. The gender difference decreased, but the SES differences remained unchanged.

Ahacic et al.[4] studied dental health between 1968 and 1992. He found great general improvement, decreased gender and regional differences as well as decreased SES differences.

[a]Address for correspondence: Marti G. Parker, Department of Social Work, Stockholm University, 10691 Stockholm, Sweden. +46 8 16 12 18 (voice); +46 8 674 73 98 (fax).
e-mail: marti.parker@socarb.su.se

TABLE 1. Odds ratios for health indicators by SES, adjusted for age and sex

	SRH less than good	Joint pain	Circulatory problems	Low peak flow
Unskilled workers	1.11	0.87	1.19	1.44
Skilled workers	1.22	1.70	1.24	1.13
Non-manual workers	0.63	0.51	0.51	0.47
Farmers and self-employed	1.18	1.32	1.33	1.31
All	1.00	1.00	1.00	1.00
p	n.s.	< 0.001	< 0.005	< 0.05

NOTE: Reference group is sample average.

INEQUALITIES AMONG THE OLDEST OLD

Why do social inequalities persist in a welfare state dedicated to universal bene-fits and access to care? One explanation is that the studied cohort lived much of their lives before the Swedish welfare system was developed. Another explanation is that many mechanisms that influence health have nothing to do with benefits or care, but are nonetheless SES related, for example, health behavior, working conditions, aspi-rations, and childhood conditions. Paradoxically, perhaps SES inequalities are seen among the oldest old because the welfare state has been able to keep both blue- and white-collar workers alive despite poor health and functional limitations.

CHANGES OVER TIME

In a welfare system that aims to reduce social inequalities, do these findings signal success or failure of the efforts of the past decades? Despite general improve-ments, social inequalities persist in many areas. The decreasing class differences in dental health may reflect the fact that dental care is so directly related to dental status, but it may also reflect the policy of targeting low-income groups for dental health programs. To decrease social inequalities, is it necessary to direct measures

TABLE 2. Odds ratios for function measures by SES, adjusted for age and sex

	ADL	Mobility	Performance
Unskilled workers	1.9[a]	1.7[a]	2.0[a]
Skilled workers	1.5	2.0[a]	1.8[a]
Non-manual workers	1.00	1.00	1.00
Farmers and self-employed	1.2	1.1	1.5

NOTE: Reference group is non-manual workers.
[a] $p < 0.05$.

towards certain groups, for example, to women and blue-collar workers, in addition to the universal benefits available in the welfare system? The pathway to mobility limitations is much more complicated and less directly related to care. Mobility reflects overall health, that is, the general improvement due to living conditions in a population.

REFERENCES

1. THORSLUND, M. & O. LUNDBERG. 1994. Health and inequalities among the oldest old. J. Aging Health **6:** 51–69.
2. PARKER, M.G., M. THORSLUND & O. LUNDBERG. 1994. Physical function and social class among Swedish oldest old. J. Gerontol. **49:** S196–201.
3. AHACIC, K., M.G. PARKER & M. THORSLUND. 1999. Mobility limitations in the Swedish population from 1968 to 1992: age, gender and social class differences. Aging Clin. Exp. Res. In press.
4. AHACIC, K., I. BARENTHIN, M. THORSLUND & O. LUNDBERG. 1999. Inequalities in Swedish dental health 1968–1991. Manuscript in preparation.

A Multivariate Model of Functional Decline in the Elderly: The Differential Influence of Income versus Education

JOYCE C. PRESSLEY[a]

College of Physicians and Surgeons, The Gertrude H. Sergieusky Center, Columbia University, New York, New York 10032, USA

INTRODUCTION

Both total and active life expectancies are increasing amidst reports that gains differ significantly across social and economic strata. Factors influencing who improves, worsens, or remains nondisabled as they age are complex and not well understood.

This study examined independent factors associated with population-level functional change in elderly who were community-dwelling at baseline, comparing those who deviated versus followed the somewhat expected trajectory of physical decline with increasing age.

METHODS

Models for assessing predictors of change in elderly functional status used longitudinal data from the 1984 National Long-Term Care Survey (NLTCS) community-dwelling population (baseline) and the 1989 NLTCS community and institutional surveys (follow-up). The NLTCS was linked to six years of Medicare claims data, 1984–1989. Socioeconomic status measures included variables for categorical annual baseline income and education measured as 0–7 years, 8–11 years, and 12 or more years completed. We then employed a disease risk classification scheme,[1] previously tested for use in community-dwelling elderly[2] to assess the hundreds of ICD-9-CM codes found in Medicare administrative data and categorize them for each individual according to population-level disease risk.[3] Functional decline was defined as more limitations in activities of daily living (ADLs) at follow-up than baseline, improved as fewer, and nondisabled as no limitations in ADLs or instrumental activities of daily living (IADLs). For final results, we ran two identical functional decline models with demographic, condition, ADL, and disease risk measures, first representing socioeconomic status by education and then by income.

[a]Address for correspondence: Joyce C. Pressley, Ph.D., M.P.H., Columbia University, The Gertrude H. Sergievsky Center, College of Physicians and Surgeons, 630 West 168th Street PH19, New York, NY 10032, USA. 212-305-4858 (voice); 212-305-2426 (fax).
e-mail: pressle@sergievsky.cpmc.columbia.edu

TABLE 1. Population characteristics at baseline and disease risk during follow-up by functional change

	Remained not disabled or improved, n (%)	Worsened n (%)
Population	882 (37.5)	1491 (62.5)
Age (median years, range)	73 (65–100)	78 (65–106)
Gender[a]		
Male	342 (46.7)	391 (53.3)
Female	540 (32.9)	1100 (67.1)
Race[a]		
White	763 (36.8)	1309 (63.2)
Black	108 (39.7)	164 (60.3)
Other	11 (37.9)	18 (62.1)
Education (mean ± sd)	9.2 ± 3.8	8.6 ± 4.0
Income (mean ± sd)	$13,137 (± 10,451)	$11,428 (± 10,069)
Private Insurance (both surveys)	464 (52.6)	558 (37.4)
Medicaid at baseline	135 (15.3)	282 (18.9)
Medicaid at follow-up	132 (15.0)	559 (37.5)
Patient-reported conditions at baseline		
Circulatory		
Cerebrovascular	165 (18.7)	308 (20.7)
Stroke	35 (4.0)	69 (4.6)
Heart attack	35 (4.0)	69 (4.6)
Other heart problem	228 (25.9)	409 (27.4)
Circulation 'trouble'	413 (46.8)	732 (49.2)
Hypertension	426 (48.3)	685 (46.0)
Musculoskeletal		
Arthritis/Rheumatism	657 (74.5)	1157 (77.7)
Broken bones	59 (6.7)	80 (5.4)
Other		
Mental	149 (16.9)	518 (34.7)
Cancer	40 (4.5)	58 (3.9)
Diabetes	110 (12.5)	229 (15.4)
Emphysema	74 (2.6)	112 (7.5)
Pneumonia	35 (4.0)	65 (4.4)
Parkinson's disease	11 (1.4)	35 (2.4)
Highest disease risk during follow-up, all conditions		
None/low	260 (29.5)	231 (15.5)
Moderate	99 (11.2)	118 (7.9)
Moderately severe	383 (43.4)	690 (46.3)
Very severe/catastrophic	140 (15.9)	452 (30.2)

[a]Percentages for race and gender are row percentages. All others are column percentages.

RESULTS

Population characteristics for elderly whose ADL status declined and those who remained nondisabled or improved are shown in TABLE 1. Education was negatively associated with the prevalence of most diseases reported during the year of the baseline survey. Diseases generally regarded as being vaccine-preventable, such as the flu and some pneumonia, were 1.3 to 1.4 times higher in the least educated elderly (21.7% vs. 16.7%, $p = 0.001$ and 4.9% vs. 3.3%, $p = 0.208$ respectively). Circulatory problems and diabetes were 1.3 times higher (56.6% vs. 40.4%, $p < 0.001$ and 16.5% vs. 13.5%, $p = 0.019$, respectively), dementia 1.4 times higher (6.4% vs. 4.5%, $p < 0.001$), and hypertension 1.2 times higher (49.8% vs. 45.4%, $p = 0.014$) in persons not completing versus completing elementary school. Furthermore, many conditions demonstrating an educational gradient had a "dose–response" pattern, with disease prevalence in intermediate educational categories falling between the lower and higher education categories.[2] Differences in disease occurrence observed across income categories were generally not as strong or consistent as those observed for educational status.

In multivariate models, among the independent predictors of worsened functional status were increased age, gender (female), lower income, higher disease risk during

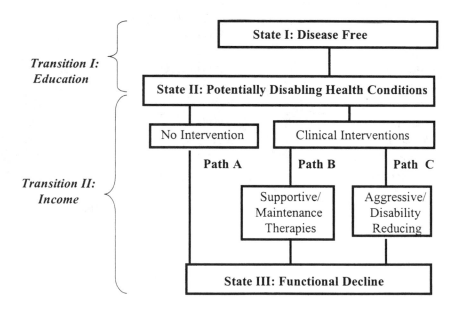

FIGURE 1. Pathways through which socioeconomic components are hypothesized to exert their strongest influence on physical functional decline. **State I:** Disease free; **State II:** Presence of diseases or conditions capable of producing disability; and **State III:** Progression of diseases and conditions to functional decline. Three paths through which income is hypothesized to influence differential population trajectories: **Path A:** Natural state, no intervention; **Path B:** Supportive or maintenance therapies; and **Path C:** Aggressive potentially disability-reducing therapies.

follow-up, dementia, injuries, and similar prevalence of diabetes but increased hospitalizations among diabetics. Education was inversely related to the prevalence of most potentially disability-producing diseases at baseline, but once disease was present, income, but not education, independently predicted declining physical function during follow-up. Correlations between income and education differed significantly by age, race, and gender; they were higher in whites, males, and younger elderly. Racial differences were greater than gender differences.

CONCLUSIONS

These findings suggest that demographic differences in population composition contribute considerable heterogeneity and complexity to the study of socioeconomic status and health outcomes. In addition, two principal components of socioeconomic status, education and income, appear to contribute to population-level active life expectancy through different mechanisms in the elderly (FIG. 1).

ACKNOWLEDGMENTS

This work is largely excerpted from the author's Ph.D. dissertation. She is grateful to her dissertation committee at Duke University and her mentors at Columbia University for their comments on this work. Partial support of this research was provided by the Department of Veteran's Affairs, Veteran's Health Administration, Health Services Research and Development Service. Dr. Pressley currently receives salary support from the National Institute on Aging.

REFERENCES

1. SULLIVAN, L.W. & G. WILENSKY. 1989. Medical Hospital Mortality Information 1987 1988 1989. Vol. 25 Technical Supplement. Health Care Financing Administration, Baltimore.
2. PRESSLEY, J.C. 1996. Factors Impacting Functional State and Health Care Utilization in the Elderly. Doctoral dissertation. Duke University, Durham, NC.
3. PRESSLEY, J.C. & C.H. PATRICK. 1999. Frailty bias in comorbidity risk adjustments of community-dwelling elderly populations. J. Clin. Epidemiol. **52:** 753–760.

Socioeconomic Status, Social Support, Age, and Health

TONI C. ANTONUCCI,[a] KRISTINE J. AJROUCH, AND MARY JANEVIC

Institute for Social Research, The University of Michigan,
426 Thompson Street, P.O. Box 1248, Ann Arbor, Michigan 48106, USA

This study examines the hypothesis that aspects of social relations moderate the relationship between SES and health; that is, this association varies with differences along four major dimensions of social relations: instrumental, emotional, and negative support, and network structure.

In 1992, 923 white and black respondents aged 40 and over were interviewed as part of the Survey of Social Relations.[1] The sample was drawn from a stratified probability sample in the Detroit metropolitan area. Social relations variables included the number of people in social network, perceived instrumental support (whether spouse and child would provide care if respondent was ill), emotional support (whether respondent confides in spouse and child), and negative support (whether spouse and child get on the respondent's nerves). Respondents rated all social support variables on a five-point scale (1, strongly agree; 5, strongly disagree). Education level was used as an SES indicator. Years of education were split into three groups: less than high school, high school, and more than high school. Health was measured by a global self-rated health question (5, poor; 1, excellent).

Following Baron and Kenny,[2] we assessed the moderating impact of the social relations variables on the relationship between SES and health by regressing health on (1) the independent SES variable (education level), (2) the social relations variable that is hypothesized to be the moderator, and (3) the interaction of (1) and (2). A significant interaction term implies that the social relations variable is moderating the impact of SES on health. Analyses were conducted separately for each of two age groups: 40–59 and 60–93.

Findings indicate that there is no interaction effect of SES and social network size on health. However, interaction effects are evident for instrumental, emotional, and negative support. These are summarized in TABLE 1. Graphs of the significant interactions suggest complex associations among SES, social relations variables, and health. For example, FIGURE 1 demonstrates that respondents aged 40–59 with more than a high school education and who confide in their spouse are healthier than those who do not. This relationship was reversed among respondents with less than a high school education. However, in the 60–93 age group, health is about the same for all respondents who confide in their spouse. Among those in this age group who do not confide in their spouse, education level has a negative effect on health: people with less than a high school education report poorer health; those with more than a high school education report better health. A consistent pattern that emerged was that respondents in the middle education group (high school) were the least likely in both

---

[a]Address for correspondence: 313-747-4575 (voice).

TABLE 1. Interactions between social relations and SES

Social relations	Age	
	40–59	60–93
Network structure		
Network size	ns	ns
Instrumental		
Spouse	$p < 0.001$	ns
Child	$p < 0.01$	ns
Emotional		
Spouse	$p < 0.001$	$p < 0.05$
Child	$p < 0.05$	ns
Negative		
Spouse	ns	$p < 0.05$
Child	$p < 0.05$	ns

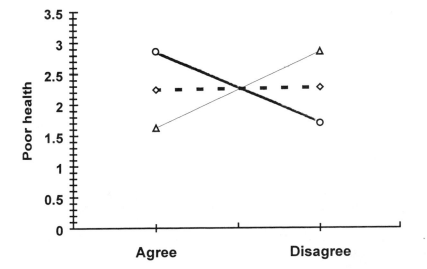

FIGURE 1. Emotional support, ages 40–59: confide in spouse ($p < 0.001$). Symbols: ◯, below high school; ◇, high school; △, above high school.

age groups and across variables to experience a moderating effect of social relations on health.

The results suggest that social relations affect the association between SES and health across age. Of special interest are those in the lowest SES group. Older, lower SES adults who do not confide in their spouse are clearly more vulnerable to health problems, but younger people who confide in their spouse are less healthy. This latter finding might speak to the special vulnerability of younger individuals who face significant health problems. Social relations are apparently more likely to exert a moderating effect on the SES–health relationship in the 40–59 age group than in the 60–93 age group, a possible life course effect. Additionally, the effect of SES on health for those considered middle aged (40–59) is moderated by both the relationship with their children and spouse, whereas only relations with the spouse had a significant moderating effect for the older (60–93) respondents.

In sum, these findings suggest that it is necessary to recognize that types of social relations differentially affect health among people of different ages and education levels. Future research should examine other SES indicators as well as other types of social relations across the life span.

REFERENCES

1. ANTONUCCI, T.C. & H. AKIYAMA. 1996. Social Relations and Mental Health Over the Life Course, Final Report. National Institutes of Mental Health, #ROIMH46549.
2. BARON, R.M. & D.A. KENNY. 1986. Moderator–mediator variable distinction in social psychological research: conceptual, strategic and statistical considerations. J. Pers. Soc. Psychol. **51:** 1173–1182.

Measurement of Social Capital

JAMES N. BURDINE,[a,b] MICHAEL R.J. FELIX,[b] NINA WALLERSTEIN,[c]
AMY L. ABEL,[b] CHARLES J. WILTRAUT,[b] YVETTE J. MUSSELMAN,[b]
AND CHRIS STIDLEY[c]

[b]Felix, Burdine and Associates, 5100 Tilghman Street, Suite 215,
Allentown, Pennsylvania 18104, USA

[c]University of New Mexico, Albuquerque, New Mexico 87131, USA

The value of social capital has been discussed extensively in the literature; however, there are few publications of efforts to measure social capital directly at the community level using quantitative methods.[1–4] The research objective for this project was to test an instrument for measuring social capital as one component of community/ population health status assessments. The instrument developed for this project included new measures, as well as measures based on previous research, modified for application in a community-based assessment.

Data were collected as part of an ongoing series of community and/or population health status assessments conducted in 1998-1999 at eight sites (in four states). A total of 5,823 valid instruments were obtained from a random digit dialing recruited/ mailed survey instrument method (overall response rates of 36% to 78%). Data elements in the surveys include social capital, functional health status (SF-12), disease prevalence, demographics/social determinants of health, community issues, health risks and preventive behavior, health and human services utilization, insurance data, and access to care measures.

Social capital has been defined as "the stock of relationship quality that exists among a group of individuals which: motivates their awareness of membership in the group, their interest in acting in the group's best interest, and facilitates their ability to do so."[5] A factor analysis of fourteen items, hypothesized to measure various dimensions of social capital, produced three factors (Social Integration, Civic Involvement, and Religiosity). Scores for these factors were created by summing the individual item scores. Conversion to Z scores allowed for summing of the three factors for each community. The resulting factor scores were rank ordered in order to be able to compare the eight sites (FIG. 1).

Physical and mental component scores (PCS and MCS) from the SF-12 were calculated for each site and the rank order of those scores compared with the social capital ranking. The rank order of sites for MCS and social capital scores were identical (FIG. 2). The rank order for PCS scores matched for only one of the eight sites. An initial conclusion is that social capital may be more closely related to mental health than physical health. The authors also conclude that a valid approach to measuring social capital is available through the instrument employed and tested in this study.

[a]Address for correspondence: James N. Burdine, Dr. P.H., President and Senior Scientist, Felix, Burdine and Associates, 5100 Tilghman Street, Suite 215, Allentown, PA 18104, USA. 610-366-1310 (voice); 610-366-1322 (fax).
e-mail: jim@felixburdine.com

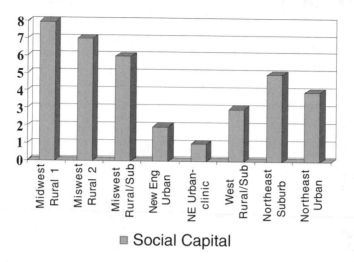

FIGURE 1. Rank order overall social capital—sum of Z-scores for social integration, civic involvement, and religiosity scores.

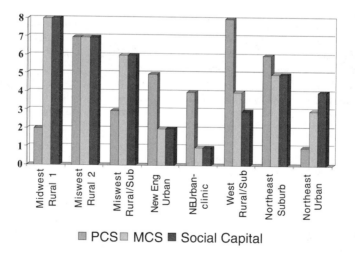

FIGURE 2. Rank order of sites for physical and mental health functioning and social capital.

As standardized measures of overall health status, PCS and MCS scores are influenced by age, income, and other social determinants of health. Additional analyses of these data will be performed to determine the extent to which other factors influence the relationships between social capital and health status measures.

REFERENCES

1. KIWACHI, I. *et al.* 1997. Social capital, income inequality and mortality. Am. J. Public Health **87:** 1491–1498.
2. PATRICK, D.L. & T.M. WICKIZER. 1995. Community and health. *In* Society and Health. B.C.Amick *et al.,* Eds.: 46–92. Oxford University Press, New York.
3. PUTNAM, R.D. 1993. The Prosperous community: social capital and economic growth. Am. Prosp. Spring: 35–42.
4. SAMPSON, R.J. *et al.* 1997. Neighborhoods and violent crime: a multilevel study of collective efficacy. Science **277:** 918–924.
5. SAFRAN, D. 1998. Personal communication.

Racism and Health: Segregation and Causes of Death Amenable to Medical Intervention in Major U.S. Cities

CHIQUITA A. COLLINS[a]

School of Public Health, 140 Warren Hall, University of California at Berkeley, Berkeley, California 94720-7360, USA

OBJECTIVES

A growing number of studies have emphasized that racism, in its multiple manifestations, has pervasive adverse consequences.[1,2] This study examines the extent to which racial residential segregation affects the health of African Americans (or blacks) and whites. The analyses reveal that residential segregation plays a significant role in accounting for elevated rates of mortality amenable to medical intervention, although the strength of the association varies by geographic region.

METHODOLOGY

Data are extracted from national mortality records from 1989 through 1991 and the 1990 US Census. Analyses are based on U.S. central cities with a total population of at least 100,000 and with an African American population of at least 10%. These criteria yielded a sample size of 107 cities. The dependent variables in this study are the adult mortality rates for blacks and nonblacks per 100,000 population.

Using a classification scheme proposed by Rutstein and colleagues,[3] only mortality amenable to medical intervention was analyzed, which includes death from infectious and parasitic diseases (e.g., tuberculosis, syphilis, and measles), specific cancers, anemia, pneumonia and influenza, appendicitis, heart diseases, viral hepatitis, diabetes, ulcers, and congenital abnormalities. Mortality rates were adjusted for the age distribution of the 1990 U.S. population using direct standardization techniques to obtain race- and gender-specific, age-standardized mortality rates. All race-specific information obtained from the U.S. Census corresponds with the racial categories of the mortality data. Race was defined as either black or nonblack.

Racial residential isolation is the primary measure of racial residential segregation used. Following the recommendation of Massey and Denton,[4] black isolation from nonblacks is calculated using an interracial exposure measure, the interaction index $_xP_y^*$. It captures the degree to which blacks have potential contact with nonblacks. Values of $_xP_y^*$ were reversed so that a high value on the isolation index represents a high level of residential segregation. The scores on the index range from zero to 100. They represent the probability that a randomly drawn black person in

[a]Address for correspondence: 510-643-1884 (voice).
e-mail: ccollin@socrates.berkeley.edu

the city interacts with a nonblack person. In contrast to prior research, which typically measures residential segregation at the census tract level, this study measured the black social isolation index based on block-group level data. Race-specific measures of low occupational status and poverty were used as indicators of socioeconomic deprivation. Occupational status was measured by the proportion of persons who are not employed in managerial and professional positions. Poverty was measured by the proportion of persons below the federal poverty line (measured in 1989 dollars).

Analyses were performed for cities in four major geographical regions in the United States: the West, Midwest, Northeast, and the South. The natural log of the total population size is used as a demographic control in all analyses. Ordinary least squares (OLS) regression is used to assess the extent to which social isolation (residential segregation) is related to mortality amenable to medical intervention.

RESULTS

This study demonstrates that after adjustment for socioeconomic deprivation, cities with high levels of black social isolation tend to be positively related to rates of mortality amenable to medical intervention for both African Americans and whites, with the pattern varying by region. That is, cities with high levels of residential segregation tend to have higher rates of mortality amenable to medical intervention. This pattern is evident particularly in the Midwest, for both African American (marginally significant) and white males. Black social isolation was also positively related to elevated rates of mortality in cities in the Northeast, but only for African American men (marginally significant) and women. Interestingly, we find that for

TABLE 1. Unstandardized (and standardized) regression coefficients for the association of the black social isolation index and mortality amenable to medical intervention, men and women (aged 15–64) by race: 1990[a]

Region	African Americans		Whites	
	Men	Women	Men	Women
West ($n = 13$)	1.93	0.93	−1.57	−0.30
Isolation index	(0.25)	(0.45)	(−0.21)	(−0.17)
Midwest ($n = 26$)	0.71[b]	0.21	0.65[c]	0.15
Isolation index	(0.36)	(0.28)	(0.46)	(0.24)
Northeast ($n = 21$)	4.55[b]	2.07[c]	0.64	0.13
Isolation index	(0.49)	(0.56)	(0.28)	(0.17)
South ($n = 47$)	1.96[c]	0.38	1.84[d]	0.33[d]
Isolation index	(0.35)	(0.17)	(0.40)	(0.33)

[a]Adjusted for population size, poverty, and occupational status.
[b]$p \leq 0.10$.
[c]$p \leq 0.05$.
[d]$p \leq 0.01$.

residents in the South, residential segregation has a positive association for causes of death amenable to medical intervention for both African American and white men, as well as for white women (TABLE 1).

In additional analyses (not shown), we attempted to assess the segregation and mortality association for cities in the South ($n = 47$) compared to those in other areas ($n = 60$). Overall, we find that a positive association between social isolation and mortality was more pronounced, for both blacks and whites, in cities in the South than in other areas in the country. This pattern is evident for men of both racial groups and only for white women.

CONCLUSIONS

Racial residential segregation affects the quality of life for most African Americans. A growing but small body of research has indicated that residential segregation also adversely impacts the health of African Americans. This study provides important additional evidence to understanding how the social environment may influence mortality, particularly for causes of death considered preventable if adequate medical care is accessible for residents in large urban areas. One of the most intriguing findings is that segregation not only affects elevated rates of mortality amenable to medical intervention among African Americans, but this relationship is also evident for white Americans as well. These findings highlight the need for research to identify the specific contextual or neighborhood characteristics of residential environments that may be consequential to health. In addition, concerted efforts to prevent premature or unnecessary deaths will require identifying specific mortality risks of living in racially segregated urban areas as well as evaluating social inequalities in access to and the quality of health care.

ACKNOWLEDGMENTS

Preparation of this paper was supported in part by the Institute for Research on Race and Public Policy at the University of Illinois at Chicago. I wish to thank David R. Williams for helpful comments on an earlier version of this paper.

REFERENCES

1. COLLINS, C. & D.R. WILLIAMS. 1999. Segregation and mortality: the deadly effects of racism? Sociol. Forum **14:** 495–523.
2. WILLIAMS, D.R. & C. COLLINS. 1995. U.S. socioeconomic and racial differences in health: patterns and explanations. Ann. Rev. Sociol. **21:** 349–386.
3. RUTSTEIN, D.D., W. BERENBERG, T.C. CHALMERS, *et al.* 1976. Measuring the quality of medical care: a clinical method. N. Engl. J. Med. **294:** 582–588.
4. MASSEY, D.S. & N. DENTON. 1988. The dimensions of residential segregation. Soc. Forces **67:** 281–315.

Identifying Social Pathways for Health Inequalities

The Role of Housing

JAMES R. DUNN[a,b] AND MICHAEL V. HAYES[c]

[b]Centre for Health Services and Policy Research, University of British Columbia,
429-2194 Health Sciences Mall, Vancouver, British Columbia, Canada V6T 1Z3

[c]Department of Geography, Simon Fraser University,
Burnaby, British Columbia, Canada V5A 1S6

To date, relatively little research has systematically investigated pathways between housing, socioeconomic status, and health status.[1] At the same time, there is a growing awareness that one of the most important research needs in health inequalities scholarship is to better elucidate those pathways by which differences in socioeconomic status manifest in everyday life, and produce, at the aggregate level, the systematic social gradient in health observed in all industrialized countries of the world.[2,3]

Existing research on the influence of social support, workplace organization, relative and absolute income inequalities, and life-course influences on health give some preliminary direction as to the possible pathways at work in producing social gradients in health. In particular, power relations, identity, social status, and control over life circumstances emerge as factors differentially shaping the everyday lives of people at different points in the social hierarchy, with consequent effects on health status.[4] Three important dimensions of housing—its materiality, meaningfulness, and spatiality—are well known to shape power relations between social actors and groups, to influence the distribution of control over individuals' life circumstances, and to differentially shape social identity and confer social status,[5] suggesting possible pathways between housing, social inequality, and population health.

In this study, we sought to investigate links between social inequality, population health, and housing using a combination of quantitative and qualitative methods. Specifically, we conducted a mail survey of 522 residents of two lower-middle income Vancouver neighborhoods (Mount Pleasant and Sunset) and collected information on material and meaningful dimensions of people's housing and neighborhood, as well as information on perceived neighborhood friendliness, social support, recent life events, work stress, self-rated health status, satisfaction with health, and mental health. TABLE 1 shows the results of nonparametric tests for significant relationships between individual explanatory variables and individual outcome variables. Asterisks in the cells indicate a statistically significant relationship, and shading of the cell indicates the relationship was a graded one in the expected direction (see FIG. 1 for example of such gradients).

[a]Address for correspondence: 604-822-1371 (voice); 604-822-4994 (fax).
e-mail: jdunn@chspr.ubc.ca

TABLE 1. Bivariate relationships: Mount Pleasant and Sunset combined

EXPLANATORY VARIABLE (* $p < .05$; ** $p < .01$; *** $p < .001$)	HEALTH STATUS	HEALTH SATISFAC.	MENTAL HEALTH
age			
gender			
income	*	***	
education			
marital status			
ethnicity			
language			
income source	***	***	*
working status	***	***	**
no. persons in hhld			
household type			
number of children at home	*		
monthly housing expense			
equity in home			
capital gains on 1st residence			
feel like you belong in hood?			
proud of neighbourhood?	***	**	***
proud of dwelling?	*	*	**
home reflects identity?	***	***	***
can't stand to be at home?			***
home a good location for life?	***	***	***
worry about having to move?			*
can buy needed items in hood?			
strain of housework	**	**	**
strain of child care			
difficulty with housing costs	**	***	***
no. of close friends	*		
no. of close relatives			
have a confiant?			*
have someone to help?	***		*
satisfaction w/ social activities	*	***	*
job - learn new things?	*		
decision latitude			
job security	**	***	
hostility & conflict at work?	*		
co-workers helpful?	*		*
overall job satisfaction	***	**	**

EXPLANATORY VARIABLE (* $p < .05$; ** $p < .01$; *** $p < .001$)	HEALTH STATUS	HEALTH SATISFAC.	MENTAL HEALTH
dwelling type			**
housing tenure	**	**	**
dwelling part of a co-op?	*	*	*
crowding index (hrs/persons)			
age of dwelling			
interior design / layout	*	*	*
exposure to sunlight		*	**
noise from inside bldg			**
noise from outside bldg			**
amount of space			*
heating			
indoor air quality	***	***	***
safety & security of dwelling	*	*	***
overall dwelling satisfaction	***	***	***
dwelling score			
parks and greenspace			
amount of traffic			
street lighting			
police protection			
recreation facilities			*
personal safety		*	***
neighbourhood as a whole		*	***
neighbourhood score		***	***
how friendly are your neighbours?			***
talk with neighbours - frequency			
help to/from neighbours - freq			
adjust routines due to safety?			**
Sense of Coherence Score	**	***	***
Feel constantly under stress?	***	***	***
lost job	*		*
divorced or separated		***	***
serious illness or injury			
spouse or partner died			*
someone close died			
worried about someone			
financial problems in hhld	***	***	***
life events score	***	***	***

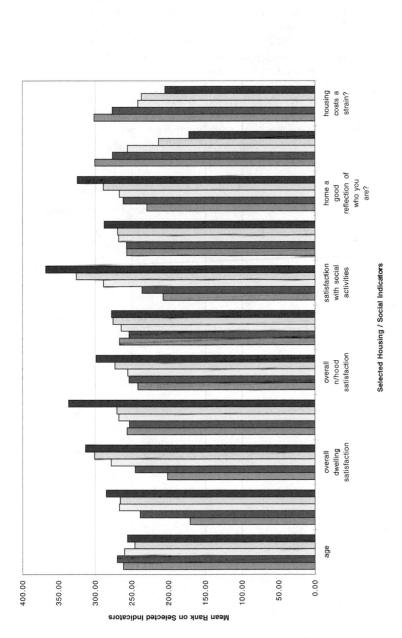
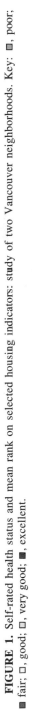

FIGURE 1. Self-rated health status and mean rank on selected housing indicators: study of two Vancouver neighborhoods. Key: ▦, poor; ▨ fair; ▢, good; ▢, very good; ▪, excellent.

The results in TABLE 1 and FIGURE 1 support the hypothesis that material, meaningful, and spatial dimensions of housing are related to health status. People who reported being proud of their dwelling, or that their dwelling was a reflection of their identity, for instance, were more likely to report better health status on all three measures. Control factors, like housing tenure (own/rent), and presence of a tenants' self-management structure (co-op), were significantly associated with health status. Those who reported difficulties in meeting their housing costs, worry about a forced move, dislike of being at home, or dissatisfaction with a number of the physical features of their dwelling were significantly more likely to report poorer health status. Factors such as household composition, crowding (persons per bedroom), and age of dwelling were not significantly associated with health outcomes.

REFERENCES

1. MACINTYRE, S., A. ELLAWAY, G. DER, G. FORD & K. HUNT. 1998. Do housing tenure and car access predict health because they are simply markers of income or self esteem? A Scottish study. J. Epidemiol. Comm. Health **52:** 657–664.
2. LYNCH, J. & G. KAPLAN. 1997. Understanding how inequality in the distribution of income affects health. J. Health Psych. **2**(3): 297–314.
3. MACINTYRE, S. 1997. The Black Report and beyond: what are the issues? Soc. Sci. Med. **44**(6): 723–745.
4. WILKINSON, R.G. 1996. Unhealthy Societies: The Afflictions of Inequality. Routledge, London.
5. DUNN, J.R. 1998. Social Inequality, Population Health, and Housing: Towards a Social Geography of Health. Ph.D. dissertation, Simon Fraser University, Burnaby, Canada.

Transitions into Poverty Following Job Loss and the Depression–Reemployment Relationship

ELIZABETH M. GINEXI,[a] GEORGE W. HOWE,[a] AND ROBERT D. CAPLAN

Center for Family Research, George Washington University,
2300 Eye Street, NW, Room 613, Washington, D.C. 20037, USA

INTRODUCTION

For many, unemployment triggers a precipitous financial decline. In a sample of 254 recently unemployed men and women recruited from unemployment offices in urban and suburban counties in Southern Maryland, only about 6% were below the poverty line before job loss, whereas nearly 40% were below the poverty line after job loss. Six months later, 21% of the families remained below the poverty line.

A substantial body of research has demonstrated a link between job loss and subsequent increases in depressive symptoms.[1-4] Longitudinal investigations have suggested further that it is the unemployment experience that causes the depressive affect rather than preexisting vulnerabilities.[3,5,6] Although some propose that reemployment may reverse the depressive effects of unemployment,[1-3] the extant evidence has not ruled out the possibility that depression may delay reemployment. Also, the role of demographic indicators in this process remains unexplored.

PRESENT STUDY

Individual growth curve modeling and discrete-time survival analyses were used to examine whether reemployment and/or demographic indicators predicted (a) declines in depressive symptoms or (b) time to reemployment. We also investigated whether these relationships were stable or changed over 12 months.

Depressive symptoms (CES-D Scale) and reemployment were assessed over the course of one year among 154 men and 100 women job seekers. Participants ranged in age from 19 to 63 ($M = 35.6$, $SD = 9.5$); 44.4% of the sample were African-American, the remainder were white.

RESULTS

Reemployment within six months was predictive of declines in average (see FIG. 1) and individual levels of depressive symptoms. This pattern did not hold for

[a]Address for correspondence: Elizabeth Ginexi or George Howe, George Washington University, Center for Family Research, 2300 Eye St., NW, Room 613, Washington, DC 20037.
e-mail: cfremg@mail.gwumc.edu

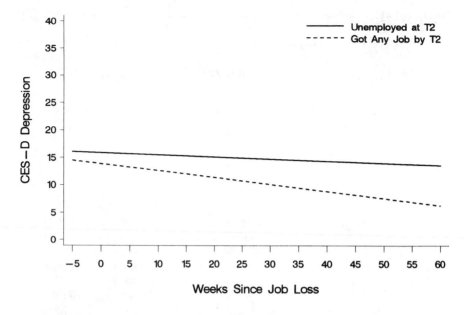

FIGURE 1. Declines in depression as a function of reemployment.

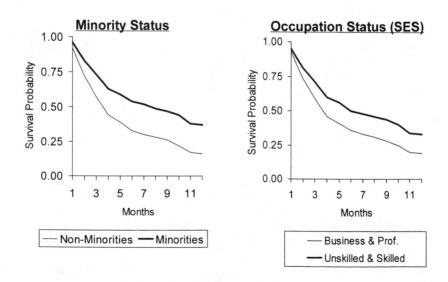

FIGURE 2. Demographic predictors of time to reemployment.

reemployment procured beyond six months. However, initial depression was completely unrelated to time to reemployment. Demographic indicators were not predictive of changes in depression during either the early or later months following job loss, but minority status, SES, and age were significant predictors of time to reemployment (see FIG. 2). Among job seekers who were still unemployed after six months, only SES remained a significant predictor of later re-employment.

CONCLUSIONS

Reemployment obtained within the first six months served to resolve post job loss depressive symptoms, and initial post job loss depression neither prevented nor aided job seekers in becoming reemployed quickly. At the same time, minorities, persons in lower SES levels, and older job seekers were less likely to procure early reemployment.

ACKNOWLEDGMENTS

This poster is based on research supported in part by funding from the Prevention Research Branch of the National Institute of Mental Health (R01-MH47292). We gratefully acknowledge the help of Thomas Wendel of the Maryland Department of Labor, Licensing, and Regulation in securing the sample. The first author was funded by a Public Health Service Grant National Research Service Award (5T32MH19833-04).

REFERENCES

1. KESSLER, R.C., J.B. TURNER & J.S. HOUSE. 1988. Effects of unemployment on health in a community survey: main, modifying, and mediating effects. J. Soc. Issues **44:** 69–85.
2. FRESE, M. & G. MOHR. 1987. Prolonged unemployment and depression in older workers: a longitudinal study of intervening variables. Soc. Sci. Med. **25:** 173–178.
3. FEATHER, N.T. & G.E. O'BRIEN. 1986. A longitudinal study of the effects of employment and unemployment on school-leavers. J. Occup. Psychol. **59:** 121–144.
4. FLYNN, R.J. 1993. Effect of unemployment on depressive affect. *In* Depression and the Social Environment: Research and Intervention with Neglected Populations. P. Cappeliez & R.J. Flynn, Eds.: 185–217. McGill–Queen's University Press, Montreal.
5. PATTON, W. & P. NOLLER. 1984. Unemployment and youth: a longitudinal study. Aust. J. Psychol. **36:** 399–413.
6. TIGGEMANN, M. & A.H. WINEFIELD. 1984. The effects of unemployment on the mood, self-esteem, locus of control, and depressive affect of school-leavers. J. Occup. Psychol. **57:** 33–42.

Longitudinal Effects of Occupational, Psychological, and Social Background Characteristics on Health of Older Workers

MESFIN SAMUEL MULATU[a] AND CARMI SCHOOLER

Section on Socio-Environmental Studies, National Institute of Mental Health, Bethesda, Maryland 20892-9005, USA

INTRODUCTION

Several studies in the United States and Britain have shown linkages between socioeconomic status and health.[1] The mechanisms through which these linkages occur, however, remain unclear. Our primary analyses explore such potential mechanisms by examining the independent and interactive effects on health outcomes, after 20 years, of three different sets of variables linked to social status: job conditions and psychological and sociodemographic characteristics.

METHODS

Sample

The primary sample used in the present analyses included all 1974 workers that were located in 1994–1995 in the Kohn and Schooler longitudinal study of occupational conditions, personality, and health outcomes.[2] There were 334 men and 181 women with mean [SD] age in 1994–1995 of 64 [9.3] years. Detailed information about the sample and measures used are presented elsewhere.[2]

Measures

Sociodemographic factors examined included age, gender, race, education, paternal education, religion, and urbaneness and region of origin. Job-related variables included 1974 occupational status, hours of work, job income, and various measures of the actual nature of work done (e.g., complexity, dirtiness, heaviness of work). Among the 1974 psychological characteristics included are authoritarianism, self-confidence, self-deprecation, morality, fatalism, and anxiety. Detailed descriptions of all 1974 job, personality, and social background characteristics are provided elsewhere.[2] Health outcomes in 1994–1995 included caseness for clinical depression, extent of ill health defined by self-rated health, number of diagnoses, number of prescription medications, and self-rated difficulties of daily life. All variables are scored in the direction their labels suggest.

[a]Address for correspondence: Mesfin Mulatu, Ph.D., SSES/NIMH/NIH, 7550 Wisconsin Avenue, Room B1A-14, Bethesda, MD 20892-9005. 301-496-3383 (voice); 301-402-0621 (fax).
e-mail: Mesfin.Mulatu@nih.gov

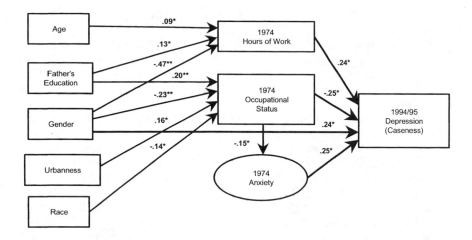

FIGURE 1. Significant paths in a longitudinal model predicting clinical depression. NOTE: χ^2/df = 393.2/184; *$p < 0.05$ and **$p < 0.01$. Indicators for the latent variable "1974 anxiety," and insignificant variables and paths are not shown. Coefficients are completely standardized βs and γs.

Analyses

The effects of the predictors on continuous (ill health, daily difficulties) and categorical (clinical depression) outcomes were systematically estimated in path analytic models using the Mplus modeling program.[3] Both direct and indirect effects were explored.

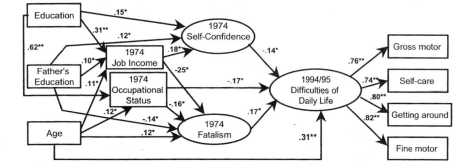

FIGURE 2. Significant paths in a longitudinal model predicting difficulties of daily life. NOTE: RMSEA = 0.048; χ^2/df = 1397.2/701; *$p < 0.05$ and **$p < 0.01$. Indicators for the latent concepts (e.g., "1974 self-confidence") and insignificant variables and paths are not shown. Coefficients are completely standardized βs and γs.

RESULTS AND DISCUSSION

We found significant relationships, in the expected directions, between 1974 sociodemographic, job-related, and psychological variables and 1994–1995 health outcomes. As expected, 1994–1995 ill-health was positively related to age ($\beta = 0.29$, $p < 0.001$) and negatively to 1974 occupational status ($\beta = -0.17$, $p < 0.05$). As shown in FIGURES 1 and 2, 1974 occupational status continued to have its pervasive effects on other health outcomes. Being in a high-status job in 1974 protected workers from clinical depression as well as difficulties of daily life in 1994–1995. Caseness for clinical depression in 1994–1995 was also predicted by longer hours of work and higher levels of anxiety in 1974. Similarly, 1994–1995 difficulties in daily activities were predicted by older age, lower self-confidence, and higher levels of fatalistic thinking in 1974.

In addition to these direct effects, interesting indirect effects on health outcomes were also found that suggest possible pathways for the impacts of socioeconomic characteristics on health. For instance, 1974 occupational status reduced 1994–1995 difficulties of daily living by decreasing 1974 fatalistic thinking; it also reduced 1994–1995 clinical depression by lessening 1974 levels of anxiety. Similarly, level of education improved health by increasing both self-confidence and occupational status (see FIGS. 1 and 2). Our findings indicate that social background, job, and psychological characteristics are predictive of health outcomes both directly and indirectly and that job conditions and psychological characteristics have these effects even after a lapse of 20 years. A fuller understanding of the dynamic interaction of these characteristics may help explain how socioeconomic status affects health.

REFERENCES

1. MARMOT, M., C.D. RYFF, L.L. BUMPASS, M. SHIPLEY & N.F. MARKS. 1997. Social inequalities in health: next questions and converging evidence. Soc. Sci. Med. **44**(6): 901–910.
2. KOHN, M. & C. SCHOOLER. 1983. Work and Personality: An Inquiry into the Impacts of Social Stratification. Ablex Publishers, Norwood.
3. MUTHÉN, L.X. & B.O. MUTHÉN. 1998. M*plus* User's Guide. Muthén and Muthén, Los Angeles.

Social Class and Social Cohesion: A Content Validity Analysis Using a Nonrecursive Structural Equation Model

CARLES MUNTANER,[a,b,c] GARY OATES,[c,d] AND JOHN LYNCH[e]

[b]Department of Psychiatric and Community Health,
University of Maryland-Baltimore, Baltimore, Maryland 21201-1579, USA

[c]National Institute of Mental Health, Bethesda, Maryland 20892, USA

[d]Department of Sociology, University of Connecticut,
Storrs, Connecticut 06269-2068, USA

[e]Department of Epidemiology, University of Michigan,
Ann Arbor, Michigan 48109-2029, USA

The psychosocial construct of "social cohesion," understood as social behaviors indicating trust, reciprocity, and concern for the well-being of the members of one's community, is the key determinant of health in the "income inequality and social cohesion model" model (Ref. 1, p. 211). Social cohesion is defined as participation in public affairs, civic responsibility or involvement in public life. Social cohesion can be measured with indicators of voting participation, newspaper readership, or number of cultural voluntary associations (Ref. 1, p. 119–120). Here we define social cohesion as the amount of individual participation in social groups in the community. Indicators of membership in civil organizations, a measure of social cohesion used in the "income inequality and social cohesion" research program,[1] would be appropriate according to that definition. But in order for a psychometric measure to have content validity, it must include a representative sample of indicators of the construct it is supposed to measure. Current measures of social cohesion downplay or do not include forms of participation in social groups that are characteristic of working class communities such as union membership.[2] Furthermore, these working class forms of cohesion can affect the health of communities through labor and political action (e.g., research on collective control[3]). However, the "income inequality and social cohesion" model does not contemplate the relation between class and social cohesion. In political sociology, research within the resource mobilization framework has revealed that members of the middle class have more time and resources to devote to civic participation than members of the working class.[4] Therefore we expect that the *forms of civic social activism tapped by current indicators*[1] *will be associated with middle class location and negatively associated with working class location.* Next, because group participation antecedes collective political participation (e.g., voting, strikes[4]), we hypothesize that Wilkinson's form of *organization membership will mediate the association between middle class and political*

[a]Address for correspondence: Carles Muntaner, Ph.D., P.O. Box 1579, University of Maryland School of Nursing, 655 West Lombard Street, Baltimore, MD 21201-1579, USA.
 e-mail: cmontane@wvu.edu

participation whereas union membership will be the mediator of political participation for working class locations. In testing these hypotheses, we take into account the role of potential confounders such as expected efficacy of individual political action, income, and education.

The study utilizes data from the American ($n = 1719$) and British ($n = 1458$) portions of the Political Action I survey, and subsample ($n = 523$) of the American portion of the Political Action II survey.[5] This subsample comprises of respondents to the Political Action I survey who were reinterviewed seven years later as part of the Political Action II project. The American portion of the Political Action I survey was conducted between June and September of 1974, and the American Portion of the Political Action II survey was conducted between May and September of 1981. Both surveys are based on multistage area probability samples of households. A structural equation model (SEM) with latent variables was used to determine the relative mediating roles of civic organization and union membership and their relation to social class. These models combine structural equation and factor modeling and directly adjust for the fact that latent variables are imprecisely measured.[6] The exogenous variables are the dichotomous *social class* indicator (working class location versus nonworking class location) and the two control variables, *income* and *education*. The explanatory variables are social cohesion (*membership in civic organizations* and *union membership*), individual perceptions of *political efficacy* and the two ultimate dependent variables are *conventional participation* and *legal protesting*. Four of the variables included in this model—organization membership, political efficacy, conventional participation, and legal protesting—are latent variables. Loadings and descriptions for these indicators are listed in TABLE 1. The model, presented in TABLE 2, is designed to remove the effects of political efficacy and organization or union membership on participation of any reciprocal relationship between the two variables. It utilizes panel data from the sample of Americans who were interviewed in 1974 and again in 1981. Identification is obtained by using the time 1 measures of organization membership, union membership, and political efficacy as instruments for their time 2 counterparts, and by excluding cross-lagged effects from the model. The RMSEA was used to assess the similarity between the observed and the estimated variance–covariance matrices.

Findings from the reciprocal effects models are both consistent with the notion that organization membership and union membership are associated with "nonworking class" (i.e., capitalist, manager, and professional locations) and working class locations, respectively, and that both forms of social cohesion are mediators of the social class–political participation relationship (see TABLE 2). Organization membership is a significant function of social class, rendered less likely by working class location. The likelihood of union membership is enhanced by working class position. In spite of the good fit of the model, a relative low sample in the analysis of reciprocal effects cautions against strong inferences and recommends replication of these results with larger samples.

These results are consistent with the conclusion that measures of social cohesion in the "income inequality and social cohesion" research program lack content validity, because they exclude forms of social cohesion emerging from working class communities. This might result in a characterization of these communities as not socially cohesive and attribute their population health experience to this alleged col-

TABLE 1. Factor loadings for each indicator in the model's four latent variables: conventional participation, legal protest, political efficacy, and organization membership[a]

| Latent variable | Reciprocal effects model | | Description |
	Time 1	Time 2	
Conventional participation[b]			
Meeting	—	0.72	[How often do you] "attend a political meeting or rally?"
Official	—	0.71	"…contact public officials or politicians?"
Campaign	—	0.69	"…spend time working for a political party or candidate?"
Work	—	0.64	"…work with other people in this community to try to solve some local problem?"
Discuss	—	0.55	"…discuss politics with people?"
Convince	—	0.41	"…try to convince friends to vote the same as you?"
Voted	—	0.36	"Did you vote in the [last general] election?"
Legal protest[c]			
Boycott	—	0.51	"Joining in boycotts."
Demo	—	0.54	"Attending lawful demonstrations."
Petition	—	0.48	"Signing a petition."
Political efficacy[d]			
Don't care	0.76	0.82	"I don't think public officials care much about what people like me think."
Notopin	0.81	0.75	"Parties are only interested in people's votes, but not their opinions."
Losetie	0.77	0.64	"Generally speaking, people we elect to congress lose touch with the people pretty quickly."
Nosay	0.58	0.61	"People like me have no say in what the government does."
Organization membership[e]			
Polorg	0.42	0.43	Political party
Polorg2	0.22	0.26	Other political organizations
Proforg	0.50	0.65	Professional associations
Intgporg	0.30	0.29	Special interest groups or hobbies
Civicorg	0.35	0.42	Civic groups
Raceorg	0.12	0.16	Racial or ethnic organizations

[a]$p < 0.01$ or $p < 0.05$ for each loading. Control variables: Z of family income—standardized (gross yearly) family income in dollars/pounds. Z of family education—respondent's education in years.

[b]The first six indicators are accompanied by the following response categories: 4, often; 3, sometimes; 2, seldom; 1, never. The seventh (voted) is a dichotomy (1, yes) (0, no).

[c]Accompanying response categories are the following: 4, often; 3, sometimes; 2, seldom; 1, never.

[d]Accompanying response categories are the following: 1, strongly agree; 2, agree; 3, disagree; 4, strongly disagree.

[e]For each item, membership is coded 1 and nonmembership 0. Class was assigned according to response: (1) working class—employees who fall within none of the four middle–upper class occupation categories (see 0 response occupation categories); (0) middle and upper class—a combination of the following occupational categories:
• capitalists—self-employed and supervising at least one person;
• self-employed—self-employed and supervising no one;
• supervisors—employed individuals who supervise others;
• professional/managerial—nonsupervisory employed individuals who hold/held jobs classified as such by the ILO.
NOTE: Classifications are based on respondents' current or last job. Respondents who had never held a paid job were excluded from the analysis.

TABLE 2. Estimates for reciprocal effects model: standardized coefficients reported[a,b]

	Political efficacy		Organization membership		Union membership		Conventional participation	Legal protest
	(T1)	(T2)	(T1)	(T2)	(T1)	(T2)	(T2)	(T2)
Working class (T1)	0.05	—	-0.17^c	—	0.23^c	—	0.09	0.02
Political efficacy (T1)	—	0.57^c	—	—	—	—	—	—
Political efficacy (T2)	—	—	—	0.03	—	0.05	0.06	-0.03
Organization membership (T1)	—	—	—	$0.84^{a,c}$	—	—	—	—
Organization membership (T2)	—	0.16^c	—	—	—	—	0.55^c	0.24^c
Union membership (T2)	—	—	—	—	—	0.71^c	—	—
Union membership (T2)	—	-0.01	—	—	—	—	0.04	0.34^c
Z of family income (T1)	0.10	—	0.17^d	—	0.14^c	—	0.10^e	0.13^e
Education (T1)	0.31^c	—	0.67^c	—	-0.07	—	0.06	0.35^c

[a]The errors between organization membership at time 1 and time 2 were allowed to correlate.
[b]RMSEA = 0.035; $\chi^2 = 870.78$; $df = 626$.
[c]$p < 0.01$.
[d]$p < 0.05$.
[e]$p < 0.10$.

lective liability. The unintended consequence of such characterization could be to fuel punitive or moralistic policies.[2]

ACKNOWLEDGMENTS

This work was supported by the funds from NIMH and CDC, project # Z01 MH02610-04, Z01 MH02610-05, U48/CCU310821 (Dr. Muntaner). The contents are solely the views of the authors and do not necessarily represent the official views of the aforementioned funding agencies.

REFERENCES

1. WILKINSON, R.G. 1996. Unhealthy Societies: The Afflictions of Inequality. Routledge, London.
2. FOX PIVEN, F. & R.A. CLOWARD. 1999. The Breaking of the American Social Compact. Vintage Books, New York.

3. JOHNSON, J.V. & G. JOHANSSON. 1991. The Psychosocial Work Environment: Work Organization, Democratization and Health. Baywood, New York.
4. JENKINS, C.J. & B. KLANDERMANS. 1995. The Politics of Social Protest: Comparative Perspectives on States and Social Movements. University of Minnesota Press, Minneapolis.
5. JORESKOG, K.G. & A.-M. AISH. 1990. A panel model for political efficacy and responsivenesss: an application of LISREL 7 with weighted least squares. Qual. Quant. **24:** 405–426.
6. JORESKOG, K.G. & D. SORBOM. 1993. Lisrel 8 User's Reference Guide. Scientific Software International, Chicago.

The Effect of Job Strain on Ambulatory Blood Pressure in Men: Does It Vary by Socioeconomic Status?

PAUL A. LANDSBERGIS,[a,b] PETER L. SCHNALL,[b,c] KATHERINE WARREN,[b] THOMAS G. PICKERING,[b] AND JOSEPH E. SCHWARTZ[b,d]

[b]Weill Medical College of Cornell University, New York, New York 10021, USA

[c]University of California, Irvine, Irvine, California 92717, USA

[d]State University of New York at Stony Brook, Stony Brook, New York 11790, USA

Job strain has consistently been shown to be a risk factor for cardiovascular disease (CVD) and for blood pressure when it is measured with an ambulatory monitor.[1] Job strain is defined as work that combines high psychological workload demands with low decision latitude or low control.[2] In addition, some studies have suggested that the effect of job strain on CVD and on CVD risk factors is greater among men with lower socioeconomic status (SES) (e.g., Johnson *et al.*[3] and Hallqvist *et al.*[4]). We tested this hypothesis in a sample of 283 healthy male employees, aged 30–60 at initial recruitment, at eight New York City work sites, 195 of whom were restudied three years after their initial participation. Mean systolic (SAmBP) and diastolic (DAmBP) ambulatory blood pressure at work, home, and during sleep were computed from 24-hour recordings and diary entries specifying location. Job characteristics were assessed by a psychosocial questionnaire. Multiple regression analysis was used to examine the cross-sectional and prospective associations of AmBP with job strain, controlling for age, body mass, race/ethnicity, smoking, alcohol consumption, and worksite. Interaction terms were computed by multiplying job strain by years of education, occupational status (Nam-Powers scale, which ranges from 1–99), occupational category (white-collar; clerical, technical or administrative; blue-collar), and personal or family income.

Initial study results had indicated a substantial association between job strain and AmBP both cross-sectionally[5,6] and prospectively.[7] We now find that the job strain–AmBP association at entry into the study (Time 1) was somewhat stronger among men with lower SES. For example, compared to men with a college degree and without job strain, the work SAmBP of men with only a high school degree or less and with job strain was 7.2 mm Hg higher, but the work SAmBP of college graduates with job strain was only 2.6 mm Hg higher. Similarly, compared to white-collar workers without job strain, the work SAmBP of blue-collar workers with job strain was 12.5 nun Hg higher, but the work SAmBP of white-collar workers with job strain was only 3.4 mm Hg higher (FIG. 1). In addition, the observed fall in AmBP over three years among men leaving job strain was somewhat greater for those with

[a]Address for correspondence: Weill Medical College of Cornell University, Division of Hypertension, 525 East 68th St., New York, NY 10021. 212-746-2166 (voice); 212-746-8451 (fax).
e-mail: palands@med.cornell.edu

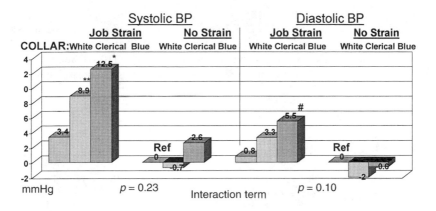

FIGURE 1. Job strain and work ambulatory BP by occupational status ($n = 283$ men, Time 1), controlling for age, body mass index, race, smoking, alcohol use, and work site. $\#p = 0.10$, $*p = 0.05$, $**p = 0.01$ (vs. reference group).

lower SES. For example, among men who entered the study exposed to job strain but were not exposed three years later, those with family income below the median ($55,000) showed a decrease of 5.5 mm Hg work DAmBP, whereas those with higher incomes had virtually no change in work DAmBP (FIG. 2). Similar findings were observed for home and sleep AmBP.

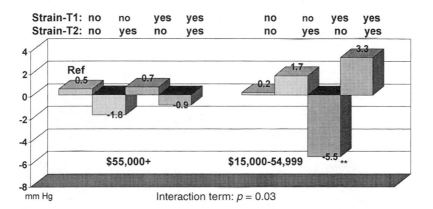

FIGURE 1. Job strain change and 3-year work diastolic ambulatory BP change by family income ($n = 195$ men, Time 1–2), controlling for age, body mass index (T1, T2), race, smoking (T1, T2), alcohol use (T1, T2), and work site. $**p = 0.01$ (vs. reference group).

In summary, men with lower SES appear to show a greater impact of job strain on blood pressure and a greater benefit when leaving a situation of job strain. SES had no consistent main effect on blood pressure. Overall, the main predictors of blood pressure in this sample are age, race, body mass index (BMI), and job strain. The main predictors of blood pressure change are BMI change and job strain change.[7]

REFERENCES

1. SCHNALL, P.L., P.A. LANDSBERGIS & D. BAKER. 1994. Job strain and cardiovascular disease. Annu. Rev. Public Health **15:** 381–411.
2. KARASEK, R. & T. THEORELL. 1990. Healthy work: stress, productivity, and the reconstruction of working life. Basic Books, New York.
3. JOHNSON, J.V., E.M. HALL & T. THEORELL. 1989. Combined effects of job strain and social isolation on cardiovascular disease morbidity and mortality in a random sample of the Swedish male working population. Scand. J. Work Environ. Health **15:** 271–279.
4. HALLQVIST, J., F. DIDERICHSEN, T. THEORELL, C. REUTERWALL, A. AHLBOM & THE SHEEP STUDY GROUP. 1998. Is the effect of job strain on myocardial infarction due to interaction between high psychological demands and low decision latitude? Results from Stockholm Heart Epidemiology Program (SHEEP). Soc. Sci. Med. **46:** 1405–1415.
5. SCHNALL, P.L., J.E. SCHWARTZ, P.A. LANDSBERGIS, K. WARREN & T.G. PICKERING. 1992. Relation between job strain, alcohol, and ambulatory blood pressure. Hypertension **19:** 488–494.
6. LANDSBERGIS, P.A., P.L. SCHNALL, K. WARREN, T.G. PICKERING & J.E. SCHWARTZ. 1994. Association between ambulatory blood pressure and alternative formulations of job strain. Scand. J. Work Environ. Health **20:** 349–363.
7. SCHNALL, P.L., P.A. LANDSBERGIS, J. SCHWARTZ, K. WARREN & T.G. PICKERING. 1998. A longitudinal study of job strain and ambulatory blood pressure: results from a three-year follow-up. Psychosom. Med. **60:** 697–706.

Socioeconomic Differences in Social Information Processing and Cardiovascular Reactivity

EDITH CHEN[a] AND KAREN A. MATTHEWS

*Department of Psychiatry, University of Pittsburgh School of Medicine,
3811 O'Hara Street, Pittsburgh, Pennsylvania 15213, USA*

Low socioeconomic status (SES) has a profound influence on children's physical health. As SES decreases, all-cause mortality rates increase linearly,[1] and rates of injury, pneumonia, and cancer mortality increase.[2] One potential explanation for the SES and health relationship may involve social information processing. Lower SES children, because of their more frequent exposure to unpredictable and stressful situations, may develop a schema about the world being a threatening place that requires constant vigilance. This schema may predispose children to interpreting a wide range of situations, including those that are ambiguous in outcome, as threatening. Children who display a bias toward interpreting ambiguous situations as threatening may also be prone to heightened cardiovascular reactivity during such situations. Over time, more frequent episodes of reactivity may place these children at risk for negative health outcomes such as cardiovascular disease (See FIG. 1).

Research has demonstrated that lower SES is associated with heightened reactivity to laboratory stressors[3] and higher resting levels of blood pressure[4] among children. Trait variables such as hostility mediate this relationship among African-American children.[3] In addition, adults in lower status occupations who also have hostile attributional styles have higher blood pressure elevations at work.[5] However, the role of situationally based variables such as social information-processing biases has not been investigated in children.

We tested the mediational role of social information processing in a sample of 198 children (ages 8–17), half Caucasian and half African-American (Time 1: T1). Ninety of these children were retested an average of three years later (Time 2: T2). At both times, children were probed about perceptions of hostile intent and anger in response to scenarios with negative or ambiguous outcomes (Social Cognition Interview). At both times, cardiovascular reactivity was averaged across three laboratory stress tasks (mirror tracing, reaction time, cold forehead). SES was measured by family and paternal Hollingshead scores (based on parent education and occupation).

At T1, among Caucasians, low-SES children responded with more hostile intent perceptions and anger than high-SES children during ambiguous, but not negative, scenarios (see TABLE 1). In addition, analyses of the reactivity data revealed that among Caucasians, lower SES was associated with greater vascular reactivity

[a]Address for correspondence: Edith Chen, Ph.D., University of Pittsburgh School of Medicine, 3811 O'Hara St., Pittsburgh, PA 15213, USA. 412-624-0946 (voice); 412-624-0967 (fax).
e-mail: chene@msx.upmc.edu

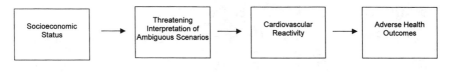

FIGURE 1.

TABLE 1. Correlations between SES and Social Cognition Interview responses by race

	Caucasian	African American
Ambiguous scenarios (Time 1)		
Hostile intent	-0.27^a	-0.13
Anger	-0.23^b	-0.19
Negative scenarios (Time 1)		
Hostile intent	0.00	-0.05
Anger	0.18	-0.15
Ambiguous scenarios (Time 2)		
Hostile intent	0.07	-0.57^a
Anger	-0.33^b	-0.21
Negative scenarios (Time 2)		
Hostile intent	-0.13	-0.19
Anger	0.23	-0.26
Ambiguous scenarios (Time 2 − Time 1)		
Hostile intent	0.19	-0.49^a
Anger	0.26	-0.01
Negative scenarios (Time 2 − Time 1)		
Hostile intent	-0.03	-0.12
Anger	0.05	-0.18
Ambiguous scenarios (Time 1 + Time 2)		
Hostile intent	-0.06	-0.55^a
Anger	0.16	-0.37^b
Negative scenarios (Time 1 + Time 2)		
Hostile intent	-0.03	-0.07
Anger	0.33^b	-0.45^b

NOTE: Higher scores reflect higher social class, and greater perceptions of hostile intent or anger.
[a]$p < 0.01$.
[b]$p < 0.05$.

[greater increases in diastolic blood pressure (DBP) and total peripheral resistance (TPR)] in response to laboratory stressors. When response to ambiguous scenarios was partialled out, the percent of variance in DBP/TPR reactivity that SES accounted for decreased by 18–43%.

At T2, among African Americans, lower SES was associated with increases in systolic blood pressure (SBP) in response to laboratory stressors. In addition, lower SES was associated with greater perceptions of hostile intent during ambiguous scenarios at T2 (see TABLE 1). Finally, when response to ambiguous scenarios was partialled out, the percent of variance in SBP reactivity that SES accounted for decreased by 31%. In addition, longitudinal analyses revealed that among African Americans, lower SES at T1 was associated with both increases in hostile intent perceptions from T1 to T2 and with consistently high hostile intent perceptions at both T1 and T2 (see TABLE 1). When increases in hostile intent perceptions were partialled out, the percent of variance in T2 SBP reactivity that SES accounted for decreased by 70%. When consistently high hostile intent perceptions were partialled out, the percent of variance in T2 SBP reactivity that SES accounted for decreased by 28%.

In sum, social information-processing biases appears to be a promising mediator explaining the SES and cardiovascular reactivity relationship in children. Although SES contributes only a small amount to the variance in cardiovascular reactivity, social information processing biases explain a substantial portion of these SES effects.

REFERENCES

1. MARE, R.D. 1982. Socioeconomic effects on child mortality in the United States. Am. J. Public Health **72:** 539–547.
2. NELSON, M.D. 1992. Socioeconomic status and childhood mortality in North Carolina. Am. J. Public Health **82:** 1131–1133.
3. GUMP, B.B., K.A. MATTHEWS & K. RAIKKONEN. 1999. Modeling relationships among socioeconomic status, hostility, cardiovascular reactivity, and left ventricular mass in African-American and White children. Health Psychol. **18:** 140–150.
4. WRIGHT, L.B., F. TREIBER, H. DAVIS, C. BUNCH & W.B. STRONG. 1998. The role of maternal hostility and family environment upon cardiovascular functioning among youth two years later: socioeconomic and ethnic differences. Ethn. Dis. **8:** 367–376.
5. FLORY, J.D., K.A. MATTHEWS & J.F. OWENS. 1998. A social information processing approach to dispositional hostility: relationships with negative mood and blood pressure elevations at work. J. Soc. Clin. Psychol. **17:** 491–504.

Social Environmental Stress in Indigenous Populations: Potential Biopsychosocial Mechanisms

MARK DANIEL,[a,b] KERIN O'DEA,[b] KEVIN G. ROWLEY,[b]
ROBYN McDERMOTT,[c] AND SHONA KELLY[d]

[b]Department of Epidemiology and Preventive Medicine,
Monash University, Melbourne, Victoria, Australia

[c]Tropical Public Health Unit, Queensland Health, Cairns, Queensland, Australia

[d]Department of Health Care and Epidemiology,
University of British Columbia, Vancouver, Canada

INTRODUCTION

The correlation of stress and socioeconomic status with health status is well documented, but our understanding of the mechanisms by which these affect health is limited.[1] Social environmental stress is of two forms. *Systemic stress,* specific to social group experiences, reflects inequalities and imbalance in society, linking lived experience to health status. *Random stress* operates with similar probability across all social groups, linking individual-level experiences (e.g., divorce) to health status.

Indigenous populations are susceptible to systemic stress. "Westernization," the process by which traditional societies are exposed to and made dependent on modern ways of living or external resources inconsistent with traditional patterns, could be inherently stressful for indigenous people.[2] Westernization may affect health not only through shifts in diet and activity patterns, but by neuroendocrine reactions to psychogenic stress.[3] Glycated hemoglobin A_{1c} (HbA_{1c}), elevated by catecholamine-mediated increases in blood glucose,[4] is a practical biomarker of stress.[5] We tested the hypothesis that HbA_{1c} concentrations are greater in indigenous than in westernized populations.

METHODS

The study contrasted three indigenous and two nonindigenous population groups (TABLE 1). Persons sampled were volunteers for community-based diabetes-screening initiatives, representative of their respective population groups. Fasting HbA_{1c} and 2-hour post-load glucose levels were determined. All participants were classified

[a]Current address for correspondence: Dr. Mark Daniel, Department of Health Behavior and Health Education, School of Public Health, University of North Carolina at Chapel Hill, CB# 7400, Rosenau Hall, Room 302, Chapel Hill, NC 27599-7400, USA. 919-843-8043 (voice); 919-966-2921 (fax).
  e-mail: mdaniel@sph.unc.edu

TABLE 1. Descriptive characteristics for population samples ($n = 611$)

	Indigenous			Non-Indigenous	
	Australian Aborigines ($n = 116$)	Torres Strait Islanders ($n = 156$)	Native Canadians ($n = 155$)	Caucasian Australians ($n = 67$)	Greek Migrants ($n = 117$)
	Mean ($\pm$ S.D.)[a]				
Age (years)	41.3 ± 18.9	36.3 ± 16.1	42.0 ± 13.8	59.6 ± 7.8	59.9 ± 6.5
Male (%)	48.3 ± 9.2	51.3 ± 7.9	34.8 ± 7.7	83.6 ± 9.1	50.4 ± 9.3
Female (%)	51.7 ± 9.2	48.7 ± 7.9	65.2 ± 7.7	16.4 ± 9.1	49.6 ± 9.2
Normoglycemia (%)	57.8 ± 9.1	75.0 ± 6.9	89.0 ± 5.1	74.6 ± 10.6	70.1 ± 8.5
Impaired glucose (%)	16.4 ± 6.9	7.7 ± 4.3	6.5 ± 4.0	16.4 ± 9.1	19.7 ± 7.3
Diabetes mellitus (%)	25.9 ± 8.1	17.3 ± 6.7	4.5 ± 3.4	9.0 ± 7.1	10.3 ± 5.7

[a]Figures given are mean ± SD, adjusted for cluster sampling.

by WHO criteria as normoglycemic or having impaired glucose tolerance (IGT) or diabetes mellitus (DM). Body mass index (BMI, in kg/m^2) was assessed. The data were analyzed for group differences, adjusting for age, gender, BMI, glycemic status, and 2-hour glucose.

RESULTS

Indigenous people had greater HbA_{1c} concentration at each glycemic status classification (FIG. 1). Mean HbA_{1c} concentration did not differ between Australian Aborigines, Torres Strait Islanders, or Native Canadians ($p > 0.119$), or between Australian Caucasians and Greek migrants ($p > 0.998$). Mean HbA_{1c} concentration was greater for indigenous relative to nonindigenous groups ($F_{1,579} = 40.3$; $p > 0.0001$). Covariate-adjusted means (95% CI) were 5.85 (5.54–6.15) for indigenous groups, and 4.95 (4.58–5.31) for nonindigenous groups, for a difference (95% CI) of 0.90 (0.58–1.22).

DISCUSSION

At the population level, mean HbA_{1c} concentration is greater by 18.2% for indigenous relative to nonindigenous groups. A greater prevalence of diabetes and glucose intolerance cannot explain greater HbA_{1c} concentration among indigenous groups: HbA_{1c} was greater at each level of glycemic status, and the overall difference was independent of age, sex, BMI, and 2-hour glucose. That differences were statistically significant for normoglycemic as well as diabetic persons is especially important.

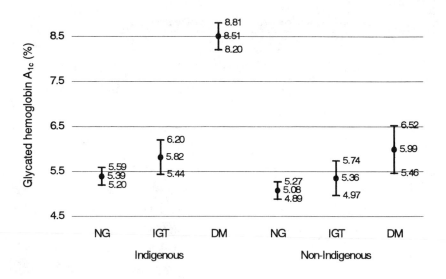

FIGURE 1. Mean glycated hemoglobin A_{1c} by ethnicity and glycemic status, with cluster-adjusted 95% confidence bounds: weighted linear contrasts of indigenous versus nonindigenous (Westernized) groups. NG, normoglycemic; IGT, impaired glucose tolerance; DM, diabetes mellitus.

Systemic stress may explain, in part, high HbA_{1c} concentrations among indigenous peoples. This may reflect dissonance related to westernization, not social change *per se*, as HbA_{1c} levels did not differ between Greek migrants and Caucasian Australians. A biological effect of westernization could be mediated by the CNS by cognitively appraised stress. Social change in association with perceived limited control is correlated with psychosocial stress and multifactorial stress responses.[6] Perceived coping inefficacy, and related depression, involve emotional arousal with neuroendocrine responses.[7] CNS modulation of expectancy learning may also occur, where the situational context itself effects emotional arousal. Causal interpretations of one's environment inducing stress reactions involve a combination of external locus of control, lack of stability, and low degree of controllability.[8]

ACKNOWLEDGMENTS

This work was supported in part by the National Health & Medical Research Council of Australia (Grant #954605) and Health Canada through the National Health Research & Development Program (Grant #6610-2022). M.D. holds a Medical Research Council (Canada) Fellowship (1998–1999).

REFERENCES

1. ANESHENSEL, C.S. 1992. Social stress: theory and research. Ann. Rev. Sociol. **18:** 15–38.
2. PEARSON, J.D. *et al.* 1990. Modernization and catecholamine excretion of young Samoan adults. Soc. Sci. Med. **31:** 729–736.
3. BRUNNER, E. 1997. Stress and the biology of inequality. Br. Med. J. **314:** 1472–1476.
4. NETTERSTROM, B. 1988. Glycated hemoglobin and physiological stress. Behav. Med. **14:** 13–16.
5. KELLY, S., *et al.* 1997. Searching for the biological pathways between stress and health. Ann. Rev. Public Health **18:** 437–462.
6. ELY, D.L. 1995. Organization of cardiovascular and neurohumoral responses to stress: implications for health and disease. Ann. N.Y. Acad Sci. **771:** 594–608.
7. BANDURA, A. 1982. Self-efficacy mechanism in human agency. Am. Psych. **37:** 122–47.
8. MICHAELA, J.L. & J.V. WOOD. 1986. Causal attributions in health and illness. *In* Advances in Cognitive-Behavior Research and Therapy. P.C. Kendall, Ed.: 179–235. Academic Press. New York.

Social Status, Anabolic Activity, and Fat Distribution

ELISSA EPEL,[a,b] NANCY ADLER,[b] JEANNETTE ICKOVICS,[c] AND BRUCE McEWEN[d]

[b]Department of Psychiatry, University of California, San Francisco, San Francisco, California 94143-0848, USA

[c]Department of Epidemiology and Public Health, Yale University, New Haven, Connecticut 06520, USA

[d]Laboratory of Neuroendocrinology, Rockefeller University, New York, New York 10021-6399, USA

Growth hormone (GH), an important anabolic hormone, may serve as a measure of positive health. GH is related to more rapid wound healing and speedy recovery from burns, whereas GH deficiency is related to mortality. Excessive exposure to stress may increase cortisol reactivity and decrease activity of the somatotropic axis, including GHRH, GH, and IGF-1. Subordinate baboons, for example, have lower levels of the anabolic hormone IGF-1, which is in part controlled by GH secretion.[1] People of lower SES may experience more stress and develop negative attitudes that may lead to lower anabolic functioning. We therefore investigated whether overnight urinary growth hormone excretion (uGH) was related to social status, central fat distribution (as measured by waist-to-hip ratio or WHR), body mass index (BMI), and reported psychological and physical health.

METHOD

Sixty healthy white women were exposed to three consecutive sessions of challenging laboratory tasks. Urinary growth hormone was measured on a night after a stressful laboratory session and seven days later, and the average uGH was calculated. Women were categorized as either high (above 0.80) or low WIM (below 0.75), and as high (BMI > 24) or low BMI (BMI ≤ 24). Given known differences in GH by weight, lean and overweight women were analyzed separately. Socioeconomic status (SES) was measured by educational degree, and childhood SES was measured by the average years of parents' education.

[a]Address for correspondence: University of California, San Francisco, 3333 California Street, Box 0848, Suite 465, San Francisco, CA 94143, USA. 415-476-7285 (voice).

TABLE 1. Correlations between average nocturnal urinary growth hormone and education

	Overweight women (BMI > 24)	Lean women (BMI ≤ 24)	Total sample
	(*n* = 30)	(*n* = 27)	(*n* = 57)
SES current (education)	−0.20	0.58[a]	0.20
SES from childhood (parent's education)	−0.24	0.47[b]	0.14

[a]$p < 0.01$
[b]$p < 0.05$

RESULTS

GH and Education

Urinary GH was significantly related to greater education (using Spearman rank order correlations), and childhood SES, although only among lean women (see TABLE 1). Women with graduate degrees had the highest uGH, whereas the women with the least education (high school degrees) had the lowest uGH (see FIG. 1).

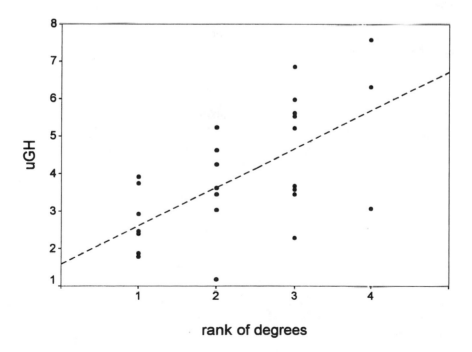

FIGURE 1. Urinary growth hormone (mg/12 h) by education degree among lean women. 1, high school; 2, B.A.; 3, M.A./M.S.W.; 4, Ph.D. or J.D.

Overweight women had lower uGH overall, and their uGH was not related to education.

GH, Central Fat, and Education

Urinary GH was negatively related to central fat across the sample [$r(54) = -0.29$; $p < 0.03$] while controlling for BMI. For lean women, education was marginally negatively related to central fat ($r = -0.36$; $p = 0.07$), and uGH appeared to mediate this relationship, as follows: A multiple regression was used to test whether uGH mediated the relationship between education and central fat. After controlling for uGH, the already weak relationship between education with central fat disappeared ($\beta = -0.19$, $p = 0.44$). Finally, across the sample, independent of BMI, uGH was related to other measures of health, such as better self-reported physical health, lower stress, lower hostility, and more active coping.

CONCLUSION

These results suggest that nocturnal GH is an important mediator of "positive health." Positive health is not simply the opposite of allostatic load but represents resilience to disease. GH is higher among lean women with more education and with higher childhood SES and is associated with a more positive psychological profile. These results also support the hypothesized pathway that low social status may lead to lower GH, which in turn influences accumulation of central fat. GH may prove to be a critical factor in explaining the SES–health gradient at higher levels of SES, at least among lean women.

REFERENCE

1. SAPOLSKY, R. & M. SPENCER. 1997. Insulin-like growth factor I is suppressed in socially subordinate male baboons. Am. J. Physiol. **273:** R1346–1351.

Socioeconomic Status as a Correlate of Sleep in African-American and Caucasian Women

MARTICA HALL,[a,b] JOYCE BROMBERGER,[b,c] AND KAREN MATTHEWS[b,c]

[b]Department of Psychiatry, University of Pittsburgh,
Pittsburgh, Pennsylvania 15213, USA

[c]School of Public Health, University of Pittsburgh,
Pittsburgh, Pennsylvania 15213, USA

INTRODUCTION

Sleep may be an important pathway between the chronic stress of lower socioeconomic status (SES) and adverse health outcomes. Stressful life events and circumstances have potent effects on subjective, as well as laboratory-assessed, measures of sleep.[1,2] Emerging evidence suggests that stress-related sleep disruptions are associated with a number of adverse health outcomes such as susceptibility to upper respiratory tract infections and immune system dysregulation.[3,4] Stress-related sleep disruptions may also be a risk factor for psychiatric morbidity, such as major depression and posttraumatic stress disorder.[5,6] To date, however, relationships among the chronic stress of lower SES, sleep, and health outcomes have not been evaluated. In the present study we focused on the first piece of the stress–sleep–health relationship, that is, the impact of the chronic stress of lower SES on subjective sleep complaints.

METHODS

Subjects were a local cohort of 462 women from the multisite Study of Women's Health Across the Nation (SWAN). Age range of subjects was 41 to 52 years, 35% of whom were African-American and the remainder were Caucasian. Due to the impact of the menopause on sleep, only women who were classified as pre- or early perimenopausal were included in these analyses.

Education was trichotomized into 12 years or less, college-educated, and greater than 16 years of education. Income was dichotomized into subjects earning less than or greater than $35,000 annually. The chronic stress of lower SES was dichotomized as moderate to severe versus no difficulty making ends meet. Sleep measures included sleep difficulties (e.g., trouble falling asleep) experienced once or more per week or not at all during the past two weeks and subjective sleep quality, defined as restless versus sound sleep.

[a]Address for correspondence: Martica Hall, Ph.D., Sleep and Chronobiology Center, E-1101 O'Hara Street, Pittsburgh, PA 15213, USA. 412-624-2246 (voice); 412-624-2841 (fax).
e-mail: hallmh@msx.upmc.edu

TABLE 1. Adjusted odds ratios for sleep quality and associated risk factors

	Adjusted odds ratio	95% Cl
Age	0.89^a	0.81–0.98
Race	0.97	0.92–1.02
Menstrual status	0.72	0.44–1.14
Education	0.98	0.68–1.41
Income	0.79^b	0.46–1.35
Meeting ends	1.92^a	1.14–3.23

NOTE: All measures entered simultaneously.
$^a p < 0.05.$
$^b p < 0.01.$

Logistic regression was used to calculate the strength of relationships among income, education, the chronic stress of difficulties making ends meet, and measures of sleep, after controlling for the effects of age, race, and menstrual status on sleep. Hierarchical logistic regression was used to evaluate mediation of the SES–sleep relationship by chronic stress.

RESULTS

After controlling for the effects of age, race, menstrual status, and education on sleep, income and difficulty making ends meet were significant predictors of subjective sleep quality (p values less than 0.05), whereas neither significantly predicted frequency of sleep difficulties. As shown in TABLE 1, women with annual family incomes below \$35,000 and moderate to severe difficulty making ends meet reported significantly more restless sleep than did women with incomes above \$35,000 and no difficulties making ends meet. Income was not a significant predictor of sleep when analyses were run with income as a more continuous variable. Menstrual status was the only significant predictor of frequency of sleep difficulties. Women classi-

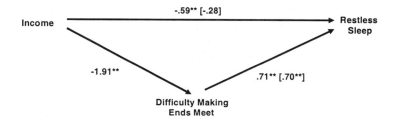

FIGURE 1. Chronic stress of low SES as a mediator of the income–sleep relationship. Values in brackets represent standardized regression coefficients with predictors entered in the same step; ** $p < 0.01$.

fied as early perimenopausal reported greater frequency of sleep difficulties than did premenopausal women ($p < 0.01$).

Tests of mediation revealed that difficulty making ends meet was a significant mediator of the income–sleep relationship. In the first equation, income was a significant predictor of subjective sleep quality ($p < 0.01$), after controlling for age. In the second equation, income and difficulty making ends meet was entered in the same step of the regression equation. In this model, difficulty making ends meet was a significant predictor of subjective sleep quality ($p < 0.01$), whereas the income–sleep relationship was no longer significant (see FIG. 1).

DISCUSSION

Results indicate that poverty is associated with subjective sleep complaints in middle-aged women, irrespective of age, race, or menstrual status. Although data were collected cross-sectionally, subjective reports of difficulty making ends meet emerged as a mediator of the relationship between income and subjective sleep quality. Thus, results are consistent with the hypothesis that the chronic stress associated with lower SES is a significant pathway between poverty and poor sleep.

SUMMARY

Sleep may be an important pathway between the chronic stress of lower socioeconomic status (SES) and adverse health outcomes. We evaluated relationships between SES and subjective sleep complaints in a sample of 462 women between the ages of 41 and 52. Stepwise logistic regression revealed that income and the subjective stress of lower SES were significant correlates of sleep, after controlling for age, race, menstrual status, and education. Lower income (below \$35,000 annually) and moderate to severe difficulty making ends meet were significantly associated with poorer subjective sleep quality. In a separate set of analyses, difficulty making ends meet was shown to fully mediate the relationship between income and subjective sleep quality. Longitudinal research on the extent to which the chronic stress of lower SES leads to sleep disruptions and predicts subsequent health outcomes is needed in order to evaluate the causal role of sleep in the SES–health relationship.

ACKNOWLEDGMENTS

This research was supported in part by the National Institute of Aging AG12546 and the National Institute of Mental Health MH01554 and MH30914.

REFERENCES

1. HALL, M., D.J. BUYSSE, M.A. DEW, H.G. PRIGERSON, D.J. KUPFER & C.F. REYNOLDS. 1997. Intrusive thoughts and avoidance behaviors are associated with sleep disturbances in bereavement-related depression. Depres. Anxiety **6:** 106–112.

2. IRONSON, G., C. WYNINGS, N. SCHNEIDERMAN, A. BAUM, M. RODRIGUEZ, D. GREENWOOD, C. BENIGHT, M. ANTONI, A. LAPERRIERE, H.S. HUANG, N. KLIMAS & M.A. FLETCHER. 1997. Posttraumatic stress symptoms, intrusive thoughts, loss, and immune function after Hurricane Andrew. Psychosom. Med. **59:** 128–141.
3. HALL, M., A. BAUM, D.J. BUYSSE, H.G. PRIGERSON, D.J. KUPFER & C.F. REYNOLDS. 1998. Sleep as a mediator of the stress-immune relationship. Psychosom. Med. **60:** 48–51.
4. COHEN, S., W.J. DOYLE, D.P. SKONER, B.S. RABIN & J.M. GWALTNEY, JR. 1997. Social ties and susceptibility to the common cold. JAMA **277:** 1940–1944.
5. ROSS, R.J., W.A. BALL, K.A. SULLIVAN & S.N. CAROFF. 1989. Sleep disturbance as the hallmark of post-traumatic stress disorder. Am. J. Psychiatry **146**(6): 697–707.
6. CARTWRIGHT, R.D. & E. WOOD. 1991. Adjustment disorders of sleep: the sleep effects of a major stressful event and its resolution. Psychiatry Res. **39:** 199–209.

The Differential Effects of Sleep Quality and Quantity on the Relationship between SES and Health

AMY E. SICKEL,[a,b] PHILIP J. MOORE,[b] NANCY E. ADLER,[c]
DAVID R. WILLIAMS,[d] AND JAMES S. JACKSON[d]

[b]Department of Psychology, George Washington University,
Washington, D.C. 20052, USA

[c]Department of Psychiatry, University of California,
San Francisco, California 94115, USA

[d]Institute for Social Research, University of Michigan, Ann Arbor, Michigan 48106, USA

INTRODUCTION

Although socioeconomic status (SES) has long been recognized as a principal determinant of health, one factor yet to be considered in the context of SES and health is the role of sleep. Individuals of lower socioeconomic status have been found more likely to experience sleep disorders,[1] and sleep disturbances have been associated with poorer health.[2] The amount of sleep people get has been found to mediate the relationship between stress-related intrusive thoughts and natural killer cell levels.[3] However, sleep has yet to be examined as a potential mediator of the impact of socioeconomic status on physical or mental health. This study tested the following three hypotheses. First, participants of higher socioeconomic status will report better psychological health. Second, participants of higher socioeconomic status will report better physical health. Third, the relationship between participants' socioeconomic status and their health will be mediated by either their quantity or quality of sleep.

METHOD

The data for the current analyses comes from the 1995 Detroit Area Study (DAS), a multistage area probability sample of adults. Face-to-face interviews were conducted on 520 Caucasians and 586 African Americans. 63% (693) were women who ranged in age from 18 to 89 years old, with an average age of 46 years.

[a]Address for correspondence: Department of Psychology, George Washington University, 2125 G. Street, NW, Washington, DC 20052, USA. 202-994-4942 (voice); 202-994-1602 (fax).
e-mail: sickel@gwu.edu

Socioeconomic Status

There were two measures of SES. First, *degree years* of education indicated the number of years associated with participants' completion of their highest degree. Second, participants reported access to *income* for 1994.

Sleep

Sleep quantity indicated participants' average hours of sleep per night during the previous month. *Sleep quality* was assessed on a 1–5 scale (1, "poor"; 5, "excellent").

Psychological and Physical Health

The index of *psychological health* combined participants' reports of depression and their overall satisfaction with their lives ($r = -0.22$, $p < 0.001$). Depression responses indicated whether participants had felt depressed for two weeks or more during the previous 12 months, ("yes" or "no"). Current life satisfaction was measured on a 1–5 scale (1, "not at all satisfied"; 5, "completely satisfied"). Both measures were standardized and combined to form an aggregate, single-item measure of psychological well being. Self-reported overall *physical health* was assessed by participants' responses on a 1-to-5 scale (1, "poor"; 5, "excellent").

RESULTS

Psychological Health

Although participants' education levels were not directly related to either their sleep quality or mental health, higher income was associated with both better sleep quality ($b = 0.11$, $p < 0.01$) and greater psychological well-being ($b = 0.21$, $p < 0.001$). Better psychological health was also associated with better sleep quality ($b = 0.18$, $p < 0.001$). Sleep quantity was unrelated to participants' education, income, or their mental health. (FIG. 1).

Physical Health

As in the model of psychological well-being, higher income was directly associated with more education ($b = 0.35$, $p < 0.001$), better sleep quality ($b = 0.11$, $p < 0.01$) and better physical health ($b = 0.13$, $p < 0.01$). Physical well-being was also directly related with more education ($b = 0.14$, $p < 0.01$) and better sleep quality ($b = 0.24$, $p < 0.001$), whereas sleep quantity was unrelated to either SES or physical health (FIG. 2).

Sleep Quality versus Sleep Quantity

Regression analyses tested the effect of the interaction between sleep quality and quantity on physical and psychological health. This interaction was a significant predictor of participants' physical health ($b = -0.34$, $p < 0.05$).

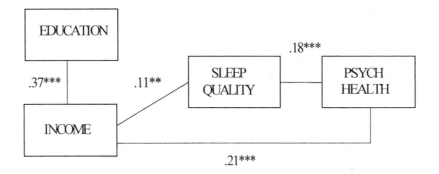

FIGURE 1. Path-analytic model (n = 928) predicting psychological health from education, income, and sleep quality. Models show standardized regression coefficients. ***$p < 0.001$; **$p < 0.01$.

DISCUSSION

Considered separately, both income and education were associated with both physical and psychological health. However, when combined to predict health, income continued to exert a direct influence on both physical and psychological well being, whereas education predicted only physical health. Sleep quality mediated the effect of income on physical and psychological health, and sleep quantity moderated the relationship between sleep quality and physical well being. These findings are consistent with previous research showing significant associations between SES and health, but also suggest that different components of socioeconomic status operate through different pathways to affect health.

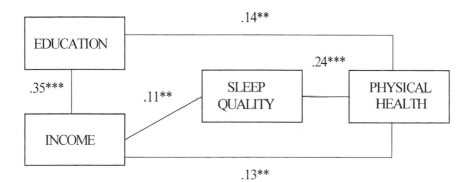

FIGURE 1. Path-analytic model (n = 928) predicting self-reported physical health from education, income, and sleep quality. Models show standardized regression coefficients. ***$p < 0.001$; **$p < 0.01$.

REFERENCES

1. HUNT, S.M., J. MCEWEN & S.P. MCKENNA. 1985. Measuring health status: a new tool for clinicians and epidemiologists. J. Roy. College Gen. Pract. **35:** 185–188.
2. SEGOVIA, J., R.F. BARTLETT & A.C. EDWARDS. 1989. The association between self-assessed health status and individual health practices. Can. J. Pub. Health **80:** 32–37.
3. HALL, M., A. BAUM, M.D. BUYSSE, H.G. PRIGERSON, *et al.* 1998. Sleep as a mediator of the stress–immune relationship. Psychosom. Med. **60:** 48–51.

Stress Responsivity and Body Fatness: Links between Socioeconomic Status and Cardiovascular Risk Factors in Youth

FRANK TREIBER,[a,b,c,d] GREGORY HARSHFIELD,[b,d] HARRY DAVIS,[d,e] GASTON KAPUKU,[b,d] AND DONNA MOORE[b,d]

[b]Department of Pediatrics, [c]Department of Psychiatry, [d]Georgia Prevention Institute, and [e]Office of Biostatistics, Medical College of Georgia, Augusta, Georgia 30912-3710, USA

Inverse associations between socioeconomic status (SES) and cardiovascular (CV) morbidity and mortality have long been established. Although pathogenesis of CV disease (CVD) has its origins in childhood, few studies have examined relationships between SES and preclinical markers of CVD risk in youth (e.g., increased systolic blood pressure [SBP] and increased left ventricular mass [LVM]). Findings have been mixed with regard to relationships between SES and resting blood pressure (BP) in youth. To our knowledge only one pediatric study has examined SES and LVM; an inverse association was observed.[1]

This study evaluated the impact of family and neighborhood indices of SES on LVM and resting BP in 549 African-American and white youth. Adiposity and exaggerated vasoconstrictive-mediated reactivity to stress were examined as possible mediating variables linking SES with the CVD risk factors.

All subjects had a verified family history of CVD (i.e., essential hypertension and/or premature myocardial infarction). All subjects were normotensive, nondiabetic, and free from acute or chronic illness. During an annual evaluation, anthropometrics (e.g., height, weight, waist/hip circumference, multiple skinfolds) were measured using established protocols.[2,3] Hemodynamics at rest and during laboratory stressors of postural change, social competence interview, and virtual reality car driving were measured using established protocols.[2,3] The anatomically validated formula of Devereaux et al.[4] was used to calculate echocardiographic-derived LVM, which was adjusted for body habitus using height$^{2.7}$ (LVM/ht$^{2.7}$).

Pearson correlations were conducted comparing SES with the CVD risk factors, adiposity, and total peripheral resistance (TPR) reactivity. Correlations were conducted separately by gender and age group (younger, 15.1 ± 1.1 years, 182 whites, 156 blacks, 151 males versus older, 19.2 ± 1.6 years, 93 whites, 118 blacks, 110 males). As shown in TABLES 1 and 2, among males, lower family SES (i.e., Hollingshead Four Factor Scale) was associated with higher resting SBP and increased LVM/ht$^{2.7}$. Among older females, lower neighborhood SES (i.e., aggregate of seven indices from 1990 Census tract data) was associated with higher resting SBP and

[a]Address for correspondence: Frank Treiber, Ph.D. Medical College of Georgia Georgia Prevention Institute, Bldg. HS1640, Augusta, GA 30912-3710, USA. 706-721-6295 (voice); 706-721-7150 (fax).
  e-mail: ftreiber@mail.mcg.edu

TABLE 1. Younger youth

	Males				Females			
	Family SES	Neighborhood SES	Resting SBP	LVM/ht.$^{2.7}$	Family SES	Neighborhood SES	Resting SBP	LVM/ht.$^{2.7}$
CV Markers								
Resting SBP (mmHg)	-0.23^a	0.01	—	—	-0.06	-0.08	—	—
LVM/ht.$^{2.7}$ (g/m$^{2.7}$)	-0.26^a	-0.09	0.21^b	—	-0.10	-0.05	0.27^a	—
Adiposity								
BMI (kg/m^2)	-0.23^a	-0.11	0.33^c	0.52^c	-0.30^c	-0.10	0.35^c	0.75^c
WHR	-0.16	0.03	0.19^b	0.39^c	-0.20^b	-0.14	0.23^a	0.50^c
Conicity	-0.18^b	0.02	0.24^a	0.28^b	-0.19^b	-0.14	0.24^a	0.41^c
Sum of skinfolds (mm)	-0.12	0.03	0.21^a	0.39^c	-0.26^a	-0.05	0.22^a	0.62^c
Vasoconstrictive responsivity ($\overline{\times}$ TPR)								
Car driving	-0.27^a	-0.09	0.02	0.05	0.03	-0.01	0.24^a	0.03
Social competence	-0.16	0.04	0.01	-0.04	0.06	0.06	0.16^b	-0.02
Postural change	-0.13	-0.01	0.17^b	0.02	0.13	0.06	0.24^a	-0.04

ABBREVIATIONS: BMI, body mass index; WHR, waist-to-hip ratio; TPR, mmHg/l/min; conicity $=$ (waist[m]/0.109$\sqrt{\text{wgt}[\text{kg}]}$/ht[m]).
$^a p < 0.01.$
$^b p < 0.05.$
$^c p < 0.001.$

TABLE 1. Older youth

	Males				Females			
	Family SES	Neighborhood SES	Resting SBP	LVM/ht.$^{2.7}$	Family SES	Neighborhood SES	Resting SBP	LVM/ht.$^{2.7}$
CV Markers								
Resting SBP (mmHg)	-0.21^a	-0.05	—	—	-0.03	-0.23^a	—	—
LVM/ht.$^{2.7}$ (g/m$^{2.7}$)	-0.37^b	-0.16	0.17	—	-0.14	-0.22^a	0.22^a	—
Adiposity								
BMI (kg/m^2)	-0.38^b	-0.13	0.19^a	0.49^b	-0.26^a	-0.15	0.10	0.76^b
WHR	-0.16	0.01	0.16	0.19	-0.31^c	-0.10	0.02	0.48^b
Conicity	-0.11	0.07	0.14	0.14	-0.31^c	-0.12	0.02	0.53^b
Sum of skinfolds (mm)	-0.24^a	-0.02	0.09	0.28^c	-0.22^a	-0.08	0.09	0.63^b
Vasoconstrictive responsivity ($\bar{\times}$ TPR)								
Car driving	-0.10	-0.24^c	0.21^a	0.09	-0.27^a	-0.10	0.43^b	-0.04
Social competence	0.05	-0.11	0.07	0.03	-0.25^a	-0.04	0.42^b	-0.09
Postural change	-0.13	-0.21^a	0.26^c	-0.01	-0.29^c	-0.03	0.33^c	-0.02

ABBREVIATIONS: BMI, body mass index; WHR, waist-to-hip ratio; TPR, mmHg/l/min; conicity $= (\text{waist}[m]/0.109\sqrt{\text{wgt}[kg]}/\text{ht}[m])$.

[a] $p < 0.05$.
[b] $p < 0.001$.
[c] $p < 0.01$.

increased $LVM/ht^{2.7}$. Examination of possible mediating effects of reactivity and adiposity indicated that in older youth, irrespective of sex and race, increased TPR stress responsivity (i.e., postural change, car driving, social competence interview) was associated with lower SES and increased resting SBP. In both age groups, increased general (i.e., body mass index) and central (i.e., waist-to-hip ratio, conicity) adiposity were associated with lower SES and increased $LVM/ht^{2.7}$.

These results are unique and important for several reasons. First, the findings provide further evidence that the influence of SES is evident long before overt manifestation of CVD. Second, the study involved a large sample of white and African-American youth and found that race was not a moderator of relationships between SES and CVD risk factors. Third, and most importantly, exaggerated vasoconstrictive reactivity and adiposity were mediating factors linking lower SES with increased SBP and/or $LVM/ht^{2.7}$. Lifestyle modification programs (i.e., physical activity, diet, stress management) are needed to reduce the CVD risk burden in lower SES youth.

ACKNOWLEDGMENTS

This study was supported in part by Grants HL35073 and HL41781 from the National Institutes of Health.

REFERENCES

1. GUMP, B.B., K.A. MATTHEWS, *et al.* 1999. Modeling relationships among SES, hostility, CV reactivity, and LVM in African American and white children. Health Psychol. **18:** 140–150.
2. JACKSON, R.W., F.A. TREIBER, *et al.* 1999. Effects of race, sex, and socioeconomic status upon cardiovascular stress responsivity and recovery in youth. Int. J. Psychol. **31:** 111–119.
3. TURNER, J.R., F.A. TREIBER, *et al.* 1997. Use of a virtual reality car driving stressor in cardiovascular reactivity research. Behav. Res. Methods Instr. Comp. **29:** 386–389.
4. DEVEREUX, R.B., D.R. ALONSO, *et. al.* 1986. Echocardiographic assessment of left ventricular hypertrophy: comparison to necropsy findings. Am. J. Card. **57:** 450–458.

Social Class Differences in Maternal Stress Appraisal During Pregnancy

MELISSA HAWKINS,[a] JANET A. DiPIETRO, AND KATHLEEN A. COSTIGAN

Department of Population and Family Health Sciences,
Johns Hopkins University, Baltimore, Maryland 21205, USA

INTRODUCTION

Well-designed prospective studies in the past 10 years have provided cumulative evidence that both maternal exposure to psychosocial stress and low socioeconomic status (SES) during pregnancy significantly increase the risk for adverse reproductive outcomes. Prenatal stress is likely to be mediated by contextual features of the environment, and the contribution of low SES to maternal appraisal of stress is currently unknown. Furthermore, studies that have investigated stress during pregnancy have typically used methods to quantify stress that do not include factors related to pregnancy and so may underestimate prenatal stress.

METHOD

This study was designed to examine the contribution of SES to maternal appraisal of pregnancy specific and nonspecific stress during the second half of pregnancy and is part of a larger longitudinal project examining the effect of each on fetal development. Two samples of healthy women with normal pregnancies, stratified by SES ($n = 52$ middle/high SES, $n = 51$ low SES), were assessed at three gestational ages (24, 30, and 36 weeks) using multiple measures of psychosocial functioning. The higher SES group consisted of employed, older, well-educated ($M = 16.3$ years education), primarily nonminority (77%) women; subjects in the lower SES group were predominantly unemployed, less educated ($M = 11.8$ yrs), and African-American. At each time, existing scales for report of daily stressors (DSI[1]) and emotional intensity, independent of hedonic tone (AIM[2]) were administered. In addition, we developed the Pregnancy Experience Scale (PES[3]) to assess negative and positive aspects of pregnancy (i.e., hassles and uplifts), which are not often operationalized in studies of prenatal stress.

Data were subject to repeated measures analyses and group comparisons. Results indicated the following: (1) Measures of pregnancy specific and nonspecific stress (PES and DSI) were highly stable over pregnancy (TABLE 1) for both groups. The correlations are comparable, although somewhat lower, than those for the AIM, which is a trait measure (AIM r values range from 0.74 to 0.90). This suggests that

[a]Address for correspondence: Melissa Hawkins, Johns Hopkins University, Department of Population and Family Health Sciences, Hampton House, Rm. 393, 624 N. Broadway, Baltimore, MD 21205. 410-614-6130 (voice); 410-955-2303 (fax).
e-mail: mhawkins@jhsph.edu

TABLE 1. **Stability of stress measures over time: correlation coefficients for DSI and Pregnancy Experience "frequency of hassles/uplifts" by SES**[a]

	High SES ($n = 52$)		Low SES ($n = 51$)	
Daily Stress Inventory	30 weeks	36 weeks	30 weeks	36 weeks
24 weeks	0.62	0.58	0.71	0.61
30 weeks	—	0.67	—	0.82
Pregnancy Experience Scale				
24 weeks	0.66	0.68	0.54	0.78
30 weeks	—	0.66	—	0.42

[a] $p < 0.001$.

"stress" scales administered during pregnancy may actually index trait characteristics. (2) Contrary to expectations, middle/high SES women reported higher levels of daily stress than low SES women ($F(1,98) = 10.79$; $p < 0.001$; FIG. 1) and there was a significant interaction: women in the lower SES group reported decreasing stress over time ($F(2,196) = 6.24$; $p < 0.05$). Despite this, women in the lower SES group described themselves as having greater emotional intensity ($t(101) = -3.79$; $p <. 0.001$). (3) Women in both SES groups endorsed similar items (e.g., clothes not fitting; feeling the baby move) as the most common pregnancy hassles and uplifts. However, women in the low SES group reported both fewer hassles ($F(1,98) = 4.37$; $p < 0.05$) and more uplifts ($F(1,98) = 5.62$; $p < 0.05$).

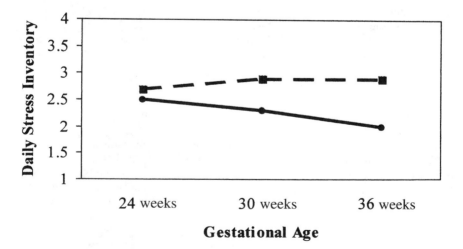

FIGURE 1. Daily Stress Inventory values during pregnancy: ●, low SES; ■, high SES.

CONCLUSIONS

The experience of pregnancy does not seem to be perceived as a negative stressor among low SES women as is often presumed. In contrast to women in the low SES group, employed and more educated women reported significantly more daily stressors, which did not decline during pregnancy. Both groups of women were similar in the features of pregnancy considered to be stressful, and both reported more pregnancy-specific uplifts than hassles. However, women in the lower SES group were more uplifted and less hassled by pregnancy, indicating that perceptions of pregnancy also differ by social class. We suggest that role strain in the high SES group may contribute to the increased appraisal of pregnancy-specific and nonspecific stress. These results highlight the role of social context in understanding the processes that mediate stress appraisal during pregnancy and related outcomes.

ACKNOWLEDGMENT

This research was support by 2R01 HD27592, NICHD, awarded to the second author.

REFERENCES

1. BRANTLEY, P.J. *et al.* 1987. A daily stress inventory: development, reliability, and validity. J. Behav. Med. **10:** 61–73.
2. LARSEN, R.J. *et al.* 1986. Affect intensity and reactions to daily life events. J. Pers. Soc. Psyol. **51:** 803–814.
3. DiPIETRO, J.A. *et al.* 1999. Psychosocial stress in pregnancy: development and validation of the Pregnancy Experience Scale. Submitted.

The Effects of Race, Gender, and Education on the Structure of Self-Rated Health among Community-Dwelling Older Adults

BETH HAN,[a] BRENT J. SMALL, AND WILLIAM E. HALEY

Department of Gerontology, University of South Florida, Tampa, Florida 33620, USA

INTRODUCTION

Would you say your health is excellent, very good, good, fair, or poor? Compared with one year ago, would you say that your health is better now, about the same, or worse than it was then? These are typical items of self-rated health that have been widely used to assess the global health. Furthermore, these measures have been consistently found to be very robust and independent predictors of functional disability and mortality among older adults.[1,2]

Self-rated health among older adults has often been considered as a function of physical illness and functional disability.[3,4,5] Self-rated health is a summary expression of the various illnesses and functional disabilities known to the individual respondent.[6,7] However, several questions still remain. For example, does depression have an impact on respondent's self-rated health? Furthermore, are there any effects of gender, ethnicity, and education on the structure of self-rated health?

METHODS

This study systematically examined the effects of gender, ethnicity, and education on the structure of subjective ratings of health. A structural equation model was developed to test hypotheses concerning the relationship between depression and the structure of self-rated health among the elderly. Furthermore, factorial invariance methods were applied to test the structure of self-rated health across different genders, ethnic groups, and educational levels. A total of 7873 community-dwelling older adults (see TABLE 1) were identified from the first wave of Assets and Health Dynamics among the Oldest Old national survey.[8] The best-fitting model ($\chi^2 =$ 676.58; $p < 0.01$; CFI = 0.97; see TABLE 2) supported the view that depression was a third significant component of self-rated health, in addition to the influence of chronic illness and functional impairment.

Using this model as a basis, differences between gender, ethnic groups, and socioeconomic status were then examined. Analyses revealed significant differences in the predictive relationship across participants of varying gender, racial groups,

[a]Address for correspondence: Beth Han, Department of Gerontology, University of South Florida, 4202 East Fowler Ave., SOC 107, Tampa, FL 33620, USA. 813-974-2414 (voice); 813-974-9754 (fax).

e-mail: hhan@luna.cas.usf.edu

and education levels. Specifically, functional impairment played a stronger predictive role for depression of Caucasian males than Caucasian females. Moreover, this relationship was stronger for elderly with fewer years of education (not more than six years) than highly educated elderly (at least 16 years). Overall, the results indicate that the predictive relationships to subjective ratings of health are a complex phenomenon and are influenced by gender, ethnic groups, and education levels.

REFERENCES

1. IDLER, E.L. & S.V. KASL. 1995. Self-ratings of health: do they also predict change in functional ability? J. Gerontol. **50:** s344–353.
2. SCHOENFELD, D.E., L.C. MALMROSE, D.G. BLAZER, *et al.* 1994. Self-rated health and mortality in the high-functioning elderly—a closer look at healthy individuals: MacArthur field study of successful aging. J. Gerontol. **49:** M109–115.
3. LIANG, J. 1986. Self-reported physical health among aged adults. J. Gerontol. **41:** 248–260.
4. LIANG, J., J. BENNETT, N. WHITELAW & D. MAEDA. 1991. The structure of self reported physical health among the aged in the United States and Japan. Med. Care **29:** 1161–1180.
5. JOHNSON, R. & F.D. WOLINSKY. 1994. Gender, race, and health: the structure of health status among older adults. Gerontologist **34:** 24–35.
6. DONABEDIAN, A. 1973. Aspects of Medical Care Administration. Harvard University Press, Cambridge.
7. TISSUE, T. 1972. Another look at self-rated health among the elderly. J. Gerontol. **27:** 91.
8. SOLDO, B.J., M.D. HURD, W.L. RODGERS & R.B. WALLACE. 1997. Asset and health dynamics among the oldest old: an overview of the AHEAD study. J. Gerontol. **52B:** 1–20.

[Tables are on the next four pages.]

TABLE 1. Percentage distribution of characteristics for white females, white males, black females, and black males who were 65 years old or older

Indicators	White females ($n = 4216$)	White males ($n = 2568$)	Black females ($n = 724$)	Black males ($n = 365$)
Age (years)				
65–74	42.77	41.94	40.06	41.37
75–84	43.52	46.57	45.99	47.12
85+	13.71	11.49	13.95	11.51
Education (years)				
0–8	22.04	24.22	46.69	55.34
9–12	51.13	44.90	41.43	33.98
12+	26.83	30.88	11.88	10.68
Number of medicines/month				
0	10.74	14.88	8.70	10.41
1	24.00	23.83	21.69	24.38
2	19.50	18.81	21.27	21.10
3	16.75	15.77	19.06	18.36
4	11.50	11.76	12.85	12.05
5	7.71	6.66	7.46	5.75
≥6	9.80	8.29	8.98	7.95
Number of current illnesses				
0	17.65	19.74	13.12	15.62
1	29.53	31.62	23.90	26.85
2	24.15	24.69	28.87	26.58
3	16.75	14.45	18.51	15.62
≥4	11.93	9.50	15.61	15.34

TABLE 1/continued.

Indicators	White females (*n* = 4216)	White males (*n* = 2568)	Black females (*n* = 724)	Black males (*n* = 365)
Number of IADL impairments				
0	70.64	73.21	61.19	63.56
≥1	29.36	26.79	38.81	36.44
Number of ADL impairments				
0	70.04	76.25	57.87	66.85
≥1	29.96	23.75	42.13	33.15
Number of depressive symptoms				
0	34.39	39.84	27.21	24.93
1	20.73	21.73	19.61	22.47
2	12.07	10.86	13.12	11.23
3	12.41	12.81	13.54	14.79
4	17.15	10.24	21.41	18.63
≥5	3.25	4.52	5.11	7.95
General health ratings				
Excellent	11.39	11.53	4.56	7.67
Very good	24.64	22.86	17.96	13.70
Good	30.12	32.13	26.80	29.04
Poor	22.51	21.11	30.80	29.59
Very poor	11.34	12.38	19.89	20.00
Comparison with health 1 year ago				
Better	13.83	11.57	16.44	15.89
Same	64.68	67.52	56.08	57.53
Worse	21.49	20.91	27.49	26.58

TABLE 2. Standardized maximum likelihood estimates of Liang's model and our hypothesized models for the total sample ($n = 7873$), females ($n = 4940$), males ($n = 2933$)

Parameters	Liang's model $n = 7873$	Our model $n = 7873$	Liang's model $n = 4940$	Liang's model $n = 2933$	Our model $n = 4940$	Our model $n = 2933$
Causal impact of chronic illness on						
Functional limitation	0.55	0.56	0.55	0.53	0.57	0.52
Self-rated health	0.56	0.56	0.55	0.57	0.55	0.58
Causal impact of functional disability on						
Self-rated health	0.32	0.28	0.35	0.30	0.30	0.26
Depression		0.67	N/A	N/A	0.63	0.74
Self-rated health						
Self-rated health	N/A	0.13	N/A	N/A	0.15	0.08
Squared multiple correlation for						
Self-Rated Health	0.61	0.68	0.64	0.59	0.71	0.65
Factor loadings:						
Chronic illness						
Number of medicines/per month	0.69	0.69	0.71	0.66	0.71	0.66
Number of current diseases	0.71	0.71	0.72	0.68	0.72	0.68
Functional disability						
Number of ADL impairment	0.76	0.68	0.78	0.73	0.71	0.62
Number of IADL impairment	0.63	0.69	0.65	0.60	0.69	0.70
Depression						
Depressive affect		0.94			0.95	0.93
"depressed" (nv307)		0.78			0.76	0.80
"lonely" (nv312)		0.73			0.71	0.77
"sad" (nv315)		0.81			0.78	0.85
Well-being		0.88			0.87	0.91
"happy" (nv311)		0.82			0.83	0.81
"enjoy" (nv314)		0.82			0.81	0.85
Somatic problems		0.93			0.92	0.94
"sleep" (nv310)		0.56			0.53	0.60
"get going" (nv316)		0.67			0.65	0.70

TABLE 2/continued.

Parameters	Liang's model $n = 7873$	Our model $n = 7873$	Liang's model $n = 4940$	Liang's model $n = 2933$	Our model $n = 4940$	Our model $n = 2933$
Self-rated health						
General health ratings (v204)	0.86	0.82	0.85	0.87	0.80	0.84
Comparison with health 1 year ago (v208)	0.33	0.35	0.33	0.34	0.35	0.36
Residual error variances in equations						
Chronic illness	1.00	1.00	1.00	1.00	1.00	1.00
Functional disability	0.70	0.69	0.70	0.73	0.68	0.73
Depression		0.55	N/A	N/A	0.61	0.45
Self-rated health	0.38	0.32	0.36	0.41	0.28	0.35
Measurement error variances						
Number of medicines/ per month	0.52	0.52	0.49	0.57	0.50	0.57
Number of current diseases	0.50	0.50	0.48	0.53	0.48	0.54
Number of ADL impairment	0.42	0.54	0.39	0.47	0.49	0.63
Number of IADL impairment	0.61	0.52	0.58	0.65	0.52	0.51
"depressed" (nv307)		0.39			0.42	0.35
"lonely" (nv312)		0.46			0.49	0.41
"sad" (nv315)		0.35			0.39	0.28
"happy" (nv311)		0.32			0.31	0.40
"enjoy" (nv314)		0.32			0.35	0.28
"sleep" (nv310)		0.69			0.72	0.64
"get going" (nv316)		0.55			0.58	0.51
General health ratings (v204)	0.27	0.34	0.39	0.24	0.36	0.30
Comparison with health 1 year ago	0.89	0.88	0.89	0.88	0.88	0.87

NOTES: All estimates of both models are significant at the $p < 0.05$ level.

Socioeconomic Differences in Measures of Hostility

ARI HAUKKALA[a]

National Public Health Institute, Department of Epidemiology and Health Promotion, Mannerheimintie 166, FIN-00300 Helsinki, Finland

INTRODUCTION

It has been hypothesized that hostility contributes to socioeconomic (SES)-differences in health in two ways. First, low SES and associated negative childhood experiences may create hostility that is then related to poor health.[1] Second, income inequalities within a society may facilitate hostility among low-income groups.[2] To understand the relationships between hostility, low SES, and poor health, the different dimensions of hostility have to be taken into account. Hostility is a broad psychological concept that includes cognitive, emotional, and behavioral aspects. Traits in hostility include cynicism, anger, mistrust, and aggression. These traits have been difficult to separate both on the theoretical level and in empirical measures.[3]

METHODS

The data is from the Finnish 1992 cardiovascular risk factor survey. A random sample of 1,547 men and 1,856 women, aged 25–64 years was stratified by gender, age group, and area. Respondents completed the Cynical Distrust Scale[4] (CynDis) from the Cook-Medley hostility scale, and the following STAXI scales,[5] trait anger (Anger), anger suppression (AX/In), control (AX/Con), and expression (AX/Out). Indicators of socioeconomic status were years of *education* and household *income*.

RESULTS

Correlation and descriptive statistics are represent in TABLE 1. Men had higher mean scores in AX/In, AX/Con, and CynDis; whereas women had significantly higher mean scores in anger, AX/Out, and years of education. Cynical distrust decreased when years of education increased among persons of both genders. Years of education had moderate positive correlation with anger expression (AX/Out), which was higher among women ($r = 0.24$) than among men ($r = 0.13$). All other correlations between SES variables and hostility measures were similar among men and women. Age correlated moderately with anger, AX/Out, and AX/Con among women; whereas among men there was no significant correlation between these variables. Older

[a]Address for correspondence: 358-9-4744 8613 (voice); 358-9-4744 8338 (fax).
e-mail: ari.haukkala@ktl.fi

TABLE 1. Correlations between trait anger (Anger), anger suppression (AX/In), control (AX/Con), and expression (AX/Out), cynical distrust (CynDis), years of education, household income, and age, including means and standard deviations (SD) among men and women

	Men							Women						
Variables	Anger	AX/Out	AX/In	AX/Con	CynDis	Education	Income	Anger	AX/Out	AX/In	AX/Con	CynDis	Education	Income
1. Anger	1.0							1.0						
2. AX/Out	0.60	1.0						0.58	1.0					
3. AX/In	0.30	0.07	1.0					0.24	−0.13	1.0				
4. AX/Con	−0.47	−0.48	0.12	1.0				−0.50	−0.55	0.15	1.0			
5. CynDis	0.27	0.08	0.23	−0.18	1.0			0.19	−0.01	0.23	−0.11	1.0		
6. Education	−0.05	0.13	0.01	0.06	−0.31	1.0		0.09	0.24	−0.06	−0.09	−0.31	1.0	
7. Income	−0.03	0.07	0.03	0.08	−0.22	0.41	1.0	0.02	0.10	−0.02	0.01	−0.22	0.38	1.0
8. Age	0.02	−0.08	0.09	−0.01	0.20	−0.41	−0.06	−0.16	−0.27	0.06	0.21	0.19	−0.46	−0.16
Mean	18.6	14.0	17.2	24.7	19.4	11.0	5.7	19.3	14.5	16.7	23.2	18.7	11.2	5.4
SD	4.7	3.6	4.3	5.0	4.4	3.9	2.0	4.5	3.8	4.4	5.1	4.6	3.7	2.0
n	1517	1514	1521	1516	1508	1544	1527	1796	1809	1807	1795	1813	1853	1802

respondents were more likely to be cynical among persons of both genders. The negative correlation between education and cynical distrust remained after adjusting for age ($r = -0.26$). Cynical distrust was not related to AX/Out, but these measures both showed a moderate correlation with trait anger.

DISCUSSION

In this study we found that the cynical component of hostility was clearly related to lower SES, whereas reported tendency to express anger was related to higher SES. This difference indicates that the general concept of hostility is too broad to use in SES studies. It may be argued that anger expression reflects higher self-confidence in an ability to express anger if necessary,[6] whereas elevated cynicism may be a consequence of cumulative negative experiences during the lifetime. Different concepts of hostility have functions in social exchange; if other people hurt you, you react with anger. Among obese persons, cynical distrust might even be functional as protection against others' negative attitudes.[7] The roots for these differences may lie in childhood, but the moderate correlation with age indicates that cynicism may rise in older age as well. Finland has had one of the most equal income distributions of Western nations during the last decades. Therefore, high correlation between education and cynical distrust was unexpected. Although anger-related emotions might have adverse health outcomes, more permanent cognitive aspects of hostility, like distrust and cynicism, would be interesting topics for future research in health inequality studies.

REFERENCES

1. WILLIAMS, R.B. 1998. Lower socioeconomic status and increased mortality: early childhood roots and the potential for successful interventions. JAMA **279:** 1745–1746.
2. WILKINSON, R.G. 1996. Unhealthy Societies: The Afflictions of Inequality. Routledge, London.
3. RUSSELL J.A. & B. FEHR. 1994. Fuzzy concepts in a fuzzy hierarchy: varieties of anger. J. Pers. Soc. Psychol. **67:** 186–205.
4. GREENGLASS, E.R. & J. JULKUNEN. 1989. Construct validity and sex differences in Cook-Medley Hostility. Pers. Individ. Diff. **10:** 209–218.
5. SPIELBERGER, C.D. 1988. Professional Manual for the State–Trait Anger Expression Inventory (STAXI). Psychological Assessment Resources, Orlando.
6. DIEKMANN, A., M. JUNGBAUER-GANS, H. KRASSING & S. LORENZ. 1996. Social status and aggression: a field study analyzed by survival analysis. J. Soc. Psycol. **136:** 761–768.
7. HAUKKALA, A. & A. UUTELA. 2000. Cynical hostility, depression and obesity: the moderating role of education and gender. Int. J. Eat. Dis. **27:** in press.

SES and Oral Health Status
in an Elderly Population

NOELLE LALLEY HUNTINGTON,[a] ELIZABETH A. KRALL,
RAUL I. GARCIA, AND AVRON SPIRO III

*Veterans Administration Normative Aging Study, Boston VA Outpatient Clinic and
Boston University School of Dental Medicine, Boston, Massachusetts 02118, USA*

INTRODUCTION

The relationship between health and socioeconomic status is well documented.[1] Less is known, however, about the relationship between oral health and SES, and most studies focus on oral health behaviors, such as brushing and flossing,[2] rather than oral health outcomes. This study explores SES differences in two measures of oral health status—number of teeth, an indicator of overall oral health status, and self-report of oral health. It also explores possible mediators, both behavioral and attitudinal, that are known to vary by SES and that may be related to oral health outcomes. These mediators include perceived economic security, possession of dental insurance, utilization of preventive services, access to care, smoking, and social support.

METHODS

Analyses were performed on data from the VA Normative Aging Study (NAS) and the Dental Longitudinal Study (DLS)—two ongoing studies that have followed community-dwelling men for more than 30 years. The NAS collects information on a variety of health and psychosocial issues. The subset ($n = 1231$) considered here also participates in the DLS, which periodically collects information on oral health. Participants were chosen because of their overall good health and geographic stability. Nearly all participants (96%) are white, and all were employed at the outset. A variety of white- and blue-collar occupations are represented. The oral health data used in this study was collected when participants were an average of 66.5 years of age (range, 47–90 years).

Socioeconomic status was defined by the Duncan Socioeconomic Index, a measure of occupational prestige that takes into account the typical income and education levels of people in those occupations. However, because many of the participants were retired at the time of this study, current income was used as a second indicator of SES.

[a]Address for correspondence: Noelle Lalley Huntington, Dept. of Health Policy and Health Services Research, Boston University School of Dental Medicine, 715 Albany St., B-301, Boston, MA 02118, USA. 617-638-4971(voice); 617-638-6381 (fax).
e-mail: nlhuntin@bu.edu

RESULTS AND CONCLUSIONS

Multiple regression of the oral health outcomes on SES were significant for number of teeth ($R^2 = 0.05$; $p < 0.001$) and self-report of oral health ($R^2 = 0.02$; $p = 0.007$). For men from lower prestige occupations, those with a lower current income (below \$40,000) had significantly fewer teeth ($\overline{X} = 19.5$) than men with a higher current income ($\overline{X} = 21.9$; $p = 0.036$). Men with a lower current income rated their oral health more poorly (40% rated it as excellent or very good; 26% as fair or poor) than did men with a higher current income (46% excellent or very good; 18% fair or poor), regardless of occupational prestige.

Each mediator was added, in turn, to the two SES/oral health models, to determine if their inclusion significantly improved the prediction of either oral health measure. For number of teeth, utilization of preventive services significantly improved the model ($R^2 = 0.13$; $p < 0.001$). For participants from higher prestige occupations, 88% had a preventive visit in the past year, compared with 75% of participants from lower prestige occupations. Those who had a preventive visit had an average of 22.4 teeth, compared with 16.1 teeth for those who did not ($p < 0.001$).

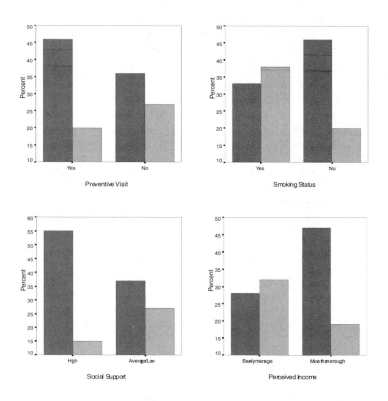

FIGURE 1. Comparing self-report of oral health status (excellent or very good versus fair or poor) by group for four mediating variables: preventive visits, smoking status, social support, and perceived income. ■, Excellent/Good; ▨, Fair/Poor.

For self-report of oral health status, several mediators were found to significantly improve the model: utilization of preventive services ($R^2 = 0.03$; $p = 0.003$); smoking status ($R^2 = 0.05$; $p < 0.001$); social support ($R^2 = 0.04$; $p < 0.001$); and perceived economic security ($R^2 = 0.03$; $p = 0.002$). Participants who did not have a preventive visit in the past year rated their oral health more poorly (36% excellent/very good; 27% fair/poor) than participants who did have a preventive visit (46% excellent/very good; 20% fair/poor). Though smoking status did not differ by either measure of SES, those who smoked rated their oral health more poorly (33% excellent/very good; 38% fair/poor) than those who did not (46% excellent/very good; 20% fair/poor) (FIG. 1).

Participants with the highest levels of social support rated their oral health better (55% excellent/very good; 15% fair/poor) than those with low to average levels of social support (37% excellent/very good; 25% fair/poor). However, they did not differ on number teeth, presenting an average of 21.8 and 21.4 teeth, respectively. For those who felt that they barely managed on their income, 28% rated their oral health as excellent or very good, and 32% rated it as fair or poor. For those who felt they had more than enough income, 47% reported excellent or very good oral health, and 19% reported fair or poor. Again, there was no difference in the number of teeth between these groups—those who "barely managed" averaged 21.8 teeth; those with "more than enough" averaged 21.6 teeth.

Path analyses (SES→mediator→outcome) were performed to determine the total effect (direct + indirect) of each predictor on the two outcomes. Compared to SES, only utilization of preventive care was found to have a larger effect, and this was true only when predicting number of teeth (FIG. 2). For all other mediators, their effect on either outcome was exceeded by the total effect of SES.

The relationship between SES and perceived oral health status appears to be mediated by a number of factors, particularly attitudinal factors (perceived income and perceived social support). In contrast, the relationship between SES and clinical oral health status (number of teeth) appears to be mediated only by behavior (preventive visits). This pattern is supported by two additional findings: (1) no difference

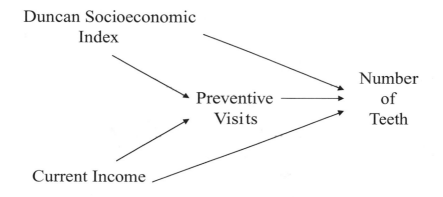

FIGURE 2. Path diagram showing the direct and indirect relationships between SES and number of teeth mediated by preventive visits.

was found in number of teeth based on varying attitudes; and (2) smokers had significantly fewer teeth ($\overline{X} = 18.6$) than nonsmokers ($\overline{X} = 21.3$; $p = 0.023$). This suggests that the relationship between SES and oral health might be explained, in part, in two different ways. The first is that there may be a cluster of dispositions that tend to vary by SES that influence both attitudes about oral health and attitudes about other life situations. The second is that there may be a cluster of behaviors that vary by SES that have an impact on clinical oral health status. Depending on the outcome (clinical status or perception of status) different factors may be influencing the relationship between SES and oral health.

ACKNOWLEDGMENT

This work was supported by the US Department of Veterans Affairs—CSP/ERIC.

REFERENCES

1. WILLIAMS, D.R. 1990. Socioeconomic differentials in health: a review and redirection. Soc. Psychol. Q. **53:** 81–99.
2. RONIS, D.L., *et al.* 1993. Tooth brushing, flossing and preventive dental visits by Detroit-area residents in relation to demographic and socioeconomic factors. J. Public Health Dent. **53:** 138–145.

Hostility, Coronary Heart Disease, and Ischemia

The Role of Socioeconomic Status

AMY R. MALKIN,[a] MICHAEL MILGRAUM, STEPHEN BOYLE,
SUSAN TOWNSEND, AND ARON W. SIEGMAN

Department of Psychology, University of Maryland,
Baltimore County, Baltimore, Maryland 21250, USA

INTRODUCTION AND METHODS

This study investigated (1) the role of SES in the hostility—coronary heart disease (CHD) relationship and (2) the role of socioeconomic (SES) in the hostility—exercise-induced ischemia relationship. One hundred and ninety six patients (101 men and 95 women) were recruited from among patients referred for thallium stress testing. On the basis of their medical history and thallium-stress scans, patients were categorized in the following groups: (1) normal (no CHD or ischemic response, $n = 44$), 2) Documented CHD (positive thallium scans or previous MI, n = 119), or (3) equivocal ($n = 33$). Participants also completed the Hollingshead Index for Social Position,[1] which classified participants as "upper-class" ($n = 27.6\%$), "middle-class" ($n = 34.7\%$), or "lower-class" ($n = 37.8\%$) and the Cook-Medley Hostility (Ho) Scale.[2]

RESULTS

Logistic regression, adjusted for age, gender, and cholesterol, revealed a significant relationship between SES and CHD ($RR = 0.427$, $p < 0.001$) (see FIG. 1). Both components of SES (income and education) were significantly related to CHD. Logistic regression, adjusted for age, gender, and cholesterol, revealed a significant relationship between the Total Ho-Scale score and CHD ($RR = 1.08$, $p < 0.04$), and borderline relationships between the hostile affect subscale and CHD ($RR = 1.29$, $p < .08$), and the aggressive responding subscale and CHD ($RR = 1.25$, $p < 0.08$). These relationships, however, were clearly not significant after adjusting for SES.

Partial correlations, adjusted for age, gender, and cholesterol, revealed a significant negative relationship between SES and exercise-induced ischemia ($r = -0.29$, $p < 0.03$) (see FIG. 2). Interestingly, when the relationships between ischemia and income and education were examined separately, ischemia was significantly related to income ($r = -0.29$, $p < 0.03$) but not to education. None of the Ho Scale scores were significantly related to exercise-induced ischemia after adjusting for traditional risk factors.

[a]Address for correspondence: Amy R. Malkin, M.A., Department of Psychology, University of Maryland, Baltimore County, 1000 Hilltop Circle, Baltimore, MD 21250, USA. 410-455-2567 (voice); 410-455-1055 (fax).

e-mail: amalki1@gl.umbc.edu

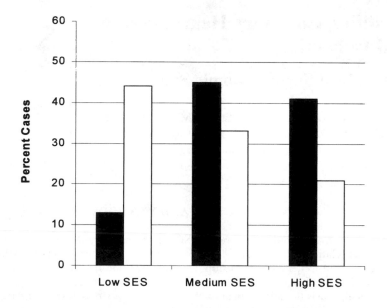

FIGURE 1. Percent CHD and No-CHD cases in low-, medium-, and high-SES groups.
■, No CHD; □, CHD.

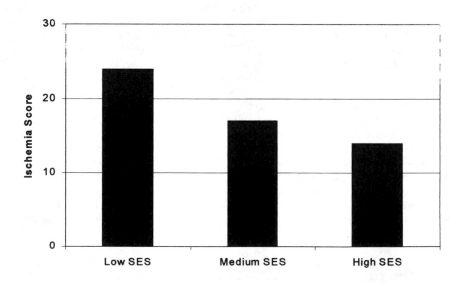

FIGURE 2. Exercise-induced ischemia scores in low-, medium-, and high-SES groups.

CONCLUSIONS

The results of the present study suggest that (1) SES is significantly related to both CHD and exercise-induced ischemia, even after adjusting for traditional risk factors; (2) of the components of SES, income is a stronger contributor to CHD and exercise-induced ischemia than is education; (3) hostility is related to CHD, but controlling for SES eliminates the hostility–CHD relationship.

REFERENCES

1. HOLLINGSHEAD, A.B. 1971. Commentary on "the indiscriminate state of social class measurement." Soc. Forces **49:** 563–567.
2. COOK, W.W. & D.M. MEDLEY. 1954. Proposed hostility and pharasaic–virtue scales for the MMPI. J. Appl. Psychol. **38:** 414–418.

Education, Infant Health, and Cigarette Smoking

ELLEN MEARA[a]

Department of Economics, Harvard University, Cambridge, Massachusetts 02138, USA

Although empirical analyses of behavior show little impact of behavior on health and mortality disparities across education and income groups, these studies have focused on older individuals.[1,2] When examining infant health and socioeconomic status (SES), behavior such as cigarette smoking emerges as an important factor. About 60 (20)% of the difference in low birth weight rates between college-educated and other white (black) women stem from differences in smoking behavior.[3] However, we know little about why disparities in smoking behavior arise between college-educated and other women.

The objective of this paper is to test several hypotheses for why smoking during pregnancy differs by education level. The analysis uses repeated cross-sectional samples of women over age 18 from the National Health Interview Surveys 1966, 1970, 1974, 1978, 1979, 1983, 1985, 1987, 1990, and 1991. These surveys are representative of the noninstitutionalized adult female population of the United States when sample weights are applied.

The first hypothesis tests whether smoking knowledge, measured as the share of correct answers to 10 questions regarding the health consequences of smoking, can explain differences in rates of smoking during pregnancy by education. The impact of education on smoking during pregnancy dropped by only 10% when controlling for smoking knowledge. Thus, knowledge cannot explain differential smoking behavior by education.

The second and third hypotheses are tested using the response to the 1964 Surgeon General's report on smoking. FIGURE 1 shows the trend in female smoking rates by education following the advent of highly publicized information on the hazards of smoking. Smoking rates were nearly identical across education groups in 1966, but by 1991 there was a 19-percentage-point difference in rates of smoking between college educated and other women. This disparity equals the difference in the rates of smoking during pregnancy during that period. The growth in differential smoking rates by education arises from trends. First, differences in smoking rates emerge when quitting behavior differs by education. Second, changes in differential smoking initiation by education level have increased disparities in smoking.

The second hypothesis tests whether education influences the way women use health knowledge. It treats differential quitting behavior by education as a response to health knowledge induced by different levels of education. As shown in TABLE 1, college-educated women quit smoking 6 percentage points faster than less-educated

[a]Address for correspondence: The National Bureau of Economic Research, 1050 Massachusetts Avenue, Cambridge, MA 02138-5398.
e-mail: emeara@fas.harvard.edu

TABLE 1. Changes in female smoking rates following the Surgeon General's 1964 report

	Quitting behavior		
	Share of who smoked in		Difference
	Pre-1964[a]	1983	1963–1983
Below high school degree	0.522	0.330	0.192[b]
Some college	0.510	0.258	0.252[b]
Difference	0.012	0.072	
Difference in quit rates			0.060[b]
	Smoking at age 16		
	Share who smoked by age 16		Difference
	Turned 16 before 1953	Turned 16 after 1983	1963–1983
Below high school degree	0.061	0.152	0.091[b]
Some college	0.041	0.063	0.022[b]
Difference	0.020	0.089	
Growth in initiation differences			0.069[b]

NOTE: Quitting behavior is based on women born in 1917–1946, Health Interview Surveys 1953.
[a]Smoking rates for 1963 are approximated using share of women who had "ever smoked."
Smoking at age 16: the "Turned 16 before 1953" sample includes women aged 17–36 in 1974.
Smoking at age 16: the "Turned 16 after 1983" sample includes women aged 18–27 in 1999.
[b]$p < 0.001$.

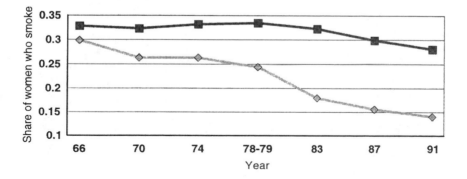

FIGURE 1. Trends in female smoking rates 1966–1991. ■, below high school degree; ◆, college degree.

women after the Surgeon General's report. Thus, when interpreting quitting behavior as the impact of education on women's response to knowledge, over 30% of the 19-percentage-point difference in female smoking occurs because education causes women to apply health knowledge differently.

The third hypothesis uses differential initiation behavior following the Surgeon General's report to indicate how much of the differential smoking behavior must be explained by factors other than education. At age 16, women have similar levels of schooling. TABLE 1 shows that the difference in smoking at age 16 between women who will eventually attend college and other women grew by 7 percentage points following the Surgeon General's report. This implies that much of the differential smoking rates by education (36%), is the result of factors other than education that differ across women and help to determine both investments in health and in education. The wide disparities in smoking behavior early in adolescence suggest that programs to reduce smoking during pregnancy should target potential mothers at younger ages.

ACKNOWLEDGMENT

The author gratefully acknowledges support from the National Institute on Aging.

REFERENCES

1. LANTZ, P.M. *et al.* 1998. Socioeconomic factors, health behaviors, and mortality. JAMA **279:** 1703–1708.
2. MARMOT, M.G. *et al.* 1991. Health inequalities among British civil servants: the Whitehall II study. Lancet **337:** 1387–1393.
3. MEARA, E. 1999. Economic determinants of health: the role of socioeconomic status, medical innovation, and managed care. Ph.D. thesis, Harvard University, Cambridge, MA.

Morbidity and Health—National Health Interview Survey, 1987

In Generalized Additive Models

JEAN C. NORRIS,[a,b] MARK VAN DER LAAN,[c] AND GLADYS BLOCK[c]

[b]*Public Health Institute, 2001 Addison Street,*
2nd floor, Berkeley, California 94704-1104, USA

[c]*School of Public Health, University of California at Berkeley,*
Berkeley, California 94720-7360, USA

INTRODUCTION AND METHODS

This study addresses the relationship of nutrition, health habits, and demographic factors to health and morbidity in the United States, using nonparametric regression (smoothed curve) models[1] and National Health Interview Survey (NHIS) data on individual morbidity and usual dietary intake.[2] To assess the relative importance of socioeconomic status (SES) and demographic factors and health habits, we built a socioeconomic–demographic model for the first outcome variable, a composite Morbidity Index (not mortality), including race, age, education, income, and an indicator combining marital status and living arrangement. We then added significant health habit terms, including smoking, alcohol, diet change, body mass index (BMI), and vitamin/mineral supplement use. To see whether and how those factors are associated with health, we used the same terms in the model with self-assessed health as the outcome. Adding health habits variables reduced estimated morbidity; nevertheless, health habits account for a fraction of the variance explained by socioeconomic and demographic variables, increasing explained variance by 47% (to 17%) and in health by 15% (to 24%).

The shape of the income term (FIG. 1, bottom) is consistent across all models; high morbidity at and below poverty decreases with increasing income to about $15,000 above poverty (approximate 1987 median), with little further benefit of income. Both higher education and higher income remain associated with self-assessed health. After controlling for income, black race does not predict the Morbidity Index (FIG. 1, top), but remains associated with lower health self-rating. Three possible SES terms—income, education, and occupation—are associated with each other and with age. Adding occupation (which included levels for "housekeeping" and "not in labor force") caused reverse curvature in the age term, an indicator of interaction.

Good health habits affect health positively, significantly, between ages 50 to 75 years. In the health model with health habits terms, there is no further worsening of health after about age 50 (FIG. 2, top). In the morbidity model with health habits

[a]Address for correspondence: 510-649-1987 (voice); 510-649-7894 (fax).
e-mail: jcnorris@phi.org

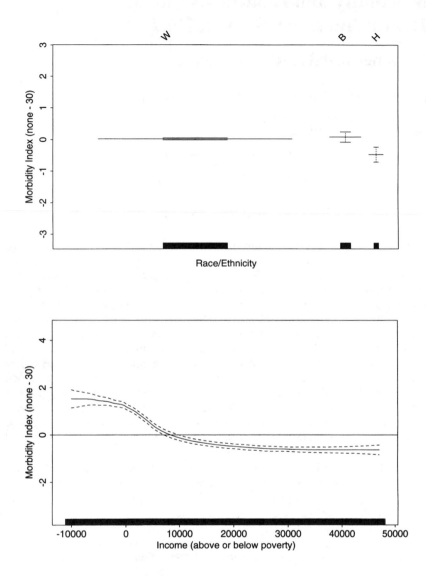

FIGURE 1. Both plotted variables were included in a 12-term generalized additive model (S-Plus GAM). Smoothed functions (*solid line*) are bounded by 95% pointwise standard errors (*dashed lines* for curves). Morbidity of blacks is different from whites (**top**) after income enters the model (**bottom**). Increased morbidity is sharply focussed below about $15,000 above poverty (approximate 1987 median). Rugs on the *x*-axis indicate data density. Data are from the NHIS 1987 Cancer Epidemiology Supplement ($n = 17,612$).

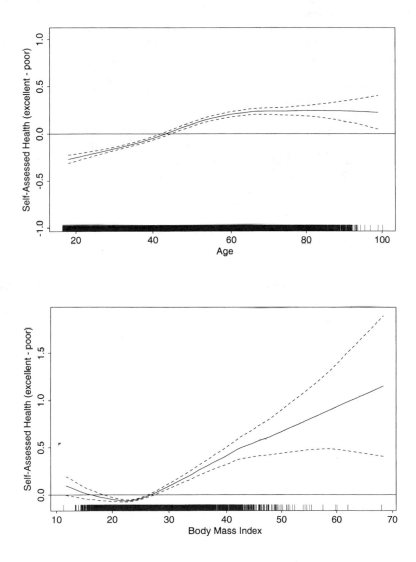

FIGURE 2. After health habit terms enter the model, self-assessed health is no longer associated with age beyond about age 50 (**top**). Body mass index (BMI) (**bottom**) shows a minimum range associated with optimum health. Both terms were included in a 12-term generalized additive model (S-Plus GAM). Smoothed functions (*solid line*) are bounded by 95% pointwise standard errors (*dashed lines*). Data are from the NHIS 1987 Cancer Epidemiology Supplement (*n* = 17,612).

terms, morbidity increases most sharply between ages 40 to 65, after which the slope is more gradual. Shapes of health habits terms are consistent with current knowledge, even when curvature is not statistically significant.[3] Smoking effects decline after about 50 to 60 pack years. The alcohol term is J-shaped, relating about 10 to 15 drinks per week to lower morbidity. The parabolic curvature of BMI (FIG. 2, bottom) reveals a narrow, optimum, range related to both lower morbidity and higher self-rated health. Diet change in the past year, like taking vitamin supplements, corresponds to worse morbidity than diet change of longer duration, suggesting change induced by onset of morbidity. Weight loss, although clearly related to morbidity, is unlikely to be intentional and may also be induced by morbidity. These models may underestimate significance of effects because of possible reverse-cause relationships. Smoothers attenuating the extremes of curvature at maxima and minima[4] would underestimate the true range of these functions.

Results of this study suggest the power of nonparametric regression to reveal meaningful curvature in exploratory analysis. Parameterized versions of GAM models, although computationally intensive, would enhance nutrition and health policy research.

REFERENCES

1. CHAMBERS, J.M. & T.T. HASTIE, Eds. 1993. Statistical Models in S. Chapman & Hall, London.
2. NCHS. 1993. 1987 National Health Interview Survey, NCHS CD-ROM, Series 10, no. 1. USDHHS/ PHS/ CDC/ NCHS. Hyattsville, MD
3. NORRIS, J.C. 1996. Nutrition, Morbidity and Lost Productive Time in the 1987 National Health Interview and Cancer Epidemiology Supplement. DrPH thesis, University of California, Berkeley.
4. HÄRDLE, W. & J.S. MARRON. 1991. Simultaneous error bars for nonparametric regression. Ann. Statistics **19**(2): 776–796.

Neighborhood Socioeconomic Context and Adult Health

The Mediating Role of Individual Health Behaviors and Psychosocial Factors

STEPHANIE A. ROBERT[a]

School of Social Work, University of Wisconsin-Madison,
1350 University Avenue, Madison, Wisconsin 53706, USA

It is not only one's own socioeconomic position that affects health—the socioeconomic context of one's neighborhood may affect one's health as well. Neighborhood socioeconomic context is associated with individual health status and mortality, over and above the effects of individual-level socioeconomic position.[1] However, we do not yet know *why* neighborhood socioeconomic context matters to health over and above one's own socioeconomic position. This study explores whether the independent relationship between neighborhood socioeconomic context and individual health is mediated by social factors—individual health behaviors, psychosocial factors, and social integration/support.

Prior analyses demonstrated independent associations between neighborhood socioeconomic characteristics (e.g., percentage of neighborhood households receiving public assistance, percentage adult unemployment, percentage of families earning $30,000 or more) and individual health status (number of chronic conditions, self-rated health), over and above individual-level socioeconomic position (income, education, assets) among a representative sample of 3,617 adults in the U.S. (from the 1986 American's Changing Lives Study (ACL)).[2] Data from 1980 census tracts and enumeration districts provided neighborhood socioeconomic information for each ACL respondent. The current research replicates those analyses (see, for example, column 1, TABLE 1) but then adds blocks of health behavior variables (smoking, physical activity, body mass index), psychosocial variables (sense of vulnerability, sense of mastery, number of life events), and social integration/support variables (informal and formal social integration, martial status) both separately and simultaneously to examine whether the health effects of the neighborhood socioeconomic variables are reduced or eliminated by these mediators (columns 2–5, TABLE 1). Analyses also examine whether neighborhood socioeconomic variables predict each of the mediating behavioral, psychosocial, and social integration/support variables, controlling for individual-level socioeconomic position and demographic variables (TABLE 2). OLS and logistic regression analyses were performed with adjustment of standard errors (using SUDAAN) to correct for design effects.

Results indicate that lower neighborhood socioeconomic context is associated with higher body mass index and less physical activity, and with lower sense of

[a]Address for correspondence: 608-263-6336 (voice); 608-263-3836 (fax).
e-mail: sarobert@facstaffwisc.edu

TABLE 1. Effects of percentage of households receiving public assistance on self-rated health (high, worse health)—mediating role of health behaviors, psychosocial factors, and social integration ($n = 3,617$)[a]

	Independent community SES effect[b]	Controlling for health behavior mediators	Controlling for psychosocial mediators	Controlling for social integration/ support mediators	Controlling simultaneously for all mediators
Intercept	3.990^c	3.195^c	3.492^c	4.124^c	3.004^c
Age	0.016^c	0.015^c	0.017^c	0.016^c	0.015^c
Race (black)	-0.076	-0.119^e	-0.040	-0.048	-0.066
Sex (female)	0.020	0.016	-0.018	0.043	-0.004
Education (years)	-0.046^c	-0.034^c	-0.038^c	-0.040^c	-0.022^e
Income (logged)	-0.187^c	-0.182^c	-0.153^c	-0.222^c	-0.193^c
Assets level					
<$10,000	—	—	—	—	—
$10,000+	-0.094	-0.045	-0.079	-0.084	-0.025
Missing	-0.152	-0.089	-0.107	-0.154	-0.050
Neighborhood SES: % households w/public assistance	0.007^d	0.006^e	0.006^e	0.007^d	0.004
Health behaviors					
BMI		0.023^c			0.022^c
Physical activity		-0.154^c			-0.152^c
Smokes now		0.173^d			0.159^d
Psychosocial factors					
Mastery			-0.110^c		-0.101^c
Vulnerability			0.117^c		0.112^c
Number of life events			0.049		0.058^e
Social integration/ support					
Informal integration				-0.016	-0.010
Formal integration				-0.055^e	-0.013
Married				0.161^d	0.184^d
R^2	0.184	0.220	0.215	0.191	0.253

[a]All data are weighted; standard errors are adjusted for design effects; unstandardized betas are presented.
[b]Results from first column were published previously.[2]
[c]$p \leq 0.001$.
[d]$p \leq 0.01$.
[e]$p \leq 0.05$.

TABLE 2. Independent effects of percentage of households receiving public assistance on body mass index, physical activity, mastery, and vulnerability (n = 3,617)[a]

	Body Mass Index	Physical Activity	Mastery	Vulnerability
Intercept	23.695^b	-0.552^d	-2.220^b	1.565^b
Age	0.026^b	-0.009^b	0.006^b	-0.006^b
Race (black)	1.295^b	-0.057	-0.000	-0.320^b
Sex (female)	-0.987	-0.201^b	-0.096^d	0.208^b
Education (years)	-0.127^c	0.040^b	0.040^b	-0.030^c
Income (logged)	0.262	0.054^d	0.153^b	-0.100^c
Assets level				
<$10,000	—	—	—	—
$10,000+	-0.489	0.223^b	0.064	-0.045
Missing	-0.976^c	0.120	0.108	-0.198^d
Neighborhood SES: percentage of households with public assistance	0.027^d	-0.007^d	-0.008^d	0.008^d
R^2	0.042	0.111	0.071	0.052

[a]All data are weighted; standard errors are adjusted for design effects; unstandardized betas are presented.
[b]$p \leq 0.001$.
[c]$p \leq 0.01$.
[d]$p \leq 0.05$.

mastery and higher sense of vulnerability, over and above individual-level socioeconomic position, age, sex, and race. However, there was no independent association between neighborhood socioeconomic context and current smoking status, number of life events, informal social integration, or formal social integration (results not shown).

Results also indicate that individual health behaviors, when considered simultaneously, mediate some, but not all of the relationship between neighborhood context and individual health, and the same is true for the psychosocial factors considered simultaneously. When health behaviors, psychosocial factors, and social integration/support measures are considered simultaneously, they explain the relationship between neighborhood socioeconomic context and individual health. TABLE 1 demonstrates one example of these analyses by first looking at the independent effects of percentage of households receiving public assistance on self-rated health (column 1)[2] and then demonstrating the mediating role of the behavioral, psychosocial, and social integration/support variables (columns 2–5). Similar results were found for the effects of neighborhood percentage of adult unemployment and percentage of families earning $30,000 or more on number of chronic conditions (results not shown).

This study suggests that health behaviors and psychosocial factors play some role in explaining why neighborhood socioeconomic context matters to health. However, the mediating factors included in this study did not *dramatically* eliminate the neighborhood socioeconomic effects on individual health, indicating that there are probably other factors that help mediate this relationship. These other factors may include access to health and social services, exposure to unhealthy physical environments, or other aspects of the social, service, and physical environments not adequately addressed in this study.

REFERENCES

1. ROBERT, S.A. 1999. Socioeconomic position and health: the independent contribution of community socioeconomic context. Ann. Rev. Soc. **25:** 489–516.
2. ROBERT, S.A. 1998. Community-level socioeconomic status effects on adult health. J. Health Soc. Behav. **39**(March): 18–37.

Goal-Striving Stress, Social Economic Status, and the Mental Health of Black Americans

SHERRILL L. SELLERS[a] AND HAROLD W. NEIGHBORS[b]

[a]*School of Social Work, Florida State University, Tallahassee, Florida 32306, USA*

[b]*School of Public Health and Institute for Social Research,
University of Michigan, Ann Arbor, Michigan 48106, USA*

INTRODUCTION

Goal-striving stress refers to the discrepancy between aspirations and achievements, hard work and accomplishment, options and opportunities, and perhaps provides a pathway linking social structure and mental health. Although a number of scholars have speculated about the relationship between blocked opportunities and psychopathology, few studies have empirically examined associations between striving efforts and mental health among black Americans.[1–5] In addition, existing studies have often used community samples, considered a single aspect of mental health, or were unable to operationalize goal-striving stress in a more nuanced fashion.[2,4] This study examines the influence of goal-striving stress on the mental health of a national sample of black Americans.

METHODS

Data

Data were drawn from the second wave of data collection of the National Survey of Black Americans (NSBA).[3] Of the original 2,107 respondents, 951 were reinterviewed in 1987 (approximately 82% of those who were located).

Dependent variables

Three dimensions of mental health were considered: well-being, self-esteem, and psychological distress. Well-being was measured by *happiness,* a single item that ranged from "very happy" to "not happy at all" on a three-point scale, and *life satisfaction,* a single item that ranged from high satisfaction to low satisfaction on a four-point scale. A *self-esteem* index was constructed from six items that assessed respondents' sense of self-worth, with high scores indicating high self-esteem. A 10-item scale of *psychological distress* was used, with high scores indicating higher levels of distress.

Independent variables

Poverty status was measured by dichotomizing an income-to-needs score. *Goal-striving stress* consisted of three items measuring the discrepancy between aspirations and achievement weighted by the level of disappointment associated with failing to achieve one's goals. Respondents were asked to imagine a ladder with 10 steps

TABLE 1. Unstandardized OM regression coefficients predicting happiness, life satisfaction, self esteem, and psychological distress

	Happiness		Life satisfaction		Self-esteem		Psychological distress	
	1A	1B	2A	2B	3A	3B	4A	4B
Age	0.004^a (0.001)	0.004^a (0.001)	0.003^c (0.001)	0.003^c (0.001)	-0.004^a (0.001)	-0.004^a (0.001)	-0.008^a (0.001)	-0.008^a (0.001)
Gender (1, women)	-0.130^a (0.032)	-0.131^a (0.032)	-0.013 (0.037)	-0.014 (0.036)	-0.006 (0.022)	-0.006 (0.022)	0.124^a (0.024)	0.124^a (0.024)
Employment (1, yes)	-0.017 (0.037)	-0.011 (0.036)	0.039 (0.041)	0.045 (0.041)	0.059^d (0.025)	0.060^d (0.025)	-0.026 (0.027)	-0.027 (0.027)
Poverty (1, poor)	0.028 (0.036)	-0.074^c (0.045)	-0.129^b (0.041)	-0.240^a (0.051)	-0.106^a (0.025)	-0.132^b (0.031)	0.075^b (0.027)	0.093^b (0.033)
Education	0.004 (0.005)	0.003 (0.005)	-0.016^b (0.006)	-0.016^b (0.006)	0.032^a (0.004)	0.032^a (0.004)	-0.016^a (0.004)	-0.016^a (0.004)
Region (1, south)	0.107 (0.031)	0.105^b (0.031)	0.109^b (0.035)	0.105^b (0.035)	-0.032 (0.021)	-0.033 (0.021)	-0.031 (0.023)	-0.031 (0.023)
Marital status								
formerly married	-0.107^b (0.034)	-0.104^b (0.034)	-0.230^a (0.039)	-0.227^a (0.039)	0.060^b (0.023)	0.061 (0.023)	0.042 (0.025)	0.041 (0.025)
never married	-0.002 (0.047)	-0.002 (0.047)	0.088^c (0.053)	0.086^c (0.053)	0.027 (0.032)	0.027 (0.032)	-0.062^c (0.035)	-0.062^c (0.035)
Goal-striving stress	-0.020^a (0.002)	-0.026^a (0.003)	-0.027^a (0.002)	-0.034^a (0.003)	-0.008^a (0.001)	-0.010^a (0.002)	0.016^a (0.002)	0.017^a (0.002)
Moderating Effects								
goal striving*poor		0.016^a (0.004)		0.017^a (0.005)		0.004 (0.003)		-0.003 (0.003)
Constant	1.985 (0.123)	2.021 (0.123)	3.388 (0.139)	3.427 (0.139)	3.198 (0.084)	3.208 (0.084)	2.242 (0.092)	2.236 (0.092)
R^2	0.085	0.092	0.115	0.121	0.152	0.153	0.136	0.136
F	19.665	19.311	26.792	25.596	37.642	34.105	33.28	30.033
R^2 change		0.007		0.006		0.001		0.000
n	1914		1873		1900		1918	

[a] $p < 0.001$.
[b] $p < 0.01$.
[c] $p < 0.1$.
[d] $p < 0.05$.

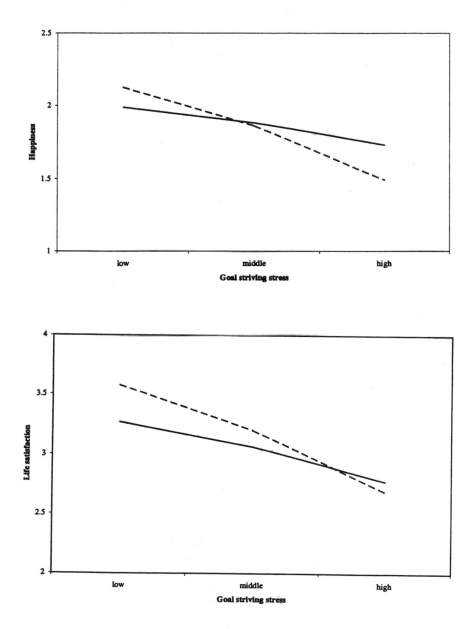

FIGURE 1. Interaction between poverty status and goal-striving stress: ————, poor; - - - -, not poor.

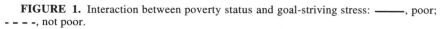

"where step 10 represents your best way of life and step 1 represents your worst way of life." Aspirations were measured by asking the step number that best described where the respondent would like to be the following year. Achievement was measured by asking the step number that best described where the respondent was at the current time. Importance of the goal was measured by asking respondents, on a four-point scale, how disappointed they would be if they could never reach the step to which they aspire.

Analytic strategy

Ordinary least squares regression was used to estimate the effects of goal striving stress on a set of mental health outcomes and to examine the moderating effects of poverty status on the relationships between goal-striving stress and mental health. In all analyses, the effects of age (years), education (in years completed), gender, and marital and employment status were controlled. Analyses were weighted up to the original 2,107 cases.

RESULTS

As shown in columns "A" of TABLE 1, goal-striving stress is strongly related to mental health: As goal-striving stress increases, levels of happiness, life satisfaction, and self-esteem decrease; and levels of psychological distress increase. The moderating effects of poverty status are presented in columns "B." Although no moderating effects were found for self-esteem and psychological distress, effects were found for well-being. Compared to poor persons, individuals above poverty had higher levels of happiness and life satisfaction at low levels of goal striving, but as levels of striving increased, individuals above poverty had significantly lower levels of happiness and life satisfaction. FIGURE 1 illustrates these findings.

DISCUSSION

Finding that goal-striving stress is negatively related to mental health among black Americans is consistent with arguments that locate the genesis of illness within the social structure. Goal striving appears to be a source of chronic stress; for blacks, perhaps it is particularly pernicious because racial prejudice and discrimination systematically block opportunities to achieve life goals. The moderating effects of poverty status support this speculation. Perhaps those above poverty attach their well-being to economic advancement and, having achieved a measure of success, assume that additional effort will yield additional reward. In a society in which rewards are often distributed inequitably, this assumption can lead to decreased well-being. Poverty status did not moderate the relationship between goal-striving stress and self-esteem or psychological distress. However, if the mismatch between efforts and rewards persists, more severe mental health problems, such as depression and suicide, may develop. It is likely that the impact of goal-striving stress varies over time and across the life course. In addition to consideration of temporal relationship between goal-striving stress and health, future research should consider racially differentiated health outcomes such as hypertension and the interplay between goal-striving stress and coping strategies such as John Henryism.

REFERENCES

1. ANESHENSEL, C. 1992. Social stress: theory and research. Annu. Rev. Sociol. **18:** 15–38.
2. DRESSLER, W. 1988. Social consistency and psychological distress. JHSB **29:** 79–91.
3. JACKSON, J. *et al.* 1996. Perceptions and experiences of racism and the physical and mental health status of African Americans: a thirteen-year national panel study. Ethnic Dis. **6:** 123–138.
4. NEIGHBORS, H. & S. LUMPKIN. 1990. The epidemiology of mental disorder in the black population. *In* Handbook of Mental Health and Mental Disorder among Black Americans. Dorothy Ruiz, Ed. Greenwood Press, New York.
5. PARKER, S. & R. KLEINER. 1966. Mental illness in the urban Negro community. Free Press, New York.

Moderating and Mediating Effects of Socioeconomic Status, Perceived Peer Condom Use, and Condom Negotiation on Sexual Risk Behavior among African-American and White Adolescent Females

CATLAINN SIONÉAN[a] AND RICK S. ZIMMERMAN

Departments of Behavioral Science and Sociology, University of Kentucky, College of Medicine, Lexington, Kentucky 40536, USA

Existing research indicates that economic disadvantage at the neighborhood and individual levels affect adolescent sexual risk behavior, yet the mechanisms though which these effects operate are less clear. We seek to elaborate the existing research by examining, at the individual level, the extent to which SES moderates the relationship between race and condom use, as well as potential mediating effects of perceived peer norms regarding condom use, condom self-efficacy (CSE), and condom negotiation on female adolescent condom use. In addition, we controlled for age at first intercourse and prescription contraceptive use. Our sample consisted of 209 sexually active African-American and white female high school students, ages 15–16. To test for moderating and mediating effects, we used three sets of general linear models, first testing for relationships between race, SES, and condom use and stepping in potential mediating variables, then running separate models for African-American and white students (TABLE 1).

The overall model indicated that SES largely accounts for race differences in condom use. In general, African-Americans used condoms more frequently than did white students; however, this was primarily due to the lower frequency of use among poor white students. Socioeconomic status did not affect condom use of African-American students (FIG. 1). Perceived peer norms, CSE, and condom negotiation were all positively related to condom use, regardless of race and SES. Tests for homogeneity of slopes across levels of race in the overall model revealed no differences. In order to best detect differences in the effects of mediating variables across levels of SES, we ran separate models for African-American and white students. For African-American young women, SES was *not* related to condom use (as in the overall model), while perceived peer condom use, condom self-efficacy, refusal of unsafe sex and age at first intercourse were all positively related (FIG. 1). The effects of the mediators did not vary across levels of SES. The strongest predictor in the model was

[a]Current address for correspondence: Catlainn Sionean, Rollins School of Department of Behavioral Sciences and Health Education, 1518 Clifton Road, Room 520, Atlanta, GA 30322, USA.

e-mail: csionea@sph.emory.edu

TABLE 1. Standardized regression coefficients for models predicting African-American and white adolescent women's condom use

	Model 1	Model 2	Model 3	Model 4	Model 5	Model 6	Model 7
Age	0.155	0.120	0.120	0.113	0.104	0.073	0.059
Race	−0.199[b]	−0.212[b]	−0.164	−0.157	−0.076	−0.020	0.054
SES		−0.098	−0.031	0.010	0.055	0.101	0.119
Race*SES			−0.103	−0.115	−0.214[a]	−0.218[a]	−0.249[c]
Age first sex				0.174[a]	0.136[a]	0.121	0.104[a]
Rx contraceptive use				−0.166[a]	−0.145[a]	−0.145[a]	−0.110[a]
Peer condom use					0.405[c]	0.323[c]	0.271[c]
Condom self-efficacy						0.329[c]	0.161[b]
Refused unsafe sex							0.518[c]
Adj. R^2	0.036	0.040	0.039	0.095	0.252	0.347	0.577

[a]$p < 0.05$.
[b]$p < 0.01$.
[c]$p < 0.001$.

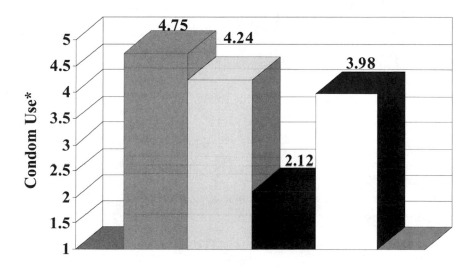

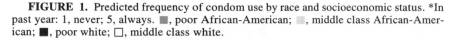

FIGURE 1. Predicted frequency of condom use by race and socioeconomic status. *In past year: 1, never; 5, always. ■, poor African-American; ▨, middle class African-American; ■, poor white; □, middle class white.

refusal behavior ($b = 0.445$, $p < 0.001$). The model for African-American young women explained 56% of the variance in condom use frequency.

For white young women, SES was negatively related and perceived peer condom use and refusal were positively related to frequency of condom use. In contrast to the findings for African-American young women, for white young women condom self-efficacy was *completely* mediated through refusal behavior; it had no significant effect after accounting for refusal behavior. The effects of the social psychological variables did not vary across levels of SES. However, the effects of two control variables did. Prescription contraceptive use was significantly related to condom use only among middle-class whites. Middle-class white young women who had more frequently used prescription birth control used condoms less than did those who infrequently used prescription birth control. For poor whites, prescription birth control was positively but non-significantly related to condom use. In addition, although the effect of age at first intercourse was not significantly related to condom use for either middle-class or poor whites, the effects were significantly different for the two groups [$t^* = 1.977$ ($df = 81$), $p < 0.05$]. For middle-class whites, the effect of age at first intercourse was positively related to condom use ($b = 0.185$) while the opposite was true for poor whites ($b = -0.406$). The model for white young women explained 64% of the variance in their condom use frequency.

Our results indicate that African-American adolescent females use condoms regardless of their SES, in part because of their beliefs in their abilities to use condoms and subsequent negotiation of safer sex with their partners. Further research is needed to examine factors that may influence condom use among working class white adolescent women.

Dissociative Disruptions—Psychological (Psychosocial) Pathways Uncovered in the Healing Process

LAUREN E. STORCK[a]

Clinical Faculty, Department of Psychiatry, Harvard Medical School,
25 Mount Auburn Street, Cambridge, Massachusetts 02138, USA

The study of clinical discourse (psychotherapy narratives) can offer information about pathways between socioeconomic disadvantages and poorer health. It is suggested that a form of psychological *dissociation* due to repression of painful experiences related to class or socioeconomic position contributes significantly to weaken defenses and make more vulnerable certain already "at risk" groups such as women with young children and cultural minorities.

Although sociologists, journalists, and public health advocates have written detailed descriptions of the chronic and complex psychological, social, and economic consequences of poverty and working-class life,[1,2] few psychotherapists and psychologists have turned their attention to the powerful psychodynamics of class injuries in individuals and groups. These psychological experiences stand out in the discourse between clinician and patient, however, if the clinician attends to the mention of socioeconomic insults rather than to intra-psychic or purely interpersonal (dyadic) experiences:

> Everybody knows about my mother's "problem." She has been spending too much for years. My sisters and brothers are fed up with her. She's probably suffering from depression. She is so full of shame! All her sisters and brothers, she comes from a big family, are better off than she is. But what do you expect?! My father died when I was three. She had four kids to raise. Most of *them* had two salaries! And no children! I'm worried about her, and I know she wants to come live with me (holds head).

Can you talk about this with anyone else?

> No...not even my sister! And I can't take a vacation, you don't understand. In my family, we didn't take vacations. You never knew if there would be enough for the next week.

This dialogue, and many related versions of similar suppressed pain, does not occur at the first meetings. The patient is well-dressed, composed, and often has a demanding job. She does not mention financial difficulties until later, when there is a modicum of trust and relief from her own acute depression or anxiety. She is usually coming into therapy for the first time. She has a complex relationship with her family of origin; a disappointing current relationship with her partner; and struggles with divided loyalties, a sense of loneliness and betrayal that has been disconnected from her class mobility, issues of trust, self-criticism, and lack of supports. It is as if the many life-long socioeconomic insults and hardships have been cut off from her day-

[a]Address for correspondence: 617-576-3919 (voice and fax).
e-mail: lstorck@hms.harvard.edu

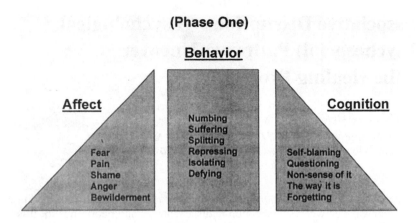

FIGURE 1. Disconnections, repressions, or unconscious injuries of membership in "lower" social groups.

to-day awareness, so that she navigates her life and relationships without needed instruments. Because our culture frequently stigmatizes the worker or professional who voices concerns about class and psychosocial issues, there are few socially acceptable words and routes to recovery from class injuries.

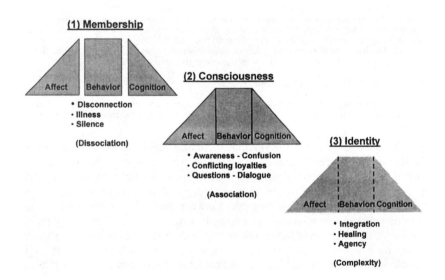

FIGURE 2. Developmental phases of individual/group experiences in lower social positions.

From the self-identified "workaholic" individual patient, to the couple who struggle over how to discipline children, to a group therapy setting where each group member resonates to the humiliation suffered when one is the target of class-prejudiced remarks (e.g., someone reports being stunned by the label "white trash" many years previously), the reality of social ordering and its deleterious effects permeates clinical discourse. These painful and hurtful social experiences are internalized, with memories dissociated from cognitive and affective processing (FIG. 1).

Psychotherapy dialogue can repair some of the psychological disconnections for individuals, families, and social groups by attentive listening and responding with patience and collaborative constructions of understanding. Bearing witness to the buried hurt and pain[3] facilitates healing. The patient can then think and plan more effectively for the future, discovering agency. Group therapy (especially group analysis, a social and cultural therapy) may be the intervention of choice,[4] since group and individual lives are continually intertwined. A three-phase psychosocial developmental process (FIG. 2) is suggested: from dissociation to capacity for meaningful association to mature identity and complexity. Future research would examine discourse of patients in treatment for mood, anxiety, and related disorders, to track the dissociative process in more detail and to design appropriate interventions.

REFERENCES

1. RUBIN, L. 1976. Worlds of Pain: Life in the Working Class Family. Basic Books, New York.
2. WILSON, W.J. 1996. When Work Disappears. Alfred A. Knopf, New York.
3. HERMAN, J. 1992. Trauma and Recovery. Basic Books, New York.
4. STORCK, L.E. 1998. Social class divisions in the consulting room: a theory of psychosocial class and depression. Group Anal. **31:** 101–115.

Does Cognitive Functioning Mediate the Well-Documented Link between Education and Functional Disability in Middle-Aged Adults?

LINDA A. WRAY[a,b] AND JOHN W. LYNCH[c]

[b]Department of Medical Education, University of Michigan Medical School,
G-1212 Towsley Center, Ann Arbor, Michigan 48109-0201, USA

[c]School of Public Health, University of Michigan,
Ann Arbor, Michigan 48109-2029, USA

Wide bodies of literature document gradients in the experience of disease and function by levels of education and other measures of socioeconomic status: The lower a person's education, the more likely the person will suffer from a greater variety and severity of diseases as well as functional disability arising from those diseases. It is unclear whether education proxies for other indicators of SES (income, net worth) or measures all the knowledge and skills accumulated over the life course that may be health protective. For example, because education and cognitive functioning are often perceived as two sides of the same coin, cognitive functioning may also measure life course knowledge and skills. The dimension of cognitive functioning that reflects a person's fluid or basic processing abilities promotes the acquisition of new information that, in turn, is reflected in the dimension of crystallized or knowledge-based abilities. Both dimensions of cognitive functioning are likely to influence the amount of education that a person achieves; conversely, the amount of education achieved (as well as other life course experiences) may influence a person's cognitive functioning. The moderate correlation between education and cognitive functioning ($r = 0.44$) in middle-aged adults suggests that although they are complementary, they may tap into different conceptual realms. Earlier research by the authors[1] demonstrated that high levels of cognitive functioning behave like high levels of education in associations with enhanced health outcomes in middle-aged adults. Further, cognitive functioning—like education—moderates the effects of some diseases on the reporting of functional disability.[2]

In this study, we examine more closely the relationships among education, cognitive functioning, and functional disability; and we hypothesize that cognitive functioning will mediate the link between levels of education and functional disability both cross-sectionally and longitudinally in middle-aged men and women. Using data from the nationally representative Health and Retirement Study (1992, 1994), we test this link in sequentially entered blocks of variables that include: (1) education; (2) cognitive functioning; (3) education and cognitive functioning; (4) education, cognitive functioning, demographic, disease, and health factors; and (5) the variables in (4) plus social and other education-related material resources. The

[a]Address for correspondence: 734-615-0273 (voice); 734-936-1641 (fax).
e-mail: wrayl@isr.umich.edu

models are tested in the full sample of middle-aged adults as well as stratified by income and sex. Results indicate that both education and cognitive functioning are significant negative predictors of functional disability in both 1992 and 1994. When tested together, the effects on functional disability of education and cognitive functioning are reduced but remain significant. Net of demographic factors, disease burden, health behaviors, and SES, higher cognitive functioning reduces the negative effect of lower education on functional disability for the full sample in 1992 (but not in 1994). Finally, cognitive functioning exerts a small negative effect on functional disability in both 1992 and 1994 over and above the effects of other measures of SES among middle-aged men in the lowest quartile for income. Here, cognitive functioning (but not education in 1994) appears to compensate for low income in reducing

TABLE 1. OLS regression estimates of functional disability in 1992 regressed on education, cognitive functioning, and selected predictors among U.S. adults age 51–61, by income quartile and sex

Characteristics		Lowest Quartile		Highest Quartile	
	All Parameter Estimate	Men Parameter Estimate	Women Parameter Estimate	Men Parameter Estimate	Women Parameter Estimate
Model 1					
Intercept	4.53^{***}	5.98^{***}	6.49^{***}	3.94^{***}	3.42^{***}
Education	-0.38^{***}	-0.18^{**}	-0.40^{***}	-0.18^{***}	-0.21^{***}
R^2	0.07	0.01	0.04	0.03	0.02
Model 2					
Intercept	4.32^{***}	5.48^{***}	6.50^{***}	3.83^{***}	3.07^{***}
Cognitive functioning	-0.11^{***}	-0.15^{***}	-0.16^{***}	-0.04^{***}	-0.07^{***}
R^2	0.03	0.02	0.04	0.01	0.02
Model 3					
Intercept	4.50^{***}	5.45^{***}	6.31^{***}	4.01^{***}	3.46^{***}
Education	-0.32^{***}	-0.10	-0.27^{***}	-0.17^{***}	-0.16^{***}
Cognitive functioning	-0.05^{***}	-0.13^{**}	-0.12^{***}	-0.01	-0.05^{**}
R^2	0.07	0.02	0.06	0.03	0.03
Model 4[a]					
Intercept	7.56^{***}	3.89^{***}	4.39^{***}	2.70^{***}	4.04^{***}
Education	-0.08^{***}	-0.01^{**}	-0.14^{***}	-0.12^{***}	-0.09^{*}
Cognitive functioning	-0.02^{***}	-0.05^{*}	-0.03^{*}	0.00	-0.01
R^2	0.42	0.41	0.41	0.27	0.37

KEY: $^*p < 0.05$; $^{**}p < 0.01$; $^{***}p < 0.001$.
[a]Net of age, sex, disease burden, self-care burden, irregular exercise, current smoker, income, net worth for overall analyses; net of all but income for stratified analyses.

functional disability among men, net of other demographic, health, and SES factors. Two potential explanations are considered: (1) compensation and (2) life course exposure.

First, it may be that for middle-aged adults with fewer socioeconomic resources upon which to draw, some resources (cognitive functioning) are drawn upon more heavily than are others (education), perhaps to compensate for the negative effects of lower income. In contrast, adults at high income levels may possess more education-related resources and experiences (higher status jobs with fewer physical demands, greater health benefits, safer living environments, longer time horizons) than do low-income men, increasing their ability to buffer the effects of disease on functional disability more successfully. Second, cognitive functioning may be less

TABLE 2. OLS regression estimates of functional disability in 1994 regressed on education, cognitive functioning, and selected predictors among U.S. adults age 51–61, by income quartile and sex

Characteristics	All Parameter Estimate	Lowest Quartile		Highest Quartile	
		Men Parameter Estimate	Women Parameter Estimate	Men Parameter Estimate	Women Parameter Estimate
Model 1					
Intercept	4.04***	5.25***	6.01***	2.32***	3.58***
Education	−0.38***	−0.19**	−0.44***	−0.17***	−0.25***
R^2	0.06	0.01	0.04	0.02	0.03
Model 2					
Intercept	3.84***	4.78***	6.17***	1.97***	3.26***
Cognitive functioning	−0.10***	−0.15***	−0.13***	−0.03	−0.05**
R^2	0.02	0.02	0.02	0.00	0.01
Model 3					
Intercept	4.04***	4.75***	5.91***	2.34***	3.61***
Education	−0.35***	−0.09	−0.38***	−0.16***	−0.22***
Cognitive functioning	−0.03***	−0.13**	−0.07*	−0.00	−0.03
R^2	0.06	0.02	0.05	0.02	0.03
Model 4[a]					
Intercept	6.33***	3.06***	4.20***	2.24***	3.61***
Education	−0.12***	−0.02	−0.25***	−0.11**	−0.12**
Cognitive functioning	−0.01	−0.08*	0.00	0.00	0.00
R^2	0.36	0.34	0.33	0.24	0.32

KEY: *$p < 0.05$; **$p < 0.01$; ***$p < 0.001$.
[a]Net of age, sex, disease burden, self-care burden, irregular exercise, current smoker, income, net worth for overall analyses; net of all but income for stratified analyses.

of an education marker in low-income men than in high-income men. In particular, low-income men may have been exposed to fewer education-related resources and experiences over their entire life course than have high-income men, disadvantaging them in middle age and forcing them to draw more heavily on the resources they do possess. This study's results suggest that the pathways from disease to functional disability and links with SES are not straightforward nor easy to interpret.

ACKNOWLEDGMENTS

This research was supported by NIA Grant No. U01-AG09740 and NIA Grant No. T32-AG00117.

REFERENCES

1. WRAY, L.A. *et al.* 1998. The impact of education and heart attack on smoking cessation among middle-aged adults. J. Health Soc. Behav. **39:** 271–294.
2. WRAY, L.A. & J. LYNCH. 1998. The role of cognitive ability in links between disease severity and functional ability in middle-aged adults. Presented at Gerontological Society of America Annual Meetings. November 1998, Philadelphia, PA.

Socioeconomic Status and Health: A New Explanation

FRANK W. YOUNG[a]

Department of Rural Sociology, Cornell University, Ithaca, New York 14853, USA

As a first step toward explaining the persistent association of socioeconomic status and health, this study reproduces the well-known monotonic relationship between education and income and health status, both self-report and doctor's assessment. This is the first fact to be explained. It then codifies the biomedical explanation of health, including its contemporary incorporation of social factors, especially socio-economic status (SES), as indirect variables that "operate through" the proximate determinants, that is, environmental threats such as disease, malnutrition, stress, and host resistance. Given this theory, the introduction of indicators of the proximate determinants in a regression equation should dissolve the relationship of SES with health, but in fact it proves to be impossible. Using data from NHANES III, TABLE 1 shows that SES holds despite a gamut of controls. From this evidence, it appears unlikely that the biomedical model contains a variable that will dissolve the SES effect. Therefore, we conclude that SES has a direct effect on health. This is the second fact to be explained.

The proposed explanation generalizes a community-level "problem-solving capacity" process to population health differentials as follows. When confronted with public health problems, communities initially apply specialized knowledge, then they debate alternatives, and sometimes mobilize behind a "reform movement." If a community has a high level of institutionalized problem-solving capacity, it will create or borrow dedicated "agencies" such as clinics, water purification, or taboos on teen-age pregnancies. The mutual reinforcement of strategies and agency tends to raise the level of health of the residents. Thus, community-level health is a function of capacity × agency, or, $h = f(C \times a)$. (Upper-case letters are used for concepts; lower-case for categories.)

The same formula holds for individuals. People with superior problem-solving capacity apply specialized knowledge, consider alternatives, and shift perspectives in order to solve the problems of daily living and to acquire the specific habits that, in combination with general problem-solving capacity, improve health. These habits are the familiar exercise, diet, safe sex, nonsmoking, and so forth; and the formula $h = f(C \times habits)$ summarizes the proposition at the individual level. The postulated causal mechanism at both levels is that participation in problem solving optimizes biological functioning, which is associated with indicators of health. Agencies and habits, even if they can be shown to promote health, are secondary to general problem-solving capacity.

[a]Address for correspondence: 607-272-0244 (voice); 607-254-2896 (fax).
e-mail: fwy1@cornell.edu

TABLE 1. Regression analysis of two measures of health, by sex, showing strength of education and income despite a wide range of controls on proximate determinants[a]

Variable	Self-reported health		Clinical assessment	
	men	women	men	women
Age	0.01ns	0.06	−0.25	−0.29
African-American	−0.02ns	−0.05	−0.02ns	−0.04
Schooling	0.18	0.20	0.06	0.06
Income	0.12	0.10	0.11	0.08
Chronic conditions	−0.17	−0.19	−0.12	−0.10
Health problems	−0.12	−0.12	−0.07	−0.04
Disabilities	−0.03	−0.03	−0.12	−0.11
Ever smoked	−0.06	−0.05	−0.02ns	0.02
BMI	−0.06	−0.08	−0.20	−0.30
Percent fat intake	0.03	0.01ns	−0.00ns	−0.01ns
Percent fiber intake	0.04	−0.02ns	0.03	0.03
Exercise score	0.13	0.14	0.04	0.00ns
Alcoholic drinks	0.03	0.08	0.04	0.05
Drinks much	−0.05	−0.03	−0.05	−0.03
Time since doctor	0.04	−0.04	−0.03	−0.03
Takes medications	−0.11	−0.10	−0.06	−0.03
R^2	0.28	0.29	0.33	0.39

[a]Data from NHANES III; $n = 18,150$.
NOTE: Numbers are regression coefficients. All are significant at the 0.05 level unless marked with an "ns."
Variable definitions: age—range of 17–90, with mean of 43.2 years; African-American—mean = 12%; schooling—number of completed years, ranging from 0–17; income—family income was compressed to 11 categories, beginning with 0 income and increasing by $5,000 intervals to $50,000+ (The mean of 6.6 corresponds to $27,000.); chronic conditions—sum of heart + arthritis + high blood pressure + cancer + cataracts + hay fever + emphysema + bronchitis + asthma + stroke (percent 1+, 51.7); health problems—1 if had to change work or housework due to health problems; disabilities—1 if respondent was observed in bed, or in wheelchair, crutches, shuffling, hands or legs paralyzed, hearing or speech impaired or with persistent cough; ever smoked—1 if respondent has smoked at least 100 cigarettes in lifetime ($M = 53\%$); BMI—percent body weight (kg)/height (m^2) calculated by NHANES ($M = 26.3$, 12–80); percent fat intake—percent kcal from fat ($M = 33.5$, 0–83; NHANES calculation); percent fiber intake—fiber (grams) consumption per day ($M = 16.7$, 0–134; from NHANES); exercise—sum of following activities in last month: jogging/running, bicycling, swimming, aerobics, dancing, calisthenics, gardening, lifting weights, or sports ($M = 1.9$; 0–8. Percent reporting one or more activity, 68.7); drinks—1 if respondent reports at least 12 alcoholic drinks in last 12 months ($M = 54\%$); drinks much—1 if respondent drank 3+ drinks on any day in previous year ($M = 26\%$); time since doctor—months since you last saw a doctor? ($M = 36.9$ months; 0–120); takes medications—1 if has taken any prescribed medicines in the last month ($M = 44\%$); self-reported health status: 1, poor; 5, excellent (20.4%); clinical appraisal, doctor's rating: 1, poor; 5, excellent (46.3%).

This theory explains the SES gradient because the school environment, regardless of content, teaches the application of specialized knowledge (the mere fact of the different "subjects" studied), weighing alternatives (student groups recognize alternative views), and the value of supporting new perspectives (team sports). The direct impact of SES is explained by the biological optimizing effect of problem-solving activity (even if problems remain unsolved) that bypasses the proximate determinants.

This explanation also applies to the well-known Whitehall findings because the civil service grades reflect the levels of problem-solving capacity. The civil service recruits people with superior problem-solving capacity, and once in a grade they quickly learn the collectively shared skills. These deal with real-world problems that call forth the kind of problem-solving capacity emphasized in this theory. The people at the top have superior problem-solving capacity that they apply to their own lives. Because of this capacity and its application to daily life, they have better health.

A Framework for Evidenced-Based Reviews of Interventions for Supportive Social Environments

L. ANDERSON,[a,b] M. FULLILOVE,[c] S. SCRIMSHAW,[d] J. FIELDING,[e]
J. NORMAND,[f] S. ZAZA,[b] L. WRIGHT-DEAGUERO,[b] AND D. HIGGINS[b]

[b]Centers for Disease Control and Prevention,
1600 Clifton Road, Atlanta, Georgia 30333, USA

[c]Columbia University, New York, New York 10032, USA

[d]University of Illinois at Chicago, Chicago, Illinois 60637, USA

[e]Los Angeles County Department of Health, Los Angeles, California 90095, USA

[f]National Institutes of Health, Bethesda, Maryland 20892, USA

BACKGROUND

A Task Force on Community Preventive Services was formed in 1996 under the auspices of the U.S. Public Health Service to develop a Guide to Community Preventive Services (Guide), which will summarize what is known about the effectiveness of selected population-based interventions to improve health. A fundamental influence on health at the macro or societal level is the social environment. It is the intent of the Guide chapter on the sociocultural environment to provide an evidence-based review of public health programs that address social determinants of health inequalities. Health care services are seen as an important, but relatively small part of the public health endeavor. Other interventions, those that focus on sharing the resources available to our society to create a supportive social environment, are considered.

METHODS

A multidisciplinary content development team (the authors) formed to develop a conceptual approach to the sociocultural environment chapter. The logic framework we have developed identifies *determinants* of health in the social environment and *linkage points* along pathways from root determinants to intermediate outcomes to health outcomes that may be amenable to *community interventions*. A priority-setting process, which considers disparities in population health status, is used to select a set of community interventions that are the subject of systematic review in the

[a]Address for correspondence: Laurie M. Anderson, Ph.D., M.P.H., Centers for Disease Control and Prevention, 1600 Clifton Rd., Mailstop Mail K-73, Atlanta, GA 30333, USA. 770-488-8189 (voice); 770-488-8462 (fax).
e-mail: LAA1@cdc.gov

published literature. This work will yield a body of evidence on intervention effectiveness and, just as notable, identify where gaps in intervention research exist.

RESULTS

The sociocutural environment conceptual framework, presented as FIGURE 1, depicts health as a product of social institutions and processes and not as restricted to individual risk factors for diseases. Public health is viewed as "what we, as a society, do collectively to assure the conditions in which people can be healthy"[1] and, thus, focuses broadly on fundamental domains for health policy and intervention programs including housing, employment, civic engagement and participation in decision-making, and opportunities for developing human capacity.

Rather than focusing on high-risk populations, a socioenvironmental approach focuses on high-risk conditions. Adequate resources are prerequisite to creating a supportive social environment for health. Standard of living, culture and history, social institutions, built environments, political structures, economic systems, and technology are all resources a population can draw upon to sustain a supportive environment for health. Equity and social justice are seen as quintessential to health.[2] They are conditions that characterize the distribution of resources among the population.

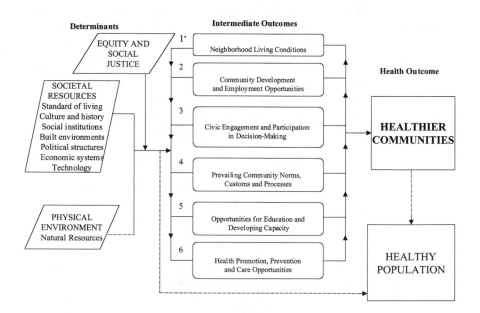

FIGURE 1. *Guide to Community Preventive Services*: sociocultural environment logic framework. SOCIETAL RESOURCES concerns the presence of essential resources, whereas EQUITY and SOCIAL JUSTICE concerns the distribution of those resources within the population. - - - -, pathways that will not be examined. * Links 1–6 indicate strategic points for intervention.

The contribution of economic, political, and social conditions to health are reciprocal; acting on any one "intermediate outcome" in the sociocultural environment logic model has consequence for all. Interventions to ameliorate underlying social causes of premature death and disability require multidisciplinary and intersectoral approaches. These interventions are the subject of evidence-based reviews to provide recommendations for population-based health promotion and disease prevention action in the Guide to Community Preventive Services, Sociocultural Environment Chapter.

REFERENCES

1. INSTITUTE OF MEDICINE. 1988. The Future of Public Health. Committee for the Study of the Future of Public Health. National Academy Press, Washington, DC.
2. WIKINSON, R.G. 1994. Unhealthy Societies: The Afflicitons of Inequality. Routledge, London.

Social Ordering in Developing Countries: Does Hierarchy Have the Same Effect as in Post-industrial Nations?

A Look at Nepal

STEPHEN BEZRUCHKA[a]

Department of Health Services, School of Public Health and Community Medicine, Box 357660, University of Washington, Seattle, Washington 98195-3576, USA

INTRODUCTION

Several studies using international data sets have shown that in both rich and poor countries the infant mortality rate (IMR) and other measures of population heath are correlated with income distribution. Less developed countries with greater equity have better health indicators than countries with a more polarized ordering.[1,2] Within rich countries, age-adjusted mortality rates are associated with income distribution.[3–5] Wilkinson[6] has suggested that after economic growth brings a country to a per capita GNP of approximately $5,000, factors other than economic development are more associated with health differences between populations. This paper examines multiple sources of published data on resource inequality in an underdeveloped country, Nepal, to identify the effects on health of basic needs (food, housing, sanitation) and inequality.

RESULTS

IMR in Nepal is associated with the caste orderings typical of a traditional South Asian society (FIG. 1). Status in Nepal is acquired through heredity in caste and social class orderings, in which Brahmin and Chhetri are the highest Hindu castes with Tamang ranking very low and Newars enjoying high status.

Nepal has begun a transition from a subsistence to a monetized economy, making it difficult to estimate income distributions. The poorest and most remote districts, where maternal education is low and access to health care difficult, have the highest infant mortality, whereas the economically more developed urban districts have the lowest values, suggesting that financial wealth and achievement are becoming more important measures of social ordering. The best health indices are in districts where there is more consistent availability of food (less chronic malnutrition) and access to clean water and latrines.

The poorest districts in Nepal appear to be the most equitable, perhaps because they have had little economic development. Land distribution is an important mea-

[a]Address for correspondence: 206-932-4928 (voice); 206-685-4184 (fax).
e-mail: sabez@u.washington.edu

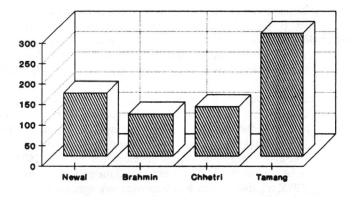

FIGURE 1. IMR for four hill population groups 1983. Estimates of IMR per 1,000 live births for four hill population groups, 1983. Source: Joint UNICEF/WHO Nutrition Support Program in Nepal—a community-based nutrition project 02/1983; as cited in CHP, 1988.

sure of equity in agrarian societies and more readily measured than income. In Nepal infant mortality is negatively correlated with the Gini Index of landholdings by district, with the highest rates found where land is most equitably held. In those districts, there are steeper plots, less off-farm income-generating activities, and few modern amenities (TABLE 1). Mugu District, an extreme example, has the most equitable land distribution, yet is one of the poorest with the highest infant mortality rate and lowest life expectancy.[7,8]

DISCUSSION

Social ordering might be expected to have the same biological effects on different populations, but the relative power of these effects may vary at different levels of development. In order for equity to be an important consideration for health in

TABLE 1. Correlation of inequality of landholding (Gini Index) with selected indicators of development for 74 districts of Nepal 1991[a]

Indicator	Correlation with Gini Index of landholding
Topography (less than 30 degree slope)	0.612
Nonagricultural population (%)	0.39
Household modernity (own bicycle)	0.585
Infant mortality	−0.367
Landownership (% self-owned)	0.513
Cultivated land (% under crop)	0.729

[a]Source: Thapa et al.[8] All values are significant at $p < 0.001$.

settings such as Nepal, basic needs such as adequate food and minimal health services must be met. Biological mechanisms through which social ordering affects health may predominate only after such conditions are met. These findings suggest that at the district level in Nepal, health outcomes are associated with absolute measures of wealth or income, much as has been found in small-area studies in the United States.[9]

In Nepal, economic development has proceeded in urban areas, where it has created greater imbalances and inequalities. Relatively small amounts of expenditure on public health—including schooling, access to safe water, sanitation, adequate food, and basic health care could produce large improvements in health outcomes. Taiwan provides an example of a country's economic development where in 1976, mortality was strongly associated with absolute household income and less with income distribution, but by 1995, relative income had become more important.[10]

REFERENCES

1. FLEGG, A. 1982. Inequality of income, illiteracy, and medical care as determinants of infant mortality in developing countries. Pop. Stud. **36:** 441–458.
2. RODGERS, G.B. 1979. Income and inequality as determinants of mortality: an international cross section analysis. Pop. Stud. **33:** 343–351.
3. KAPLAN, G.A. *et al.* 1996. Inequality in income and mortality in the United States: analysis of mortality and potential pathways. Br. Med. J. **312:** 999–1003.
4. KENNEDY, B.P. *et al.* 1996. Income distribution and mortality: cross sectional ecological study of the Robin Hood index in the United States. Br. Med. J. **312:** 1004–1007.
5. LYNCH, J.W. *et al.* 1998. Income inequality and mortality in metropolitan areas of the United States. Am. J. Public Health **88:** 1074–1080.
6. WILKINSON, R.G. 1996. Unhealthy Societies: The Afflictions of Inequality. Routledge, London.
7. THAPA, S. 1996. Infant mortality and its correlates and determinants in Nepal: a district-level analysis. J. Nepal Med. Assoc. **34:** 94–109.
8. THAPA, S. *et al.* 1997. Inequality of landhold in Nepal: some policy issues. Contrib. Nepalese Stud. **24:** 133–145.
9. FISCELLA, K. *et al.* 1997. Poverty or income inequality as predictor of mortality: longitudinal cohort study. Br. Med. J. **314:** 1724–1728.
10. CHAING, T.-I. 1999. Economic transition and changing relation between income inequality and mortality in Taiwan: regression analysis. Br. Med. J. **319:** 1162–1165.

SES, Medicare Coverage, and Flu Shot Utilization among Vulnerable Women in the Women's Health and Aging Study

KEVIN D. FRICK[a,b] AND ELEANOR M. SIMONSICK[c]

[b]Department of Health Policy and Management, School of Hygiene and Public Health, Johns Hopkins University, Baltimore, Maryland 21205-1901, USA

[c]National Institute on Aging, Epidemiology, Demography, and Biometry Program, Bethesda, Maryland 20892, USA

The link between socioeconomic status (SES) and health may derive, in part, from a link between SES and the utilization of health care and prevention services. Both economic theory and a health services research paradigm of access suggest that both monetary and nonmonetary constraints affect the utilization of health care and prevention services. Economic theory suggests that individuals make decisions based on their preferences but are limited in time, money, and other resources. One description of access focuses on five domains, including affordability, acceptability, accessibility, availability, and accommodation.[1]

Medicare coverage of specific services has the potential to diminish monetary constraints on utilization. However, the population covered by Medicare may still face nonmonetary *and* monetary constraints to the utilization of health care and preventive services. In particular, Medicare did not initiate coverage of such services until relatively recently. Increasing the affordability of these services will not necessarily eliminate all disparities in utilization among individuals of different SES. One's SES may be correlated with the nonmonetary constraints and remaining monetary constraints one faces. Policy can be informed by an examination of whether Medicare coverage of a preventive service changes the association between measures of SES and utilization of that service.

This study focuses on changes in the association between SES measures and flu shot utilization in a population of older, moderately to severely disabled women before and after Medicare coverage. The analysis first assesses the relationship between SES measures and flu shot utilization generally and separately, before and after the implementation of Medicare flu shot coverage. The analysis then compares the associations between SES measures and flu shot utilization in separate multivariate models before and after coverage. Non-SES measures are included in the model to avoid confounding by variables (such as health) that might be correlated with SES but more directly related to flu shot utilization. The differences in the associations between SES variables and flu shot utilization before and after Medicare coverage will be tested for statistical significance.

[a]Address for correspondence: Johns Hopkins University, School of Hygiene and Public Health, 624 N. Broadway, Rm. 606, Baltimore, MD 21205-1901, USA. 410-614-4018 (voice); 410-955-0470 (fax).
e-mail: kfrick@jhsph.edu

The Women's Health and Aging Study baseline data are used in this analysis and have been described in detail elsewhere.[2] The data were collected from November 1992 to February 1995, spanning the introduction of Medicare coverage of flu shots in May 1993. These data are representative of the moderately to severely disabled, community-dwelling, older female population living primarily in eastern Baltimore, Maryland. Each woman had limitations in at least one task in each of at least two of the following four domains: upper extremity, mobility, self-care, and higher functioning. The last two categories are similar to ADLs and IADLs, respectively.

Two sets of analyses implement the steps described above. First, simple logistic regressions were run using one measure of SES at a time. The simple regressions were run in order to look for general relationships between each variable and flu shot utilization and relationships before and after coverage. January 1, 1994 is the date after which all individuals interviewed were assumed to have flu shot coverage at a time that was relevant to when they would have obtained their most recent flu shot. This leads to conservative conclusions about the impact of coverage. TABLE 1 shows the results from the simple logistic regressions. Each line shows the SES variable, the number of categories that were used to describe the variable, an indication of the significance and direction of associations in simple regressions including all observations and separated into before and after regressions, and an indication of whether the before and after models were significantly different. Relationships suggested by the results in TABLE 1 were tested in multivariate logistic regression analyses that

TABLE 1. Signs and significance levels in simple logistic regressions

SES Measure (Categories)	Significance and signs of simple logistic regression associations		
	Total	Pre-coverage	Post-coverage
Zip code (12)	NS	NS	$p < 0.10$ (mixed)
Education (4)	$p < 0.01$ (+)	$p < 0.10$ (+)	$p < 0.01$ (+)
Income (continuous)	$p < 0.01$ (+)	$p < 0.01$ (+)	$p < 0.01$ (+)
Pension income (Y/N)	$p < 0.01$ (+)	$p < 0.05$ (+)	$p < 0.01$ (+)
Investment income (Y/N)	$p < 0.01$ (+)	$p < 0.05$ (+)	$p < 0.10$ (+)
Social security (Y/N)	NS	NS	NS
Job income (Y/N)	NS	NS	NS
SSI (Y/N)	$p < 0.01$ (−)	$p < 0.10$ (−)	$p < 0.10$ (−)
Food stamps (Y/N)	NS	NS	NS
Cash—children[a] (Y/N)	NS	$p < 0.10$ (−)	NS
No driver (Y/N)	$p < 0.05$ (−)	NS	$p < 0.05$ (−)
Medigap (Y/N)	$p < 0.01$ (+)	$p < 0.10$ (+)	$p < 0.01$ (+)
Medicaid (Y/N)	NS	NS	NS

[a]Coefficients are significantly different ($p < 0.10$) pre- and post-.

also included measures of health status and race. The data include insufficient observations to test all source-of-income variables; only income was included in the multivariate logistic regression. TABLE 2 shows the odds ratios from the multivariate regressions before and after coverage with an indication of the significance of each odds ratio. None of the odds ratios were significantly different before and after coverage. Income and having a usual source of care other than a physician's office are significantly related to flu shot utilization at $p < 0.10$ before coverage but not after. Measures of health are associated with flu shot utilization both before and after coverage. Living alone, Medigap coverage, and not having a driver in the household are significantly related to flu shot utilization only after coverage.

Medicare coverage changed the magnitude and significance of several associations between SES variables and flu shot utilization. Multivariate analyses suggest that while the effect of income was mitigated by coverage, other SES effects were accentuated. Coverage does not affect all constraints older individuals face. Using coverage to change prices and address affordability is unlikely to mitigate all SES-based differences in utilization. Without addressing other domains of access, for example, acceptability and availability, and information, differences in nonfinancial constraints and preferences will remain. With these differences, gaps in utilization and health status will remain.

TABLE 2. Results of logistic regressions with samples from before and after medicare flu shot coverage

Variable	Pre-coverage odds ratios	Post-coverage odds ratios
Excellent—good health	0.688^a	0.769
Cardiopulmonary disease	1.236	1.427^a
Age	1.066	1.278
Age-squared	1.000	0.998
At least some college	1.298	1.478
Lives alone	1.331	1.613^b
Married	1.424	1.091
Income (10,000s)	1.228^b	1.124
Medicaid	1.186	1.488
Medigap	1.261	1.590*
Usual source not physician's office	1.436^a	1.148
No driver in househhold	0.972	0.646^a
Black	0.863	0.495^c
	$n = 453$	$n = 512$

$^a p \leq 0.10.$
$^b p \leq 0.05.$
$^c p \leq 0.01.$

REFERENCES

1. PENCHANSKY, R. & J.W. THOMAS. 1981. The concept of access: definition and relationship to consumer satisfaction. Med. Care **19**(2): 127–140.
2. GURALNIK, J.M., L.P. FRIED, E.M. SIMONSICK, J.D. KASPER & M.E. LAFFERTY, Eds. 1995. The Women's Health and Aging Study: Health and Social Characteristics of Older Women with Disability. National Institute on Aging, Bethesda.

The Association of Race/Socioeconomic Status and Use of Medicare Services

A Little-Known Failure in Access to Care

MARIAN E. GORNICK[a]

Georgetown Public Policy Institute, Washington, D.C. 20007, USA

Before Medicare was enacted in 1965, public policy experts were concerned over the fact that the use of health care services was inversely related to income.[1] Disparities in health care were attributed to the fact that only about one-half of the population aged 65 and over had health insurance. By enrolling virtually the entire elderly population in the program, Medicare was expected to make health care services equally accessible to all. Studies based on data available in the first two decades of the program suggested that Medicare was successful in closing the gaps in health care.[2] However, studies based on more detailed data that became available during the 1990s show that the use of specific Medicare services differs substantially by race and socioeconomic status.[3] When health status measures for vulnerable subgroups of the elderly are juxtaposed against patterns of Medicare utilization, the results are paradoxical because utilization patterns are often dramatically at odds with the major indicators of health status.

As examples, at age 65, life expectancy is lower for blacks compared to whites. Mortality rates are higher for the least affluent of the elderly compared to the most affluent, especially for the least affluent white men. Elderly blacks, Hispanics, and the least affluent in all racial/ethnic minority groups tend to have higher rates of chronic conditions such as diabetes and hypertension.[4] Elderly blacks have the highest death rates for heart disease, cancer, and stroke. For every major cancer site, the percentage of blacks with localized cancer at the time of diagnosis is lower than the percentage of whites (TABLE 1). Yet, data from the Medicare program broken out by race and income show that blacks and the least affluent of the elderly have substantially lower rates of physicians' office visits, influenza immunizations, mammography, diagnostic testing, cancer screening, and common surgical procedures (but more emergency room visits) compared to white beneficiaries and the most affluent of the elderly (TABLE 2).

These patterns of utilization by race and socioeconomic status indicate that the most plausible explanations for disparities in Medicare utilization involve the characteristics of the beneficiaries and the health care delivery system. The lower use of self-initiated services—such as physicians' office visits, influenza immunizations, and mammograms—by minorities and the poorest of the elderly may be explained, at least in part, by the "culture of poverty." Yet, the culture of poverty cannot explain

[a]Address for correspondence: 3704 N. Charles Street, Suite 401, Baltimore, MD 21218, USA. 410-467-5118 (voice); 410-243-1960 (fax).
e-mail: mgornick@aol.com

disparities in the use of services such as colonoscopy, coronary artery bypass surgery, or hip replacement—which must be recommended by physicians. These disparities are more probably explained by the "culture of advantage,"[5] which influences individuals to expect high-quality medical care and to learn to work through the maze of the health care system to obtain information about the best practitioners and the newest tests and procedures.

Certain characteristics of the health care system are likely to reinforce the effects of the cultures of poverty and advantage. Physicians are likely to be more comfortable interacting with patients who are advantaged like themselves. Moreover, providers may be influenced by stereotypical beliefs that poor and minority patients miss appointments, do not understand the complexities of medical science, and do not adhere to orders. These perceptions may affect the decision-making processes and lead physicians to refrain from ordering procedures that require patient compliance or a middle class life style for effective aftercare in the home. Only a few studies have been undertaken to examine this issue from the perspective of care delivered to population subgroups.[6]   Rather, the health care system is evaluated on the care provided individual patients, leaving policy-makers largely unaware of disparities in the use of many covered services. The Medicare experience underscores the reality that health insurance alone is not sufficient to assure equal access to health care. There is a critical need to understand why socioeconomic status and race are associated with the use of Medicare services so that policy-makers can initiate new approaches to assure equity in health care.

TABLE 1. Cancer death rates for persons aged 65 and over, all sites,[a] and specific sites[b] and percent of patients (all ages) with localized cancer at time to diagnosis, by race, 1986–1991

Site of cancer	Deaths per 100,000		Percent of patients with localized cancer at time of diagnosis	
	White	Black	White	Black
All sites	1070	1336	—	—
Colon and rectum	132	157	38	32
Lung and bronchus	296	328	15	13
Breast	128	125	59	48
Corpus and uterus	22	40	74	52
Prostate	220	476	58	52
Urinary bladder	26	26	74	58

NOTE: Source is SEER (Surveillance, Epidemiology, and End Results) Cancer Statistics Review, 1973–1992. National Institutes of Health, National Cancer Institute. C.L. Kosary, L.A.G. Ries, B.A. Miller, B.F. Hankey, A. Harras & B.K. Edwards, Eds. NIH Pub. No. 96-2789.
  [a] 1991–1992.
  [b] 1988–1992.

TABLE 2. Medicare: use of selected services by race and income, 1993[a]

Race and Income	Ambulatory physician visits		Emergency Room physician visits		Magnetic Resonance Imaging		Mammography	
	AR	RR	AR	RR	AR	RR	AA	RR
White beneficiaries								
Total	8.1		35.0		4.3		26.0	
$20,501 and over	9.0	1.00	29.6	1.00	5.5	1.00	31.0	1.00
$16,301 to $20,500	8.3	0.92	34.6	1.17	4.4	0.81	27.2	0.88
$13,101 to $16,300	7.6	0.85	36.8	1.24	3.8	0.69	24.1	0.78
less than $13,001	7.3	0.82	39.9	1.35	3.4	0.62	20.8	0.67
Income adjusted	8.1		35.4		4.3		25.7	
Black beneficiaries								
Total	7.2		50.6		3.5		17.1	
$20,501 and over	8.0	1.00	44.2	1.00	4.5	1.00	20.4	1.00
$16,301 to $20,500	7.4	0.92	45.8	1.04	4.3	0.94	19.9	0.98
$13,101 to $16,300	7.7	0.97	52.2	1.18	4.3	0.94	21.1	1.03
less than $13,001	7.1	0.88	51.6	1.17	3.3	0.72	16.0	0.79
Income adjusted	7.6		48.6		4.1		19.2	
Black/White Ratio								
Total	**0.89**		**1.45**		**0.81**		**0.66**	
Income Adjusted	**0.93**		**1.37**		**0.95**		**0.75**	

[a]AR is rate per 100 beneficiaries, adjusted for age and sex except that ambulatory visits is rate per person; RR is the ratio of the rate in the income quartile to rate for the highest income.

NOTE: Source is Monitoring the Impact of Medicare Physician Payment Reform on Utilization and Access; 1995 report to Congress. Health Care Financing Administration, 1995. (HCFA Pub.No. 03358). Baltimore, MD.

ACKNOWLEDGMENTS

This work was supported by funding from The Century Foundation and The Commonwealth Fund. The views presented here are those of the author and should not be attributed to The Century Foundation or The Commonwealth Fund, their staff, officers, or directors.

REFERENCES

1. STARR, P. 1982. The Social Transformation of American Medicine. Basic Books, New York.
2. MCBEAN, A.M. & M. GORNICK. 1994. Differences by race in rates of procedures performed in hospitals for Medicare beneficiaries. Health Care Financ. Rev. 15(4): 77–90.
3. GORNICK, M.E., P.W. EGGERS, T.W. REILLY, R.M. MENTNECH, L.K. FITTERMAN, L.E. KUCKEN & B.C. VLADECK. 1996. Effects of race and income on mortality and use of services among Medicare beneficiaries. N. Engl. J. Med. 335: 791–99.
4. NATIONAL CENTER FOR HEALTH STATISTICS. 1998. Health, United States, 1998 with Socioeconomic Status and Health Chartbook. National Center for Health Statistics. Hyattsville, MD.
5. RAINWATER, L. 1969. The problem of lower-class culture. In On Understanding Poverty: Perspectives from the Social Sciences. D.P. Moynihan, Ed. Basic Books, New York.
6. FOX, S.A. & J.A. STEIN. 1991. The effect of physician–patient communication on mammography utilization by different ethnic groups. Med. Care 29: 1065–1081.

Index of Contributors

501